Military and Veteran Mental Health

Laura Weiss Roberts
Editor

Christopher H. Warner
Associate Editor

Military and Veteran Mental Health

A Comprehensive Guide

Springer

Editor
Laura Weiss Roberts
Department of Psychiatry and Behavioral Sciences
Stanford University School of Medicine
Palo Alto, CA, USA

Associate Editor
Christopher H. Warner
US Army Medical Department Active Duty
Fort Stewart, GA, USA

ISBN 978-1-4939-7436-8 ISBN 978-1-4939-7438-2 (eBook)
https://doi.org/10.1007/978-1-4939-7438-2

Library of Congress Control Number: 2017960431

Printed on acid-free paper

This Springer imprint is published by Springer Nature
The registered company is Springer Science+Business Media, LLC
The registered company address is: 233 Spring Street, New York, NY 10013, U.S.A.

With heartfelt gratitude to veterans and members of the military who serve, sacrifice, and often deserve better.

—Laura Weiss Roberts

To the brave men and women who have served before, serve now, and will serve in the future and to the amazing professionals who help them deal with the consequences of their sacrifices.

—Christopher H. Warner

Foreword

The wars in Southwest Asia over the past fifteen years were not the first encounters with the psychological impacts of armed conflict. Emotional turmoil and illness have undoubtedly been attending warfare since the invention of the stick and the rock; they have been the subjects of important accounts of battle since antiquity, even punctuating the Homeric tales during a preliterate era. But the wars in Afghanistan and Iraq have been characterized by pivotal changes in the nature of conventional warfare that have brought the importance of proactively addressing these issues to the forefront.

In contrast to the majority of earlier wars waged by the US forces, Operations Enduring Freedom (OEF) in Afghanistan and Iraqi Freedom (OIF) have been fought with a much smaller force of volunteer military members—many of whom have been deployed repeatedly for extended periods of time with little "dwell" at home between deployments. Exposure to direct combat has marked the experience for a larger proportion of these deployed warriors, especially the ground combatants. Fighting has been conducted across a dispersed battlespace without a "front" and "rear," leaving combatants without a clear sense of sanctuary in the combat zone. Support troops such as truck drivers, aircraft mechanics, and cooks, who in other wars would have expected relative safety on deployment, do not enjoy this ease of mind in a war where the enemy targets our troops wherever and whenever possible—often with suicide bombers or remotely detonated explosive devices. Even troops and others providing critical support functions in locations far removed from the battlefield—some back home in the USA—have been privy to the direct images and sounds of combat as they assist in targeting enemy forces or advise those flying in the air over the ground fighting or those on the ground engaged in the kinetic battle.

Families are more intimately involved in the daily stresses and potential harmful exposures resulting from deployments for their loved ones than in past conflicts. Communications are continuous and ubiquitous. In contrast to those eras in which a handwritten letter may have taken weeks to months to arrive back home or from the home to the front lines, advances in electronic communications and the ready availability of these tools have changed the experience of family members back home. Cell phone calls are sometimes even made at the point of injury or wounding to families back home. And when the soldier, sailor, airman, Marine or coastguardsman is ready to return home, rather than the long trip by train and ship that might have occurred in past wars, during which decompression and sharing of stories aimed at normalizing the experience might have occurred, the participants in modern wars can be home within hours of leaving an active combat zone.

Finally, the nature of injuries and wounds and the survival from many of these potentially life-threatening events have changed in important ways. Blasts from explosive devices such as "improvised explosive devices" (IEDs) and "explosive formed projectiles" (EFPs), from rocket-propelled grenades (RPGs), surface to surface and mortars have become the preferred weapons of enemy combatants. Survival from combat wounds is higher than ever before in history as a result of active in-theater research to find the best combination of caregiver training and competence, medical equipment, optimal treatment protocols, timely and swift evacuation by ground and air, and forward placement of surgical and other medical capabilities that ensure the best chance at survival. Too many of these blasts result in concomitant mild traumatic brain injuries or concussions. Coupled with pain from wounds and injuries, the complex comorbidity of the modern medical battlefield is closely intertwined with psychological wounds that make diagnosis and effective treatment more challenging.

All of these factors have been subjected to a level of intense interest by the nonmedical leadership of the US military and investigation by military medical scientists. Armed with emerging technology, the capacity to amass and analyze large datasets and the availability of robust funding to find answers and apply them to patients have resulted in many improvements in the prevention, mitigation, early recognition, and comprehensive management of many of the most resistant forms of psychological trauma evident during and/or resulting from military service. But research insights are worthless without intelligent application.

The editors of this textbook have gathered some of the leading names in military and veteran psychiatry to unravel the complex array of mental health issues accompanying military service, modern combat, and their lasting effects. Each is an expert in their field and has contributed seminal insights into the nature of military service and its impact on the human psyche. As a former commanding general of the US Army Medical Research & Materiel Command whose scientists were instrumental in outlining and performing many of these investigations; later as a leader of a large number of military hospitals and clinics charged with applying optimal diagnostic and therapeutic instruments; and finally as the US Army Surgeon General and Commanding General of the US Army Medical Command responsible for advising the senior Army, military, and Congressional leadership about the nature of psychological wounds and the best approaches to understanding and mitigating the effects of the past fifteen years of war on our men and women in uniform, I am very familiar with the authors of this manual. The respect they garnered for their work and for military and veteran medicine during this period is without peer. You have an extraordinary compilation of lessons on military and veteran mental health gathered by the best in the field today. Their labors are of value only if applied with vigor, respect, and compassion—a level of enlightened understanding to which every veteran of America's wars is entitled for the sacrifices they have made.

Eric B. Schoomaker, MD, PhD
Lieutenant General, US Army (Ret)
Professor and Vice Chair for Leadership, Centers & Programs
Department of Military & Emergency Medicine
F. Edward Hebert School of Medicine
Uniformed Services University of the Health Sciences
Bethesda, MD, USA

Preface

The wars in Iraq and Afghanistan have endured for over a decade and a half. More than 2.5 million members of the US Army, Navy, Air Force, and Marines have deployed to those countries in voluntary service. More than 60,000 service members were killed or injured in those conflicts to date, with many surviving injury that would have killed them in prior wars. These high survivability rates can be attributed to equipment technology advances such as body armor and helmets, as well as outstanding medical advances in battlefield and trauma care.

High survivability rates, combined with an asymmetric battlefield where there are no safe zones and the requirement for service members to complete multiple deployments in order to continue the effort with an all-volunteer force, have brought to the forefront the psychological consequences of war. These consequences are often exacerbated by co-occurring mental health or substance abuse disorders. Moreover, the reliance of enemy forces on improvised explosive devices has generated thousands of concussive injuries, which have expanded our knowledge of traumatic brain injury at a terrible cost. Further, the loss of life due to suicide among our country's veterans is an immense tragedy with immeasurable repercussions.

Our country's Department of Defense and Veterans Administration medical services downsized in the 1990s in conjunction with the drawdown of the US military. This transition has resulted in both Department of Defense and Veterans Administration medical resources being overwhelmed with demands. This transition also created a need to ensure that medical resources are focused on the best clinical practices to care for our service members and veterans. Further, with the increased awareness and recognition of post-traumatic stress disorder, addiction, and cognitive changes associated with aging, many Vietnam veterans are now coming forward, seeking assistance for symptoms and conditions that they previously did not discuss. As such, there is a growing reliance on the civilian medical system to care for both our military and veteran population, especially with our continued use of Reserve and National Guard forces who live throughout our nation's communities.

This book is dedicated to those brave men and women who have raised their right hand and promised to support and defend the Constitution of the United States and to those phenomenal men and women who care for them on a daily basis. It is our intent that this textbook will serve as a key reference for all of those providers who care for this growing population and provide an increased level of understanding of this unique culture.

The textbook is organized into four sections. The first section covers foundational information on the culture and context of health care for members of the US military and veteran population. The second section focuses on systems of care for mental health needs of military and veteran populations. The third section characterizes best practices as well as ethical issues in clinical care for mental health needs of members of the military and veterans. Guidance in relation to a wide range of topics is provided, such as mood disorders, post-traumatic stress disorder, combat and operational stress, military sexual assault, psychosis, and sleep disorders. The last section is intended to assist readers in reinforcing their learning through a set of clinical cases with accompanying questions for deeper consideration.

The contributors and editors have attempted to ensure that all information that has been presented in this textbook is correct, that is, accurate at the time of writing and congruent with general psychiatric and medical standards. Information and expert guidance may evolve, however, as medical research and clinical practice approaches progress. In addition, specific clinical circumstances may necessitate a response not covered by or recommended in this book. The authors and editors cannot assume legal liability for mistakes or misuse of this text.

We offer our heartfelt thanks to Kendra Dority for her extraordinary work in orchestrating and assisting with the editing of this text. We also express our appreciation to Ann Tennier, Gabrielle Termuehlen, Katie Ryan, and Kevin Wright for their contributions to the development of this project.

Palo Alto, CA, USA — Laura Weiss Roberts
Fort Stewart, GA, USA — Christopher H. Warner

Contents

Contributors

Amy B. Adler Center for Military Psychiatry and Neuroscience, Walter Reed Army Institute of Research, Silver Spring, MD, USA

John C. Bradley Harvard Medical School, Boston, MA, USA

Mental Health Service (116-a), VA Boston Health Care System, Boston, MA, USA

Jill E. Breitbach U.S. Public Health Service, US Northern Command, Colorado Springs, CO, USA

Pamela J. Broderick Wright-Patterson Medical Center, Wright-Patterson Air Force Base, Dayton, OH, USA

Wright State University Boonshoft School of Medicine, Dayton, OH, USA

Kim Bullock Stanford University, Palo Alto, CA, USA

Robert Joel Bush William Beaumont Army Medical Center, Fort Bliss, Fort Bliss, TX, USA

Carl Andrew Castro Suzanne Dvorak Peck School of Social Work, University of Southern California, Los Angeles, CA, USA

Danielle K. Clauss Philadelphia College of Osteopathic Medicine, Philadelphia, PA, USA

Charles Drebing Bedford VA Medical Center, Bedford, MA, USA

Laura B. Dunn Stanford University, Palo Alto, CA, USA

Ellen Edens Yale School of Medicine, New Haven, CT, USA

Carol S. Fullerton Uniformed Services University of the Health Sciences, Bethesda, MD, USA

Stuart Gilman Veterans Health Administration, Washington, DC, USA

Jeremy Goldbach Suzanne Dvorak Peck School of Social Work, University of Southern California, Los Angeles, CA, USA

Thomas Allen Grieger Department of Psychiatry, Uniformed Services University, Bethesda, MD, USA

Jeffrey Guina Wright-Patterson Medical Center, Wright-Patterson Air Force Base, Dayton, OH, USA

Wright State University Boonshoft School of Medicine, Dayton, OH, USA

Ronald J. Gurrera VA Boston Health Care System, Harvard Medical School, Boston, MA, USA

Aazaz Ul Haq VA Palo Alto Health Care System, Palo Alto, CA, USA

Charles W. Hoge Center for Psychiatry and Neuroscience, Walter Reed Army Institute of Research, Silver Spring, MD, USA

Honor Hsin Stanford University, Palo Alto, CA, USA

John D. Hunsaker Fort Belvoir Community Hospital, Ft. Belvoir, VA, USA

Uniformed Services University of the Health Sciences (USUHS), Bethesda, MD, USA

David E. Johnson Center for Forensic Behavioral Sciences, Walter Reed National Military Medical Center, Bethesda, MD, USA

Lantie Jorandby-Quinones Yale School of Medicine, New Haven, CT, USA

Joshua Jordan California School of Professional Psychology at Alliant International University, San Francisco, CA, USA

Stanford University School of Medicine, Palo Alto, CA, USA

Makoto Kawai Stanford University School of Medicine, VA Palo Alto Health Care System, Palo Alto, CA, USA

Elizabeth Klingaman Department of Psychiatry, U.S. Department of Veterans Affairs Capitol Health Care Network (VISN 5) Mental Illness Research, Education, and Clinical Center (MIRECC), University of Maryland School of Medicine, Baltimore, MD, USA

Daniel J. Lee Division of Psychiatry Drug Products, Center for Drug Evaluation and Research, U.S. Food and Drug Administration, Silver Spring, MD, USA

Alan K. Louie Stanford University School of Medicine, Palo Alto VA Health Care System, Palo Alto, CA, USA

Daniel R. May 65th Medical Brigade, Camp Humphreys, Pyeongtaek, South Korea

Margaret May Stanford University, Palo Alto, CA, USA

Holly B. Herberman Mash Uniformed Services University of the Health Sciences, Bethesda, MD, USA

Shannon McCaslin National Center for PTSD Dissemination & Training Division, VA Palo Alto Health Care System, Menlo Park, CA, USA

Eric G. Meyer Department of Psychiatry, Uniformed Services University of the Health Sciences (USUHS), Bethesda, MD, USA

Joshua C. Morganstein Uniformed Services University of the Health Sciences, Bethesda, MD, USA

Lisa Mueller Bedford VA Medical Center, Bedford, MA, USA

James A. Naifeh Uniformed Services University of the Health Sciences, Bethesda, MD, USA

Ruth O'Hara Department of Psychiatry and Behavioral Sciences, Stanford University School of Medicine, Palo Alto, CA, USA

Stanford University School of Medicine, VA Palo Alto Health Care System, Palo Alto, CA, USA

Kile M. Ortigo Palo Alto Veterans Institute for Research (PAVIR), Palo Alto, CA, USA

National Center for PTSD Dissemination & Training Division, VA Palo Alto Health Care System, Palo Alto, CA, USA

Claudia B. Padula Psychiatry and Behavioral Sciences, Stanford University School of Medicine and MIRECC VA Palo Alto Health Care System, Palo Alto, CA, USA

Ajit Pai, MD Mental Health Service, Hunter Holmes McGuire Veterans Affairs Medical Center, Richmond, VA, USA

Departments of Physical Medicine and Rehabilitation, Virginia Commonwealth University, Richmond, VA, USA

Nicholas Pastorek Michael E. DeBakey VA Medical Center, Rehabilitation and Extended Care Line, Baylor College of Medicine, Department of Physical Medicine and Rehabilitation, Houston, TX, USA

Ryan P. Peirson US Air Force School of Aerospace Medicine, Wright-Patterson Air Force Base, Dayton, OH, USA

Wright State University Boonshoft School of Medicine, Dayton, OH, USA

Walter Penk Bedford VA Medical Center, Bedford, MA, USA

Nicole L. Perry VA Boston Health Care System, Boston, MA, USA

Treven Pickett McGuire VA Medical Center, Richmond, VA, USA

Department of Psychology, Virginia Commonwealth University, Richmond, VA, USA

Department of Psychiatry, Virginia Commonwealth University, Richmond, VA, USA

Departments of Physical Medicine and Rehabilitation, Virginia Commonwealth University, Richmond, VA, USA

Sophia Pirog Stanford University School of Medicine, Alto Health Care System, Palo Alto, CA, USA

Rebecca I. Porter United States Army Medical Command, San Antonio, TX, USA

Samuel L. Preston US Army, Regional Health Command-Atlantic, Washington, DC, USA

Michelle Primeau Stanford University School of Medicine, Palo Alto, CA, USA

Palo Alto Medical Foundation, Sunnyvale, CA, USA

Yaron G. Rabinowitz Marine Special Operations School, Camp Lejeune, Jacksonville, NC, USA

Laura Weiss Roberts Department of Psychiatry and Behavioral Sciences, Stanford University School of Medicine, Palo Alto, CA, USA

Robert A. Rosenheck Veterans Affairs New England Mental Illness Research, Education, and Clinical Center, West Haven, CT, USA

Yale University School of Medicine, New Haven, CT, USA

Josef I. Ruzek National Center for PTSD Dissemination & Training Division, VA Palo Alto Health Care System, Menlo Park, CA, USA

Department of Psychiatry and Behavioral Sciences, Stanford University, Palo Alto, CA, USA

Patcho N. Santiago Uniformed Services University of the Health Sciences, Bethesda, MD, USA

Brett J. Schneider Uniformed Services University of the Health Sciences, Bethesda, MD, USA

Erica Simon Palo Alto Veterans Institute for Research (PAVIR), Palo Alto, CA, USA

National Center for PTSD Dissemination & Training Division, VA Palo Alto Health Care System, Menlo Park, CA, USA

Walter J. Sowden Center for Military Psychiatry and Neuroscience, Walter Reed Army Institute of Research, Silver Spring, MD, USA

Lillian Stevens, PhD Department of Psychology, Virginia Commonwealth University, Richmond, VA, USA

Departments of Physical Medicine and Rehabilitation, Virginia Commonwealth University, Richmond, VA, USA

Lisa Talbot Stanford University School of Medicine, Palo Alto, CA, USA

Jack Tsai Department of Psychiatry, VA New England MIRECC; Yale University School of Medicine, West Haven, CT, USA

Robert J. Ursano Uniformed Services University of the Health Sciences, Bethesda, MD, USA

Alicia B. Vanden Bussche Palo Alto University, Palo Alto, CA, USA

Christopher Waltrous Bedford VA Medical Center, Bedford, MA, USA

Christopher H. Warner US Army Medical Department Activity – Fort Stewart, Fort Stewart, GA, USA

Chase Warren Stanford University, Palo Alto, CA, USA

Randon S. Welton Wright State University Boonshoft School of Medicine, Dayton, OH, USA

Leanne M. Williams Psychiatry and Behavioral Sciences, Stanford University School of Medicine, Palo Alto, CA, USA

Gary H. Wynn Department of Psychiatry, Uniformed Services University of the Health Sciences (USUHS), Bethesda, MD, USA

Stephen N. Xenakis Uniformed Services University of Health Sciences, Arlington, VA, USA

Jennifer Yeaw Benesh & Yeaw Consulting LLC, Upper Marlboro, MD, USA

Part I

Foundations of Military and Veteran Mental Health Care

Modern History of Military and Veteran Mental Health Care

1

Thomas Allen Grieger

Introduction

The past century has seen vast changes in the nature of warfare, the selection of service members, and the nature and delivery of health-care services to active duty members and veterans. In the first half of the twentieth century, the USA entered into two world wars with the massive mobilization of citizen soldiers. By the end of the century, an all-volunteer force was in place. The nature of warfare evolved with the introduction of automatic weapons, highly accurate artillery, mechanized and armored units, aircraft, long-range missiles, "smart" bombs, drones, and satellites. The nature of mental health care for active duty members and veterans evolved as well. Psychiatrists at the beginning of the twentieth century were a rarity and practiced almost exclusively in institutional settings. Over time their direct role in combat theaters became commonplace. The Veterans Administration was created and grew with each war to become what is now the largest health-care operation in the USA. Our understanding of traumatic responses to war and deployment led to the development of a new category of psychiatric diagnosis. Research on patterns and treatments of war-related illness has fostered effective and evidence-based approaches.

T.A. Grieger, MD (✉)
Department of Psychiatry, Uniformed Services University, Bethesda, MD, USA
e-mail: thomas.grieger@gmail.com

World War I

In the early years of the twentieth century, modern psychiatric concepts had not been established. There was no system of diagnostic classification, no psychiatric pharmacological treatments, no specific psychotherapies tailored to specific disorders, and no system charged with care of returning war veterans. For the most part, the few psychiatrists practicing at the time were relegated to institutional settings housing severely ill patients. Lessons from World War I paved the way for advances in each of these areas.

Active Duty

As hostilities persisted in Europe, the USA prepared to enter into war. The Selective Service Act was passed on May 18, 1917. The draft began, and by the end of the war, 19 months later, 25% of males between the ages of 18 and 31 were in military service. The Army grew from 189,674 to 3,664,000. Casualties were high with 53,160 deaths and 179,625 wounded. The Army had 80

L.W. Roberts, C.H. Warner (eds.), *Military and Veteran Mental Health*,
https://doi.org/10.1007/978-1-4939-7438-2_1

fully equipped hospitals in the USA and 135 hospitals in Europe. The stateside hospitals cared for 1,407,191 patients and those in Europe, 755,354 patients. Nineteen hospitals provided rehabilitation to the wounded with Walter Reed Hospital specializing in prosthetic limbs for amputees much as it does to this day (United States War Department 1918; DeBruyne and Leland 2015). Returning veterans were treated primarily in military and state hospitals (United States Department of Veteran Affairs).

WWI saw the first large-scale use of modern artillery, automatic weapons, armored vehicles, and the physical and psychological threat of chemical weapons. What is now known as posttraumatic stress disorder (PTSD) was at that time labeled "shell shock" or "neurasthenia" and for a time was thought to be a concussion-like disorder caused by the close proximity of artillery explosions. Later in the war, physicians developed the understanding that the symptoms were the result of exposure to terrifying or prolonged combat (Jones and Wessely 2014; Pols and Oak 2007).

High attrition rates for psychiatric disorders motivated the principle of "forward psychiatry," designed to restore soldiers to service in theater and, if possible, in combat roles. The concept did not provide for medications or psychotherapy. Rather, fatigued and fearful soldiers could be restored to duty through basic temporary rest, food, respite, and light duties. Ultimately this concept was described as treatment in *proximity* to the front, *immediately* following the trauma, with an attitude of *expectation* of return to duty, and using only *simple* supportive methods (a concept often referred to as PIES). These principles have persisted to this day. As will be discussed later in this chapter, the ultimate effects of this approach on retention at the front lines, and later on veteran health, have been the subject of debate since its inception. Its overall goal was to maintain forward combat strength. Success at the time was measured in terms of retention at the front in comparison to return to the front for soldiers who had previously been evacuated to the rear. Experience showed that once service members were evacuated to a safe, warm, and friendly hospital environment, they had an incentive to maintain active symptoms to avoid returning to the harsh and dangerous front lines. Subsequent analysis of the outcome of forward treatment during World War I revealed that only 16.9% of such soldiers returned to their original units. Others were placed in supportive roles away from combat (Jones and Wessely 2014). The concept of forward treatment is taught to military mental health professionals and lay support personnel to this day.

Since posttraumatic symptoms were not well understood at the time, psychiatrists and military leaders believed that there must be some preexisting personality profile, such as "a heavy incidence of those varieties of mental shipwreck that we call psychoses and neuroses" (Army Medical Command 1929). The understanding was that vulnerable individuals would show a pattern of limited adaptive capacity and that such a profile could be screened out. Medical leaders therefore developed a plan to detect such personality features. All newly inducted service members were to be screened at entry, and those already on active service would be evaluated when showing signs of a mental disorder. Screening was conducted at many of the training camps, but the logistics of screening large numbers of personnel and the lack of clear screening criteria produced a negligible effect on wartime casualties (Pols and Oak 2007; Jones and Wessely 2014; Jones et al. 2003; Army Medical Department 1929; Army Medical Department n.d.). In fact, by 1927, nearly 47% of ex-service men in Veterans Administration hospitals had neuropsychiatric illnesses (Army Medical Department 1929).

The Army Surgeon General's "Division of Sanitation" organized the planning and management of psychiatric matters. This division solidified the beginning of modern military psychiatry. The Army Medical Department published Volume X Neuropsychiatry in 1929 (Army Medical Department 1929), which details the medical personnel, provision of care, detection of mental diseases, observation and treatment, and disposition of mental cases. Chapter V lays out a detailed assessment capturing the soldier's past history, family background, preservice adaptation, history of present illness, and detailed mental status and neurological examinations. This diagnostic approach, as described, closely matches diagnostic intakes conducted today. Chapter IX of the report includes 51 tables including details such as presence of a family history of disorders, age of onset, education level, time of onset of illness, state of residence, and racial distribution. Lack of standardized diagnostic criteria makes the data difficult to assess in terms of modern diagnoses.

Veterans

At the beginning of the war, services to veterans were divided among three agencies, the Veterans Bureau, Bureau of Pensions, and the National Home for Disabled Volunteer Soldiers. A number of states also had state-run veteran hospitals. The concept that the Federal government should handle the medical needs of all war-disabled veterans did not exist prior to World War I. The first consolidation of veterans programs was in 1921 when the Veterans Health Bureau was established. Former Public Health Service hospitals were turned over to the bureau, and new hospitals for veterans were constructed. Public Law 384 provided $18.6 million for constructing new and remodeling existing facilities. By the end of 1932, amazingly, 64 hospitals for veterans had been established, and some 30,000 veterans were hospitalized at government expense (Department of Veterans Affairs). Prior to this time, hospitalization was primarily a matter of warehousing the disabled, but that practice began to shift to a focus on cures. This in turn spurred the development of research to clarify diagnoses and treatment approaches, including treatment of psychiatric patients. Veterans Administration medical research reports at the time were primarily case reports or case series reports. That early entry into research set the stage for an extensive Veterans Administration research network that is still active in assessing pharmacological and psychotherapeutic treatments for trauma-related disorders as well as a myriad of other medical conditions (Hays 2010).

World War II

World War II in some ways ushered in the modern era of psychiatry. Faced with thousands of psychiatric casualties, the services needed some means of better classifying them in order to determine proper disposition. The services concluded that all diagnoses should include type of disturbance, precipitating stressors, extent of predisposition, and degree of impairment. This multiaxial diagnosis scheme paralleled that of the future *Diagnostic and Statistical Manuals* (*DSM*). General Menninger further developed Technical Bulletin 203, which further elaborated on disease characteristics; this was adopted by all services and the Veterans Administration and formed the foundation for Diagnostic and Statistical Manual, DSM I (Committee on Nomenclature and Statistics 1952).

Active Duty

World War II was a massive endeavor, with 16,112,566 service members on duty, 291,557 battle deaths, and 670,846 nonfatal wounds (DeBruyne and Leland 2015). The Army's account of the war, "Neuropsychiatry in World War II" (Army Medical Department n.d.), outlines the lessons learned from World War I and then describes the distribution of medical personnel, special education and training, use of psychiatric consultants, liaison with other agencies, public relations, and selection and induction. Part III presents Military Psychiatry in Practice with chapters on hospitalization and disposition, regional and general hospitals, troops in transit, mental hygiene consultation, preventative psychiatry, women's health, forensic psychiatry, and psychiatry in the correctional system. Perhaps the most interesting is Chapter XXVIII, "Lessons Learned" by Colonel Albert Glass, not actually added to the volume until 1965. With the benefit of hindsight, Colonel Glass outlined the conceptual errors in understanding the effects of war on service members and the impracticality and limited effectiveness of screening efforts.

Medical planners still believed that pre-entry screening was a viable means of reducing psychiatric casualties in war. Their belief was that the screening done during World War I was simply not adequate to achieve the goals. Dr. Harry Stack Sullivan was appointed as psychiatric consultant to the Selective Service. On November 7, 1940, Medical Circular No. 1 of the Selective Service outlined "Minimum Psychiatric Inspection" to aid the medical examiners of the 6043 local draft boards (Army Medical Department n.d.). Subsequent review indicated that 1,750,000 men, 12% of all examined, were rejected due to neuropsychiatric conditions (Appel 1946). Psychiatric casualties from combat were not lessened, and there is some evidence that many who were screened out could actually function at an effective level if allowed to serve (Jones et al. 2003). As war broke out, most of these screening programs were abandoned due to the high throughput of inductees into active service and the limited number of examiners. By the end of the war, it was clear that screening had limited value, that "normal" men would succumb to stress under extreme conditions, that psychiatric casualties closely paralleled other battle casualties, and that severity and duration of combat were directly associated with casualty rates (Ferrell and Appel 1994). It was also recognized that the long duration and high intensity of the war overall contributed to the increasing psychiatric casualties (Appel et al. 1946).

In 1940 there were only 20 Regular Army physicians with some training and experience in psychiatry. When the possibility of entry into another war became evident, the American Psychiatric Association formed a committee on military mobilization and met with the Surgeons General of the Army and Navy. The committee contacted 100 physicians certified by the American Board of Psychiatry and Neurology, but no psychiatrists were actually brought into service. There were so few qualified psychiatrists at the onset of war that those with any training were classed into four groups, ranging from "outstanding specialist" to "required constant supervision" with associated grades of potential assignment. At the end of 1942, there were 1235 listed psychiatrists on active duty, but only 194 held certification in psychiatry or psychiatry and neurology (Army Medical Department n.d.). To meet the shortage, the School of Military Neuropsychiatry enrolled its first class on December 20, 1942, and by the end of the war, it had graduated 1000 physicians. The training consisted of 190 h of instruction delivered over 4 weeks, similar to a rotation in psychiatry in the third or fourth year of medical school. It was not advertised as providing sufficient training for board certification but was considered "adequate for its purpose." Due to the lack of practical clinical experience, new graduates of the school required extensive supervision from experienced psychiatrists (Army Medical Department n.d.; Porter 1943). By 1944 the Army Surgeon General was authorized to redistribute physicians by qualifications between commands, which brought about the use of the psychiatric consultants in personnel assignments, a practice still in effect today. Further attempts were made to procure (induct by draft) more civilian psychiatrists into active service; such efforts met with little success.

It was common for a psychiatrist to be responsible for 100 or more patients on his wards at any given time. General medical officers were often forced to designate inexperienced medical officers as the division psychiatrist. Other units and facilities were similarly understaffed with psychiatrists. A survey in November 1944 found 1885 psychiatrists on duty, but fewer than 400 were capable of independent or supervisor status. At the end of hostilities in Europe, there were 55,000 psychiatric patients in Army hospitals, in comparison to 250,000 surgical patients and 254,000 medical patients.

Forward treatment (PIES principles as previously outlined) was again employed as a means to maintain adequate forces at or near the front. In the theater of battle, roughly 40% of neuropsychiatric casualties were actually returned to forward duty, according to Army records. Only 35% of such frontline admissions were evacuated away from the front lines, and only 1 man in 10 was sent stateside. Those kept in theater who were not sent back to the line were placed in support positions (Ferrell and Appel 1994; Appel et al. 1946).

During early periods of mobilization, psychiatric treatments were for the most part absent. If a soldier did not adjust to duty, they were referred to hospital for evaluation and disposition. Problems paralleled those seen in civilian settings, ranging from psychosis to more "neurotic" disorders (adjustment and mood disorders), immaturity, "mentally defective" (presumably intellectually impaired), and personality or character disorders. Similar to today's practice of military psychiatry, distinctions had to be made between "mental disease" and personality or intellectual disorders. Those with "illness" were given medical discharges; others were separated through administrative means by line commanders. The distinction between "neurotic symptoms" and simple lack of adjustment was not always clear.

As the war progressed, an increasing number of soldiers were evacuated who were "not as cooperative... irritable … tense and restless, subject to emotional outbursts, and admittedly unwilling to continue to serve." There was no consensus about whether such soldiers suffered from "illness" or were "maladjusted" (Army Medical Department n.d.). Among psychiatrists there was a general sense that "poor motivation and morale" were important factors in determining rates of neuropsychiatric casualties (Appel et al. 1946). The term "psychoneurosis" was poorly defined, and there was little inter-rater reliability with regard to the diagnosis.

The problem of "disposing" of noneffective personnel plagued the Army during the entire duration of the war. The infamous Section VIII of Army Regulation 615-360 ("Section Eight Discharges") proved problematic for line commanders who were not familiar with the administrative procedure or felt that it represented an acknowledgment of their failure to rehabilitate such individuals. Line commanders often pressured medical officers to medically separate individuals with primarily personality or character problems. This tension between line commanders and medical officers and between behavioral versus "medical" discharges exists to this day.

In December 1942 another category of discharge emerged, "Discharge for the Convenience of the Government," outlined in Section X of Army Regulation 615-360. That section described discharge for being physically incapable of performing skilled military work, having insufficient intelligence to absorb instructions, or being incapable of performing manual labor day after day. Complaints arose from overseas commanders that too many men were arriving "mentally unsuited for ordinary military duties." Directives were issued in March and April of 1943 requiring "greater care ... to do everything possible ... to prevent all individuals predisposed" to mental illness from entering military service and to "increase their efforts to detect individuals … with a view to the discharge of those who cannot be expected to render full military duty" (Army Medical Department n.d.).

By 1943 there were increasing numbers of "limited duty" personnel who were rated as incapable of deployed duty. In July 1943 the War Department eliminated the category "limited service," and all such men were to be discharged. Total discharges due to psychiatric disorders were 8.8 per thousand in 1942; this number peaked at 21.9 per thousand in 1943 and dropped to 17.9 per thousand by 1945. The peak discharge rate was 35.6 per thousand in September 1943. This pattern of discharges and impact on available manpower did not go unnoticed, and in November 1943 all previous instructions were rescinded, and men were reassigned to any useful service in an overseas theater (Army Medical Department n.d.).

The pendulum again swung by June 1944 when commanding officers reported that, among men returned to forward service, 26% presented excellent adjustment, while 42% presented as adequately adjusted and 32% as poorly adjusted. By September 1944, any degree of psychoneurosis was considered below minimum induction standards. There was pressure to discharge "for the convenience of the Government" rather than with a certificate of disability. Behind this pressure was a concern that disability ratings encouraged service members to "stay sick" because of disability payments.

Much of the problem with selecting the most appropriate discharge can be attributed to the fact that the psychiatric and psychological impact of warfare was not fully understood and often attributed to a lack of "moral conviction" or resentment of being forced into service. The range of treatments, even in major hospitals, was limited to rest, light duty, exercise, and "activities" therapies. The posttraumatic syndrome had not yet been recognized, there were no effective medications, and psychotherapies were not routinely practiced and were clearly not available on a mass scale (Army Medical Department n.d.).

With the advantage of 20 years of hindsight, Colonel Glass outlined the major limitations of military psychiatry during World War II. In his view military and medical leaders failed to appreciate the inevitability of large-scale psychiatric disorders under conditions of modern warfare. There was too much faith in psychiatric screening at entry with no reliably proven methods or outcome measures. Hospitalization, rather than ambulatory care, perpetuated illness and disability. Most importantly, the lack of trained and experienced military psychiatrists during the war perpetuated the problem. Glass' summary is supported by a postwar report from the Surgeon General's Office that cited 1,750,000 men rejected for service—and yet there were approximately 1,000,000 psychiatric admissions to military hospitals. That report demonstrated that most of those admitted would not have met admission criteria for civilian hospitalization but that, without an appropriate ambulatory treatment setting, service members simply could not return to their units; hospitals became the only available option (Appel 1946).

Veterans

The Veterans Administration (VA) greatly expanded during and following World War II. In the 1930s there were 60 Veteran Administration hospitals in operation. By the end of World War II, there were 34 new facilities in operation, and 43 military hospitals were transferred to the Veterans Administration from the armed services. In 1944, 76 new hospitals were authorized for construction (Office of Construction and Facilities Management n.d.). The postwar transformation was even more remarkable. Much of the modernization was driven by the newly appointed Administrator of Veterans Affairs, General Omar Bradley. At the time of his selection, the VA was in dismal condition; in January 1946 there were fewer than 1000 physicians to take care of 100,000 hospitalized patients. Following the passage of Public Law 293, the ability to hire physicians became less tedious, and within 6 months the VA physician staffing grew to over 4000 physicians. VA hospitals soon established affiliations with civilian medical schools, and by 1947, 1000 residents staffed these newly designated teaching hospitals. In their role as faculty of medical schools, VA physicians were encouraged to engage in research. Dr. Paul Magnuson became the first Assistant Chief Medical Director for Research and Education. By 1952 the VA had research programs at 66 hospitals, and the Chicago VA Research Hospital was built (Hays 2010). In addition to the hospitals, the VA also opened free-standing mental hygiene clinics across the country. The staffing of these clinics was similar to that of current interdisciplinary clinics with psychiatrists, psychologists, and psychiatric social workers in a ratio of 1:1:2. Screening intakes were conducted by the social workers, and the psychiatrist assigned providers to new patients (Futterman et al. 1947).

One of these veteran clinics reported on a case series of patients with war neuroses. The syndrome they observed included "intense anxiety, recurrent battle dreams, startle reaction to sudden or loud noises, and a tendency to sudden, explosive, aggressive reactions." They also experienced "a tendency to avoid people, fear of exposure to any type of criticism, difficulty in making decisions, and various types of sleep disturbances." They viewed this pattern as a result of "the threat of annihilation and destruction … under combat conditions" and noted that "the patient reacts to seemingly minor stimuli and seemingly innocuous situations in civilian life as if he were still under combat conditions." In addition to the description that aligns with current diagnostic criteria for posttraumatic stress disorder (PTSD), their treatments also closely approximated the current approach of prolonged exposure psychotherapy: "The monotonous repetition of the traumatic events is so characteristic of the true traumatic war neurosis. … We have also noted in many cases that after numerous repetitions, the character of the account has subtly changed so that it tends to become less devastating to the patient" (Futterman and Pumpian-Mindlin 1951).

Korean War

Active Duty

The USA had little time to settle from World War II before the onset of hostilities in Korea in 1950. At this time, the draft was still in place, and nearly 6 million served during the period between 1950 and 1953. There were 33,739 battle deaths and 103,284 non-mortal wounds (DeBrune and Leland 2015). The Korean War was challenging for combatants and for the delivery of medical and psychiatric care. The climate and geography ranged from hot and humid rice paddies to bitterly cold and barren mountainous regions. The lines of combat were constantly shifting along with the locations of frontline medical facilities. At times, the number of psychiatric casualties rose to 250 men per thousand, per annum. To some advantage, the lessons of WWII had not been completely forgotten. Once again, very low return rates from the soldiers and marines who were sent to the comforts and safety of hospital ships and nearby hospitals in Japan demonstrated the problem of evacuation away from theater (Ritchie 2002). Division psychiatrists held the responsibility for "rigid economy" in preserving fighting forces at the line. Their role was now much more sophisticated than it had been previously. In addition to providing diagnosis and treatment, they were expected to educate other medical officers and commanders regarding psychiatric principles in a combat setting and to make specific recommendations that could mitigate emergence of psychiatric problems (Edwards and Peterson 1954).

Veterans

By 1953 the workload at the Veterans Administration had greatly expanded, and the agency was reorganized into the three departments: Medicine and Surgery, Veterans Benefits, and Department of Insurance. By 1956 there were 70,000 neuropsychiatric patients in VA hospitals. There were still no "evidence-based" treatments for combat-related psychiatric conditions, but the VA began to conduct research in psychopharmacology and electroconvulsive therapy in veteran patients. During the 1950s new classes of medications, including chlorpromazine, barbiturates, benzodiazepines, tricyclic antidepressants, and monoamine oxidase inhibitors, were coming into use. Surgical treatments were still being explored, and one early "randomized-control" study involved a demonstration of the effectiveness of the lobotomy and included 188 surgical subjects and 185 controls. The value of that research to future studies included the use of matched controls and the use of the Multidimensional Patient Rating Scale as a measure of outcome. A multicenter VA study in 1956 demonstrated superiority of chlorpromazine over other agents and placebo in patients with schizophrenia. By 1957 half of all VA patients with schizophrenia were receiving tranquilizing medications, and of these the majority was prescribed chlorpromazine (Hays 2010).

Vietnam War

Active Duty

The Vietnam conflict spanned more years than any prior United States war, beginning in 1964 and extending into 1973. Roughly 8,744,000 persons served overall, with approximately half in the army. Fewer than 1 million marines fought and the navy and air force totaled 3.5 million. There were 58,220 deaths and 153,303 non-mortal casualties requiring hospitalizations (DeBruyne and Leleand 2015). Early reports indicated that the rates of psychiatric casualties from combat exposure were low, similar to those seen in stateside forces. Only 6% of all medical evacuations were for psychiatric reasons. Attribution for such low numbers includes better command planning, better training and equipment, periods of recuperation, and the "1-year tour." It has also been suggested that the availability of material goods and bars provided mitigation for the effects of combat (Bourne 1970). The concepts of proximity care in theater were still in practice but later called into question on ethical grounds (Camp 1993). The long-term psychiatric outcomes did not align with early findings.

The end of the Vietnam War in 1973 also ended the draft. The USA now relied on a totally voluntary force that included routine use of reserve forces and the National Guard. The experience of Vietnam left a bad taste for warfare among the American people. In essence, it was a war that pulled young men from their families and lives and sent them to fight in a distant land, potentially to die for theoretical strategic political goals that most people never understood or agreed with. The 1970's drawdown in forces was massive, of similar proportions to that following World War I.

Ethics of the "PIES" Concept

By the end, the war in Vietnam was extremely unpopular among the general population in the USA and also among psychiatrists, some whom had served in Vietnam. They believed the war to be unethical and, by extension, any physician who participated in promoting its execution similarly to be unethical. Ambulatory treatment near the front lines clearly met its objective of maintaining troop strength, but did it meet the psychiatric needs of the individual? To summarize the ethical debate, some argued that sending a soldier from safety to a danger zone violated general medical ethics. A balanced consideration is more complex. Is it better to send a recently exhausted but recovered, well-experienced soldier back to his unit or to send an inexperienced replacement to a strange unit? There has been no prospective study of outcomes of these two scenarios, and no such study could be conducted. Therefore, there is no way to know definitively if the evacuated soldier would fare better in the long run or if the inexperienced replacement would be at greater risk of death (Camp 1993; Grieger 1994). One small naturalistic study among Israeli Defense Force personnel provides some insight into this question. In a 20-year follow-up of several hundred soldiers, researchers found that, among soldiers with combat stress reactions, those who received classic PIES treatment fared slightly better psychologically than similar soldiers with combat stress reactions treated in a rear echelon (Solomon et al. 2005).

Post-Vietnam War Period

Veterans and Posttraumatic Stress Disorder

From 1960 to 1980, there were remarkable advances in psychiatry that influenced treatment of veterans as well as the general population. In addition to the pharmacological advances that began in the 1950s, there were unprecedented efforts to better characterize and define psychiatric illness. The *Diagnostic and Statistical Manual, Second Edition* (*DSM-II*), was published in 1968. It was 136 pages in length, with 11 chapters on categories of illness. The neurosis chapter discussed categories ranging from phobias and anxiety to depression, but there was no mention of any disorder related to trauma (Committee on Nomenclature and Statistics of the American Psychiatric Association 1968). In contrast, *DSM-III*, published in 1980, was 507 pages in length and included very specific diagnostic criteria for each disorder. It was also the first classification manual to employ field trials to assess usefulness and discrimination between diagnoses. It was the first diagnostic manual to outline the diagnosis of posttraumatic stress disorder (PTSD) in its chapter on anxiety disorders (Committee on Nomenclature and Statistics of the American Psychiatric Association 1980). The criteria are remarkably similar to those described by VA psychiatrists 30 years previously (Futterman and Pumpian-Mindlin 1951). In the pre-internet era, new revisions to the DSM were not as open to public and professional scrutiny. The inclusion of this new (and yet old) diagnostic category was seemingly not based on recently published scientific reports or field trials. Dr. Spitzer published a review of the changes to *DSM* just prior to the release of *DSM-III*. In discussing PTSD he references only a book chapter dating back to 1968 (Spitzer et al. 1980). Despite the lack of prior systematic study, criteria have remained relatively stable during the following 35 years of research.

The National Vietnam Veterans Readjustment Study and the VA National Center for PTSD

Public Law 98–160 ordered a study of the problems facing veterans of the Vietnam War. As part of the mandate, the Veterans Administration contracted a consortium of researchers to study the causes, manifestations, and long-term impact of wartime experiences (Congress of the United States 1983). Their report of the National Vietnam Veterans Readjustment Study was published in November 1988 (Kulka et al. 1998). Using a complex technique of interlinking databases, they were able to identify and interview a representative sample of 3016 Vietnam-era veterans using a combination of well-established diagnostic instruments. Researchers found that 15.2% of all male and 8.5% of all female Vietnam theater veterans suffered from PTSD at the time of the study. An additional 11.1% of male and 7.8% of female theater veterans experienced "partial PTSD" symptoms at the time of the study. That is, they had clinically significant stress reaction symptoms but did not meet full diagnostic criteria. Analysis of lifetime prevalence of PTSD was 30.6% for men and 26.9% for women among those who served in theater.

The National Center for PTSD was created in 1989 within the Department of Veteran Affairs in response to Public Law 98–528 to address the needs of veterans and other trauma survivors with PTSD (Congress of the United States 1984). Its current organization includes Headquarters in White River Junction, VT, and a research division in Boston, MA; West Haven, CT; Palo Alto, CA; and Honolulu, HI. The center maintains and makes available to clinicians, veterans, family members, and the general public a vast array of research, educational, and clinical materials as well as a treatment referral guide. One of their major achievements is the compilation of Published International Literature on Traumatic Stress (PILOTS).

Desert Shield/Desert Storm

In an effort to shape the role of war for the USA, Secretary of Defense for President Reagan, Casper Weinberger, used the lessons of the Vietnam War to develop a "doctrine for warfare." In summary, it examined the following factors: whether vital national interests are at stake, entering war with the intent of winning, force must be decisive and with clear intents, Congress and the public sentiment should be in support, entering warfare should be only done as a last resort, and such efforts should be constantly reassessed. The Iraq invasion of Kuwait met the criteria (Dubois 1991). It was determined that the USA and its allies had the force needed to overcome an adversary on foreign soil, a steady supply of oil from an ally was in the nation's interest, there were clear endpoints to the use of force, and the American people were supportive.

In contrast to World War I, World War II, and the Korean and Vietnam Wars, the war in Kuwait was of much smaller scale and duration. Roughly 2,225,000 service members were involved, with 148 battle deaths and 467 nonlethal wounds (Debruyne and Leland 2015). As the USA prepared for war, there were many uncertainties: the Iraqi Army had a reputation of ferocious performance during its battles with Iran, there was a threat of widespread use of chemical weapons (previously used against its own population during periods of unrest), and the USA's tactics and forces had not been battle-tested in 20 years. Some estimates called for tens of thousands of

American battle casualties. In contrast to prior wars, there had been considerable planning prior to the consideration of entry into war. Public Law 97–174 called for establishment of the Department of Defense-Department of Veterans Affairs Contingency Plan. Under this plan, the VA would provide up to 25,000 receiving beds at 77 primary receiving and 82 secondary receiving hospitals (Blank and Lehmann 1996). The plan was never activated.

In view of limited exposure to combat and the short duration of the war, there were few reports of posttraumatic stress symptoms and no broad-scale population studies. Some small studies among demobilized reserve units showed very low levels of PTSD symptoms in about 10% of those sampled (Southwick et al. 1993). In contrast to clear psychological disorders, veterans began to present with a multitude of physical symptoms following the completion of Desert Shield/Desert Storm. The complaints that were initially referred to as "Gulf War Syndrome," the VA now categorizes as "chronic multi-symptom illness" and approves presumptive service connection and compensation for the following: chronic fatigue syndrome, fibromyalgia, functional gastrointestinal disorders, and several other undiagnosed illnesses with symptoms (Veterans Administration n.d.).

Operations Iraqi Freedom and Enduring Freedom

In 2001 the USA was attacked on its own soil without warning, and calls for retaliation became common. In contrast with the liberation of Kuwait a decade before, the public backing and ultimate goals of the conflicts that ensued were less uniform. Much like the legacy of the Vietnam War, the American public has become highly divided about the USA's goals in the conflict and its role in the region. In contrast to Desert Shield/ Desert Storm, there have been over 2300 American deaths in Afghanistan and its surrounds and over 4000 deaths in Iraq with ongoing deaths at the time of this writing (DeBruyne and Leleand 2015).

In advance of ground hostilities, the Veterans Administration and the Services planned jointly for the assessment and management of psychiatric casualties. The Iraq War Clinician Guide, first published in 2004, is an invaluable tool for anyone working with combat veterans and was written and compiled by the National Center for Posttraumatic Stress Disorder and the Walter Reed Army Medical Center (2004).

Early surveys of returning troops using well-validated screening tools showed rates of PTSD between 12% and 20% and presence of depression in roughly 15% (Hoge et al. 2004). In light of these findings, the services implemented the Post Deployment Health Assessment program to detect service members at risk at the time of return from deployment (Appenzeller et al. 2007). Subsequent programs provided for similar screening a few months later and again prior to the next deployment. In prior wars, reporting psychiatric symptoms provided "gain," protection from return to combat. In a volunteer force, however, minimizing symptoms could preserve a career with attendant medical and retirement benefits. This logic was clearly demonstrated in one study in which screening was conducted with an "identifiable screener" and then repeated by the same individuals in an anonymous setting. The rates of PTSD and depression were nearly two to four times higher in the anonymous setting compared to the identifiable setting, presumably because of concern over career impact or other stigma (Warner et al. 2011). There is also evidence that some cases of PTSD develop months after return from combat, demonstrating the need for ongoing monitoring (Grieger et al. 2006).

Military suicide rates were traditionally lower than matched civilian suicides. This statistic began to change with the newest conflicts, and by 2008 the military rates exceeded civilian rates. The rates tripled among previously deployed members, increasing from roughly 13 per 100,000 person years in 2005 to roughly 33 per 100,000 person years in 2010. The causes for this trend are not clear but are now under close examination as part of a collaboration between the Army and the

National Institute of Health (Schoenbaum et al. 2014; Kessler et al. 2015). Increased rates of suicide in veterans have also become a concern, with rates of suicide death 60% higher than in nonveterans (Hoffmire et al. 2015).

Summary

Over the past century, each epoch of warfare has brought unique challenges and solutions. The casualties of war have forced psychiatrists, political leaders, and American society at large to recognize the terrible toll that combat has taken from some of those who fight for their country. The impact of war has pushed forward the development of systems of health-care delivery and even the very nature of diagnostic criteria and nomenclature. Stress reactions, once thought to be the physiologic products of explosive blast pressure, are now known to be complex disorders involving multiple neural networks. The unified network of Veterans Administration hospitals now provides a foundational substrate for research to develop better treatments. Service members and veterans provide naturalistic cohorts for observation over time; patterns of reactions and behaviors have been seen repeatedly following combat exposure. From these observations, the category of trauma-related disorders was born. The practice of psychiatry has gradually migrated from psychiatric institutions to general hospitals, community clinics, and the battlefield; much of this migration was born of necessity related to war casualties. Military psychiatrists have evolved beyond treatment of patients, as they now serve routinely as organizational consultants to command leaders, where they promote command actions to ameliorate the conditions that lead to psychological problems.

Key Concepts

1. Efforts to "screen out" those at risk for adverse psychological reactions to combat have proved to be minimally effective.
2. Psychiatric casualty rates correlate closely with the intensity and duration of combat exposure, making the profile of casualties unique to each war.
3. Service members are not prone to report psychological problems if doing so may impact their career.
4. Suicide rates among active duty and veterans have increased dramatically during and following service in the recent conflicts.

References

Appel JW, Beebe GW, Hilger DW (1946) Comparative incidence of neuropsychiatric casualties in World War I and World War II. Am J Psychiatr 103(2):196–199

Appenzeller GN, Warner CH, Grieger T (2007) Postdeployment health reassessment: a sustainable method for brigade combat teams. Mil Med 172(10):1017–1023

Army Medical Department (1929) 'The Medical Department of the United States Army in the World War.' Available from: http://history.amedd.army.mil/booksdocs/wwi/Neuropsychiatry/default.htm

Army Medical Department. (n.d.) 'Neuropsychiatry in World War II.' Available from: http://history.amedd.army.mil/booksdocs/wwii/NeuropsychiatryWWIIvolI/default.htm

Blank AS, Lehmann LS (1996) Preparation for psychiatric casualties in the Department of Veterans Affairs medical system. In: Ursano RJ, Norwood AA (eds) Emotional aftermath of the Persian Gulf war: veterans, families, communities, and nations. American Psychiatric Press, Washington, DC

Bourne PG (1970) Military psychiatry and the Viet Nam experience. Am J Psychiatr 127(4):123–130

Camp NM (1993) The Vietnam war and the ethics of combat psychiatry. Am J Psychiatr 150(7):1000–1010

Committee on Nomenclature and Statistics of the American Psychiatric Association (1952) Diagnostic and statistical manual of mental disorders, Second edn. American Psychiatric Association, Washington, DC

Committee on Nomenclature and Statistics of the American Psychiatric Association (1968) Diagnostic and statistical manual of mental disorders, Second edn. American Psychiatric Association, Washington, DC

Congress of the United States – 98, Public Law 98-160 (1983) 'Veterans' health care amendments of 1983.' Available at: https://www.gpo.gov/fdsys/pkg/STATUTE-97/pdf/STATUTE-97-Pg993.pdf

Congress of the United States – 98, Public Law 98-528 (1984) 'Veterans' health care act of 1984,' Available at: https://www.gpo.gov/fdsys/pkg/STATUTE-98/pdf/STATUTE-98-Pg2686.pdf

DeBruyne NF, Leland A (2015) 'American war and military operations casualties: lists and statistics, Congressional Research Service,' RL32492, pp. 1–29.

Available at: https://fas.org/sgp/crs/natsec/RL32492.pdf
Dubois TR (1991) 'The Weinberger doctrine and the liberation of Kuwait,' Parameters, pp. 24–38. Available at: http://strategicstudiesinstitute.army.mil/pubs/parameters/Articles/1991/1991%20duboise.pdf
Edwards RM, Peterson DB (1954) Korea: current psychiatric procedure and communications in the combat theater. Am J Psychiatr 110(10):721–724
Ferrel MJ, Appel JW (1994) Current trends in military neuropsychiatry. Am J Psychiatr 101(1):12–19
Futterman S, Pumpian-Mindlin E (1951) Traumatic war neuroses five years later. Am J Psychiatr 108(6):401–408
Futterman S, Kirkner FJ, Meyer MM (1947) First year analysis of veterans treated in a mental hygiene clinic. Am J Psychiatr 104(5):298–305
Grieger TA (1994) Ethics of combat psychiatry. Am J Psychiatr 151(6):949
Grieger TA, Cozza SJ, Ursano RJ, Martinez PE, Engel CC, Wain HJ (2006) Posttraumatic stress disorder and depression in battle-injured soldiers. Am J Psychiatr 163(10):1777–1783
Hays MT (2010) A historical look at the establishment of the Department of Veterans Affairs research and development program. Government Printing Office. Available at: http://www.research.va.gov/pubs/docs/ORD-85yrhistory
Hoffmire CA, Kemp JE, Bossarte RM (2015) Changes in suicide mortality for veterans and non-veterans by gender and history of VHA service use, 2000–2010. Psychiatr Serv 66(9):959–965
Hoge CW, Castro CA, Messer SC, McGurk D, Cotting DI, Koffman RL (2004) Combat duty in Iraq and Afghanistan, mental health problems and barriers to care. N Engl J Med 351(1):13–22
Jones E, Wessely S (2014) Battle for the mind: world was 1 and the birth of military psychiatry. Lancet 384:1708–1714
Jones E, Hyams KC, Wessely S (2003) Screening for vulnerability to psychological disorders in the military: an historical survey. J Med Screen 10(1):40–46
Kessler RC, Warner CH, Ivany C, Petukhova MV, Rose S, Bromet EJ, Brown M, Cai T, Colpe LJ, Cox KL, Fullerton CS, Gilman SE, Gruber MJ, Heeringa SG, Lewandowski-Romps L, Li J, Millikan-Bell AM, Naif JA, Nock MK, Rosellina AJ, Sampson NA, Schoenbaum M, Stein MB, Wessely S, Zaslavsky AM, Ursano RJ (2015) Predicting suicides after psychiatric hospitalization in US Army soldiers. J Am Med Assoc Psychiatry 72(1):49–57
Kulka RA, Schlenger WE, Fairbank JA, Hough RL, Jordan BK, Marmar CR, Weiss DS (1998) Contractual report of the findings from the National Vietnam Veterans Readjustment Study. Research Triangle Institute, Research Park Triangle, pp 1–644. Available at: http://www.ptsd,va.gov/professional/articles/article-pdf/nvvrs_vol1.pdf
National Center for Post-traumatic Stress Disorder and Walter Reed Army Medical Center (2004) Iraq war clinicians guide, Second edition. Available at: http://www.va.gov/professional/materials/manuals/iraq-war-clinician-guide.asp
Office of Construction and Facilities Management. (n.d.) Veterans Administration. Available at: http://www.cfm.va.gov/about/history.asp
Pols H, Oak S (2007) War and military mental health: the US psychiatric response in the 20th century. Am J Public Health 97(12):2132–2142
Porter WC (1943) The school of military neuropsychiatry. Am J Psychiatr 100(1):25–27
Ritchie EC (2002) Psychiatry in the Korean war. Mil Med 167(11):898–903
Schoenbaum M, Kessler RC, Gilman SE, Colpe LJ, Heeringa SG, Stein MB, Ursano RJ, Cox KL (2014) Predictors of suicide and accidental death in the Army study to assess risk and resilience in servicemembers (ArmySTARRS). J Am Med Assoc Psychiatry 71(5):493–503
Solomon Z, Shklar R, Mikulincer M (2005) Frontline treatment of combat stress reaction; a 20-year longitudinal evaluation study. Am J Psychiatr 162(12):2309–2314
Southwick SM, Morgan A, Nagy LM, Bremner D, Nicolaou AL, Johnson DR, Rosenheck R, Charney DS (1993) Trauma related symptoms in veterans of operation desert storm: a preliminary report. Am J Psychiatr 150(1):1524–1528
Spitzer RL, Williams JBW, Skodel AF (1980) DSM III: the major achievements and an overview. Am J Psychiatr 137(2):151–164
Taskforce on Nomenclature and Statistics (1980) Diagnostic and statistical manual of mental disorders, Third edn. American Psychiatric Association, Washington, DC
United States Department of Veterans Affairs. Gulf war veterans medically unexplained illnesses. Available at: http://www.publichealth.va.gov/exposures/gulfwar/medically-unexplained-illness.asp
United States Department of Veterans Affairs. History of CFM. Office of construction and facilities management, pp. 1–5, Available: http://www.cfm.va.gov/about/history.asp
United States War Department (1918) Annual report of the Secretary of War. Available at: https://archive.org/details/annualreportsec27deptgoog
Warner CH, Appenzeller GN, Grieger T, Belenky S, Brietbach J, Parker J, Warner CM, Hoge C (2011) Importance of anonymity to encourage honest reporting in mental health screening after combat deployment. Arch Gen Psychiatry 68(10):1065–1071

The Importance of US Military Cultural Competence

2

Eric G. Meyer and Gary H. Wynn

Introduction

Patients in the military[1] are trained, identified, rated, promoted, and retained based on their occupation and how well they perform at that occupation. This identity frames their perception of self, their illness, and their treatment. The principle that a patient's identity can influence treatment has been embraced for centuries (Hippocrates and Jones 1923). Since the term "cultural competence" was coined in 1982 (Green 1982), this belief has largely been subsumed as part of a culturally competent approach. Military service, to include being a dependent of a service member, dramatically shapes and defines a person's culture. Despite the proliferation of cultural competence work over the past 20 years, literature on military cultural competence was scant until Hobbs' (Hobbs 2008) and Reger's (Reger et al. 2008) respective publications in 2008. In 2011, Hoge underscored that improved military cultural competence was necessary for improved mental health outcomes in military personnel (Hoge 2011). A 2012 letter aptly titled "The Unasked Question" exposed the need for a military history in all clinical encounters (Brown 2012). With assistance from the White House's Joining Forces Program, the notion that military cultural competence is critical for improved care of military members has gained national attention.

In partnership with Joining Forces, the Association for American Medical Colleges (AAMC) completed an assessment of its member schools' military-specific curriculum. Of the 104 respondent schools, only 21.2% included any material on military culture. Discussion of traumatic brain injury (TBI) or posttraumatic stress disorder (PTSD) in the context of the military was limited to 56.7% and 47.1%, respectively (Association of American Medical Colleges 2012). A 2014 RAND report revealed that 70.5% of mental health providers working at a Veterans Affairs (VA) or Department of Defense (DoD) facility demonstrated military cultural competence. In contrast, a meager 23.7% of TriCARE affiliate providers and 7.7% of nonaffiliated providers evidenced such competencies (Tanielian et al. 2014). Another study

[1]For simplicity, the term "military" will be used rather than the combination of military/veteran. When there is a difference between these two terms, it will be explicitly stated. It should also be noted that this text refers to the US Military, not all militaries.

E.G. Meyer (✉) • G.H. Wynn
Department of Psychiatry, Uniformed Services University of the Health Sciences (USUHS), 4301 Jones Bridge Rd, Bethesda, MD 20814, USA
e-mail: Eric.meyer@usuhs.edu

L.W. Roberts, C.H. Warner (eds.), *Military and Veteran Mental Health*,
https://doi.org/10.1007/978-1-4939-7438-2_2

revealed that only 39% of providers outside of the VA/DoD were screening for military service (Pankow et al. 2013). According to a recent PEW survey (Parker 2011), civilian understanding of the military continues to wane as fewer serve in the military. Even through this is longest period of continuous war in US history, less than 0.5% of the US population has been on active duty at any point in the last 10 years. The same study reported that 77% of veterans have lost confidence that the general public understands the unique problems they experience. This is an especially sobering statistic considering that, in 2006, 66% of veterans received care completely outside of the VA (The Health Care System for Veterans: An Interim Report 2007), which may increase since Congress passed the Veterans Access, Choice, and Accountability Act in 2014 (Veterans' Access to Care through Choice, Accountability, and Transparency Act of 2014).

There are indeed a significant number of individuals whose identity, and thus care, is influenced by military culture. For example, 6% of the US population has served in the US military (U.S. Census Bureau 2010), and 33% of the US population is directly related to someone who has served (Parker 2011). Of those who have served in Iraq or Afghanistan, 12–18% are reported to have PTSD (Hoge et al. 2004). Leaders in the field of military traumatic stress contend that PTSD in the military cannot be understood, and hence effectively treated, without an appreciation that many of the symptoms can be advantageous in combat (Cozza et al. 2014; Hoge 2010). Recent findings demonstrate that military service members' negative perception of mental healthcare delivery is associated with a larger adverse impact on healthcare utilization than stigma (Kim et al. 2011). However, to better understand the importance of military cultural competence and the current efforts to improve such competencies, a review of cultural competence and military culture is required.

Case Study

A request for psychiatric consultation was placed by neurosurgery for "psychosis" in a 40-year-old male service member, currently on active duty in the US Air Force. Lieutenant Colonel (LtCol) Kevin Franks (pseudonym) had endured a 3-month history of unremitting headaches eventually attributed to a cystic septum cavum pellucidum. Over the past 3 months, numerous providers had evaluated his headaches with no abnormalities noted on exam, lab work, or imaging studies. Several pharmaceutical therapies for presumed migraines had failed. Evaluation for a cerebrospinal fluid leak was negative on multiple occasions. After steroid treatment failed, repeat imaging revealed a possible cystic septum cavum pellucidum. Surgical fenestration of the membranes was scheduled, but the neurosurgery team desired a second opinion from a neighboring hospital given the rare nature of the diagnosis and the inconsistency between the onset of the headache and imaging findings. The neurosurgical team reported that in response to their desire for a second opinion, the patient threatened to leave against medical advice unexpectedly and "fix it himself."

Upon examination, LtCol Franks explained that the delay of care caused him a great deal of frustration. He could not understand why "everyone was so comfortable with [his] being 'out of commission' given that [he was] an expensive and hard to replace asset for the military." He went on to explain that in his line a work, as an aircraft maintenance officer, if a plane was not operational everyone on the maintenance team worked around the clock to get that asset back in the air. He understood that medicine is not aircraft maintenance, but he had a difficult time appreciating the neurosurgical team's rationale for requesting a second opinion. He characterized himself as "useless" during his hospitalization and verbalized a preference for immediate surgery to expedite "getting back to doing what the military paid him to do."

LtCol Franks' frustration was primarily related to a cultural difference in the approach to his care. Neurosurgery re-explained the care plan in the patient's terms: "It's as if you had to disassemble a plane, knowing that a possible consequence was irreparable." In terms that resonated with him, the patient appreciated the neurosurgical team's conservative approach. A second opinion confirmed the diagnosis and his headache resolved hours after surgery. LtCol Franks was discharged from the hospital and quickly returned to active duty status.

Overview of Military Culture

The above case illustrates a consideration that military providers are confronted with on a daily basis. The military has a "language, a code of manners, norms of behavior, belief systems, dress, and rituals" (Reger et al. 2008). Military culture is, in fact, more delineated than most cultures, as many of its tenants are clearly defined by law. The constitutional requirement that service members relinquish their personal privacy has a dramatic influence on their approach to patient privacy. Looking beyond such foundational influences, the experience of being in the military is also palpable. Service members "develop camaraderie, esprit de corps, group cohesiveness, and a set of idealistic honorable tenets that make up the glue that hinges [them] together with common bonds" (Krueger 2000). For some, the military provides an escape that may represent a predictable, sheltered life they did not have growing up (Wertsch 1991). For others, it stands as a final bastion as a rite of initiation into manhood (Nash and Figley 2011). For many, the desire to embody the warrior mindset drives membership (Harrison 2006).

Through indoctrination, military culture overlays and often replaces previous cultural beliefs (Fenell 2008) while reducing—but not eliminating (Foynes et al. 2013)—many disparities that exist in civilian culture (Harris 2011; Hobbs 2008; Lundquist 2008). Immersion in military culture can be such an indelible experience that veterans will identify with it more than any other cultural influence even decades after leaving active duty service. Preferential military association can occur after only short times of service (de Burgh et al. 2011) and can take precedence over other common identities such as race, gender, sexual orientation, political party, or socioeconomic status. However, for some members, military culture can be a source of conflict. Some women have described military culture as negatively impacting their experience and recovery from military sexual trauma (Bell et al. 2014). Good or bad, indoctrination into military culture is so profound that it can fundamentally change a service member's worldview, often impeding transition back to civilian life (Brewin et al. 2010).

Mission oriented (Reger et al. 2008), expected to make sacrifices (Dahn 2008), and defined by their ability to function, service members have a wary relationship with mental health. Many (Hoge et al. 2004) equate having a mental health diagnosis with being "broken" or "weak" (Lande 2014), while seeking care is perceived as selfish and mission-compromising (Malmin 2013; Vogt 2011). Others fear it will damage their career (Langston et al. 2007). As early as 1967, military psychiatrists recognized that psychiatric diagnoses could pathologize normal, adaptive stress responses in the military (Dubey 1967). Similarly, current advice recommends framing military mental health concerns occupationally (Castro and Adler 2011; Hoge 2011) or in the context of performance enhancement (Lunasco et al. 2010). Despite efforts to strike a balance between keeping military patients operational while still treating them (Singh 2003), service members have reported a negative perception of mental health care that may be more disruptive than stigma (Kim et al. 2011). Looking beyond help-seeking behaviors, military culture also influences illness and treatment itself. Military culture has been cited as contributory to alcohol misuse (Ames et al. 2007; Jones 2011), family violence (Harrison 2006), sexually transmitted infection rates, and military sexual violence (Cameron et al. 2011). This is especially alarming, as military sexual trauma combined with combat exposure is associated with a twofold increase in the rates of new onset PTSD and difficulties transition to civilian life (Katz et al. 2007). Military culture has also been implicated in suppressing key elements needed for trauma recovery, including adaptive emotional resilience, behavioral flexibility, and impaired emotional communication (Greene et al. 2010; Keats 2010). It has even been argued that military culture may be the real patient when dealing with stress in the military (Singh 2003).

Deployments are a routine part of military life and have a marked impact on service members and their families (Erbes et al. 2008). Having a spouse deployed can increase parent stress, child behavioral problems, healthcare utilization, child maltreatment (Trautmann et al. 2015), and mental health problems—a risk that increases with tour length (de Burgh et al. 2011). Combat exposure can further alter family dynamics, as it places service members at increased risk of social exclusion, criminality, homelessness, self-harm, substance misuse, unexplained medical complaints, and mental illness (Deahl et al. 2011). For some families, the reintegration process after a deployment can be more difficult than the deployment itself (Rosen et al. 1993) and often requires increased support (Danish and Antonides 2013; Lester and Flake 2013). While these examples show the impact that the service member and deployments can have on a family, research also shows that family health impacts service member health (Cozza et al. 2014). Indeed, the military culture of the service member and one's family, and the bidirectional impact of military events with the family dynamic, are all salient considerations when providing care to military patients or their families.

Military Subcultures

Cultural identity is a dynamic process that intertwines varying levels of acculturation with multiple subcultures that can dramatically shift based on situational factors. Military cultural identity has thus far been presented as a homogenous experience, but like other cultures, it is more accurately understood as an amalgamation of related, and even conflicting, subcultures (Goodale et al. 2012). Service members often identify with their specific occupation—whether it be infantryman, pilot, or mechanic—more than their parent service (Meyer 2013; Wood 1988). Military medical providers are notable for the duality of their cultural orientation (Scannell-Desch 2000; Singh 2003) that instructs "officer first, doctor always." Women in the military often have a unique experience that can alter their perception of traumatic stress (Street et al. 2009) and other medical conditions (Levander and Overland 2015). Active duty culture is different than reserve or veteran subcultures. Examination of the directory of Veterans' Service Organizations (www.va.gov/vso), community-based organizations that support veterans, quickly reveals the diversity of subcultures present among veterans, with significant differentiation by branch of service, combat era, and (more recently) signature wounds of war (amputation, TBI, etc.).

To appreciate the richness associated with military cultural identity, a better understanding of the component subcultures is required. A brief description of a small collection of military subcultures is provided in this chapter, underscoring how a service member can be a member of several subcultures at the same time. These subcultures are organized within the parent culture in several ways: duty type (job), time period when the patient was on active duty, reserve status, veteran status, and the military family. Specific implications for the perception of illness, providers, and mental health are provided for duty subcultures to further illustrate the overlap and differences between these groups.

Duty Type

Naval Warfare (Capt James C. West, USN)

Background The ship represents the most meaningful paradigm for understanding naval culture. For hundreds of years, the mission of navies has been to control the seas through the regular deployment of warships. Even with modern automation, typical ships' crews include several hundred sailors and officers. A ship at sea operates as a closed social system with the captain as the ultimate authority. This leads to a culture in which authority and decision-making tend to be centralized. In addition to deference to authority, shipboard life indoctrinates a respect for systems and procedures. Warships are complex engineering systems that can most successfully operate only when all crewmembers adhere to proper operating procedures. Nowhere is this more evident than in the nuclear submarine force where the presence of both a nuclear reactor and hundreds of pounds per square inch of seawater represents a constant danger. All crewmembers are taught to respect these dangers, pay attention to details, and adhere to procedures lest they put themselves or their shipmates at risk are another perspective deeply shaped by shipboard life. A ship at sea has only the supplies that are loaded once it leaves port. Crews need to be ready to operate for long periods of time without the possibility of resupply. Thus the mentality of sailors emphasizes proper planning and provisioning and management of resources.

Navy families live around underway cycles. Most people automatically think of navy deployments as the only time sailors are away. The typical sailor assigned to a ship spends up to 50% of their time at sea. This includes routine periods at sea training and testing systems in addition to regular extended deployments. Families have to adapt to a constant cycle of separation and reunion. Spouses tend to become independent in these relationships and run the household. This is a common source of friction in navy relationships as sailors return home with the expectation of taking charge of a system used to functioning in their absence. Technology has changed the family dynamic significantly in the last two decades, as increased communications capability has in many cases connected the Internet to warships at sea. Where previously sailors would only find out events at home via Red Cross emergency notifications, now they get regular family updates via social media. This has the potential to create situations in which the sailor is able to receive worrisome information but feel unable to control the outcome of events at home. A vivid example of this is a sailor who stops receiving emails from his girlfriend while at sea who then starts finding social media posts of her photographed with other men. Clinically, this may emerge as increased distress and result in increased need for mental health care around the time of underways. Most naval hospitals are familiar with a surge in patient volume around the deployment of ships.

Perception of Illness and Treatment Perception is a product of the sea-duty screening process and appreciation of additional hazards related to service at sea. Seemingly minor illnesses such as kidney stones can be severely debilitating at sea. Urgent evacuation of acute medical problems takes away from time dedicated to missions and exposes ships and their crewmembers to additional risk. The sea-duty screening process is intended to minimize the likelihood of medical crises at sea by precluding sailors with conditions considered to be high risk. Another consideration is that the average sailor requires advanced technical training of up to a year in order to be able to fulfill job responsibilities. Loss of personnel due to illness or injury can generate significant gaps in manpower or capability of a ship. For this reason, there is a cultural tendency toward minimizing health problems and "pushing through" to meet the mission.

Perceptions of Medical Providers The perception of healthcare personnel on naval vessels is related to the proximity and level of health care available. Most US Navy vessels do not have their own physician but rather a specifically trained independent-duty corpsman (IDC). Larger ships may have a physician assigned. The independent-duty corpsman on a ship is given the title "Doc" and serves a typical population of 150 sailors. Independent-duty corpsmen have limited knowledge to diagnose and treat routine problems and prescribe a limited range of medications. This level of care is acceptable due to prescreening of all sailors for serious medical conditions before assigning them to duty aboard ships.

Attitudes Toward Mental Health Attitudes toward mental health and mental health care emphasize the ability of the individual and crew to accomplish the mission. Commanders tend to view mental health in terms of suitability to go to sea and ability to perform an assigned mission (Westphal 2007). If a sailor's mental health conditions allow them to serve safely at sea and perform an assigned mission, then commanders will view them favorably and accommodate any needs for mental health care. Malingering is a common concern, particularly that sailors will feign suicidality for purposes of getting out of time at sea. As mentioned earlier, it is common for emergency departments and behavioral health clinics to see a surge in distressed and suicidal sailors near the time of a ship's underway date. The net result is that seeking mental health care is encouraged and accepted so long as the affected sailor continues to meet mission requirements.

Aviation (Maj Christopher E. Backus, USAF)

Background Aviation is dangerous, and aviators are chosen to be highly competent and medically fit in order to mitigate that danger. They are the product of a stringent selection process in which many peers were excluded due to minor medical concerns. After selection, aviators undergo exacting training with further eliminations. The result is a community that is well aware they "made the cut" and that is highly aggressive regarding professional competence. They uncompromisingly focus on mission accomplishment and do not respect those who appear unmotivated. Flying is a fast-paced environment. Most fixed-wing aircraft must fly forward, and all aircraft have limited fuel, so making timely decisions is a hallmark of a competent aviator. Confidence is also prized, often at the expense for a tolerance for uncertainty.

Perceptions of Illness and Treatment Instead of abnormal pathology, the focus of aviator care is often normal physiology subjected to abnormal environments, such as heat/cold, vibration, high G-force exposure, and low oxygen. Fatigue and unusual sleep cycles lead to the need for go/no-go pills, one of the rare uses of medication in this population. Travel medicine requires proficient use of medications for gastrointestinal infections, malaria prophylaxis, and extensive immunizations for illnesses rarely seen in the United States.

Aviators remain aware they can be removed from aviation duty for a wide variety of medical issues, which can result in "reverse malingering," where aviators hide medical problems in order to avoid removal from aviation duty. In this sense, illness represents one of the most significant threats to continued aviation service.

Perception of Medical Providers Aviators have dedicated physicians for screening and specialized occupational health needs. It is these same physicians that may also remove their flight status due to illness. Thus, despite having access to specialized care, physicians represent the "enemy."

At the same time, physicians are evaluated as if they were fellow aviators. Physicians are seen as professional peers, responsible for a portion of mission accomplishment, a "human maintenance officer." Professional competence is assumed, as pilots are aware that physicians also have undergone extensive training. If this competence is questionable, the physician enters the mental category assigned to incompetent aviators, someone whose faults pose a risk to safety and mission accomplishment. Aviators will aggressively address this, either directly or indirectly, by avoiding and/or seeking a more competent replacement. Extended uncertainty and slow decision-making may be seen as signs of incompetence, lack of confidence, or lack of knowledge.

The threats that these unique demands can pose to good rapport and effective care can be mitigated if understood. Aviators respect a physician focused on returning them to the mission and only removing them from duty per a consistent process. Knowledge and understanding of the aviation mission are appreciated, as personal context is important to all patients. Decision-making that is slow or includes uncertainty needs to be clearly explained to avoid aviators' bias for fast, certain decision-making from tainting the physician-patient rapport.

Attitudes Toward Mental Health The stigma associated with mental health is extreme among aviators. Repercussions for mental health diagnoses can be significant, such as the almost universal disqualification for recurrent major depressive disorder. Thus, mental health symptoms like fatigue or difficulty in concentrating are not likely to be treated as a mental health condition or by a mental health provider. Instead, they will be viewed as "part of the job" and treated as an occupational issue versus a biopsychosocial one.

Special Forces (LTC Scott Moran, USA)

Background The culture of Special Operations Forces (SOF) is based on the idea of extreme performance. The ability to do one's job better than anyone else is the core of SOF. Every piece of equipment, from backpacks to aircraft, is the best. Even the training for SOF is unmatched: personnel assigned to SOF units will shoot thousands of rounds at a range to gain that performance advantage. Every component of SOF is designed to enhance the performance of the mission.

The process begins with assessment and selection. SOF operators are the equivalent of professional athletes. Operators are selected for their ability to complete the mission under any circumstance. Physical and psychological assessment selects operators who are highly resilient and determined individuals, with an unwavering focus on mission completion. Each service (Army, Navy, Air Force, Marine Corps) has a different method of assessing and selecting service members for its SOF, but the core idea remains the same: select people who are physically stronger and mentally tougher than general-purpose force. Once a service member has passed the assessment phase, they then begin the qualification phase—relentless training for over a year. Even support personnel assigned to SOF are expected to meet the same high level of performance, although they may not be assessed and selected. For example, a communications expert is expected to be able to physically keep up with "operators" and be able to get communication links working 100% of the time.

Perception of Illness and Treatment When a service member in Special Operations Forces (SOF) has an illness, their focus is on getting back to their pre-injury level of performance. Injury and illness are an expected part of being in SOF, but it is perceived to be something to be overcome. The primary focus of a SOF member is getting the mission accomplished. Any physical or mental injury or illness that "takes them out of the game" is viewed as an impediment to be fixed. Each unit has a Human Performance Training Center (HPTC), which is designed to maintain and return operators to their level of performance. This is a coordinated program of strength training and psychological training to increase performance. If a service member is injured, they will return to the HPTC once cleared by medical. There are strength coaches, athletic trainers, physical therapists, and sports psychologists who rehabilitate the service member and work to get them back to their previous high level of performance. SOF members often have difficulty with being medically separated from the military. They often will attempt to avoid disclosing to providers the extent and severity of their illness. This is not an uncommon behavior in other elite athletes.

Perceptions of Medical Providers Special Operations Forces service members expect their physicians and other providers to work just as hard as they do in getting them back to the fight. Medical providers are viewed as part of the team and are expected to excel at their profession skills. Medical providers deploy with SOF units and are often close to combat rather than remaining in deployed medical facilities as general-purpose forces medical providers often do. Providers are expected to be competent not only in their medical skills but also in combat skills such as weapons, airborne operations, and prolonged field care. Medical providers are often viewed as mentors to the 18D (SOF Medical Sergeants) and 68WW1 (SOF Medics). The providers will train these operators in advanced techniques and procedures to enable medical care to accompany the team. Medical providers earn great respect from SOF operators when they get them back to the mission.

Attitudes Toward Mental Health With behavioral health, the focus is similar: getting people back to their prior performance levels. When an operator has a behavioral health issue, the unit and the individual work hard to find the right treatment and get that person back. SOF members seeking behavioral health are thus highly motivated to get better.

Behavioral health providers in SOF are relatively new phenomena. Prior to 2012 there were no clinical behavioral health personnel assigned to SOF units. Senior leadership at Special Operations Command (SOCOM) recognized the need for this capability in SOF units and began to hire behavioral health providers for assignment with SOF units. Also in 2012, the Army launched the Comprehensive Behavioral Health System of Care, which added active duty behavioral health officers, along with Medical Command (MEDCOM) civilian and contract behavioral health providers.

Over the past several years, and due to the efforts of the SOF behavioral health community, there has been a tremendous shift in the perception of behavioral health among SOF operators. SOF personnel are more likely to seek treatment for behavioral health issues because the behavioral health providers are part of the team and are easily accessible. Senior leaders have worked hard to mitigate stigma and increase acceptance of behavioral health as an asset working to preserve the force.

Intelligence (CDR Joshua Morganstein, USPHS)

Background Intelligence personnel perform highly detailed analyses of vast quantities of extremely sensitive information. As a result, this work requires a high-level security clearance, such as top secret/sensitive compartmented information (TS/SCI), which must be maintained through frequent reevaluation procedures. Intel personnel are perpetually tasked to obtain information about individuals and organizations that conduct mass killing and disruption, including large-scale attacks and the overthrow of nations. Consequently, members of the Intelligence Community often perceive their work as being of profound importance to national security.

Intelligence work is often conducted independently, with limited outside contact. These personnel may work in bunkers or windowless rooms behind a series of locked doors. The sensitive nature of this information requires that Intelligence personnel maintain secrecy about nearly all work-related information to which they are exposed. As a result, military members of the Intelligence Community are not able to discuss their work with friends, family, or other non-Intel military personnel. Limited contact with others and the requirement to maintain secrecy may create a sense of isolation for personnel involved in Intelligence.

Those working "Intel" are often repeatedly exposed to graphic material over extended periods of time. These materials may detail or show violent and disturbing images in the aftermath of terrorist and other disaster-related activity as well as covert operations and interrogations. As a result of their recurrent and prolonged exposures to graphic material, Intelligence personnel may be at increased risk of traumatic stress.

Perception of Illness and Treatment Intelligence personnel generally perceive the presence of illness as a liability and the need for treatment as an indicator of weakness. The requirement for high intelligence and strong military entrance scores on the Armed Services Vocational Aptitude Battery (ASVAB), the qualification test for enlistment, contributes to a perception of Intel personnel as elite and mentally fit. Consequently, injury or illness that is perceived to be the result of mental weakness is particularly unacceptable. Routine health conditions viewed as commonplace as perceived in a neutral manner. Physical injury sustained in the line of duty may be esteemed and viewed as honorable. Though combat-related injuries, such as amputations or traumatic brain injury, may be associated with significant internal grief and loss, there may also be an associated sense the Intel member has truly given the most they can in the line of duty. Healthcare providers can support the well-being of service members in the Intelligence Community by appreciating the elite mentality and desire to avoid being perceived as mental weak inherent in this population.

Perceptions of Medical Providers Perception of medical providers by members of the Intel community is largely determined by providers' understanding of unique operational requirements and desire to collaborate and support the service member in maintaining their operational readiness. Providers who have experience with remote and overseas contingency operations, particularly in the Intel field, will be perceived in a more positive manner. Providers who lack specific knowledge about the Intel community can enhance rapport by asking Intel personnel about their particular medical needs. Care should be taken to avoid excessive or detailed questions about the specific work duties of Intel personnel, which can result in suspicion, guardedness, and worsened rapport. Though certain medical conditions necessitate the use of duty restrictions, deployment limitations, or alterations to a member's security clearance, these are generally experienced as highly undesirable to Intel personnel. Rapport is enhanced when providers demonstrate efforts to minimize these interventions while delivering appropriate care.

Attitudes Toward Mental Health Intelligence personnel are often hesitant to seek care for mental health symptoms, such as anxiety or depression, for several reasons. Mental health disorders may impact an individual's ability to retain top secret/sensitive compartmented information clearance. Loss of this clearance prevents Intelligence personnel from performing their duties and may result in a reassignment or relocation. It also prevents them from being able to perform their duties of safeguarding national security, which can be a significant psychological loss. Another reason Intelligence personnel avoid mental health care is the fear of inadvertently revealing sensitive information during the course of treatment. This diligence in safeguarding national security, an asset in the performance of routine work duties, frequently serves to limit help-seeking behavior. The stigma associated with being unable to perform work duties critical to national security, along with anxiety about revealing sensitive information during treatment, serve as significant barriers to the use of mental health care. In addition, Intelligence personnel that present for mental health care may require special consideration when determining the most effective interventions. Members of the Intelligence Community frequently have a strong analytical thought process and may benefit from talk therapies that emphasize a cognitive approach, particularly at the beginning of treatment during the early stages of building therapeutic rapport.

Conflicts (LTG (Ret) Eric Schoomaker, USA)

Persian Gulf War

The Persian Gulf War (Operation Desert Shield/Desert Storm; 2 August 1991–28 February 1992) was arguably the last time that US and allied coalition forces fought a large-scale armed conflict in a "linear" fashion with recognized frontline and rear areas. This war in many regards had been planned and was executed in a fashion that was anticipated by 40-plus years of preparation in central Europe for an attack by the Soviet Union and its Warsaw Pact allies. Service members prepared for large-scale casualties and for the defense against weapons of mass destruction (WMD), especially chemical weapons, by a foe that had employed them liberally during the Iran-

Iraq War (1980–1988) and against dissident ethnic groups. In reality, this war was won quickly and decisively, with minimal loss of American life—leading to an overwhelming sense of confidence in the capabilities of the US Military.

Despite the overwhelming military success of this war, unexpected aspects of the conflict dramatically impacted service members. First was the heavy reliance on the Reserves and National Guard to reflect engagement of the American people ("The Weinberger Doctrine" and "The Powell Doctrine"). The deployment of service members from disparate locations resulted in veterans experiencing post-conflict difficulties in isolation from others. Another aspect was exposure to desert dust, burning oil wells, burn pits, antidotes to nerve agents, and vaccines against potential biologic weapons of mass destruction. Such a gamut of exposures contributed to a variety of unclear somatic symptoms grouped together as Gulf War Syndrome.

Yugoslavia/Balkans

US military involvement in the ethnic conflict surrounding the implosion of the former Yugoslavia in the Balkans (1993–2004) was a harbinger of many elements of twenty-first-century armed conflict, most notably, dispersed combat and peacekeeping on a discontinuous battlefield with complex geopolitical, religious, and ethnic elements. While casualties from these operations were low, the continued employment of reserve elements, confusion about the nature of "the enemy," and the deep involvement of the media in framing the perceptions of both the warrior and the public foreshadowed wars to come. These all compounded the subcultural factors described in the above sections that characterize the Special Operations Forces (SOF), Air Force and ground forces, and especially the Active Army, Army Reserve, and Army National Guard.

Post 9/11

The September 11, 2001 attacks on the World Trade Center and the Pentagon, and the attempted attack on another target in Washington, DC, heroically foiled by the passengers of United Airline Flight 93, set into motion a series of reactive and preemptive military operations culminating in 15 years of continuous armed conflict in two major theatres. These operations mirrored many of the smaller scale experiences in the Balkans: dispersed combat and peacekeeping on a discontinuous battlefield with complex geopolitical, religious, and ethnic elements. There was no "rear" or "forward" area. Soldiers deployed in support roles, such as truck drivers, found themselves targets of directed attacks on supply lines with improvised explosive devices (IEDs). Even conventional line units were employed in roles they were psychologically unprepared for, even if given additional skills training. Naval medical and other personnel were deployed into facilities and environments far removed from their maritime mission. Airmen were exposed to direct combat through indirect fire and ambushes during resupply and other movements. In short, very few deployed soldiers, sailors, airmen, marines, and coastguardsmen were spared engagement in direct combat operations.

In addition, the past decade and a half of military engagements in Afghanistan (Operation Enduring Freedom), Iraq (Operation Iraqi Freedom and Operation New Dawn), and now Syria, in the war against the Islamic State of Iraq and the Levant or Syria (ISIL or ISIS), have seen the impact of a 30-year-old transition from a conscripted military to an all-volunteer force. While earlier generations of service members might have experienced a single long deployment (in excess of 6 months) or a predictable cycle of sea duty for 3–6 months, a large number of the active duty force, especially ground combatants in the Army and Marine Corps and Special Operations Forces, were deployed repeatedly for tours from 7 to 15 months into combat zones (contrast even the Persian Gulf War, which lasted less than 1 year). This reflects both the realities of prolonged conflict employing a relatively small Active and Reserve force and the longer enlistments of many volunteers. Compounding this "operational tempo" (OPTEMPO) is the fact that many more service members in the all-volunteer force have families than their counterparts in the conscripted force of the 1950s–1970s, in which there were far more single men, far fewer women, and a force that turned over regularly as short-term enlistments were completed and new service members replaced them.

Finally, dramatic continuous improvements occurred in the care of combatants from the Point of Injury or Illness (POI) to the sites of recovery and rehabilitation within the Military Health System of Department of Defense hospitals or the Veterans Health Administration facilities. A concerted multifactorial, multidisciplinary, tri-service effort to improve every step of casualty care from the point of injury, far-forward life-saving surgical resuscitation, intra-theater and inter-theater evacuation—usually by helicopter and specially outfitted aircraft, respectively—and comprehensive recovery and rehabilitation was undertaken. These measures led to unprecedented survival from battlefield wounds and injuries and the retention of wounded, ill, and injured combatants who could be returned to duty, including a large number of grievously wounded amputees and others.

Reserves/National Guard (MAJ (Ret) Dale Russell, USA)

Since 2001, reservists have been employed in an unprecedented and unusually prolonged manner. Reservists served key roles in supporting active duty operations; for example, during Operation Enduring Freedom/Operation Iraqi Freedom combat operations, nearly half of the active Army's ground forces were National Guards (Eaglen 2006). This increased utilization of reservists creates new social stressors, such as prolonged departures from regular civilian employment and healthcare challenges unique to its population (Griffith 2011). These stressors can generate adjustment problems (e.g., difficulty reintegrating at home), lack of social support (e.g., inability of family/friends to relate to military experiences), negative health outcomes (e.g., suicidal ideation and substance use), and higher levels of self-reports about their mental health concerns following a deployment and combat exposures compared to their active duty peers (Defense Science Board Task Force 2007; Lane et al. 2012; Riviere et al. 2011; Thomas et al. 2010). Unlike active duty personnel, reservists lack the daily peer support afforded by fellow Service members as they matriculate back into their civilian lives.

Negative health outcomes vary across reserve service branches and components (Russell et al. 2014; Schaller et al. 2014). Although the source of such variance is not specifically known, it is likely due to the military's multilayered cultural composition. Within the overarching military culture, numerous subcultures exist that affect not only military operations but also how said operations in turn affect service member subpopulations (Howard 2006). Each service branch (i.e., Army, Air Force, Navy, and Marines), service component (i.e., active and reserve), and occupational specialty (e.g., combat arms and service support) presents distinct cultural values and characteristics. Furthermore, the reserves are split between the federal force and each state's National Guard force, which not only embodies the Guard's larger culture but also each state's. In addition, the National Guard often faces additional stressors due to state mobilizations (e.g., natural disasters), which present additional health concerns that active duty missions can compound.

Veterans (Glenda Wrenn, MD, MSHP)

The nuances of military subculture, combat exposure status, and extent of military acculturation influence veteran culture. In addition to sources of cultural identification gained during service, reintegration after service is equally important in understanding veteran subculture. Reintegration often refers to post-deployment transitions but is a useful construct to apply to post-military life transitions for veterans. In both cases, reintegration includes adjustments to work and relational expectations and, if maladaptive, a reassessment of values and beliefs. A survey of veterans seeking care from the VA following deployment to Iraq or Afghanistan found that 40% of the respondents reported perceiving some to extreme difficulty reintegrating into civilian life within the past 30 days (Sayer et al. 2010). The process of reintegrating into "civilian life" can be difficult for a variety of reasons. Indeed, even the title "civilian" can be demoralizing, as is often used in a derogatory manner by service members toward those without appropriate training. Furthermore, although some barriers to mental health treatment among veterans are alleviated by reintegration, such as concerns about adverse impact on military career progression, many veterans are interested in civilian career paths for which mental health diagnoses are disqualifying (i.e., police, firefighters, and other careers that involve use of firearms) (Farmer et al. 2011).

Suspicions of being a burden can be especially painful for veterans transitioning out of their occupational military identity. The United States has long held a tradition of providing health benefits and compensation in response to disability incurred from military service. Such entitlements can raise concerns about malingering and misaligned incentives related to disability. Veterans of the Korean and Vietnam War faced intense negative societal response, often compared to idealized World War II narratives. However, World War II veterans, often dubbed the "greatest generation" (Brokaw 1998) who fought and won "the good war," were not without scrutiny. Critics of the 1944 GI Bill dubbed an unemployment benefit the "52-20 Club," indicating that veterans would avoid working to obtain the $20/month benefit for the maximum of 52 weeks. Less than one-fifth of the potential benefits were claimed (U.S. Department of Veterans Affairs). Such concerns may be misguided, as one recent study found that veterans seeking additional compensation for PTSD have equivalent treatment outcomes (Belsher et al. 2012). Indeed, the post-service experience of veterans can be just as influential in their cultural identity as their active duty experience.

Identifying patients as veterans is critical in increasing a clinician's awareness to such cultural influences and facilitating engagement with community resources to support mental health and well-being. Standard assessment for veteran status in healthcare settings is lacking (Farmer et al. 2011), placing the burden of disclosure on the veteran who may not see this as relevant to their health. Identifying veteran status and exploring that aspect of their identity can mitigate risk for a range of mental health conditions among veterans (Sripada et al. 2016). The "warrior ethos," for example, can be a barrier for mental health help-seeking, or leveraged to engage adherence to treatment (Westphal and Convoy 2015). Indeed, understanding military culture in veterans includes understanding and leveraging adaptive aspects (seeking support and guidance from other veterans in the waiting room, or the camaraderie that can augment cohesion in group therapy) as well as appreciating and mitigating maladaptive aspects (mistrust toward providers perceived as undermining military values).

Families (COL (Ret) Stephen Cozza, USA)

Military families comprise another critical subculture. The sacrifice made by service members requires a related sacrifice by their entire family, thus instilling a set of values and norms specific to military families. Before the start of the all-volunteer force, spouses and children were fewer in number and, when present, were typically those of officers or senior enlisted members. Today, military family members outnumber service members and reflect an essential part of the military community.

In fact, more than half of current active duty and selective reserve service members are married, and nearly half have children, most of whom are very young. These young military families reside throughout the continental United States, Hawaii, Alaska, and at overseas locations. While many live on or near military installations, many others also reside in geographically remote areas. They live in the communities where all of us live, but they are not always identified for who they are or their connections to military life or challenges. Leaving the military can pose its own set of challenges because the family not only loses its military identity but also its supportive military community, transitioning to civilian communities that may not recognize their experiences or needs.

Not until recent media attention have military children and families come to the broader attention of the public and scientists around the country. As a result, the experiences and life course of military children and families have largely gone unstudied. They are as different from each other as they are alike and reflect the broad socioeconomic, racial, cultural, and ethnic dimensions of the United States. In contrast to their diverse demographics, they share common values and experiences that come with military-related duty. These characteristics include a sense of meaning and purpose, military community connectedness, and service-related pride, in addition to shared experiences such as frequent residential moves, combat and noncombat-related deployments, and possible service member combat-related sequelae. Of all youth groups in the United States, military children are most likely to choose military careers themselves, reflecting the culture, traditions, and pride associated with growing up military.

Most recently, combat deployment impact has been profound for military families. Since 2001, over two million military service men and women have deployed to combat operations in Iraq and Afghanistan. They come from every military service branch, hail from every state in the country, and represent the active duty, National Guard, and reserve components of the military. Many families have faced repeated deployments, some as many as five or more. Since the start of combat operations, over 6000 service members have died in combat theater, tens of thousands have suffered combat injuries, and hundreds of thousands continue to suffer with traumatic brain injury (TBI) and posttraumatic stress disorder (PTSD) of varying severity. Managing with these combat-related changes has been one of the greatest challenges posed to military families since the Vietnam War.

Clinical Versus Research Considerations

Thus far, the focus has been on the impact military culture has on clinical encounter and the need for improved cultural competency in clinical settings. Research in military medicine also requires a similar level of appreciation for military culture. Consideration of how the research will impact the mission of the military is critical. Military members are a highly studied group, and researchers must be diligent in demonstrating how their work will ultimately serve the people being studied without compromising the mission. The military exists for a clear reason, and any research that does not improve mission effectiveness—or worse, compromises that mission—is not likely to be approved. Similarly, research that might hurt the overall image of the military (Ben-Ari and Levy 2014) may also be viewed as a threat to morale and discipline, making approval unlikely. Lastly, researchers must respect the fact that commanders are required to protect their soldiers, and may be leery of any research study, given historical events like Tuskegee. As such, researchers' questions that can be answered in civilian populations are rarely approved in military settings (McManus et al. 2007).

Importance of Military Cultural Competence

In 2008, Reger commented that psychologists not fluent with the Army's language could struggle to provide effective treatment. Indeed, given the key role that organizational culture plays in performance within civilian organizations (Martinez et al. 2015; Schein 1990), understanding the multifaceted nature of military culture is not only relevant to enhancing combat effectiveness but also to helping improve service members' overall health and well-being. With nearly 99% of US counties reporting residents that deployed to Operation Iraqi Freedom/Operation Enduring Freedom in the 2010 Census, 70% of service members seeking care outside of the military (Kuehn 2009), 40% of National Guard members meeting criteria for a mental health disorder (Gorman et al. 2011), and less than 30% of civilian providers knowledgeable on how to refer to the VA (Kilpatrick et al. 2011), Abb appropriately asked "Is your practice ready?" (Abb and Goodale 2015). Hoge further underscored the importance of "meeting soldiers where they're at" when treating PTSD (Hoge 2011), and Hall succinctly noted: "Unless we understand their language, their structure, why they join, their commitment to the mission, and the role of honor and sacrifice in military service, we will not be able to adequately intervene and offer care to these families" (Hall 2011).

A 2008 RAND report recommended increased training programs and instituting a national certificate program for providers to increase healthcare competency of TBI, PTSD, and depression in the military (Tanielian et al. 2014). Joint Veterans Affairs/Department of Defense PTSD treatment guidelines echoed this concern by calling attention to the need for improved military cultural competence (Management of Post-Traumatic Stress Working Group 2010). Around this time, the Association for American Medical Colleges published how few medical schools and residencies were covering military culture and recommended expansion of programs at medical schools nationwide. A 2012 Institute of Medicine report on PTSD further recommended greater understanding of military culture (Institute of Medicine Committee on the Assessment of Ongoing Efforts in the Treatment of Posttraumatic Stress 2014). Gleeson described the curriculum on military culture at the Uniformed Services University, America's military medical school, and recommended that all medical students be provided with similar, abbreviated, military cultural competence training (Gleeson and Hemmer 2014). It has also been suggested that military health histories be added to the electronic medical record, medical textbooks, and licensing exams (Lee et al. 2014; Meyer 2015).

Great strides have been made in response to these concerns and recommendations over the past few years. Several articles have been published on the common concerns, stressors, cultural considerations, and verbiage of service members (Cole 2014; Luby 2012; Strom et al. 2012). More robust education materials have also been produced (Table 2.1). A primer on military culture was distributed via MedEdPortal (Goldenberg et al. 2012). After 4 years of development, the Center for Deployment Psychology released an 8-h, online, peer-reviewed, interactive training curriculum (Center for Deployment Psychology). To date, more than 8,000 providers have completed the course in person, with another 16,000 completing the course online (Center of Deployment Psychology, unpublished data). The Citizen Soldier Support Program also created a well-received online training program (Thomas et al. 2010). The National Coordinator for Health information Technology put forth a proposal to include a military history in the new national electronic heath record (Office of the National Coordinator for Health Information Technology (ONC) 2014). The VA has produced a comprehensive online course on military culture (U.S. Department of Veterans Affairs 2017) and has published a brief military members, veterans, and family members (Cozza et al. 2014), which supplements preexisting efforts to highlight military specific concerns in mental health (Benedek et al. 2005). Additionally, tools for assessing military cultural competence have recently been developed (Meyer et al. 2015; Tanielian et al. 2014).

Conclusion

The concept that the military is a culture and requires the same culturally competent care as other cultures has only recently been widely accepted. Now, experts from a variety of fields have unanimously declared that military cultural competence is a critical part of providing care to military patients. To some extent, historically poor treatment outcomes have even been attributed to the inadequate cultural competence of providers and to non-culturally informed approaches to the care of military personnel and veterans. As a result of these declarations, numerous efforts have been put forth to improve the

Table 2.1 Overview of military culture resources for providers (websites active at time of publication)

Name	Website	Description
Basic training: A primer on military life and culture for health care providers and trainees Goldenberg M, Hamaoka D, Santiago P, McCarroll J	www.mededportal.org/publication/9270	This computer-based, self-guided tutorial provides a high-yield overview of military life and culture to enhance healthcare providers' ability to provide culturally competent care to service members. An excellent reference for those in need a brief overview. It can be accessed through the Association for American Medical Colleges (AAMC) MedEdPortal
Overview of military culture Center for Deployment Psychiatry	deploymentpsych.org	This extensive online training program uses a variety of teaching modalities and includes video vignettes to enhance providers' skills, knowledge, and attitudes in the area of military culture. The course is broken into four modules: Self-Assessment and Introduction to Military Ethos; Military Organization and Roles; Stressors and Resources; and Treatment, Resources and Tools. Each module requires 2 h to complete
Citizen Soldier Support Program (CSSP)	www.citizensoldiersupport.org/initiatives/education.php	In addition to their own online and in-person courses (described below), the CSSP maintains a database of helpful resources (right column)
North Carolina Area Health Education Centers	www.aheconnect.com/citizensoldier	To prepare civilian providers to address post-deployment issues facing Operation Iraqi Freedom/Operation Enduring Freedom veterans and their families, CSSP has partnered with Area Health Education Centers and medical providers from the Department of Veterans Affairs, US Navy, and US Public Health Service to create on-site and online courses for PTSD and traumatic brain injury
Military history pocket card US Dept. of Veterans Affairs	www.va.gov/oaa/pocketcard/	This double-sided card can be easily printed or saved as a pdf. It provides a series of questions that providers might consider when working with a patient who is a veteran. The questions can be also be used for active duty patients
Care of military service members, veterans and their families Cozza SJ, Goldenberg MN, Ursano RJ	Available on Amazon at goo.gl/fKQGQh	This comprehensive text (339 pages) provides civilian medical and nonmedical care providers with practical information and guidelines to effectively understand, support, and address the needs of this important population. The editors, who are experts in treating patients from all service branches, provide an overview of what it means to be part of a military family as well as an inside look at the military and Veterans Administration healthcare systems. Promoting family resilience is a fundamental theme and one that is emphasized throughout chapters on traumatic brain injury (TBI), substance use disorders, suicidal thoughts and behaviors, illness, injury, and bereavement. The book offers many features useful to the clinician who is unfamiliar with military culture, and the frequent use of tables, figures, and summary points makes information easily digestible for busy practitioners (from inside flap)

military cultural competence of all providers, including the development and distribution of curricula, clinical tools, and assessments.

There is still a great deal of work to be done. Tools focused on the cultural aspects of military service versus the occupational components are required. Assessments of efforts to improve military cultural competence demonstrating enhanced clinical outcomes are needed. With such evidence, requirements for military cultural competence would be defensible, and, more importantly, the care of service members and veterans would improve.

Key Concepts

1. The military is a culture, and, like other cultures, this culture can influence service members' perception of illness and treatment.
2. Asking about military status is a good first step to assessing whether a patient's illness is influenced by their military culture.
3. The military is comprised of different services, ranks, and occupations. These subcultures can often be a large part of the patient's military cultural identity.
4. Veterans were influenced by military culture and may still adhere to it. Assessing their integration back into civilian society is critical.
5. Family members of active duty members are also influenced by military culture. Asking them about the timing of moves and deployments and how they are handling military life can be a critical part of their assessment and treatment.
6. There are several tools available for providers interested in knowing more about military culture, many of which are listed in Table 2.1.

Disclaimer Portions of this chapter have been adapted from a recent publication by the author:

Meyer EG (2013) Military sub-cultural competency. J Mil Med 178(7):e848–50. [PMID: 23820363]

Meyer EG, Writer BW, Brim W (2016) The importance of military cultural competence. Curr Psychiatry Rep 18(3), 1–8. [PMID: 26830884]

The opinions expressed in this document are solely those of the author and do not represent an endorsement by or the views of the Department of Defense, the Department of Veterans Affairs, the Veterans Health Administration, or the US Government.

References

Abb W, Goodale R Is your practice prepared to identify or treat post deployment problems? http://www.citizensoldiersupport.org/lib/resources/The Importance of Understanding Military Culture for Civilian Health Providers.pdf. Accessed Sept 2015

Ames GM, Cunradi CB, Moore RS, Stern P (2007) Military culture and drinking behavior among U.S. navy careerists. J Stud Alcohol Drugs 68(3):336–344

Association of American Medical Colleges (2012) Serving those who serve America – joining forces: results of an AAMC survey. https://members.aamc.org/eweb/upload/ServingThoseWhoServeAmerica.pdf. Accessed May 2015

Bell ME, Turchik JA, Karpenko JA (2014) Impact of gender on reactions to military sexual assault and harassment. Health Soc Work 39(1):25–33

Belsher BE, Tiet QQ, Garvert DW, Rosen CS (2012) Compensation and treatment: disability benefits and outcomes of U.S. veterans receiving residential PTSD treatment. J Trauma Stress 25(5):494–502. https://doi.org/10.1002/jts.21747

Ben-Ari E, Levy Y (2014) Getting access to the field: insider/outsider perspectives. In: Soeters J, Shields PM, SJH R (eds) Routledge handbook of research methods in military studies. Routledge, Abingdon, Oxon, pp 9–18

Benedek DM, Ursano RJ, Holloway HC (2005) Military and disaster psychiatry. In: Kaplan & Sadock's comprehensive textbook of psychiatry, 8th edn. Lippincott Williams & Wilkins, Philadelphia

Brewin CR, Garnett R, Andrews B (2010) Trauma, identity and mental health in UK military veterans. Psychol Med 41(8):1733–1740. https://doi.org/10.1017/s003329171000231x

Brokaw T (1998) The greatest generation. Random House, New York

Brown JL (2012) The unasked question. JAMA 308(18):1869. https://doi.org/10.1001/jama.2012.14254

de Burgh HT, White CJ, Fear NT, Iversen AC (2011) The impact of deployment to Iraq or Afghanistan on partners and wives of military personnel. Int Rev Psychiatry 23(2):192–200. https://doi.org/10.3109/09540261.2011.560144

Cameron RP, Mona LR, Syme ML, Cordes CC, Fraley SS, Chen SS, Klein LS, Welsh E, Smith K, Lemos L (2011) Sexuality among wounded veterans of

Operation Enduring Freedom (OEF), Operation Iraqi Freedom (OIF), and Operation New Dawn (OND): implications for rehabilitation psychologists. Rehabil Psychol 56(4):289–301. https://doi.org/10.1037/a0025513
Castro CAE, Adler AB (2011) Reconceptualizing combat-related posttraumatic stress disorder as an occupational hazard. In: Adler AB, Bliese PD, Castro CA (eds) Deployment psychology: evidence-based strategies to promote mental health in the military. American Psychological Association, Washington, DC. https://doi.org/10.1037/12300-000
Center for Deployment Psychology (Online Course) Military Cultural Competence. http://deployment-psych.org/online-courses/military-culture. Accessed Sept 2015
Cole RF (2014) Understanding military culture: a guide for professional school counselors. Prof Couns 4(5):497
Cozza SJ, Goldenberg M, Ursano RJ (2014) Care of military service members, veterans, and their families, vol 1. American Psychiatric Publishing, a division of American Psychiatric Association, Washington, DC
Dahn V (2008) Silent service in the soldier's shadow. Couns Today 51(4):55–57
Danish SJ, Antonides BJ (2013) The challenges of reintegration for service members and their families. Am J Orthopsychiatry 83(4):550–558. https://doi.org/10.1111/ajop.12054
Deahl MP, Klein S, Alexander DA (2011) The costs of conflict: meeting the mental health needs of serving personnel and service veterans. Int Rev Psychiatry 23(2):201–209. https://doi.org/10.3109/09540261.2011.557059
Defense Science Board Task Force (2007) Deployment of members of the National Guard and reserve in the global war on terrorism. Office of the Under Secretary of Defense for Acquisition, Technology, and Logistics, Washington, DC
Dubey J (1967) The military psychiatrist as social engineer. Am J Psychiatry 124(1):52–58. https://doi.org/10.1176/ajp.124.1.52
Eaglen MM (2006) Equipping the Army National Guard for the 21st century. Background 1983 http://www.heritage.org/defense/report/equipping-the-army-national-guard-the-21st-century
Erbes CR, Polusny MA, MacDermid S, Compton JS (2008) Couple therapy with combat veterans and their partners. J Clin Psychol 64(8):972–983. https://doi.org/10.1002/jclp.20521
Farmer C, Schell TL, Jaycox LH, Tanielian T, Wrenn G (2011) Qualitative needs assessment of New York state veterans. In: Schell TL, Tanelian T (eds) A needs assessment of New York state veterans: final report to the New York State Health Foundation. RAND Corporation, Santa Monica
Fenell D (2008) A distinct culture: applying multicultural counseling competencies to work with military personnel. Couns Today 50:8–9
Foynes MM, Shipherd JC, Harrington EF (2013) Race and gender discrimination in the marines. Cult Divers Ethn Minor Psychol 19(1):111–119. https://doi.org/10.1037/a0030567
Gleeson TD, Hemmer PA (2014) Providing care to military personnel and their families. Acad Med 89(9):1201–1203. https://doi.org/10.1097/acm.0000000000000368
Goldenberg M, Hamaoka D, Santiago P, McCarroll J (2012) Basic training: a primer on military life and culture for health care providers and trainees. MedEdPORTAL Publications 8:9270
Goodale R, Abb WR, Moyer BA (2012) Military culture 101: not one culture, but many cultures. http://www.citizensoldiersupport.org/lib/resources/ORNC Military Culture 101 Workshop 14 Sep 12.pdf. Accessed Sept 2015
Gorman LA, Blow AJ, Ames BD, Reed PL (2011) National Guard families after combat: mental health, use of mental health services, and perceived treatment barriers. Psychiatr Serv 62(1):28–34. https://doi.org/10.1176/appi.ps.62.1.28
Green JW (1982) Cultural awareness in the human services. Prentice Hall, Englewood Cliffs
Greene T, Buckman J, Dandeker C, Greenberg N (2010) The impact of culture clash on deployed troops. Mil Med 175(12):958–963
Griffith J (2011) Decades of transition for the US reserves: changing demands on reserve identity and mental well-being. Int Rev Psychiatry 23(2):181–191. https://doi.org/10.3109/09540261.2010.541904
Hall L (2011) The importance of understanding military culture. Soc Work Health Care 50(1):4–18. https://doi.org/10.1080/00981389.2010.513914
Harris GL (2011) Reducing healthcare disparities in the military through cultural competence. J Health Hum Serv Adm 34(2):145–181
Harrison D (2006) The role of military culture in military organizations' responses to woman abuse in military families. Sociol Rev 54(3):546–574
Hippocrates, Jones WHS (1923) On decorum and the physician. In: Hippocrates, vol 2. Heinemann/Harvard University Press, London/Cambridge, MA
Hobbs K (2008) Reflections on the culture of veterans. AAOHN J 56(8):337–341
Hoge CW (2010) Once a warrior—always a warrior: navigating the transition from combat to home—including combat stress, PTSD, and mTBI, vol 1. Rowman & Littlefield, Lanham
Hoge CW (2011) Interventions for war-related posttraumatic stress disorder. JAMA 306(5):549–551. https://doi.org/10.1001/jama.2011.1096
Hoge CW, Castro CA, Messer SC, McGurk D, Cotting DI, Koffman RL (2004) Combat duty in Iraq and Afghanistan, mental health problems, and barriers to care. N Engl J Med 351(1):13–22. https://doi.org/10.1056/NEJMoa040603
Howard JL (2006) The role of culture in shaping perceptions of discrimination among active duty and

reserve forces in the US military. Employ Responsib Rights J 18(3):171–187. https://doi.org/10.1007/s10672-006-9015-x
Institute of Medicine Committee on the Assessment of Ongoing Efforts in the Treatment of Posttraumatic Stress D (2014) Treatment for posttraumatic stress disorder in military and veteran populations: final assessment
Jones E (2011) The military and its psychiatric challenges. Int Rev Psychiatry 23(2):125–126. https://doi.org/10.3109/09540261.2011.562010
Katz LS, Bloor LE, Cojucar G, Draper T (2007) Women who served in Iraq seeking mental health services: relationships between military sexual trauma, symptoms, and readjustment. Psychol Serv 4(4):239–249. https://doi.org/10.1037/1541-1559.4.4.239
Keats PA (2010) Soldiers working internationally: impacts of masculinity, military culture, and operational stress on cross-cultural adaptation. Int J Adv Couns 32(4):290–303. https://doi.org/10.1007/s10447-010-9107-z
Kilpatrick D, Best C, Smith D, Kudler H, Cornelison-Grant V (2011) Serving those who have served: educational needs of health care providers working with military members, veterans, and their families. Medical University of South Carolina Department of psychiatry. National Crime Victims Research & Treatment Center, Charleston
Kim PY, Britt TW, Klocko RP, Riviere LA, Adler AB (2011) Stigma, negative attitudes about treatment, and utilization of mental health care among soldiers. Mil Psychol 23(1):65–81. https://doi.org/10.1080/08995605.2011.534415
Krueger GP (2000) Military culture. In: Encyclopedia of psychology, vol 5. American Psychological Association, Washington, DC
Kuehn BM (2009) Soldier suicide rates continue to rise. JAMA 301(11):1111. https://doi.org/10.1001/jama.2009.342
Lande RG (2014) Stress in service members. Psychiatr Clin North Am 37(4):547–560. https://doi.org/10.1016/j.psc.2014.08.007
Lane ME, Hourani LL, Bray RM, Williams J (2012) Prevalence of perceived stress and mental health indicators among reserve-component and active-duty military personnel. Am J Public Health 102(6):1213–1220. https://doi.org/10.2105/ajph.2011.300280
Langston V, Gould M, Greenberg N (2007) Culture: what is its effect on stress in the military? Mil Med 172(9):931–935
Lee J, Sanders KM, Cox M (2014) Honoring those who have served. Acad Med 89(9):1198–1200. https://doi.org/10.1097/acm.0000000000000367
Lester P, Flake E (2013) How wartime military service affects children and families. Futur Child 23(2):121–141
Levander XA, Overland MK (2015) Care of women veterans. Med Clin North Am 99(3):651–662. https://doi.org/10.1016/j.mcna.2015.01.013
Luby CD (2012) Promoting military cultural awareness in an off-post community of behavioral health and social support service providers. Adv Soc Work 13(1):67–82
Lunasco TK, Goodwin EA, Ozanian AJ, Loflin EM (2010) One shot-one kill: a culturally sensitive program for the warrior culture. Mil Med 175(7):509–513
Lundquist JH (2008) Ethnic and gender satisfaction in the military: the effect of a meritocratic institution. Am Sociol Rev 73(3):477–496. https://doi.org/10.1177/000312240807300306
Malmin M (2013) Warrior culture, spirituality, and prayer. J Relig Health 52(3):740–758. https://doi.org/10.1007/s10943-013-9690-5
Management of Post-Traumatic Stress Working Group (2010) VA/DoD clinical practice guideline for management of post-traumatic stress. Veterans Health Administration, Department of Defense, Washington, DC
Martinez EA, Beaulieu N, Gibbons R, Pronovost P, Wang T (2015) Organizational culture and performance. Am Econ Rev 105(5):331–335. https://doi.org/10.1257/aer.p20151001
McManus J, McClinton A, Gerhardt R, Morris M (2007) Performance of ethical military research is possible: on and off the battlefield. Sci Eng Ethics 13(3):297–303. https://doi.org/10.1007/s11948-007-9022-9
Meyer E (2013) Case report: military subcultural competency. Mil Med 178(7):e848–e850. https://doi.org/10.7205/milmed-d-13-00027
Meyer EG (2015) The importance of understanding military culture. Acad Psychiatry 39(4):416–418. https://doi.org/10.1007/s40596-015-0285-1
Meyer EG, Hall-Clark BN, Hamaoka D, Peterson AL (2015) Assessment of military cultural competence: a pilot study. Acad Psychiatry 39(4):382–388. https://doi.org/10.1007/s40596-015-0328-7
Nash WP, Figley CR (2011) Combat stress injury: theory, research, and management. Routledge, New York
Office of the National Coordinator for Health Information Technology (ONC), Department of Health and Human Services (2014) Voluntary 2015 edition electronic health record (EHR) certification criteria; interoperability updates and regulatory improvements, vol 79. Federal Register 10880
Pankow SH, Dill MJ, Navarro AM, Jones KC, Prescott JE (2013) Health care provider awareness of the military status of patients: asking the question. AAMC Anal Brief 13(5) https://www.aamc.org/download/358546/data/oct2013analysisinbrief-awarenessofmilitarystatusofpatients.pdf
Parker K (2011) The military-civilian gap: fewer family connections. Pew research social and demographic trends. http://www.pewsocialtrends.org/2011/11/23/the-military-civilian-gap-fewer-family-connections/
Reger MA, Etherage JR, Reger GM, Gahm GA (2008) Civilian psychologists in an Army culture: the ethical challenge of cultural competence. Mil Psychol 20(1):21–35. https://doi.org/10.1080/08995600701753144

Riviere LA, Kendall-Robbins A, McGurk D, Castro CA, Hoge CW (2011) Coming home may hurt: risk factors for mental ill health in US reservists after deployment in Iraq. Br J Psychiatry 198(2):136–142. https://doi.org/10.1192/bjp.bp.110.084863

Rosen LN, Teitelbaum JM, Westhuis DJ (1993) Children's reactions to the desert storm deployment: initial findings from a survey of Army families. Mil Med 158(7):465–469

Russell DW, Cohen GH, Gifford R, Fullerton CS, Ursano RJ, Galea S (2014) Mental health among a nationally representative sample of United States military reserve component personnel. Soc Psychiatry Psychiatr Epidemiol 50(4):639–651. https://doi.org/10.1007/s00127-014-0981-2

Sayer NA, Noorbaloochi S, Frazier P, Carlson K, Gravely A, Murdoch M (2010) Reintegration problems and treatment interests among Iraq and Afghanistan combat veterans receiving VA medical care. Psychiatr Serv 61(6):589–597. https://doi.org/10.1176/appi.ps.61.6.589

Scannell-Desch E (2000) The culture of war: a study of women military nurses in Vietnam. J Transcult Nurs 11(2):87–95

Schaller EK, Woodall KA, Lemus H, Proctor SP, Russell DW, Crum-Cianflone NF (2014) A longitudinal comparison of posttraumatic stress disorder and depression among military service components. Mil Psychol 26(2):77–87. https://doi.org/10.1037/mil0000034

Schein EH (1990) Organizational culture. Am Psychol 45(2):109–119. https://doi.org/10.1037/0003-066x.45.2.109

Singh JA (2003) American physicians and dual loyalty obligations in the "war on terror". BMC Med Ethics 4(1):E4. https://doi.org/10.1186/1472-6939-4-4

Sripada RK, Lamp KE, Defever M, Venners M, Rauch SAM (2016) Perceived social support in multi-era veterans with posttraumatic stress disorder. J Nerv Ment Dis 204(4):317–320. https://doi.org/10.1097/nmd.0000000000000476

Street AE, Vogt D, Dutra L (2009) A new generation of women veterans: stressors faced by women deployed to Iraq and Afghanistan. Clin Psychol Rev 29(8):685–694. https://doi.org/10.1016/j.cpr.2009.08.007

Strom TQ, Gavian ME, Possis E, Loughlin J, Bui T, Linardatos E, Leskela J, Siegel W (2012) Cultural and ethical considerations when working with military personnel and veterans: a primer for VA training programs. Train Educ Prof Psychol 6(2):67–75. https://doi.org/10.1037/a0028275

Tanielian T, Farris C, Epley C, Farmer CM, Robinson E, Engel CC, Robbins MW, Jaycox LH (2014) Ready to serve: community-based provider capacity to deliver culturally competent, quality mental health care to veterans and their families. RAND Corporation. doi:https://doi.org/10.7249/j.ctt14bs1qk

The Health Care System for Veterans: An Interim Report. (2007) Congressional Budget Office. http://www.cbo.gov/sites/default/files/cbofiles/ftpdocs/88xx/doc8892/12-21-va_healthcare.pdf. Accessed Sept 2015

Thomas JL, Wilk JE, Riviere LA, McGurk D, Castro CA, Hoge CW (2010) Prevalence of mental health problems and functional impairment among active component and National Guard Soldiers 3 and 12 months following combat in Iraq. Arch Gen Psychiatry 67(6):614. https://doi.org/10.1001/archgenpsychiatry.2010.54

Trautmann J, Alhusen J, Gross D (2015) Impact of deployment on military families with young children: a systematic review. Nurs Outlook 63(6):656–679. https://doi.org/10.1016/j.outlook.2015.06.002

U.S. Census Bureau (2010). http://www.census.gov. Accessed Aug 2015

U.S. Department of Veterans Affairs, National Center for PTSD: Military Culture and PTSD. https://www.ptsd.va.gov/professional/continuing_ed/military_culture.asp. Accessed Sept 2017

United States Department of Veterans Affairs VA History. http://www.va.gov/about_va/vahistory.asp. Accessed Mar 2016

Veterans' Access to Care through Choice, Accountability, and Transparency Act of 2014

Vogt D (2011) Mental health-related beliefs as a barrier to service use for military personnel and veterans: a review. Psychiatr Serv 62(2):135–142. https://doi.org/10.1176/appi.ps.62.2.135

Wertsch JV (1991) A sociocultural approach to socially shared cognition. In: Resnick LB, Levine JM, Teasley SD (eds) Perspectives on socially shared cognition. American Psychological Association, Washington, DC, pp 85–100. https://doi.org/10.1037/10096-004

Westphal RJ (2007) Fleet leaders' attitudes about subordinates' use of mental health services. Mil Med 172(11):1138–1143

Westphal RJ, Convoy SP (2015) Military culture implications for mental health and nursing care. Online J Issues Nurs 20(1):4

Wood FR (1988) At the cutting edge of institutional and occupational trends: the U.S. Air Force Officer Corps. In: Moskos CC, Wood FR (eds) The military: more than just a job? Pergamon-Brassey's International Defense Publishers, Washington, DC, pp 27–30

The Commitment of the Veterans Health Administration to Mental Health Care for Veterans: Historical Overview and Context

3

Stuart Gilman and Ruth O'Hara

Care for Veterans: A Timeline

The modern American sense of societal responsibility toward active duty service members and veterans can perhaps trace its beginnings to 1636, when Plymouth Colony established a pension for those disabled in battles with Native Americans. In 1776, the Continental Congress likewise established financial benefits for disabled veterans but required the states to fund and administer them. Payment for such benefits became a federal government responsibility in 1789. These benefits expanded, first for veterans themselves in 1816 and then in 1818 for family members of soldiers and sailors who died during the War of 1812. Another change in 1818 was the expansion of pension eligibility to include financial need in addition to the previously established eligibility for physically disabled veterans. The first federal office devoted solely to veterans' needs was the Bureau of Pensions, established in 1833 in the Department of War, which continued in various administrative alignments until it was located within the Department of the Interior by 1849.

By 1861, at the outbreak of the Civil War, there were about 80,000 veterans. By the end of the Civil War, in 1865, this number grew to over 1.9 million. This number includes only veterans of the Union forces, as Confederate soldiers were not afforded federal veterans' benefits until 1958, by which time there was only a single eligible surviving Confederate veteran. The basis of the modern veterans' pension system was established by the Dependent Pension Act of 1890, which expanded definitions of disability and created a regulatory framework that was useful for veterans of the Spanish-American War of 1898 and the Philippine Insurrection (1899–1901). Prior to World War I, the Sherwood Act of 1912 allowed pensions for all veterans of the Civil War and the US-Mexican War to receive a pension at age 62, regardless of whether or not they had disability (Table 3.1).

World War I led to an innovation in veterans' benefits: vocational rehabilitation. The War Risk Insurance Act Amendments of 1917 created authority for rehabilitation and vocational rehabilitation for veterans with permanent disabilities. Shortly thereafter, the Vocational Rehabilitation Act of 1918 created the Federal Board for Vocational Rehabilitation, but the determination of eligibility for those benefits remained with the

S. Gilman
Veterans Health Administration,
Washington, DC, USA
e-mail: stuart.gilman@va.gov

R. O'Hara (✉)
Department of Psychiatry and Behavioral Sciences,
Stanford University School of Medicine, Palo Alto
Health Care System, Palo Alto, VA, USA
e-mail: roh@stanford.edu

L.W. Roberts, C.H. Warner (eds.), *Military and Veteran Mental Health*,
https://doi.org/10.1007/978-1-4939-7438-2_3

Table 3.1 Key dates in the establishment of benefits and support for US veterans

Date	Event in support of veterans benefits
1636	Plymouth Colony established a pension for physically disabled veterans
1776	Continental Congress established benefits for physically disabled veterans
1779	Responsibility for benefits for physically disabled veterans transferred to federal responsibility
1818	Addition of pension benefits for direct family member survivors of a veteran's death and addition of financial need independent of physical disability as an eligibility criterion for veteran benefits
1833	Establishment of the Bureau of Pensions, first federal office devoted to veterans' needs
1853–1855	Commitment to veterans health benefits with establishment of two facilities in Washington, DC: Soldier's Home and St. Elizabeth's Hospital
1890	Modern veterans' pension system established by the Dependent Pension Act
1912	The Sherwood Act allows all veterans of the Civil War and US-Mexican War to receive pensions at age 62, independent of disability status
1917	The War Risk Insurance Act Amendments create authority for rehabilitation and vocational rehabilitation for veterans with permanent disabilities
1918	The Vocational Rehabilitation Act creates the Federal Board for Vocational Rehabilitation
1918	The Bureau of War Risk Insurance moves to 810 Vermont Avenue NW, Washington, DC, current Headquarters of the Department of Veterans Affairs
1921	Congress creates the Veterans Bureau
1930	Congress creates the Veterans Administration, consolidating the Veterans Bureau, the Bureau of Pensions, and the National Homes for Disabled Volunteer Soldiers
1945	General Omar Bradley appointed by President Truman to head the Veterans Administration
	Bradley appoints Major General Paul Hawley to serve as VA Medical Director
1945–1947	Bradley and Hawley leadership oversaw (a) new VA hospitals to be colocated and affiliated with academic institutions, (b) establishment of VA research programs in medicine, mental health, and rehabilitation, (c) inclusion and expansion of psychiatric units and services, and (d) establishment of the VA office of Academic Affiliations
1945	George A. Kelly appointed as VA's first psychology consultant
1946	James Grier Miller appointed chief of VA's new Clinical Psychology Program

Bureau of War Risk Insurance. In 1918, the Bureau of War Risk Insurance moved to what is now the current headquarters of the Department of Veterans Affairs in Washington, DC.

Creation of the Veterans Bureau

By 1918, the responsibilities for federal services to veterans involved a confusing patchwork of agencies. Warren Harding was elected president in 1921, in part on a platform of improving the administration of veterans' benefits. Subsequently, in 1921 Congress created the Veterans Bureau, which consolidated oversight of the Public Health Service, the Department of Treasury's Bureau of War Risk Insurance, and the Federal Board of Vocational Rehabilitation. This new Veterans Bureau did not include the Bureau of Pensions of the Interior Department or the National Homes for Disabled Volunteer Soldiers, which was fortunate for those agencies as events unfolded.

President Harding appointed Charles Forbes to be the Director of the newly established Veterans Bureau. Forbes was a US Army colonel and a recipient of the Congressional Medal of Honor. Forbes, in turn, appointed Charles F. Cramer to be the Bureau's General Counsel. Forbes convinced President Harding to issue an executive order transferring to him responsibility for new facility construction (previously a responsibility of the Army) and control of all of the Bureau's supplies and equipment. In addition to those substantial assets, the new Bureau had an annual appropriation of over $500,000, which was a considerable amount in 1922 dollars. Forbes and Cramer proceeded to systematically plunder these assets by selling them for their own profit and receiving kickbacks from contractors interested in pursuing new construction projects. This came to President Harding's attention in February 1923 (*The New York Times* 1923a, b), and although he is reported to have berated Forbes, Harding allowed Forbes to flee the country before he would be arrested. Charles Cramer committed suicide on March 15, 1923 (*The New York Times* 1923c). Forbes later was arrested and convicted, serving 2 years at Leavenworth.

This scandal was widely reported and emphasized the problems with not just authorizing benefits for veterans but also fulfilling them. The 1924 War Adjustment Compensation Act established pay bonuses to WWI combat veterans to compensate for inadequate pay during their active duty. This was a politically contentious bill, which overrode President Coolidge's veto (*The New York Times* 1924). Unfortunately, in order to reduce the impact of a massive one-time charge to the Treasury, the bonus payments were structured by the ill-conceived mechanism of certificates that would mature to full value over 20 years. Perhaps this strategy would have worked had the Great Depression not taken hold in 1929. But the federal government's relationship with veterans was about to change dramatically.

First, the Veterans Bureau did not go far enough to efficiently consolidate the federal administration of veterans' benefits. By 1930, Congress created the Veterans Administration, finally consolidating the Veterans Bureau, the Bureau of Pensions, and the National Homes for Disabled Volunteer Soldiers. For the first time, this new consolidated agency could coordinate various types of pensions and other financial benefits, health-care benefits, and long-term care benefits for veterans.

The next major change in the federal government's relationship to veterans occurred as a result of the 1924 bonus payments and the impact of the Great Depression. Many veterans holding their bonus certificates were resentful that they were unable to receive their payments during this period of severe financial hardship. By early 1932, many veterans began to demand that their certificates be paid immediately rather than be allowed to mature, a proposal that would place a significant strain on the federal budget at a peak of the depression. Several hundred veterans set out from Oregon to Washington, DC, in order to bring attention to their demands (*The Washington Post* 1931). Ultimately, these demonstrators, called either the "Bonus Expeditionary Force" or the "Bonus Army," were estimated to number between 6,500 and 40,000 and camped on the mall in the nation's capital (*The New York Times* 1932a). In some cases, they occupied empty government buildings in the area. In an interesting parallel to the Occupy Wall Street movement of 2011, Walter W. Waters, the commander of the Bonus Expeditionary Force, asserted that the veterans should be given the "same consideration as bankers" (Waters 1932).

This occupation by such a large number of people caused concerns about public health for those participating in the occupation as well as for others in Washington, DC. Their occupation also caused significant political pressure. On August 2, 1932, the police attempted to break up the encampment, resulting in the death of two of the protesters (*The New York Times* 1932b). US Army troops then came to disburse the protestors, using bayonets, tear gas, and tanks, under the oversight of General Douglas MacArthur and then Majors Dwight D. Eisenhower and George S. Patton (*The New York Times* 1932c). Although the Army's actions largely succeeded in dispersing the protesters, many in the nation were appalled at the image of the Army turning on its own veterans with such force. The political fallout of this action contributed to Hoover's reelection loss to Franklin D. Roosevelt. However, Roosevelt was also opposed to early payment of the bonuses, instead preferring to offer employment through the Civilian Conservation Corps. Ultimately, in 1936 Congress overrode President Roosevelt's veto of the Adjusted Compensation Payment Act authorizing the immediate payment of the $2.4 billion in WWI bonuses (*The New York Times* 1936).

General Omar Bradley Leads the Veterans Administration into the Modern Era

The USA entered World War II in December 1941. By 1945, as Allied victory in the war in Europe was looking assured, the US federal government recognized the need to care for more than 100,000 veteran patients. The Bonus Expeditionary Army fiasco of 1932 remained memorable, and there was a will to assure the public that the government would properly address veterans' needs. President Truman accomplished this assurance by naming a unique leader to become administrator of the Veterans Administration (VA): General Omar Bradley.

Omar Bradley participated in planning the invasion of France, as well as the assault on Normandy. He was rapidly promoted, ultimately being named commander of the US Twelfth Army Group which, at 1.3 million troops, was the largest force ever placed under an American group commander (Kirkpatrick 1992). Bradley's appointment accomplished several goals: first, he was unquestionably a distinguished planner for high-stakes, complex interventions; second, he would be viewed by the public as a credible person to take on the challenge of creating an effective response to these new veterans' needs; and lastly, he was a very popular leader among service members and veterans. Congress passed legislation allowing Bradley to retain his four-star general status as active duty while he served at VA.

Perhaps the most important thing that Bradley did was to immediately bring in Major General Paul Hawley, a surgeon with combat medical experience in the 334th Infantry in France at the end of World War I. During the peacetime interval, he alternated between population health, surgical, and academic positions, including teaching epidemiology and biostatistics (Engert 1966). Through these experiences, he developed skills in what are now called health systems. Between 1918 and 1937, Hawley maintained the rank of Major. His attendance at Army War College and achievement of general officer status facilitated his engagement in high-level military health systems planning. As the USA took on an advisory role to England, Hawley was assigned to be chief surgeon with the Special Operations Group in London in September 1941. It was just weeks later that the USA entered the war, after the USA's fleet at Pearl Harbor was attacked by the Japanese on December 7, 1941 and Germany declared war on the USA on December 11, 1941. In January of 1942, Hawley became the chief surgeon of the US Armed Forces of the British Isles, European Theater of the US Army. The media referred to his role as "surgeon general" of the European theater. It was in this office that the Allied forces planned the D-Day invasion of Europe. Hawley's role was to design the combat health systems to support the invasion. Ultimately, it would link him to General Omar Bradley and provide him the experience of combat command of over 250,000 health professionals involved in the European theater (*The New York Times* 1965).

The public was aware that the VA hospital system they knew at the time was incapable of meeting the needs of the returning veterans. In this environment, Hawley and Bradley were ideal choices for leading the VA. Bradley was admired by the public for his contributions to war victories, and he was beloved by soldiers. Bradley needed a medical professional to take on the invigoration of the VA's health-care system. Hawley had developed tremendous respect from the medical profession for his role in improving survival of the battlefield wounded.

The challenges they faced were formidable: at the time of Bradley's appointment, there were about 6,700,000 living veterans. Within 6 months of his appointment, the demobilization caused that number to double and would rise to about 20,000,000 over the next 15 months. Bradley and Hawley stayed with VA for a short time, both leaving in 1947. However, what they accomplished in their months at VA was nothing short of a "Big Bang"—foundational changes accomplished in a short time that have shaped every aspect of VA health care, including mental health services, to the present day.

More specifically, Bradley and Hawley began to closely associate physician staffing with academic medical centers in order to take advantage of the existing medical staff at schools of medicine and the potential productivity leverage provided by resident physicians. Likewise, they fought to have physician appointments handled through a new mechanism unshackled by the existing civil service requirements, creating Title 38 hiring authorities in the process. They changed the direction of the construction program, in order to colocate new VA hospitals near the affiliated academic medical centers. They designed the hospitals to include psychiatric services, changing the concept of how psychiatric services relate to medical and surgical services within a hospital setting. They also reorganized the medical programs, for the first time elevating the chief medical official to report directly to the VA administrator. They also established VA research programs in medicine, mental health, and rehabilitation. These steps were interdependent and provided the basis for addressing the emerging clinical needs of returning veterans, including mental health needs in particular.

The Emergence of the Research and Educational Role of VA

The historical record is not clear about exactly who originated the idea of academic affiliations for VA. The strategic idea of using academic affiliations to assist VA had already been circulating among prominent civilian advocates, including the financier Bernard Baruch, who was engaged in advising on veterans affairs at the request of President Roosevelt, and Paul Magnuson, an academic orthopedic surgeon at Northwestern University. Prior to the arrival of Bradley and Hawley, there had been very modest training of health professionals in VA facilities, and VA leadership had been opposed to expanding VA's academic relationships. However, it is clear that Bradley and Hawley fully supported the shift, and academic affiliations proved to be the foundational assumption on which further innovations were based.

Bradley and Hawley recognized that they had core problems, including insufficient physician staffing, that academic affiliations could help address. The VA physicians who were on staff prior to and during WWII were often not specialty trained and were not well regarded by either the profession or the public; likewise, the VA facilities and their physicians were in the wrong places. With the exception of several public health hospitals operated by VA in urban areas, VA hospitals had largely been placed in rural areas. Bradley and Hawley determined that it would not be possible to recruit enough new full-time physicians to practice in VA to meet the needs of the returning veterans. For one thing, VA's reputation for quality of care was poor, and it was not a desirable place for physicians to work—and there were just not enough practicing physicians to be recruited. Even if there had been a pool of applicants, VA did not have time to do background checks and other appropriate assessments necessary to physician hiring. Once VA did identify suitable physicians, civil service regulations resulted in slow and inefficient recruitment actions, impeding the ability of VA to increase its medical staff. Academic affiliations offered a solution to these problems: schools of medicine had faculty who were already vetted and were perceived by veterans and the public to be quality physicians.

In a speech to the American Medical Association's House of Delegates in December 1945, Hawley emphasized the importance of education as a link to quality of care (Hawley 1945). Indeed, he attributed the markedly improved survival of the combat wounded in Europe to the "better education of doctors" between WWI and WWII, minimizing the importance of triage and transportation systems (Hall 1993) and of medical advances (such as the use of plasma). In the same speech, Hawley also noted that VA's physicians were so poorly regarded by the public and by the medical profession that they were not even allowed to join the American Medical Association (AMA), which was at that time selective, and the membership to which was touted as an indicator of quality. He also presented a stark forecast of the staffing problem from the available numbers: "unless we get new blood and get it fast, by the spring of 1946 we are going to only have one-third of the number of doctors as we require." Hawley said he needed a way to bring 1,300 physicians on board nationwide within a few months.

Basing the new VA on academic affiliations could address several problems simultaneously: it could lead to recruitment of a large number of attending physicians that veterans and the public respected, and it allowed for the expansion of physician residency programs that could leverage the productivity of those attending physicians. There were two main barriers to this goal, however. First, the civil service employment processes were not geared to part-time federal employment, which was thought to be necessary to recruit academic attending physicians, and those employment processes were exceptionally slow to hire and to terminate. Bradley, Hawley, and other advocates of academic affiliations were certain that they needed much more nimble human resource processes in order to succeed. This led to the development of Title 38, which not only created the position of the Chief Medical Director—later changed to the Under Secretary for Health when VA became a Cabinet Department—but also allowed for more flexible hiring, firing, and pay determination for physicians.

There was significant opposition to this latter aspect of Title 38 from unions and opposition politicians, but with Baruch lobbying from the "outside" and Bradley and Hawley lobbying from within, they were able to both have the law passed and convince the President to sign the bill. Public Law 79–293 became Title 38 of the US Code, creating the Department of Medicine and Surgery. Shortly thereafter, Bradley issued VA Policy Memorandum Number 2, establishing academic affiliations as the basis for the VA expansion.

The second barrier to realizing the full benefits of academic affiliations was geographic: the VA hospitals of the early twentieth century were largely rural, and only a few public health hospitals were available for VA to use. In response, Bradley and Hawley secured congressional support to begin a massive construction effort to create new VA hospitals closely located to existing academic medical centers. This construction would facilitate the ability of part-time academic physicians and their residents to circulate between the VA and the academic centers.

A Growing Emphasis on VA Mental Health Care

The vast new construction effort implemented by Bradley and Hawley had a major impact on mental health services, as Hawley insisted that these new VA hospitals include facilities for mental health treatment. The result was what was described as the "largest hospital building program in history," with 69 hospitals created that each had a neuropsychiatric unit, as well as 16 more predominantly psychiatric hospitals (Haun and Lebensohn 1948). Hawley insisted that approximately 30% of beds in the new hospitals be devoted to psychiatric care, establishing a precedent for psychiatric care to be a significant component of a modern hospital. Bradley and Hawley also recognized that many veterans required integrated care for physical and emotional trauma, and they sought to create amenities that would facilitate such care (Haun and Lebensohn 1948).

While the physician staffing and physical infrastructure of these new VA hospitals were being established, Hawley addressed further key elements for mental health treatment in the emerging health-care system. In 1946, Hawley wrote in the *Journal of Clinical Psychology* that about 40% of discharges for disability were due to neuropsychiatric conditions. To address this issue, he announced the establishment of "a definite program for the utilization of psychologists in the rehabilitation of veterans." He further explained, "This program calls for the use of clinical psychologists in connection with the diagnosis and study of veterans needing medical care. Psychologists are also being employed in connection with the vocational rehabilitation activities as vocational advisors. They have a very definite place in the program being carried on by the Administration" (Hawley 1946). To lead this effort, George A. Kelly was appointed as the VA's first psychology consultant in December 1945. James Grier Miller was recruited to become the first full-time chief of the new Clinical Psychology Program in the spring of 1946 (Baker and Pickren 2007).

As Baker and Pickren (2007) describe in their excellent history of psychology in VA, Miller faced an acute problem when recruiting psychologists. Not only were there too few psychologists in practice to recruit to meet VA's needs, but Miller also viewed most training programs of the time to be inadequate to prepare new psychologists for VA practice (Baker and Pickren 2007). His solution was to aggressively develop training programs within VA. While the importance of physician education in the development of VA's authorities for academic affiliations had become obvious, Miller was able to convince Bradley that language in Policy Memorandum Number 2 also applied to psychology.

As World War II was ending, the visionary leadership for VA had both immediate and strategic mechanisms to entirely revise VA's system of care. The physical infrastructure was overhauled by a massive hospital building program, which largely placed new VA hospitals near established academic medical centers and led to the development of academic affiliations so that medical staff could be efficiently shared, the creation of educational programs so that the efforts of staff practitioners could be leveraged by resident physicians and other trainees, and the investment of the health professions such as clinical psychology, rehabilitation, and many others in meeting the needs of returning veterans with injuries both visible and not. Lastly, Bradley and Hawley also recognized and invested in the research needed to foster further improvement in this comprehensive system of medical and mental health care.

Key Concepts

1. The US has had financial commitments to military veterans since the earliest colonial settlements.
2. The US Civil War saw an explicit commitment to financial support for veterans.
3. Relative underpayment to troops in World War I led to a political crisis about veterans benefits during the Great Depression, with large-scale demonstrations by the "Bonus Expeditionary Force" or "Bonus Army."
4. Corruption in the 1930s shook the public's confidence in the federal government's commitment to fulfilling veterans' benefits.
5. World War II created a major strain on the Veterans Administration's ability to meet veterans' health needs, due to the massive demobilization that occurred.
6. General Omar Bradley and Major General Paul Hawley provided key leadership in the expansion of VA Hospitals, improving medical and mental health care and staff.
7. General Bradley and Major General Hawley oversaw the alignment of VA Hospitals with academic institutions and medical and mental health education, impacting mental health care and education across the nation.
8. The VA integrated inpatient psychiatric wards in their massive postwar hospital construction effort, developed psychology services, and began investments in psychology services and education.
9. The VA Office of Academic Affiliations oversees multiple VA programs aimed at training physicians, psychologists, and associated health professionals, through residencies, internships, and postdoctoral fellowships, in medical and mental health care.
10. The integration of education, research, and clinical services has been necessary to the success of the reimagined VA.

References

Baker RR, Pickren WE (2007) Psychology and the Department of Veterans Affairs: a historical analysis of training, research, practice, and advocacy. American Psychological Association, Washington, DC

Engert RM (1966) A concise biography of Major General Paul Ramsey Hawley. General reference and research branch, Army Medical Department Center and School (US Army), Washington, DC

Hall D (1993) We were ready: health services support in the Normandy Campaign. US Army Medical Department. http://history.amedd.army.mil/booksdocs/wwii/Overlord/Normandy/HallNormandy.html. Accessed 13 Mar 2017

Haun P, Lebensohn ZM (1948) New trends in hospital design. Am J Psychiatr 104(8):555–564

Hawley PR (1945) Address by Major General Paul R. Hawley. JAMA 129(17):1192–1194

Hawley PR (1946) Psychological services in the Veterans administration. J Clin Psychol 2(2):107–109

Kirkpatrick CE (1992) Omar Nelson Bradley: the centennial. In: JP Moran (ed). US Army Center of Military History, Washington, DC

The New York Times (1923a) Col. Forbes Quits Post: gives ill health as cause of resigning Veterans' Bureau Directorship. New York Times (1923–Current file); 17 Feb 1923; ProQuest Historical Newspapers:The New York Times. p 12

The New York Times (1923b) 03/15/1923 Worried by critics, Cramer takes life: former counsel for veterans'… special to The New York Times. New York Times (1923-Current file); 15 Mar 1923; ProQuest Historical Newspapers: The New York Times, p 1

The New York Times (1923c) Worried by critics, Cramer takes life: former counsel for veterans'…special to The New York Times. New York Times (1923-Current file); 15 Mar 1923; ProQuest Historical Newspapers: The New York Times

The New York Times (1924) 06/14/1924 Coolidge presses for paying bonus: authorizes war, navy and veterans'. Special to The New York Times. New York Times (1923–Current file); 14 Jun 1924; ProQuest Historical Newspapers: The New York Times, p 15

The New York Times (1932a) Trouble at capitol. Special to The New York Times. New York Times (1932–Current file); 17 Jul 1932; ProQuest Historical Newspapers: The New York Times, p 16

The New York Times (1932b) Seven B.E.F. sites offered to waters 08/06/1932

The New York Times (1932c) Bombs and sabres win capital battle: cavalry, infantry and tanks, ... special to The New York Times. New York Times (1923–Current file); 29 Jul 1932; ProQuest Historical Newspapers: The New York Times, p 1

The New York Times (1936) Bonus bill becomes law; repassed in senate, 76–19. Special to The New York Times. New York Times (1923–Current file); 28 Jan 1936; ProQuest Historical Newspapers: The New York Times, p 1

The New York Times (1965) Gen. Paul Hawley, physician, 74, dies: army officer reorganized V.A. Medical Services. Special to The New York Times. New York Times (1923–Current file); 26 Nov 1965; ProQuest Historical Newspapers: The New York Times, p 37

The Washington Post (1931) Leaders of bonus march arrive here from Oregon 12/05/1931. The Washington Post (1923–1954); 5 Dec 1931; ProQuest Historical Newspapers: The Washington Post, p 24

Waters WW (1932) *The New York Times* "Defends bonus army: leader says it should have same consideration as bankers" Walter W. Waters, Commander of "Bonus Expeditionary Forces" at Washington. New York Times (1923–Current file); Jun 10, 1932; ProQuest Historical Newspapers: The New York Times, p 12

Resilience in the Military: The Double-Edged Sword of Military Culture

4

Amy B. Adler and Walter J. Sowden

Introduction

Service members are uniquely prepared to organize and execute missions and to perform a wide range of difficult tasks under the most challenging conditions—skills that have the potential to serve them well in any context—but that need some adjustment and fine-tuning to facilitate an effective transition to the civilian world. These skills are the product of the military's *culture of resilience*.

Case Study

Army Sergeant First Class (SFC) (ret.) Christopher Peterson (pseudonym) entered college after 20 years of military service. Before classes started, he reconned the classrooms so he knew where to go, and on the first day he arrived 30 min before classes started. He had to fight the urge to stand at attention when the professor walked in, but otherwise thought he would blend in pretty well in his college uniform of jeans and a t-shirt. He figured out the chain of command: professors, graduate students, and undergraduates. He focused on the objective: graduate. Still, it was a strange environment. The other students did not have the life experience that he had had. The questions they asked—"Did you kill anyone?" "What was it like?"—highlighted the gulf between their experiences and his own. He kept his distance, thinking they just didn't get it. He worked hard, but his grades were not top-notch, and he wondered if he belonged. He felt like he was always behind in his reading and got a B- in statistics. He had been through so much—completed Jumpmaster School, led soldiers in Iraq—and wondered why this transition was so difficult. Sometimes he looked around the classroom and wished his classmates were his old unit—where they were all in it together. In the Army, challenges belong to the group; they are the responsibility of the leadership. Here, when there was a problem, he felt like he was on his own. He had no battle-buddy, and no one had his back.

A.B. Adler (✉) • W.J. Sowden
Center for Military Psychiatry and Neuroscience, Walter Reed Army Institute of Research, Silver Spring, MD, USA
e-mail: amy.b.adler.civ@mail.mil

L.W. Roberts, C.H. Warner (eds.), *Military and Veteran Mental Health*, https://doi.org/10.1007/978-1-4939-7438-2_4

The case study describes a typical and real transition that military personnel encounter when adjusting to the civilian world. While the military culture equips them with tools to succeed, the culture also challenges them when it comes to this transition. This chapter reviews how the military's acculturation process transforms civilians into service members and how it develops their capability to withstand stress and recover from adversity (Bonanno et al. 2012; Cornum et al. 2011). This *culture of resilience* is described in a framework borrowed from organizational anthropology to highlight the artifacts, values, and assumptions that permeate military culture (Schein 2010).

Next, this chapter shows how resilience manifests within the individual service member and how this manifestation can be adaptive. It also discusses the limits of resilience. As evidenced in the opening vignette, these resilience skills—as valuable as they can be to service members—have neither a total nor a universal benefit. As with any virtue, resilience has its limits, and these limits have the potential to manifest as maladaptive responses. In addressing each of these topics, the purpose of this chapter is to provide insight into the military's[1] *culture of resilience*, how service members are imbued with this culture, and how this acculturation process can both promote and sabotage service member health, well-being, and happiness.

The Army's Culture of Resilience

Like any society, the military has its own distinct culture. It is distinguished by the specific language shared by its members; its unique set of customs, traditions, rituals, and norms; and, importantly, its values. Other organizations—like Google or Apple—may have a particular organizational culture, but in the case of the military, the organizational culture is a *Greedy Institution* (Segal 1986). While it does not control every single aspect of an individual's life, it does demand a great deal from the individual in terms of "commitment, loyalty, time, and energy" (p. 9).

Military culture is distinguished by a profound commitment to a larger goal. People who join the military have to be willing to put their own desires on hold in order to meet the needs of a demanding organization—an organization that determines what service members do, what they learn, where they live, and what risks they will be asked to take. In exchange, the military culture can offer individuals a strong community, a sense of meaning, and the feeling that they are a part of something larger than themselves. The underlying psychological contract maintains that, in exchange for the individual's committed service, the military will provide training, support, and leadership (Adler and Castro 2013). In the event a service member is wounded, the expectation is that the service member will be provided care; in the event a service member is killed, the expectation is that the service member's family will be cared for financially.

In order to understand the way in which military culture operates, this chapter borrows from organizational theory and explains the military's occupational culture through the lens of Schein's (2010) three levels of culture. Artifacts, the first and most visible element of organizational culture, can be recognized by those both inside and outside of the organization. They include such tangible signs of the culture as building architecture and dress code, as well as language and stories. Values, the second level of organizational culture, are regarded as the organization's official norms, rules, and regulations. While these statements reflect a vision for the organization and serve as the explicitly stated goals to which members of the group should aspire, they may or may not jive with the implicit underlying beliefs of the organization. The third level of culture entails the deeply embedded attitudes, or shared basic assumptions, that serve as an organization's nor-

[1] This chapter primarily describes US Army culture and data from studies with soldiers. The authors have primarily worked with the Army, but believe that this chapter's analysis will apply to the other branches after taking into account nuanced cultural distinctions.

mative bedrock. Although these attitudes and behaviors are invisible to the outsider, they profoundly impact the members of the organization.

Cultural Artifacts While all facets of military culture cannot be described here, some key elements that have significance in terms of resilience can be addressed, as well as implications for adjusting to civilian life. First, in terms of artifacts, the military uses language in a distinct way. There are so many specialized terms, abbreviations, and expressions that military language can appear foreign to the outside listener. The use of novel terminology is endemic to military life and describes everything from entering the military (Initial Entry Training, or IET) and relocation (Permanent Change of Station, or PCS) to knowing what the mission requires (Mission Essential Task List, or METL). This use of shorthand provides an immediate sense that you have stepped through the looking glass into a new world. A service member's identity also becomes linguistically coded. Young officers become "L-T"; company first sergeants become "TOP." These terms are not derogatory but indicate camaraderie and can be taken as a sign of accomplishment. "Joe" isn't one's name, but rather a moniker representing the average soldier, the everyman. These examples demonstrate how the language and terminology used—whether it is an acronym or a turn of phrase—can be nearly indecipherable to the outside observer. This in-group language can bolster the sense of belonging by clearly marking the boundary between the in and out group.

The military uses signs and symbols to mark everything including service members themselves. The uniform is not only a way to create a regimented group identity but is also replete with history and information about what matters within the culture. For example, a soldier's personal record is visible on the uniform—rank, combat experience, certain training accomplishments, and unit. How the individual wears the uniform is another sign of individual readiness—is the uniform correctly laid out (e.g., are badges measured to an eighth of an inch in terms of placement on the uniform)? Attention to detail can serve as a beacon of competence—and signals whether others can trust you. Units also have their own symbols, from mascots to flags. These symbols are carefully selected to reflect a sense of lineage, which reinforces an individual's sense that they've joined the larger military family and now have a larger group identity.

Cultural Values The culture also has a particular set of values. In the Army, these values even spell LDRSHP (which sounds right given a liberal pronunciation). LDRSHP stands for Loyalty, Duty, Respect, Selfless service, Honor, Integrity, and Personal courage. Even though reducing values to an acronym can sound trite, the actual words are valued in the military context and have deep meaning (this is addressed further later in the chapter; see also http://www.army.mil/values/index.html). The acronym emphasizes leadership, which in and of itself is one of the most highly valued aspects of military culture. Due to the hierarchical structure of the military, quality leadership is needed at each level of the organization. For example, in the Marines, the expectation is that any time two Marines are together, one is a leader.

While these values are important in influencing "what right looks like" for the soldier, another huge influence on the life of a service member is the role of rank. Rank is more than an artifact on a uniform, pay grade, and a title; it represents where the individual fits into the large, explicit hierarchy. That hierarchy determines priorities and responsibilities. It takes special skill to work effectively within this hierarchy—what the business world terms "followership" and what the military terms "subordination." The term subordination may appear to be pejorative, but in the military context, it takes on a special and important meaning. Subordination means that individuals are able to set a lower priority for their own needs and desires, in order to contribute to the good of the group and the functioning of the team. While the military requires individuals to function within this strict hierarchy, this concept is not the same as blind followership. Despite the stereotype that military members robotically follow orders, the reality is that blind loyalty is not only discouraged but that "just following orders" is not an excuse for unethical or illegal behavior. Service members are expected to exercise discretionary judgment.

Basic Underlying Assumptions There are also underlying assumptions and unwritten cultural norms. One of them involves how time is treated. Being on time is a sign of respect. Ironically, to be on time does not mean arriving on time; it means arriving 10–15 min early (if not earlier). Service members learn quickly that timeliness is one of the most important ways to judge someone's basic military bearing. Another underlying assumption is that effective military personnel plan and prepare. These skills are markers of competence. In addition, there is an unwritten rule that service members are able to manage their emotions; stoic leaders are respected, while hotheads are not. Nevertheless, some emotions are encouraged, such as pride, anger, and even love. The underlying assumption related to love reflects what Barsade and O'Neill term "companionate love": it is the intense bond forged between close teammates (also called battle-buddies) and between good leaders and their team members (Barsade and O'Neill 2014). This love can be seen during a change of command ceremony at a Company, when the outgoing commander gets choked up, or even in the official correspondence of the military. In the 39th Chief of Staff of the Army's Initial Message to the Army, General Mark A. Milley (2016) writes "Our Soldiers are the crown jewel of the Nation; we must love them, protect them, and always keep faith in them."

The Indoctrination Process

Just as individuals learn about their own culture from both explicit and implicit cues, military culture is also taught at both levels. Individuals who enter the service go through an explicit period of training in which they are taught practical skills and inculcated in military values (McGurk et al. 2006). This period of indoctrination includes adopting the artifacts of the culture, from getting a haircut to being issued a set of clothes and job-specific gear. Service members are trained in cultural traditions such as the Army's song, and new recruits are expected to master what amounts to a rule book (TRADOC Publication 600-4, IET Soldier's Handbook, i.e., the "Smart Book") and to memorize and live up to the Soldier's Creed, an explicit description of a standard of behavior.

The daily routine of a new recruit is structured. Individuals are not allowed to go anywhere on their own—not even to the latrine—but must always be accompanied by a "battle-buddy," thus reinforcing the reality and value of interdependence. Individuals are also taught to approach higher-ranking individuals with a specific physical stance ("at attention," with hands at the side and legs together, or "at ease," with hands behind the back and legs slightly apart) and to repeat the leader's role in every exchange (e.g., "yes, Drill Sergeant" or, for officers, "yes, Sir" or "yes, Ma'am"), thus reinforcing the acceptance of and respect for the organizational hierarchy in every interaction. Soldiers are also required to carry their weapon with them at all times or have it held by a battle-buddy. They are shamed or penalized if they forget it somewhere or leave it unattended, reinforcing the cultural expectation that the military requires responsibility and readiness at all times.

The work itself is a testament to building confidence and those who make it through have demonstrated their own resilience. New service members are required to build themselves physically through fitness training and foot marches and to test their resolve and mastery through simulations and field exercises. Through a series of explicit training phases that increase in difficulty and complexity, their confidence and professional identity are shaped until they are ready to graduate and continue on to their next assignment. There are, of course, numerous exceptions and subtleties to the cultural context of military life that go beyond this chapter. Without reducing the military to stereotypes, it is important to acknowledge the strong cultural forces at work in helping an individual transition to the role of service member. These cultural forces have an impact on the development of resilience.

Resilience can be defined in many ways. This chapter adopts the definition used by the

Department of Defense: "the ability to withstand, recover, and grow in the face of stressors and changing demands" (Chairman of the Joint Chiefs of Staff Instruction 3405.01, 2011). Note that the definition reflects both recovering from stress and the potential to improve as a result of that experience. The definition also implies that resilience is something that can be developed; it is not a fixed quality but rather a malleable ability. The underlying concept of resilience is a cornerstone of military culture and is reinforced explicitly both through tough, realistic training and through classroom education designed to teach a variety of skills. Resilience, or the expectation of resilience, is also reinforced implicitly through the artifacts, values, and underlying assumptions of military culture.

The Impact of Military Culture on Service Members

This chapter has reviewed the essentials of military culture and how service members are indoctrinated. This section examines what role this cultural experience plays in how service members adapt to life back in the civilian world. In reviewing the implications of culture on service member adjustment, it is important to acknowledge that there are both positive and negative consequences associated with military culture.

Balancing Values

Borrowing from Aristotle (trans. 1999; Grant and Schwartz 2011), "being resilient" has both positive and negative aspects that can be depicted as a type of "virtue curve," reflecting the concept that there is an optimal level of resilience at the asymptote of the curve. Understanding the concept of the *resilience curve* is important in the current context for several reasons. First, understanding how the inculcation of military culture serves as the impetus for both psychological strength and failure should provide the practitioner with valuable insight into the psychology of the service member during counseling. Second, while clinicians are likely to see significant levels of mental health problems in service members, they are also likely to see profound strength. Understanding how the same process could be simultaneously beneficial and detrimental may prove useful during both diagnosis and treatment. As with any strength, there is a shadow side to resilience (Adler 2013), and as clinicians become aware of the balance between the strength and the shadow side, they may be able to leverage the strengths to assist individuals. Third, teasing apart the adaptive and maladaptive resilience skills that are influencing the service member could help the clinician accentuate the effects of the adaptive resilience-oriented skills while attenuating the maladaptive effects. Without adapting these resilience skills, service members will find transitioning to civilian life more challenging. In order to meet the needs of the military service member, providers must consider the profound influence of military culture in shaping the individual's perception, attitudes, and behaviors.

This chapter's treatment of the positive and negative effects of military resilience-related skills is influenced by the US Army's Battlemind Training program. This program, originally launched in 2007, was based on evidence from randomized trials conducted with soldiers at post-deployment (Adler et al. 2009; Castro et al. 2012). Although the effect sizes were small, they were consistent with results found in universally applied early intervention programs (Bliese et al. 2011). At the core of post-deployment, Battlemind Training was the concept of a shadow side to resilience. The training emphasized the idea that the very skills that help service members survive in combat need to be adjusted in order for them to transition home successfully. This chapter adapts this framework and considers more broadly how military skills need to be adjusted as service members leave the military and transition back to civilian life. The values outlined in LDRSHP provide an organizing structure for a review of how each of the seven values help service members adapt to military life (see the "adaptive expression" column in Table 4.1) and how these same values could impede adaptation (see the "maladaptive expres-

Table 4.1 Military values as adaptive and maladaptive in a civilian world

Military value	Description	Adaptive expression	Maladaptive expression	Clinical presentation
Loyalty	Believe in and devote oneself to something or someone above and beyond oneself	Develop close bonds; trust and commitment; desire to sacrifice one's own prosperity and well-being for the good of the group; teamwork and citizenship	Blind/unquestioning loyalty; allowing loyalty to trump other virtues such as honesty and fairness; shutting out others; feeling others don't understand; sense of disconnection and loss in post-military life; secretiveness	Depression; social isolation; grief; paranoia
Duty	Fulfill obligations; accomplish tasks as part of a team; be accountable	Reliable; disciplined; task-focused; achievement-oriented; situationally aware both in garrison and in high-risk situations; high in military readiness	Lack of work-life balance; rigid; overcontrolling; quick to be upset if questioned (if the implication is they failed to fulfill a duty); impatient; uncomfortable in public spaces; tracking points of egress; physically on edge; feeling the need to be armed in safe environments	Obsessive-compulsive behaviors; hypervigilance; sleep problems; intolerance of others
Respect	Treat others with dignity; rely on team members to put forth their best effort	Successful; high performer, especially in hierarchical structures; competent	Demanding; expects clear-cut direction; impatient with disorganization or lack of clarity; easily insulted; doesn't assimilate into flat or egalitarian structures	Interpersonal conflict; aggression
Selfless service	Put welfare of the nation, Army, and subordinates before personal welfare	Sense of meaning and purpose; contributing to the greater good	Unable to find meaning outside of military; disengaged from trivial tasks; a sense of entitlement	Anhedonia; feeling disenfranchised; uneven employment record
Honor	Act in accordance with Army values; proper behavior	Stoic vision of self; deep sense of personal responsibility; self-disciplined; able to engage in emotion regulation	Limited emotional range; numb; self-blame	Emotionally controlling; restricted affect; guilt
Integrity	Do what's right, legally and morally; be honest	High standards; strong personal ethic	Interpersonal difficulties; "I'll do it myself" attitude; black-or-white thinking	Aggression; uncompromising; easily frustrated
Personal courage	Endure duress; risk personal safety	Bravery; heroism; willingness to go into high-stress situations; prefer to self-manage problems rather than rely on others	Fear of being seen as weak; self-defeating pride; meddling; avoidance of care	Becoming mired in the role of sentinel; treatment dropout

sion" column in Table 4.1). At the extreme, these values could lead to clinical symptoms (see the "clinical presentation" column in Table 4.1).

Loyalty The first value, loyalty, reflects the close relationships that service members build with their fellow unit members. How this bond is recognized may vary by branch of service or occupational specialty, but overall, it is acutely recognized that those who serve together share an important bond of trust and mutual understanding. These strong bonds help individuals to be resilient in the face of profound stress and as well as in the face of everyday stressors. The team provides support and is an important source of comfort and humor. Individuals who do not adapt this value successfully, however, may end up struggling to build and maintain close, committed ties to their family and friends outside of the military context. This reaction then cuts off systems of support and disrupts an important source of resilience—social connections. These service members may feel like guarding themselves against these "outside" connections, and this tendency may slide toward secretiveness and, at the extreme, paranoia. Ultimately, this social disconnection might involve clinical symptoms that are associated with depression, social isolation, and grief. One way to encourage individuals caught in such isolation is to remind them of past success in building strong connections and to emphasize that loyalty is not always a zero-sum transaction—one can have multiple strong, loving, and committed relationships at the same time.

Duty The second value, duty, reflects degree of trustworthiness: if service members say they will do something, they will do it. They are reliable, focused on accomplishing a mission or task, and take their responsibilities seriously. When this profound sense of professionalism is not adapted to the civilian context, however, service members might come across as rigid, demanding, bossy, and impatient. For example, when asked whether they have completed a task, service members may have a disproportionately negative reaction because they may feel that their adherence to a core value is being questioned. This overreaction may have its roots in the deeply held belief in the importance of accountability and of fulfilling one's duty. At the extreme, this reaction might involve obsessive-compulsive behaviors.

Similarly, duty is associated with military readiness, being aware of potential threats, and being ready to respond. Maintaining situational awareness is critically adaptive in the military context but may result in hypervigilance and sleep problems if not adapted. In addition, service members may feel more comfortable if they have access to weapons, and this preference could potentially place individuals at risk if their unfettered access coincides with other interpersonal problems (e.g., Selby et al. 2010). One can cast this value of duty and accountability in a positive light, and emphasize that this value can be beneficial if expressed in a targeted manner.

Respect The third value, respect, reflects a belief that service members must respect those above them and, in turn, can expect to receive respect from those below them. In a strong hierarchical structure like the military, this value is associated with success. Outside of the military, however, this value may not align with more egalitarian, less hierarchical, and/or chaotic circumstances. Service members may feel on edge about managing without clear guidelines and may appear overly deferential, thus setting themselves apart from their civilian peers. In contrast, as leaders in a civilian context, they may come across as demanding or unyielding in interpersonal relationships. These characteristics are not signs of failure but rather reflect the ability to adapt within the military environment. At the extreme, this problem with adaptation can involve repeated interpersonal conflict.

Selfless Service The next value, selfless service, reflects the willingness of service members to make sacrifices—from relinquishing their freedom to make decisions, like where to live or how long to be away from family, to potentially risking their own safety. This identity allows service members to feel part of something greater than themselves. As a skill, adhering to this value can provide motivation and a strong sense of direction in life. If this skill is not adapted for the civilian context, however, individuals may find that they are unable to discover meaning in their day-to-day tasks. They may also feel a sense of entitlement given that they have spent years serving their country, and service members are routinely treated as special by the civilian world (e.g., receiving a special salute during the Super Bowl, receiving discounts at theme parks, being offered free meals by grateful strangers). Taken to the extreme, service members integrating into civilian life may feel that they are owed something, and this sense of entitlement may block their ability to adjust to other kinds of jobs.

Honor The value of honor can be seen in how service members are expected to comport themselves. Behaving in an honorable way can encourage prosocial behavior but may also imply a level of stoicism. This ability to self-regulate can serve individuals well when responding to highly stressful situations that require immediate action (Adler et al. 2008), but may also result in restricted emotional range. Individuals who do not learn to adapt this skill may find themselves responding with muted emotions, or a sense of numbness. Alternatively, they may find themselves responding with anger, given that it is an acceptable emotion in the military context. Indeed, in one study, about 50 % of soldiers surveyed reported that anger helped them focus and be more productive (Adler et al. under review). Relying on anger, although sometimes adaptive in the military context, is less accepted in the civilian context and may lead to difficulties. Acknowledging this emotion for what it is—a vestige of military culture that was useful in that context—may help put an angry reaction into perspective. In addition, the value of honor may place some service members at risk for significant feelings of guilt. They may have done everything right on a particular mission, but the combination of loyalty, sense of duty, and honor can lead them to feel regret and guilt.

Integrity The value of integrity involves the expectation that service members should perform at a high standard and "do the right thing" in terms of moral and ethical decision-making. At its best, this value can help guide service members through a myriad of choices and allow them to focus on behaving in ways that ultimately benefits others and their units. When this value is not adapted to civilian life, interpersonal difficulties can result. Individuals may feel that no one else lives up to their standards, and thus they need to do things themselves to avoid being disappointed by others. They may also engage in all-or-none thinking, as an extension of their focus on right or wrong. Taken to the extreme, this value can result in service members feeling impatient with others who do not share this value and who do not live up to their high standards, reinforcing a sense of separation or isolation.

Personal Courage The final value, personal courage, reflects skills fundamental to military service: the willingness to go into high-risk situations knowing there may be a threat to personal safety. Together with selfless service, personal courage is at the cornerstone of resilience during the most extreme moments of military life. When adapting this value to civilian life, however, personal courage could potentially get in the way of acknowledging the need for help, for fear of being seen as weak. Service members generally prefer to take care of their problems on their own and drop out of treatment rather than seek out care from professionals (Adler et al. 2014; Hoge et al. 2014). Unless this belief is adapted, it may hinder service members' ability to effectively manage mental health-related problems or gain relief from mental health symptoms. Personal courage can also inspire service members to stand up against what they perceive as an injustice, but this quick response to intervene can slide into meddling in the lives of others (e.g., aggressively confronting someone on the bus who doesn't stand up for an elderly person) and even, at the extreme, becoming locked into the role of sentinel.

Integrating Values

These various values overlap and supplement one another, and military culture reinforces them in persistent ways. Take, for instance, the real case of the senior noncommissioned officer in a brigade who signs his emails with the following signature block:

> 'You must hurt to win!' We are all fit and strong, what makes the difference is your willingness to suffer! – Yasotay (Mongol Warlord), 1314

The statement is an artifact, something visible that all can see and identify as part of the culture. The sentiment reflects the stated values of the military, a combination of self-sacrifice and personal courage. Underlying this statement is the message that senior leaders in the organization expect individuals to strive beyond endurance, and without that willingness, danger lurks for all. In effect, this senior noncommissioned officer is calling for resilience, and this resilience may serve the organization well but may need to be adapted outside of the occupational context. Without adaptation, this kind of sentiment sets unrealistic expectations that may encourage an unhealthy level of endurance and prevent an individual from seeking professional help for mental health or even physical health problems. Taken to the extreme, an individual may begin engaging in self-destructive behaviors. Adapted successfully, resilience can sustain valuable members of society who contribute to their community while balancing their own needs for respite.

For clinicians, family members, and even service members themselves, it may be helpful to see "maladaptive" behaviors as signaling one of these military values. Understanding that these characteristics are a reflection of a set of values that are highly prized may help individuals to situate these behaviors, understand their source, and become more aware of their complexity. How can clinicians use this information? When service members are experiencing difficulty adjusting to the civilian context, this difficulty may be, in part, a reflection of the very skills that served them well during military service. Perhaps this difficulty could be rephrased as such. Perhaps clinicians can help service members to recognize that, just as it took them a while to learn these kinds of skills, it will take time to learn how to adapt those skills for the civilian context. Moreover, although this chapter has discussed the adaptive and maladaptive qualities associated with these values, the reality is not so black-and-white. There is a spectrum, and the goal is not to abandon the values that the military has emphasized but to find a workable place for them instead.

Although this chapter has largely emphasized how military resilience can interfere with adaptation, military resilience can also be a major factor in healthy and happy adjustment. First, the military culture provides a core set of principles from which an individual can build a meaningful life. Second, service members have tremendous strength from which to draw and that can serve to inspire others. Third, service members, particularly those who have deployed under harsh conditions, have perspective about the little things. Numerous studies from our team and others have documented that these service members learn to value what's truly important. In one study, for example, soldiers who recently returned from combat deployment reported that they "appreciate the little things in life more" (74.5 %), "appreciate my family and friends more than before I deployed" (66.9 %), and "have matured as a result of the deployment" (64.9 %) (Adler et al. 2011). Thus, military experience itself can bring about a heightened sense of prioritization and can also bring military families closer together. Finally, military culture is likely to influence individuals to varying degrees. The degree of influence is likely a function of length of service, the extent to which the individual's military assignments are relatively traditional, and, of course, individual differences in responding to the acculturation process.

Formal Resilience Training

Besides the influence of military culture on the development of resilience, it is important to acknowledge that there are also formal educational classes on resilience. In the US Army's Comprehensive Soldier and Family Fitness (CSF2) program, for example, resilience is taught during professional military education (e.g., formal military schools) and as part of unit training. Anonymous assessments are also conducted through the Global Assessment Test (GAT; Peterson et al. 2011), and these assessments, based largely on measures from positive psychology, are supposed to inform an individual's choice of self-study in succeeding resilience training modules. The resilience training classes have their roots in cognitive behavioral therapy and typically rely on the basics of the ABC model (for a discussion, see Reivich et al. 2011).

Sometimes the terminology is adjusted to make sense for service members and for application as a universal (rather than targeted) intervention. For example, in the Army, the ABC model is known as the ATC model and stands for Activating events, Thoughts, Consequences. Thus, when clinicians are working with service members, these concepts may be familiar to service members but may be known by different terminology.

Currently, Resilience Training in the Army also leverages findings from the field of positive psychology and performance psychology. In one training module, soldiers are taught how to Hunt the Good Stuff and reflect on gratitude (akin to a gratitude diary); in another module, they are taught how to prolong the joy of others close to them by engaging in active constructive responding (Gable et al. 2004). In yet another module, soldiers are taught to understand their strong emotional reactions by uncovering their "icebergs," or deeply held core beliefs. A problem-solving module encourages individuals to identify the proportion of a problem that is under their control, while a module on "Putting it in Perspective" walks individuals through the worst-case scenario (taken to the extreme), the best-case scenario (taken to the extreme), and the most-likely case scenario.

This training is adapted from the Penn Resiliency Program (Reivich et al. 2011) and currently used with soldiers as part of the Army Resiliency Directorate's resilience program. While there is no compelling evidence among military personnel that the training is effective, the material is evidence-informed. Other training has been adapted from the performance psychology tradition and includes skills related to relaxation (called "energy management"), imagery, self-talk, and goal setting. This training has been found effective in a group randomized trial with new soldiers (Adler et al. 2015). Currently, the training uses a one-size-fits-all model and is conducted primarily by mid-level noncommissioned officers (e.g., staff sergeants). Deployment cycle resilience training (previously called Battlemind) has also been integrated into this larger program (Hoge et al. 2015).

Clinicians may find it useful to identify common resilience training terms and to leverage service members' familiarity with these terms when working in a clinical setting. Clinicians have also adapted resilience-building courses for use in group therapy, provided as part of intensive outpatient programs (Toblin and Adler 2016). By casting these skills in terms of resilience, clinicians can leverage service member preference for self-management and also demonstrate the immediate practical utility of interventions that are also found in mental health treatment.

Conclusion and Future Directions

The vignette of SFC (ret.) Peterson, the nontraditional college student at the start of this chapter, can be considered against the backdrop of military culture. The student-vet has strengths and a core set of values that can guide him through college. He may bring excellent organizational skills to bear on college tasks. These skills should serve him well, assuming they don't get him mired in rigid thinking, make him angry with teachers who don't follow the syllabus or who change plans at the last minute, or cause him to be intolerant of his own imperfect performance. The cultural context of college life may also be jarring: the culture is individualistic, whereas military culture is collectivistic. The student is used to the loyalty associated with teamwork and may find the isolation of college life disorienting. He may feel unprotected, and feeling this lack of support may reinforce his isolation, taking its toll on him over time.

This chapter has reviewed the role of organizational culture, how it informs the way resilience is conceptualized and reinforced within the military, and the implications for adjustment to civilian life. There are many questions that should be explored to fully understand these inter-relationships.

First, this chapter has primarily focused on combat deployments, but other deployments impact service members as well, including humanitarian and peacekeeping deployments. To what extent do these deployments differ in their influence on service member resilience and post-military adjustment?

Second, this chapter has focused on resilience and has not specified mental health problems. Although posttraumatic stress disorder (PTSD) is a common focus of much research with service members, other topics such as anger and aggression and risk-taking should also be considered. Research into these areas has noted that they are particularly salient for men and may be behaviors through which men express their emotional stress (Martin et al. 2013).

Third, this chapter has taken a relatively US-centric view of the military experience. While several studies have examined how resilience is addressed across other nations (e.g., Adler et al. 2013; Britt et al. 2016), it is not clear how the impact of military values and organizational culture might influence post-military life differently across nations.

Finally, this chapter has not focused on military families. Military families are in the unique position of representing both part of the military culture and the civilian world. They are potential assets that can be leveraged for understanding how to best help service members adjust. Similarly, previous unit members and leaders are a potentially powerful set of allies that remain largely untapped when helping service members adjust in post-military life. Both types of families (the traditional military family and the organizational family) might be useful for supporting successful adaptation.

Whether presenting in a clinical setting or as a part of a casual interaction, service members bring with them an historical context. By remembering to consider the larger military culture, clinicians can begin to appreciate the task of adapting military skills to civilian life and the strengths and challenges implicit in that transition.

Key Concepts

1. Organizational Culture
   (a) The military promotes a distinct culture through cultural artifacts, cultural values, and basic underlying assumptions.
   (b) Culture is taught during indoctrination.
   (c) Resilience is valued and taught implicitly and explicitly.
2. Balancing Values
   (a) Military values can benefit service member quality of life and meaning.
   (b) Without adapting military values, adjustment after leaving the military can be challenging.
3. Integrating Values
   (a) Clinicians can restructure how veterans understand adjustment challenges.
   (b) Adjustment challenges can be framed as difficulty adapting military values to the civilian context.

Disclaimer The views expressed in this chapter are those of the authors and do not reflect the official position of the Walter Reed Army Institute of Research, the US Army, or the Department of Defense.

References

Adler AB (2013) Resilience in a military occupational health context: directions for future research. In: Sinclair RR, Britt TW (eds) Building psychological resilience in military personnel: theory and practice. American Psychological Association, Washington, DC, pp 223–235

Adler AB, Castro CA (2013) The occupational mental health model for the military. Mil Behav Health 1:1–11. https://doi.org/10.1080/21635781.2012.721063

Adler AB, Wright KM, Bliese PD, Eckford R, Hoge CW (2008) A2 diagnostic criterion for combat-related posttraumatic stress disorder. J Trauma Stress 21:301–308

Adler AB, Bliese PB, McGurk D, Hoge CW, Castro CA (2009) Battlemind debriefing and Battlemind training as early interventions with soldiers returning from Iraq: randomization by platoon. J Consult Clin Psychol 77:928–940. https://doi.org/10.1037/a0016877

Adler AB, Zamorski M, Britt TW (2011) The psychology of transition: adapting to home after deployment. In: Adler AB, Bliese PB, Castro CA (eds) Deployment psychology: evidence-based strategies to promote mental health in the military. American Psychological Association, Washington, DC, pp 153–174

Adler AB, Delahaij R, Bailey SM, Van den Berge C, Parmak M, van Tussenbroek B, … Castro CA (2013) NATO survey of mental health training in Army recruits. Mil Med, 178, 760–766

Adler AB, Britt TW, Riviere LA, Kim PY, Thomas JL (2014) Longitudinal determinants of mental health treatment seeking by US soldiers. Br J Psychiatry, 1–5. https://doi.org/10.1192/bjp.bp.114.146506

Adler AB, Bliese PD, Pickering MA, Hammermeister J, Williams J, Harada C, Csoka L, Holiday B, Ohlson C (2015) Mental skills training with Basic Combat Training soldiers: A group randomized trial. J Appl Psychol. Advance online publication. https://doi.org/10.1037/apl0000021

Adler AB, Brossart DF, Toblin RL (under review) Can Anger Be Helpful? Soldier Perceptions of the Utility of Anger

Aristotle (trans. 1999). Nicomachean ethics (W.D. Ross, trans.) Kitchener, Batoche Books, Ontario

Barsade SG, O'Neill OA (2014) What's love got to do with it? A longitudinal study of the culture of companionate love and employee and client outcomes in the long-term care setting. Adm Sci Q 59:551–598

Bliese PB, Adler AB, Castro CA (2011) Research-based preventive mental health care strategies in the military. In: Adler AB, Bliese PB, Castro CA (eds) Deployment psychology: evidence-based strategies to promote mental health in the military. American Psychological Association, Washington, DC, pp 103–124

Britt TW, Crane M, Hodson SE, Adler AB. Effective and ineffective coping strategies in a low-autonomy work environment. J Occupational Health Psychol. 2016 Apr;21(2):154.

Bonanno GA, Mancini AD, Horton JL, Powell TM, Leardmann CA, Boyko EJ, Wells TS, Hooper TI, Gackstetter GD, Smith TC, Millennium Cohort Study Team (2012) Trajectories of trauma symptoms and resilience in deployed U.S. military service members: prospective cohort study. Br J Psychiatry 200:317–323. https://doi.org/10.1192/bjp.bp.111.096552. Epub 2012 Feb 23

Castro CA, Adler AB, McGurk D, Bliese PD (2012) Mental health training with soldiers four months after returning from Iraq: randomization by platoon. J Trauma Stress 25:376–383. https://doi.org/10.1002/jts.21721

Cornum R, Matthews MD, Seligman ME (2011) Comprehensive soldier fitness: building resilience in a challenging institutional context. Am Psychol 66:4–9

Gable SL, Reis HT, Impett EA, Asher ER (2004) What do you do when things go right? The intrapersonal and interpersonal benefits of sharing positive events. J Pers Soc Psychol 87:228–245. https://doi.org/10.1037/0022-3514.87.2.228

Grant AM, Schwartz B (2011) Too much of a good thing the challenge and opportunity of the inverted U. Perspect Psychol Sci 6(1):61–76

Hoge CW, Grossman SH, Auchterlonie JL, Riviere LA, Milliken CS, Wilk JE (2014) PTSD treatment for soldiers after combat deployment: low utilization of mental health care and reasons for dropout. Psychiatr Serv 65(8):997–1004. https://doi.org/10.1176/appi.ps.201300307

Hoge CW, Ivany CG, Brusher EA, Brown MD, Shero JC, Adler AB, Warner CH, Orman DT (2015) Transformation of mental health Care for U.S. soldiers and families during the Iraq and Afghanistan wars: where science and politics intersect. Am J Psychiatry. https://doi.org/10.1176/appi.ajp.2015.15040553

McGurk D, Cotting DI, Britt TW, Adler AB (2006) Joining the ranks: the role of indoctrination in transforming civilians to service members. In: Adler AB, Castro CA, Britt TW (eds) Military life: the psychology of serving in peace and combat, Operational Stress, vol 2. Praeger Security International, Westport, pp 13–31

Martin LA, Neighbors HW, Griffith DM. The experience of symptoms of depression in men vs women: analysis of the National Comorbidity Survey Replication. JAMA psychiatry. 2013 Oct 1;70(10):1100–6.

Milley MA (2016) 39th Chief of Staff Initial Message to the Army. Available at https://www.army.mil/article/154803/39th_Chief_of_Staff_Initial_Message_to_the_Army/

Peterson C, Park N, Castro CA (2011) Assessment for the U.S. Army Comprehensive soldier fitness program: the global assessment tool. Am Psychol 66:10–18. https://doi.org/10.1037/a0021658

Reivich K, Seligman EPM, McBride SA (2011) Master resilience training in the U.S. Army. Am Psychol 66:25–34. https://doi.org/10.1037/a0021897

Schein EH. Organizational culture and leadership. John Wiley & Sons; 2010 Aug 16.

Segal MW (1986) The military and the family as greedy institutions. Armed Forces Soc Fall 13:9–38. https://doi.org/10.1177/0095327X8601300101

Selby EA, Anestis MD, Bender TW, Ribeiro JD, Nock MK, Rudd MD, ..., Joiner TE (2010) Overcoming the fear of lethal injury: evaluating suicidal behavior in the military through the lens of the interpersonal–psychological theory of suicide. Clin Psychol Rev 30(3):298–307

Toblin RL, Adler AB (2016) Resilience training as a complementary treatment for PTSD. In: Benedek DM, Wynn GH (eds) Complementary and alternative medicine for PTSD. Oxford University Press, New York, pp 243–268

Psychiatry Graduate Medical Education in Military and Veterans Affairs Training Facilities

5

Daniel R. May, Patcho N. Santiago, Alan K. Louie, and Laura Weiss Roberts

Introduction to Psychiatry Graduate Medical Education in Military Facilities

All graduate medical education programs in psychiatry must meet the requirements of the psychiatry residency review committee of the Accreditation Council for Graduate Medical Education (ACGME), and residents must meet these standards for successful graduation (Accreditation Council for Graduate Medical Education). This requirement is true regardless of whether the program is offered through a civilian or military training institution. Military psychiatry residencies nevertheless possess additional programmatic components that differ from their civilian counterparts in order to prepare their residents for future careers as military medical corps officers (Hill et al. 2007; Ritchie and White 1993). At the same time, many civilian graduate medical education (GME) programs also recognize the importance of having clinical exposure to patient populations that include retired military personnel and other veterans, such as through initiatives like Joining Forces (Lehrmann and Roberts 2009; Roberts 2015; Scaturo and Huszonek 2009; The White House). While more than half of US clinicians have worked with retired military personnel through the Department of Veteran Affairs (VA) (Roberts 2015; Veterans Health Administration & Office of Academic Affiliations), there remains a common misconception about military medicine that active duty service members receive most of their care through the VA. However, the majority of service members and their family members receive their care through the Military Health System (MHS) in military treatment facilities (MTFs) on military installations, which are separate from the VA. In addition to working at MTFs, many military psychiatrists work in positions outside of hospitals, serving with combat units in preventive, public psychiatry roles.

Beyond learning about the fundamentals of psychiatry and caring for patients, military psychiatrists are groomed to become leaders in a military environment and learn how to communicate

D.R. May
65th Medical Brigade, Camp Humphreys, Pyongtaek, South Korea
e-mail: daniel.r.may.mil@mail.mil

P.N. Santiago
Uniformed Services University of the Health Sciences, Bethesda, MD, USA
e-mail: patcho.santiago@usuhs.edu

A.K. Louie
Stanford University School of Medicine, Palo Alto VA Health Care System, Palo Alto, CA, USA
e-mail: louiemd@stanford.edu

L.W. Roberts (✉)
Department of Psychiatry and Behavioral Sciences, Stanford University School of Medicine, Palo Alto, CA 94305, USA
e-mail: robertsl@stanford.edu

L.W. Roberts, C.H. Warner (eds.), *Military and Veteran Mental Health*,
https://doi.org/10.1007/978-1-4939-7438-2_5

mental health concerns to military commanders (Warner et al. 2005). Trainees are immersed in the culture of the military and must develop an understanding of the myriad of experiences of a military officer. The culture and experiences associated with the military consist of not only combat deployments but also the nuanced experience of being "in garrison" and the impact of military life on families, which can affect the mental health of service members. Civilian psychiatrists will inevitably encounter current or former service members and may increase their own military cultural competency from understanding the unique GME training that military psychiatrists go through to more effectively treat this patient population (Meyer 2012; Meyer et al. 2016).

This chapter begins with a review of military psychiatry GME: historical context, mission, unique curriculum, learning environment, paths to becoming a military psychiatrist, and contributions to society. Subsequently, VA psychiatry GME will be discussed: historical context, mission, collaborations with medical schools, faculty, learning environment, and the future.

The Mission of Military Psychiatry Graduate Medical Education

It is important to reiterate here that the Department of Defense (DoD) and the Department of Veterans Affairs (VA) are two distinct organizations in the executive branch of the US government, each with a distinct mission. The mission of the Department of Defense is to provide military forces to protect the country and deter war, with its primary headquarters at the Pentagon (Department of Defense 2015; Gates 2010). The DoD consists of elements of the seven armed forces, particularly the Army, Navy, and Air Force. The Marine Corps is also under the authority of the DoD, however resides under the Department of the Navy. Additionally, the Coast Guard can be transferred to the control of the DoD during times of war and is otherwise under the auspices of the Department of Homeland Security in times of peace. The Department of Health and Human Services and the Department of Commerce maintain authority over the Public Health Services and the National Oceanic and Atmospheric Administration, respectively. In contrast to the Department of Defense, the VA's mission is to care for those who formerly served in one of the seven armed forces as well as eligible family members (Shinseki 2014). This care is provided through numerous benefits and services, including the provision of medical services.

Initially, the Army and Navy trained psychiatric providers at St. Elizabeth's Hospital in Washington DC, starting around 1909 (Heaton et al. 1966). However, due to the need to improve the retention of capable psychiatric providers, the Army and Navy planned numerous psychiatric training programs in the 1940s. Initially, however, only the Army residencies at Walter Reed and Letterman were accredited in 1948, and the Navy residencies at Bethesda, Great Lakes, and Philadelphia were accredited in 1946. After the Air Force separated from the Army Air Corps in 1947, they continued to recruit psychiatrists from the Army. It was not until 1965 that Wilford Hall started the first Air Force psychiatry training program (Wise 1987). Military psychiatry has had a profound impact on modern psychiatry, dating back to Brigadier General William Menninger's development of the War Department Technical Bulletin, Medical 203 in 1945, which laid the foundation for the subsequent formation of the *Diagnostic and Statistical Manual-I* (*DSM-I*) (Menninger 2004).

Military GME programs perform an essential role of ensuring that lessons from past wars and conflicts are not forgotten. For instance, an important lesson learned from World War I and subsequent wars was the importance of "forward psychiatry," or the importance of being close to those who need mental health support, especially in deployed settings (Jones 1995). This is often taught through the acronym "PIES," or *providing* care in close proximity to those in need, providing them *immediate* care, conveying a sense of *expectancy* of healing, and keeping interventions *simple*, while subsequent mnemonics ("BICEPS") included *brevity* and *centrality* as guides for initial elements of treating stress reactions.

At the core of military service resides a sense of duty to country and to other service members and their families, and this sense stems from the mission of military medicine "to conserve the fighting strength" (Carter 1993). For military mental health providers in particular, there is a sense of urgency to address the behavioral health needs of the more than 2 million active duty service members (Defense Manpower Data Center 2016) and 21 million veterans (United States Census Bureau 2015). In any given 30-day period, Kessler and colleagues found that a quarter of non-deployed service members met criteria for a mental disorder (Kessler et al. 2014). Additionally, many of the mental health needs of soldiers, sailors, Marines, and airmen go unseen. Furthermore, the mental health of a service member rarely occurs in isolation, and their families are frequently affected (Cozza et al. 2005; Lester et al. 2016; McFarlan 2009; Meyer 2012; Park 2011; Ursano et al. 1989). During times of greater utilization of the military, there can be greater stress on the service members and their families, and mental health providers must be appropriately trained to meet their needs (McNulty 2005; Ursano et al. 1989). Changing military demands not only result in fluctuations in the pathology that trainees see but can result in shifts in teaching staff as some are deployed to theater (Groom et al. 2015).

The primary mission of military GME is to provide future psychiatrists who are skillfully trained to address the mental health needs of the military. In doing so, military GME must achieve dual objectives: to train fully competent physicians in accordance with ACGME standards as well as to prepare physicians to serve in an evolving military operational environment (Groom et al. 2015). With regard to meeting ACGME accreditation standards, a study by De Lorenzo in 2008 showed that military GME programs generally were awarded longer accreditation cycle lengths than their civilian counterparts (De Lorenzo 2008). These high-quality training programs also have among the highest board pass rates in the country (usuhs.edu).

As the military is at the forefront of an evolving geopolitical landscape, psychiatrists must be able to adapt to the demands of the military (Warner et al. 2007). Military psychiatry training programs not only prepare psychiatrists for these demands, but the programs themselves must also adapt to meet the needs of the armed services during war, as various training faculty get deployed (Diebold et al. 2015; Groom et al. 2015). Military mental health providers must be prepared to work in a myriad of different treatment settings or "operational environments" with fluctuating periods of demands or "operational tempos." An operational environment can have many different characteristics, depending on the branch of service, the location of services rendered, and the needs of the military (Hill et al. 2007; Ritchie and White 1993). The stressors experienced by a Marine aboard an amphibious assault ship are different than those experienced by a soldier in an infantry unit. The wartime footing has become even more heterogeneous since 2001, and sailors can be found manning a 0.50 caliber machine gun in the convoy of a Provincial Reconstruction Team in landlocked Afghanistan (Myers 2008). Military psychiatrists must therefore understand how the stress of the operational environment and operational tempo can affect patients and must also recognize that they can be subjected to similar stressors themselves.

Military Graduate Medical Education Accession Pathways

There are a number of paths to becoming a trained military psychiatrist (Diebold et al. 2015), and one does not need to complete a psychiatry residency in a military program to become a military medical corps officer. Nevertheless, the vast majority of the uniformed service psychiatrists have been trained through military residency programs. There are three primary approaches to becoming a military psychiatrist which this chapter will discuss: joining the military prior to or during medical school, joining the military after medical school, or joining after residency.

Most commonly the journey begins when an aspiring medical student applies to medical school. Applicants may consider the F. Edward Hébert School of Medicine at the Uniformed Services University of the Health Sciences

(USUHS) in Bethesda, Maryland. "America's Medical School," USUHS, is the nation's federal medical school and trains 172 medical students annually. The students are active duty officers in four uniformed services: the Army, Air Force, Navy, and Public Health Service (PHS). Upon matriculation, they are commissioned as second lieutenants or ensigns, and while they are full-time students, they are paid a salary and allowances equal to that of other military officers of the same rank. USUHS, like any other medical school, must meet accreditation standards set by the Liaison Committee on Medical Education, and aside from the military uniforms worn daily by the students, these programs have few differences from civilian medical schools (usuhs.edu).

Prospective medical students may also consider applying for the Health Professions Scholarship Program (HPSP) offered by the Army, Navy, and Air Force. This scholarship pays for the tuition at an American civilian medical school, as well as for mandatory expenses such as books. In addition, HPSP students receive a monthly stipend and a signing bonus for joining the program. HPSP students receive a commission as a junior officer in the reserves and go on active duty for 45 days every year, which can be used for basic military officer training, clinical rotations at military hospitals (McCroskey and Nieves 2016), or for "home orders" where they continue work at their medical schools (without any need to wear the uniform). An important decision for applicants for both USUHS and HPSP is to consider what branch of the military to serve with, and while a recruiter can assist with this process, most prospective students also find mentors with prior service who often provide much more specific guidance about the lives of physicians in the three branches.

At USUHS, the service commitment is typically 7 years after residency training, while for a 4-year HPSP agreement, a psychiatrist will typically serve a total of 8 years—4 years in residency and 4 years as a staff psychiatrist. Both USUHS and HPSP students pursuing a career in psychiatry must apply to military residencies offered by their service branch. The Army and Navy have a joint program at the Walter Reed National Military Medical Center in Bethesda, Maryland. The Army has a second program at Tripler Army Medical Center in Honolulu, Hawaii. The Navy also has programs at Naval Medical Centers in Portsmouth, Virginia, and San Diego, California. The Air Force is unique in having dual civilian-military programs in San Antonio, Texas, and Dayton, Ohio (Welton et al. 2015). Occasionally, a medical student may be granted a full deferment to attend a civilian residency, though this is dependent on the needs of the military.

There are other avenues to becoming a military psychiatrist as well, such as through other programs with the National Guard, the reserves, or joining after medical school and during residency through the Financial Assistance Program (FAP), which offers an annual grant and monthly stipend to residents, while they continue to receive their salary from their residency program. Physicians also have the opportunity to join the military after residency as a "direct accession," and if their specialty is a critical need for the armed forces (such as psychiatry), then they may be considered for the Health Professions Loan Repayment Program (HPLRP), which provides an annual loan repayment in return for serving on active duty. Physicians who desire to complete a second residency training program might prefer to do this through the military, particularly as residency programs tend to pay more than their civilian counterparts. Additionally, a number of contractors and other federal employees work at military facilities and also contribute to the training of psychiatry residents.

While the length of commitment, locations of training programs, and amount of financial remunerations are important factors to consider, in the end, many military medical students do not cite the financial benefits as their primary reason for joining the armed forces but instead report a desire to serve their country as their principal motivator (Holmes et al. 2009).

The Military Graduate Medical Education Learning Environment

Upon completion of medical school, trainees are promoted to the rank of captain (in the Army or Air Force) or lieutenant (in the Navy) prior to starting the intern year of residency training. Most psychiatry residents will be granted continuous contracts which will give them the opportunity to complete all 4 years of their psychiatry residency as long as they remain in good academic standing. However, some interns, particularly in the Navy, may receive contracts that will enable them to serve as general medical officers (GMO) after completing their internship. After serving as a general medical officer, typically for 2 years, they may decide to return to complete the psychiatry residency as a PGY-2 (postgraduate year 2) or pursue another career path. Additionally, a number of trainees switch to a military psychiatry residency program as a PGY-2 after completing a transitional year or primary care internship.

The learning curve can be steep for residents as they become acclimated to military culture—that is, to the social norms, expected behaviors and attitudes, communication styles, and the seemingly countless military acronyms and other terminologies (Department of Defense 2016). This mastery of the culture is, obviously, in addition to learning the fundamentals of their medical specialty. Military psychiatry residencies consist of both on-site rotations at the primary medical treatment facility (MTF) and other off-site rotations at other military, VA, and civilian facilities associated with the program. Residents will wear the uniform of the day while at military hospitals, or occasionally a white coat and scrubs if indicated by their clinical duties, but when rotating at civilian locations, they will wear civilian clothes despite being on active duty.

Civilian rotations are a critical part of a trainee's learning experience. These "outside rotations" expose residents to the differences and similarities in how civilian healthcare models operate. In addition to the differences in patient demographics between military and civilian clinical environments, residents learn about how differences in healthcare management can influence patient care. These off-site rotations can be synergistic, in that they allow ideas and resources to be exchanged between military and civilian programs. Civilian and military institutions have a lengthy history of collaboration, which have been beneficial to all parties involved. Notably, the two Air Force psychiatry residencies are built upon civilian-military partnership models, with both civilian psychiatry residents and their military counterparts collaborating in the same program (Welton et al. 2015).

Residents are prepared throughout their residency to work in numerous different environments depending on their future job assignments. However, residents may also consider extending their training by pursuing a fellowship after residency. There are many such programs offered through the military, including fellowships in child and adolescent psychiatry, geriatric psychiatry, psychosomatics, pain, forensic psychiatry, and addiction psychiatry, although sometimes they may be selected to conduct fellowship training at civilian institutions. When conducting civilian fellowship training, fellows typically remain on active duty and continue to receive active duty pay and allowances but wear civilian clothes throughout the time period.

The forensic psychiatry fellowship has a unique military-specific curriculum, as trainees must become familiar with how principles of forensic psychiatry relate to the Uniform Code of Military Justice (UCMJ). An additional program that is unique to the military is the Disaster and Preventive Psychiatry Fellowship offered at Uniformed Services University of the Health Sciences (USUHS), which consists of 1 year of training in the Master in Public Health program, followed by a year of practicum experience at federal institutions that are implementing public psychiatry concepts into policy and practice. As of this writing, there have not been any fellows enrolled in the Disaster and Preventive Psychiatry Fellowship program for the last 4 years.

The Military Unique Curriculum

While military residencies must adhere to standards of the professional accrediting body, the Accreditation Council for Graduate Medical

Education, the military GME curriculum is structured with additional training to prepare residents to be mental health leaders in the military environment. The military psychiatrist must understand the importance of making accurate diagnoses and identifying effective therapeutic interventions. Once patients leave the psychiatric setting, they will be placed in job roles that are an integral part of the military mission. Trainees must recognize that a service member who is struggling from significant mental illness may pose a potential danger to other military members if they are unable to effectively perform their job duties or defend from potential enemy threats. Psychiatrists who are deployed may find that they are living in close proximity with their patients. All told, the core competency of interpersonal and communication skills is uniquely tested by the mission of military medicine and the GME curriculum is designed to prepare residents to confront these challenges.

Military psychiatrists must maintain a public health mind-set, as psychiatrists are frequently in charge of the mental health and well-being of whole communities, whether that community is a Marine Corps division or the sailors and family members stationed at an overseas naval base. Didactics in the training programs incorporate public health concepts so that residents are ready to engage in program planning and development to "conserve the fighting strength"—the mission of the military medical corps.

This idea of training to the mission is evident in some of the unique experiences military residents participate in. The Combat Casualty Care Course (C4) is a weeklong operational medicine course for officers that prepares them to understand the operational environment in a deployed setting, which can oftentimes be an environment with limited resources and potential dangers that need to be prepared for. It is important for physicians to understand the roles and responsibilities of medics and corpsmen, as they are at the forefront of providing medical and psychiatric care on the battlefield before a patient reaches a military treatment facility (MTF). Mental health providers must recognize that battlefield care not only includes combat triage and casualty evacuation but also preventive combat and operational stress control measures, as noted elsewhere in this book.

Combat stress control doctrine is so critical to military medicine, that it is an integral part of the operational capstone field exercise conducted at Uniformed Services University of the Health Sciences (USUHS), Operation Bushmaster (West et al. 2015). Here, not only are fourth-year medical students run through graded training exercises in the application of medical and surgical clinical skills in an operational environment, but there is also a specific, graded evolution that all students must go through as the Combat Stress Control officer. Further, there are graded rotations in leadership in charge of the platoon, an experience that can really resonate with students as they are exposed to the idea that they are not simply to become physicians, but they must also become leaders. At Operation Bushmaster, psychiatry residents serve as "Observer/Controllers," the faculty for the Combat Stress Control Rotation, and in this role, they must balance being clinician-educators while modeling the physician-officer for these impressionable student-doctors.

Perhaps one surprise of the military-unique curriculum is the emphasis on developing superior skills in psychotherapy. Military psychiatrists are taught to develop comprehensive biopsychosocial formulations and identify appropriate interventions accordingly. Some military programs maintain close ties to local psychoanalytic institutes when available, and some programs offer training psychotherapy, which allows residents to experience the patient role. In allowing residents the opportunity to reflect on their own mental processes and the dynamic forces in their minds, residents experience for themselves how a therapist gleans interpretations from their sessions with their training psychotherapist. This opportunity is offered in a safe environment outside of the program in order to maintain the trainee's privacy while encouraging the resident to process difficult challenges during their residency (Gray 2004). Also in preparation for their year of outpatient psychiatry training, the Center for Deployment Psychology at USUHS offers 2-day courses on prolonged exposure and cognitive processing therapy, as the Department of Defense requires that a substantial cohort of behavioral health providers receive training in evidenced-based treatments for post-traumatic stress disorder (PTSD).

The Clinical Learning Environment

In most ways, the clinical environment in military residencies is no different than what would be encountered in civilian residencies, but at the same time, a trainee's experience is shaped by the system of healthcare delivery and the patient population characteristics. Military healthcare beneficiaries not only include active duty service members but also family members (both spouses and children) and eligible retirees. One of the differences between military and civilian training environments is the approach to healthcare utilization management. Specifically, military service members and authorized family members (called "dependents") receive health insurance through TRICARE. Therefore, access to care is primarily authorized by TRICARE, and residents have little exposure to other healthcare insurances when working within military treatment facilities.

Trainees must also learn about differences in the limits of confidentiality as it is applied to civilian populations versus military patients. Specifically, the Health Insurance Portability and Accountability Act (HIPAA) provides, under the Military Command Exception, for circumstances when privacy may be broken in circumstances where military missions could be compromised, and military psychiatry residents must learn how and when to titrate the release of protected health information to their patients' commanding officers, which is not otherwise acceptable with civilian populations. In addition, while the process of involuntary commitment of active duty service members to inpatient psychiatric facilities differs from state laws, this process is also regulated to ensure service members can exercise personal rights. However, contrary to what some might assume, military psychiatrists cannot order patients to take prescribed medications. That is, despite any differences, trainees are taught to respect patient rights, autonomy, and the limitations of military authority with regard to treatment.

An important component of the clinical environment is the resources that are available to military service members and their families. There is a vast array of resources available to service members and retirees, such as the Fleet and Family Support Center or Army Community Services frequently found on military bases. Oftentimes, the limiting variable in accessing these resources is not their availability, but rather a lack of awareness. As such, trainees learn about the importance of these auxiliary resources and how to effectively refer patients. These resources can vary depending on the specific military installation, branch of the military, or VA facility.

Military demographics are not equivalent to the general civilian population. As such, military mental health professionals must be familiar with the unique culture that they will work with after leaving training and must keep this in mind when reading nonmilitary-based research. Military service members tend to be young and healthy and must undergo screening to ensure medical and mental health fitness prior to enlisting or commissioning. Additionally, entry-level training camps further assess the resiliency of the service member. However, despite this screening process, it is important for mental health providers to learn about particular susceptibilities of the military population. For instance, it is important for trainees to understand the role of stigma and shame, which can be impediments to service members accessing care (Hoge et al. 2004).

While an extensive review of the factors influencing risk for mental health issues is outside of the scope of this discussion, it is important for trainees to become familiar with the voluminous literature related to military psychiatry. Important topics consist of (but are not limited to) suicide (Castro and Kintzle 2014; Cazares et al. 2015; Lee 2012), combat trauma (Hoge et al. 2014; Marmar et al. 2015; Toblin et al. 2012), military sexual trauma (MST) (Mercado et al. 2015), traumatic brain injury (TBI) (Wilk et al. 2012; Stein et al. 2015), and substance use disorders (Kelsall et al. 2015), in addition to other common conditions such as depression, bipolar, anxiety, and schizophrenia which can often first present in this population. Trainees must also recognize that the service member's family system may be susceptible to stress from the demands of the military. For example, young children may be at higher risk of abuse and neglect following the return of a parent from deployment (Taylor et al. 2016). An important task that is accomplished by military mental health GME is to acclimate trainees to the numerous interventions that will help them to create solutions to problems that their patients will be facing.

Another critical role of military psychiatrists is to monitor a service member's fitness for duty. Service members are generally expected to be "worldwide deployable" and need to be prepared to receive orders to new military assignments. However, when physical or psychiatric illness affects a service member, trainees must learn the mechanisms for placing duty limitations, which are different for each branch of service.

Providers must be conscientious of the impact that different diagnoses and treatments can have on a service member's career. For instance, service members may be denied deployment opportunities if they are not stable on their medications or are taking medications that cannot be adequately monitored in theater. Pharmacies in a deployed environment may only have a limited formulary. It may not be feasible to obtain the necessary routine lab monitoring for other medications. Some medications may also lead to withdrawal symptoms if the service member is unable to get access to their medications due to unanticipated circumstances.

The deployment environment may have additional factors that can influence a service member's treatment plan, which might not otherwise be a concern while in the continental United States. For instance, extremes in temperature can predispose patients to dehydration, and in a reciprocal fashion, some medications can influence thermoregulation, which could lead to hyperthermia in a desert environment. Additionally, service members may not have the same level of access to medical care while in theater, which can pose a risk for conditions such as psychosis, substance addictions, and even those with chronic infectious disease such as HIV, which could otherwise be well controlled with optimal access to medical care. Given these considerations, some psychiatric conditions are incompatible with further military service and may require an administrative separation or a medical board at the recommendation of the psychiatrist. An accurate diagnosis is also important to ensure that the patient can receive the correct treatments as they transition to the VA or to civilian care.

Beyond Military Psychiatry Training

Upon completion of residency, trainees can continue to advance their education as they become leaders in the field (Ritchie and White 1993). Graduating trainees will have been exposed to a number of major research efforts that will continue to contribute to the scientific understanding of military mental health. While the Department of Veterans Affairs and Department of Defense's clinical practice guidelines on suicide, depression, post-traumatic stress disorder (PTSD), and bipolar disorder provide clear direction on treating the active duty and veteran populations, large-scale psychiatric epidemiologic research including the Land Combat Study, the Millennium Cohort Study, and the Study to Assess Risk and Resilience in service members (STARRS) continue to add to our knowledge and understanding of public mental health issues. The integration of behavioral health in primary care, such as in the RESPECT-MIL (Re-Engineering Systems of Primary Care Treatment in the Military) project, has been showing residents to recognize the growing importance of integrating psychiatry at the "front lines" of healthcare to proactively reach patients even before being referred by their primary care physician (Higgins and Lacy 2006).

Military cultural competency remains important for anyone treating military service members, whether in a military treatment facility, in the VA, or in a civilian practice (Meyer et al. 2016). However, one survey of 52 residents in a residency program not affiliated with a military hospital revealed that the majority desired additional training in treating those who have been impacted by war but none of them felt completely prepared to do so (Munshi et al. 2010). Further collaboration between civilian and military training programs could prove beneficial to both patients and trainees, as veterans of war will always return home and receive their healthcare in their communities. Another study has suggested that adding a trauma curriculum for psychiatry residents may increase resident awareness of the high prevalence of experiencing potentially traumatic events and lead to increased screening for stressor-related disorders of all types (Ferrell et al. 2014). Continued efforts to develop effective academic affiliations across institutions have been recognized as a mutually beneficial solution to some of the challenges that the VA has recently been facing (Bakaeen et al. 2014), and military facilities could experience similar benefit from such collaboration.

The Mission of Veterans Affairs and Psychiatric Graduate Medical Education

The Department of Veterans Affairs' (VA) mission, in contrast to the mission of the Department of Defense, is, "…To care for him who shall have borne the battle, and for his widow and his orphan," as taken from President Lincoln's second inaugural address (Lincoln 1865). The early seeds for the current day VA system go back at least as far as World War I, when, in anticipation of many disabled soldiers, Congress enacted the War Risk Insurance Act of 1917 to provide for "rehabilitation." While the current VA service for veterans and their families is, of course, not limited to rehabilitation medicine, much of the initial impetus was to rehabilitate soldiers to be once again employable, not only for their own good but also to mitigate the great financial burden of disability pensions on the federal government observed since the Civil War (Linker 2016). This thinking established the VA not only as a major healthcare entity but also as a conduit for social action and conscience to address the obligations of a society after armed conflict. In 1921, the Veteran Bureau was federally funded for the care of veterans, and in 1930, Executive Order 538 under President Hoover created the US Department of Veterans Affairs, originally with 54 hospitals. This number has now grown about threefold across 23 regional networks, with almost 9 million enrollees (National Center for Veterans Analysis and Statistics 2016).

Tasked by society with this serious obligation of providing the highest quality of care for veterans, the VA was also mandated to be involved in the education of health professionals by Title 38 U.S.C. Over the years, the VA has embraced this mandate with a vast clinical training portfolio, encompassing most specialties of medicine as well as many domains of psychology, nursing, pharmacy, and other health professions. In 2014, the VA system provided some training for each of over 41,000 (20 %) physician residents and almost 23,000 (35 %) medical students (Congressional Research Service 2016). Approximately two-thirds of all physicians have received at least some training in the VA system (Office of the Administrative Assistant to the Secretary of the Army 2016). The VA pays "direct costs" for resident stipends and fringe benefits and "indirect costs" including program overhead and higher costs of care in teaching hospitals. In fiscal year 2015, the VA budget for graduate medical education was about $1.5 billion (Congressional Research Service 2016). Thus, not only is the VA now the biggest integrated delivery system of healthcare in the United States, but it is also "the Nation's largest integrated provider of health care education and training for physician residents and other health care trainees" (Department of Veterans Affairs 2014) (Fig. 5.1).

The current importance and complexity of GME in the VA system were highlighted in "The Report of the Blue Ribbon Panel on VA-Medical School Affiliations: Transforming a Historic Partnership for the 21st Century." A number of recommendations propound the continuation and even strengthening and expanding of GME in the VA. Training is viewed as vital to "prepare an appropriately skilled healthcare workforce."

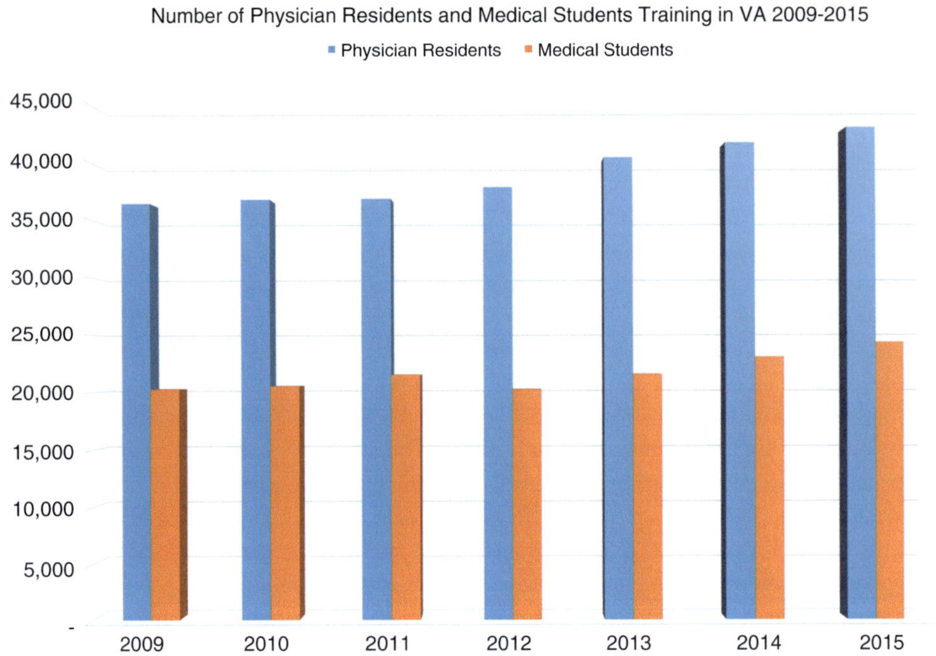

Fig. 5.1 Statistics: Health Professions Trainees, Veterans Health Administration (Office of the Administrative Assistant to the Secretary of the Army 2015)

The panel made a call for special efforts with regard to mental health, along with diversity and cultural sensitivity, geriatric care, polytrauma, and rural health. They also urged "design and testing of innovative new education models with the potential to transform the content and process of medical education." One example of this would be creative ways to promote interprofessional training, between physicians and non-physicians. All of this is not without accountability. The report recommends an inventory of VA educational assets, fiscal analysis, management of indirect cost, and productivity measures. In sum, the panel's report gives GME education in the VA system enthusiastic support into the twenty-first century, at or above current levels of support.

The Veterans Affairs Learning Environment in Psychiatry Graduate Medical Education

Rotations for residents at VA medical centers make a unique and uniquely important contribution to psychiatry graduate medical education. In addition to the broad spectrum of psychiatric disorders, the veteran population allows for an educational focus on post-traumatic stress disorder (both combat- and sexual assault-related), addiction, traumatic brain injury and polytrauma, spinal cord injury, severe mental illness, suicide (Pheister et al. 2014), and more. Of note, the VA has created multisite centers with independent funding streams to concentrate on priority disorders, like the War Related Illness and Injury Study Center, National Center for PTSD, and the Mental Illness Research Education Clinical Centers. These centers often include rigorous and intensively resourced training components. Looking to future specialization of training, a large percentage of the veterans seeking care engaged in military service during the Vietnam War, and this population is aging. The VA has been anticipating an increasing need for geriatric psychiatry, and the VA system has been able to allocate funds to meet expanding geriatric needs and training, along with Centers for Excellence in geriatrics and Parkinson's disease. Commitment to the field of geriatric psychiatry is especially important since many university hospitals have struggled in this arena because of limited funding for geriatric services.

VA rotations offer a particular healthcare culture that is valuable for trainees to experience, in its own right and in contrast to the cultures in other systems. A multidisciplinary team approach is especially emphasized on psychiatric inpatient units in the VA, including the collaboration between clinical psychologists and psychiatrists (Scaturo and Huszonek 2009). This is partly because the VA has invested in strong training programs for clinical psychologists, like predoctorate internships and postdoctoral fellows. In fact, approximately one-half of clinical psychologists in the United States have had some education in a VA (Office of the Administrative Assistant to the Secretary of the Army 2016).

Also influencing the trainees is the military culture of service, inherent to the VA and embodied by the sacrifices and disabilities of the patients. Now, with veterans returning from the more recent conflicts (e.g., Operation Enduring Freedom, Operation Iraqi Freedom, Operation New Dawn), the stories of sacrifice have even more immediacy and realism for medical students and residents, who are often similar in age and readily empathize. This identification and empathic connection engage the trainees in playing their own authentic role in "caring for those who served." This experience, in turn, dovetails with the long tradition of VA rotations having fewer layers of trainees and providers than university hospitals, thus allowing trainees to feel more of the responsibility of being on the frontline of care. Thus, there is a special opportunity for teachers and clinical supervisors at the VA to align with and strengthen instruction and modeling of the ACGME competency of professionalism. No less important is the VA's culture for serving the most vulnerable populations and underserved among veterans, including a Homeless Initiative.

An unmistakable feature of the VA culture is its massive size. This size may equate to bureaucratic frustrations, but it also provides opportunities, including educational ones, to design a high-quality system of care of unusual scale. The VA has focused on this with Centers of Excellence in Research, Quality, and Patient Safety. Going forward, teaching residents about different healthcare delivery systems will be crucial for assembling the best attributes of each into the healthcare of the future. A strength for education in particular is the system of care at the VA with relative continuity, from inpatient to outpatient treatment and across all intensity levels of care, from community outreach teams to psychiatric inpatient units. The VA is a "classroom laboratory" for learning the real-life challenges of providing psychiatric care of high quality and value. For example, the National Center for PTSD in the VA endorsed prolonged exposure as an evidence-based treatment for PTSD. This endorsement has allowed this treatment to be incorporated into some psychiatry residencies as part of the training in cognitive behavioral treatments. Subsequently, the VA disseminated this treatment across the VA system. This endorsement thus afforded a unique opportunity to learn about how to disseminate and scale a treatment protocol with high fidelity in a massive healthcare system. Residents ideally will be trained to take on these types of system-based practice challenges.

While research in the VA is not the subject of this chapter, the interface of research and education deserves quick mention. The VA is a major contributor to academic research, and research generally enhances clinical care and education in the VA by infusing a scholarly standard of basing treatment on evidence and awareness of the latest therapeutics. And, research is specifically important to GME training with regard to research methodologies, design, data analysis, and basic and clinical studies. Even if a resident does not plan a career including research, participation in scholarly activities is an ACGME requirement for all residents. The VA is emerging as an excellent place for residents to do scholarly work, for instance, in quality improvement and patient safety, and to pursue treatment services research. For residents who are considering academia, they may want to continue on after residency in one of the VA post-doctorate research fellowships. Subsequently, a VA career path in academia has the benefit of career development awards and research grants funded by the VA, in addition to National Institutes of Health (NIH) and other non-VA grant monies.

Integration and Its Challenge

The first affiliation agreements between the VA and medical schools were in 1946, under Policy Memorandum No. 2 (Department of Veterans Affairs 1946). By 2014–2015, 135 allopathic medical schools were affiliated with VA medical facilities—successful and sustained collaboration between the VA and academic psychiatry has been part of this affiliation (Lehrmann and Roberts 2009). The integration of GME into a VA healthcare is complex because medical schools and VA medical centers are different types of organizations and operate in divergent ways (Mohl et al. 2009). The VA is the second largest federal entity represented in the President's Cabinet since 1989 and accountable to Congress and the public. An academic medical school may be public or private, may be affiliated with a university or not, and may have many different leadership structures. Decision-making processes within the VA and within a medical school may differ radically, and yet a constructive relationship involving mutualism and shared benefit is important to VA-medical school collaborations. Faculty appointments illustrate some of the challenges faced across the VA and medical school systems. Even though about 70 % of VA staff clinicians hold appointments in medical schools (Congressional Research Service 2016), VA faculty members are often employees of the VA, unlike the non-VA faculty members who are usually employed by the medical school or its hospital. The VA and medical school have different salary structures, benefits, and bonuses, which may or may not be similar. Employment expectations may also differ, like the length of the workweek. VA employment is usually calculated on a 40-hour workweek, while medical school employees may assume longer hours. Confusion may occur when referring to percentage-time effort since the absolute number of hours involved, of course, depends on the length of a workweek. Furthermore, the VA refers to a one-eighth system for part-time efforts, with eight-eighths representing full-time work. All these differences make it difficult to fairly institute guidelines or policies, which might incentivize teaching across the whole faculty, e.g., a bonus for educational work might be possible in one organization but not in another.

The relationship between the VA hospital and the medical school thus often requires coordination by a "Dean's Committee" consisting of the medical school dean, relevant departmental chairs, and VA leaders. The Dean's Committee often reviews issues, such as the number of resident stipends, faculty staffing considerations, and the appropriateness of program expansion.

Balancing imperatives of the VA, the needs of the medical school and its trainees, and the demands of relevant accrediting bodies can be challenging. The VA allocates funding that primarily goes toward paying stipends for residents' salary and benefits associated with training at VA facilities. These funds are substantial and essential to the fiscal health of many GME programs. Educational considerations are also important and intersect with pragmatic resource issues. In psychiatry residencies, for instance, the available number of inpatient versus outpatient resident slots must be reconciled with the VA's patient flow, staffing, and space requirements. And though the number of women who are veterans is increasing, VA rotations will typically have a much higher percentage of male patients, which shapes the training experience. Similarly, a VA psychiatric consult/liaison service may be an excellent teaching site, but the diagnoses are going to have a disproportionate number of some diagnoses (e.g., traumatic brain injury, spinal cord injury). Thus, ongoing communication and sometimes negotiation are important between the VA and the medical school at every level—top leadership as well as program directors and faculty overseeing residents on their individual rotations.

Not uncommonly, the VA is geographically separated from the medical school, and this circumstance can bring about many challenges—which may be overcome through intentional efforts by leaders at the VA and the medical school. For example, the residency training director may not have a VA appointment, and the VA may be considered an affiliated site. Barriers to communication and lack of attunement across the clinical training sites may result in the VA rotation(s) seeming to be relatively disconnected from the program—and even perceived as less valued. For instance, the perception may develop that, when the residency is short a resident due to an unexpected leave, the VA rotation will be more likely than the university hospital rotation to be asked to bear the shortfall in staffing or that, in general, VA rotations are less likely to be filled to capacity or to be required. Worse yet is a situation in which residents begin to devalue the VA rotation in their education. Such perceptions and hard realities may be prevented by fortifying channels of communication and representation between the VA rotation educators/administrators and the training director with regularly scheduled feedback sessions. The establishment of a local, on-site education committee is one positive strategy for overcoming challenges that arise across training sites, including the VA.

Recruitment of high-quality new physicians to the VA is advantaged by having VA GME-partnered programs, since residents often apply after their training and many physicians are looking for positions with opportunities to teach. In psychiatry, 76 % of VA trainees say they would be willing to work in a VA after they graduate, and 94 % of clinical psychologists say the same (Office of the Administrative Assistant to the Secretary of the Army 2015). The recruitment of faculty members as VA employees occurs through the human resource department of the VA and must follow VA regulations, with regard to hiring protocols like posting of jobs and salary negotiations. Of note, only some VA clinicians teach residents and have faculty appointments, and VA salaries and benefits may not differ depending on inclusion or exclusion of teaching duties. In other words, extra pay or time protected from clinical duties is not generally provided for teaching done in addition to the regular clinical duties carried out by all VA physicians. Some may argue that the trainees assist (e.g., progress note writing) the faculty member who teaches and this saves him or her time in exchange for teaching effort, but this is not always the case or quantifiable. While it may be true that teaching in the medical school settings also does not garner extra pay, at least all physician faculty members in the medical school generally teach and there is not the perception of teaching and nonteaching positions being paid similarly. Furthermore, some non-VA teaching settings do provide bonuses or other systems to incentivize teaching that the VA does not offer. One must be sensitive to these employment perceptions with regard to recruitment and maintenance of a teaching faculty in a VA.

One should note that not all VA faculty members are, strictly speaking, VA employees. Examples of exceptions are faculty members who work at the VA but who are paid through the medical school and are under medical school employment. In these cases, the VA reimburses the medical school for the faculty member's time during the week at the VA, which might be a part-time or even full-time effort. Faculty members who work for the medical school receive salary and benefits under a different system and have other expectations with regard to space and time for research activities. Adding these faculty members to the mix results in the existence of at least three types of VA physicians working side by side: those who teach and are VA employees, those who teach and are medical school employees, and those who do not teach and are VA employees. This is generally not a problem, but it does complicate the management of the clinical learning environment and the associated faculty members. Leaders should be sensitive to possible friction between academic and nonacademic physician staff and between faculty physicians who are employed by the VA and employed by the medical school.

Veterans Affairs and Graduate Medical Education in the Future

For the foreseeable future, the VA system will continue to play an important and unique role in graduate medical education in this country, and it has a central role in psychiatry residency training. This role may be reinforced if Medicare and other sources of funding for physician training are reduced, as has been threatened. For the relationship between the VA and medical schools to continue to flourish, benefits need to be perceived by both from education and research at VA medical centers. This has certainly been the case since World War II and throughout the major conflicts of recent decades.

With inevitable changes in the economics of medicine, academic departments of psychiatry will be called upon to strengthen their partnerships and to sustain and deepen their relationships with VA affiliates. Departments will need to stay in close communication with VA leadership and anticipate changing challenges and opportunities. In psychiatry, for example, telehealth and other technological innovations in health delivery will be a growth area for education and research at the VA. The high percentage of veterans living in more rural areas make this a high priority and worth the investment in technology infrastructure for the VA, compared to other health systems with more localized populations. Similarly, the VA is well positioned to teach and research the integration of psychiatry into primary care, including the development of measurement-based care in psychiatry.

In sum, VA support and involvement have become vital to graduate medical education (GME) and will probably grow. Ongoing evidence of this is the Veterans Access, Choice, and Accountability Act of 2014 that adds 1,500 VA GME positions, particularly primary care and mental health, between 2015 and 2019. Psychiatric GME will continue to rely on the VA system for an important part of training. A practical reason for this continued reliance is that the VA finances a large number of psychiatric resident stipends and fringe benefits from "specific purpose funds" allocated centrally and greatly contributes to the psychiatric curricula on a local level at residency programs. It also provides unique strengths including educational and research preeminence in PTSD, substance use disorders, suicide prevention, traumatic brain injury and polytrauma, rural care, a comprehensive and seamless treatment system, and a culture of service and duty. And, the list is still expanding with the VA investing in integration of behavioral health and primary care, telepsychiatry, geriatric mental healthcare of Vietnam-era veterans, interprofessional training, and so on. The VA will be a noted leader in these and other realms in research and GME education.

Key Concepts

1. Military psychiatry residency training programs have the same requirements as their civilian counterparts but add significant elements of public psychiatry and preventive psychiatry to the curriculum in order to prepare active duty military physicians to serve in operational units with the Army, Navy, and Air Force.
2. There are several pathways to service as a military medical corps officer, and most involve financial assistance for medical school while incurring an active duty service obligation after residency training is complete.
3. The clinical learning environment in Department of Defense (DoD) and Department of Veterans Affairs (VA) hospitals is enriched by the organizations' culture of "serving those who serve" and a commitment to treat the mental health consequences of war.
4. The collaboration between the VA and Psychiatric Graduate Medical Education (GME) in the United States is mutually beneficial and will continue.
5. Psychiatric GME relies on the VA financially for a significant portion of resident stipends.
6. Veteran Affairs greatly benefits from the presence of psychiatric residents in VA facilities with regard to service and recruiting staff psychiatrists.
7. The VA offers unique training opportunities to psychiatry residencies, including but not

limited to experience with post-traumatic stress disorder (PTSD), substance use disorders, suicide prevention, traumatic brain injury and polytrauma, rural care and telehealth, the embedding of behavioral health into primary care, a comprehensive and seamless treatment system, and a culture of service and duty.

Disclaimer The views expressed in this chapter are those of the authors and do not reflect official policy or position of the Department of the Navy, the Department of the Army, the Department of Defense, the Department of Veterans Affairs, the US Government, or any of the institutional affiliations listed.

References

Bakaeen FG, Blaustein A, Kibbe MR (2014) Health care at the VA: recommendations for change. JAMA 312(5):481–482

Carter BS (1993) The military physician and conservation of force. Mil Med 158(6):374–375

Castro CA, Kintzle S (2014) Suicides in the military: the post-modern combat veteran and the Hemingway effect. Curr Psychiatry Rep 16(8):460

Cazares PT, Santiago P, Moulton D, Moran S, Tsai A (2015) Suicide response guidelines for residency trainees: a novel postvention response for the care and teaching of psychiatry residents who encounter suicide in their patients. Acad Psychiatry 39(4):393–397

Congressional Research Service (2016) The veterans health administration and medical education: a fact sheet, 2016. Available online: https://digital.library.unt.edu/ark:/67531/metadc824415/m2/1/high_res_d/R43587_2016Jan19.pdf. Accessed 14 Oct 2016

Cozza SJ, Chun RS, Polo JA (2005) Military families and children during operation Iraqi freedom. Psychiatry Q 76(4):371–378

De Lorenzo RA (2008) Accreditation status of U.S. military graduate medical education programs. Mil Med 173(7):635–640

Defense Manpower Data Center (2016) Active duty military strength by service, 2016. Available online: https://www.dmdc.osd.mil/appj/dwp/dwp_reports.jsp. Accessed 2016 Apr 11

Department of Defense (2015) About the department of defense (DoD). Available online: http://www.defense.gov/About-DoD. Accessed 20 May 2016

Department of Defense, United States, Joint Chiefs of Staff (2016) Department of Defense dictionary of military and associated terms joint publication 1–02

Department of Veterans Affairs (1946) Policy memorandum No. 2, Policy in association of veterans' hospitals with medical schools. Available online: https://www.va.gov/oaa/Archive/PolicyMemo2.pdf. Accessed 20 May 2016

Department of Veterans Affairs (2014) FY 2014–2020 Strategic plan. Available online: https://www.va.gov/op3/docs/StrategicPlanning/VA2014-2020strategicPlan.PDF. Accessed 14 Oct 2016

Diebold CJ, Leong SL, Zuchowski S, Gibson RT (2015) Pathways to a career in military psychiatry. Acad Psychiatry 39(4):402–409

Ferrell NJ, Melton B, Banu S, Coverdale J, Valdez MR (2014) The development and evaluation of a trauma curriculum for psychiatry residents. Acad Psychiatry 38(5):611–614

Gates R (2010) Functions of the department of defense and its major components. United States Department of Defense, Washington, DC

Gray SH (2004) A training psychotherapy elective for military psychiatry residents. J Am Acad Psychoanal Dyn Psychiatry 32(3):429–439

Groom RM, Carr RB, Leong SL, Hornbaker-Park MB (2015) Impact of an enduring war on two military psychiatry residency programs. Acad Psychiatry 39(4):354–359

Heaton LD, Anderson RS, Glass AJ, Bernucci RJ, United States Department of the Army, Office of the Surgeon General (1966) Neuropsychiatry in World War II. Office of the Surgeon General, Department of the Army, Washington, DC

Higgins MJ, Lacy TJ (2006) The role of psychiatry in U.S. Air Force primary care: research-based models for clinical consultation and education. Mil Med 171(11):1117–1122

Hill JV, Lange C, Bacon B (2007) Becoming a successful division psychiatrist: the sequel. Mil Med 172(4):364–369

Hoge CW, Castro CA, Messer SC, McGurk D, Cotting DI, Koffman RL (2004) Combat duty in Iraq and Afghanistan, mental health problems, and barriers to care. N Engl J Med 351(1):13–22

Hoge CW, Riviere LA, Wilk JE, Herrell RK, Weathers FW (2014) The prevalence of post-traumatic stress disorder (PTSD) in US combat soldiers: a head-to-head comparison of DSM-5 versus DSM-IV-TR symptom criteria with the PTSD checklist. Lancet Psychiatry 1(4):269–277

Holmes SL, Lee DJ, Charny G, Guthrie JA, Knight JG (2009) Military physician recruitment and retention: a survey of students at the uniformed services university of the health sciences. Mil Med 174(5):529–534

Jones F (1995) Psychiatric lessons of war. In: Zajtchuk R (ed) War psychiatry. Office of The Surgeon General, Washington, DC, pp 1–33

Kelsall HL, Wijesinghe MS, Creamer MC, McKenzie DP, Forbes AB, Page MJ, Sim MR (2015) Alcohol use and substance use disorders in Gulf War, Afghanistan, and Iraq War veterans compared with nondeployed military personnel. Epidemiol Rev 37:38–54

Kessler RC, Heeringa SG, Stein MB, Colpe LJ, Fullerton CS, Hwang I, Naifeh JA, Nock MK, Petukhova

M, Sampson NA, Schoenbaum M, Zaslavsky AM, Ursano RJ (2014) Thirty-day prevalence of *DSM-IV* mental disorders among non-deployed soldiers in the US army: results from the Army study to assess risk and resilience in Servicemembers (Army STARRS). JAMA Psychiat 71(5):504–513

Lee EA (2012) Complex contribution of combat-related post-traumatic stress disorder to veteran suicide: facing an increasing challenge. Perspect Psychiatr Care 48(2):108–115

Lehrmann JA, Roberts LW (2009) U.S. Department of Veterans Affairs and academic departments of psychiatry: a substantive, enduring, and promising collaboration. Acad Psychiatry 33(1):1–3

Lester P, Aralis H, Sinclair M, Kiff C, Lee KH, Mustillo S, Wadsworth SM (2016) The impact of deployment on parental, family and child adjustment in military families. Child Psychiatry Hum Dev 47:938

Lincoln A (1865) Second inaugural address. Inauguration. United States Capital, Washington, DC

Linker B (2016) The great war and modern health care. N Engl J Med 374(20):1907–1909

Marmar CR, Schlenger W, Henn-Haase C, Qian M, Purchia E, Li M, Corry N, Williams CS, Ho CL, Horesh D, Karstoft KI, Shalev A, Kulka RA (2015) Course of posttraumatic stress disorder 40 years after the Vietnam war: findings from the National Vietnam veterans longitudinal study. JAMA Psychiat 72(9):875–881

McCroskey A, Nieves JE (2016) Psychiatry clerkships in active duty military installations: a medical student experience. Acad Psychiatry 40(2):394–395

McFarlane AC (2009) Military deployment: the impact on children and family adjustment and the need for care. Curr Opin Psychiatry 22(4):369–373

McNulty PA (2005) Reported stressors and health care needs of active duty Navy personnel during three phases of deployment in support of the war in Iraq. Mil Med 170(6):530–535

Menninger WW (2004) Contributions of Dr. William C. Menninger to military psychiatry. Bull Menn Clin 68(4):277–296

Mercado R, Foynes MM, Carpenter SL, Iverson KM (2015) Sexual intimate partner violence as a form of MST: an initial investigation. Psychol Serv 12(4):348–356

Meyer E (2012) Developing military cultural competency in health care providers. Acad Med 87(1):3

Meyer EG, Writer BW, Brim W (2016) The importance of military cultural competence. Curr Psychiatry Rep 18(3):26

Mohl PC, Hendrickse W, Orsak C, Vermette H (2009) Veterans affairs and academic medical center affiliations: the North Texas experience. Acad Psychiatry 33(1):17–22

Munshi A, Woods N, Hodges B (2010) Psychiatry, war, and the learning needs of residents. Acad Psychiatry 34(3):208–210

Myers N (2008) Sailors take on nontraditional roles in Afghanistan, 2008. Available online: http://archive.defense.gov/news/newsarticle.aspx?id=50970. Accessed 20 May 2016

NCVAS (2016) Department of veterans affairs statistics at a glance, 2016. Available online: https://www.va.gov/vetdata/docs/Quickfacts/Homepage_slideshow_06_04_16.PDF. Accessed 14 Oct 2016

Office of the Administrative Assistant to the Secretary of the Army (2015) 2015 Statistics: health professions trainees, 2015. Available online: https://www.va.gov/oaa/docs/OAA_Statistics.pdf. Accessed 14 Oct 2016

Office of the Administrative Assistant to the Secretary of the Army (2016) Mission of the office of academic affiliations, 2016. Available online: http://www.va.gov/oaa/oaa_mission.asp. Accessed 14 Oct 2014

Park N (2011) Military children and families: strengths and challenges during peace and war. Am Psychol 66(1):65–72

Pheister M, Kangas G, Thompson C, Lehrmann J, Berger B, Kemp J (2014) Suicide prevention and postvention resources: what psychiatry residencies can learn from the veteran's administration experience. Acad Psychiatry 38(5):600–604

Ritchie C, White R (1993) Becoming a successful division psychiatrist: guidelines for preparation and duties of the assignment. Mil Med 158(10):644–648

Roberts LW (2015) Sacrifice and service, protectors and teachers: the role of military and veteran patients in training early-career psychiatrists. Acad Psychiatry 39(4):349–350

Scaturo DJ, Huszonek JJ (2009) Collaborative academic training of psychiatrists and psychologists in VA and medical school settings. Acad Psychiatry 33(1):4–12

Shinseki E (2014) Department of veterans affairs, FY 2014–2020 Strategic Plan, 2014. Available online: http://www.va.gov/op3/docs/StrategicPlanning/VA2014-2020strategicPlan.PDF. Accessed 14 Oct 2016

Stein MB, Kessler RC, Heeringa SG, Jain S, Campbell-Sills L, Colpe LJ, Fullerton CS, Nock MK, Sampson NA, Schoenbaum M, Sun X, Thomas ML, Ursano RJ (2015) Prospective longitudinal evaluation of the effect of deployment-acquired traumatic brain injury on posttraumatic stress and related disorders: results from the army study to assess risk and resilience in servicemembers (Army STARRS). Am J Psychiatry 172(11):1101–1111

Taylor CM, Ross ME, Wood JN, Griffis HM, Harb GC, Mi L, Song L, Strane D, Lynch KG, Rubin DM (2016) Differential child maltreatment risk across deployment periods of US Army soldiers. Am J Public Health 106(1):153–158

Toblin RL, Riviere LA, Thomas JL, Adler AB, Kok B, Hoge CW (2012) Grief and physical health outcomes in U.S. soldiers returning from combat. J Affect Disord 136(3):469–475

United States Census Bureau (2015) How do we know? A snapshot of our nation's veterans. Available online: http://www.census.gov/library/infographics/veterans.html. Accessed 14 Oct 2016

Ursano RJ, Holloway HC, Jones DR, Rodriguez AR, Belenky GL (1989) Psychiatric care in the military community: family and military stressors. Hosp Community Psychiatry 40(12):1284–1289

Warner CH, Bobo WV, Flynn J (2005) Early career professional development issues for military academic psychiatrists. Acad Psychiatry 29(5):437–442

Warner CH, Appenzeller GN, Barry MJ, Morton A, Grieger T (2007) The evolving role of the division psychiatrist. Mil Med 172(9):918–924

Welton RS, Hamaoka DA, Broderick PJ, Schillerstrom JE (2015) The best of both worlds: psychiatry training at combined civilian-military programs. Acad Psychiatry 39(4):360–364

West JC, Woodson JT, Benedek DM (2015) Large-scale simulation for teaching combat and operational stress control: operation bushmaster. Acad Psychiatry 39(4):398–401

Wilk JE, Herrell RK, Wynn GH, Riviere LA, Hoge CW (2012) Mild traumatic brain injury (concussion), posttraumatic stress disorder, and depression in U.S. soldiers involved in combat deployments: association with postdeployment symptoms. Psychosom Med 74(3):249–257

Wise MG (1987) The past, present, and future of psychiatric training in the U.S. armed services. Mil Med 152(11):550–553

Ethical Considerations of the Practice of Psychiatry in the Military

6

Brett J. Schneider and John C. Bradley

Introduction: Dual Agency of Military Physicians

Service as a military psychiatrist requires an appreciation of—and adherence to—strict ethical principles. Military medical officers are bound by the ethical codes of both the profession of medicine and profession of the military. These professional ethics may frequently come into conflict and must be reconciled in daily practice. A military psychiatrist's acceptance of the role of "dual agent" is necessary in order to understand the duties and responsibilities, including fiduciary and legal responsibilities, associated with their dual roles, and to serve the interests of the patient as well as those of the military service to the best of one's ability.

Military physicians are unique in that they are members of two professions. They are medical professionals who are required to adhere to the ethical guidelines for medicine and their specific specialty, and they are military officers who must adhere to the regulations, ethical requirements, and command structure within the military. As such, situations may arise in which adherence to both requirements may be in conflict. This tension of adhering to two sets of guidelines, which can at times be at odds, is usually referred to as "dual agency." Dual or mixed agency refers to the conflicts and potential unethical breaches of the fiduciary relationship between a provider of services and a consumer of those services. Dual agency is not unique to medicine and, in fact, can exist in any profession where a fiduciary relationship exists—including law, for example. This chapter addresses the issue of dual agency by discussing how this potential tension may be similar to and different from other settings where psychiatrists practice.

Section 8 of the American Psychiatric Association's (APA) 2013 "The Principles of Medical Ethics with Annotations Especially Applicable to Psychiatry" is especially relevant to this chapter's discussion of dual agency:

> **Section 8** A physician shall, while caring for a patient, regard responsibility to the patient as paramount.

1. Psychiatrists' relationships with companies, organizations, the community, or larger society can affect their interactions with patients.
2. When the psychiatrist's outside relationships conflict with the clinical needs of the patient, the psychiatrist must always consider the impact of such relationships and strive to resolve conflicts in a manner that the psychiatrist believes is likely to be beneficial to the patient.

B.J. Schneider (✉)
Uniformed Services University of the Health Sciences, Bethesda, MD, USA
e-mail: brett.schneider@usuhs.edu

J.C. Bradley
Harvard Medical School, Boston, MA, USA

Mental Health Service (116-a), VA Boston Health Care System, Boston, MA 02130, USA
e-mail: john.bradley7@va.gov

L.W. Roberts, C.H. Warner (eds.), *Military and Veteran Mental Health*,
https://doi.org/10.1007/978-1-4939-7438-2_6

3. When significant relationships exist that may conflict with patients' clinical needs, it is especially important to inform the patient or decision-maker about these relationships and potential conflicts with clinical needs.
4. In informing a patient of treatment options, the psychiatrist should assist the patient in identifying relevant options that promote an informed treatment decision, including those that are not available from the psychiatrist or from the organization with which the psychiatrist is affiliated. (American Psychiatric Association 2013)

In order to address the inherent dual agency issues described in Section 8, this chapter will discuss the ethical principles and the frameworks for applying them and will relate these principles and frameworks to other areas of potential conflict as illustrated in several case studies from military contexts. This chapter also demonstrates how the guidelines of Section 8 provide a framework of informed consent and transparency that allows for these tensions to be dealt with honestly and for the candid identification of potential ethical conflicts. The practices of transparency and informed consent allow the clinician to honor the patient's autonomy by informing them of potential conflicts, ethical or otherwise, which may arise and which may come into conflict with any other ethical principles. The principles of autonomy and beneficence are the most likely ethical principles to be potentially compromised by a system that requires dual agency in its routine functioning.

Balancing Patient Safety, Patient Autonomy, and Duty to Others

In the military context, a psychiatrist not only has a fiduciary responsibility to the patient but also has a responsibility to military commanders to ensure the readiness of the service member for military duty, to maximize the availability of personnel for the mission, and to detect cases of malingering. These "duties to others" often require a treating psychiatrist to perform a balancing act to maintain the most ethically tenable position.

Case Study 1

While stationed on a Forward Operating Base in Iraq, Army Sergeant John Smith (pseudonym) becomes suicidal due to anxiety, repeated trauma, loss of comrades-in-arms in battle, and a sense of survivor guilt. He reports these thoughts to a fellow soldier. They both know there is a combat stress control (CSC) unit stationed nearby and are able to arrange to have Sergeant Smith evaluated for his suicidal thoughts and the many symptoms he is now reporting. The behavioral health provider has many clinical decisions to make in determining the appropriate management, and all of these clinical decisions must occur in consideration of the ethical principles that guide medical care and military operations.

In the above case study, how would the considerations be similar or different if Sergeant Smith were simply Mr. Smith and if the same set of circumstances were present in a civilian setting, in which Mr. Smith might have been witness to a mass casualty by an active shooter? This case study presents a number of ethical dilemmas over and above those of a civilian case due to the dual agency of the military psychiatrist.

In any scenario—whether in a civilian or military context—the first determination both clinically and ethically is to maintain the suicidal patient's safety. This means that in any scenario, if the suicidality is such that the patient has intent and plan, and there are active psychiatric symptoms that increase the possibility of the patient acting in an impulsive manner, the clinical and ethical "right" decision is to get the patient to a level of care where his safety can be maintained and the appropriate treatment can be provided. In a combat zone, however, the availability of such a location is less certain than in most similar civilian situations. For example, there may be a military hospital with the capability of managing acute suicidality just like a stateside hospital, but referral would require evacuating the patient to this location over dangerous terrain through a combat zone. Nevertheless, the clinical *and* ethical responsibility, under the ethical principle of beneficence, is to ensure the patient's safety. There also may be scenarios where the capability to hospitalize does not exist in the theater of operations, and this situation would require evacuation of this patient to a military hospital in Europe or the United States.

When inpatient psychiatric hospital level of care does not exist, a military psychiatrist might need to put a patient under supervision by members of their own unit. In practice, this so-called "unit watch" presents several ethical dilemmas related to safety and confidentiality. This culturally accepted practice gradually changed over time as clinicians considered how ethical principles aligned with standards of care (Payne et al. 2008). Specifically, the ethical principle of nonmaleficence gradually moved the dial on this practice as the risk of suicide in service members rose statistically during the period of wartime. Prior to the ongoing operations starting in 2003, the military had a suicide rate half of that in civilian practice (Department of Veterans Affairs and Department of Defense 2013). As the suicide risk was relatively low, practitioners felt that patients could be safely managed in a nonclinical setting and "unit watch" seemed an appropriate risk management strategy. The ethical principle of beneficence guided this practice, as many suicidal crises were the result of interpersonal issues that could be fixed at the unit level. Therefore, it was felt that avoiding a psychiatric hospitalization to impact a transient situation was in the patient's best interest.

Another distinction between civilian and military practice is that managing the access to lethal means, which is part of the standard of care for managing the suicidal patient, has a completely different set of considerations for the hypothetical patient Sergeant John Smith in a combat zone. All military personnel are armed and have ready access to lethal means. Even physicians are armed in order to provide protection to themselves and their patients if needed. Service members who have their access to weapons restricted for their safety are easily spotted by others and become identified as mental health patients. This necessary safety intervention causes a de facto breach of confidentiality by publicly labeling the soldier as a patient at risk and in need of additional supervision. The potential stigmatization creates additional concerns about the negative consequences of help-seeking behavior and may have the unintended public health consequence of creating a barrier to care for others in need (Weisfeld et al. 2008).

One could also ask the practical question of whether it is ethical to disarm someone in a combat zone and deprive them of their right to protect themselves from attack. How should one manage the clinical and ethical balancing act of keeping the patient safe—often a very paternalistic intervention—and allowing the patient to maintain autonomy and avoid stigma? Ensuring the patient's safety is the foremost concern, but one may have to compromise by allowing the patient to keep their weapon and "disabling" it in some way.

In situations such as this one, the nuances involved in clinical practice and ethics in a military setting may be different from a similar situation in a civilian or even a stateside military setting. Here, the two ethical principles of beneficence and autonomy—which appear simpler to quantify in "normal" practice—become more difficult to parse due to changes in the circumstances of the situation. In effect, this example demonstrates that the applicability of ethical concepts is, in reality, a dynamic rather than static process.

To continue the same case study with a slightly different scenario, this time Sergeant Smith and his civilian counterpart Mr. Smith present with suicidality, but now, after clinical evaluation, the suicidality does not require hospitalization. The behavioral health provider learns that the active symptoms, especially the sense of loss and the repeated trauma, are the precipitators of the suicidality, and the risk of repeated exposure is anticipated to be a perpetuating factor for the suicidality.

In the civilian scenario with Mr. Smith, the trauma that was the precipitator is not a perpetuating factor because presumably he will not be at high risk to encounter another situation in the foreseeable future in which an active shooter harms people he knows. In the military situation, however, Sergeant Smith will very likely be subject to traumatic exposures again. This creates a dilemma for the military clinician that presumably does not exist for the civilian clinician. Is it ethical to return Sergeant Smith to his unit and subject him to possible re-traumatization? As is often the case in determining an ethical dilemma, the answer may be "it depends." For example, a military psychiatrist may choose to have Sergeant Smith taken off of combat duty for a limited time, receive treatment, and see if Sergeant Smith's symptoms and suicidality stabilize. This would be in line with a more paternalistic view aligned with the ethical principle of beneficence over autonomy.

Occasionally, the service member will not want to be placed on limited duty, and then the clinician needs to determine what is in the patient's *and* the unit's best interest. The clinician must be sure that the patient can function in his or her duties and not put themselves and others at risk due to the level of symptomatology demonstrated. The situation becomes more complex when taking into account the concept of the military psychiatrist's duty to others, which must be considered for a psychiatrist who is also a dual agent. A civilian psychiatrist treating Mr. Smith may allow for more patient autonomy if Mr. Smith were demanding to go back to work, because presumably, he would not be putting other people at risk in his job. If there were a risk to others, perhaps the civilian psychiatrist would err on the side of being more paternalistic.

There may sometimes be a situation in which, ethically speaking, the better choice may be to override patient autonomy and act in the best interest of the larger group (Weisfeld et al. 2008). This is a utilitarian ethical argument, which is a type of ethical consideration pertinent to providers who are dual agents and that may not often apply to clinicians who do not frequently deal with dual agency situations. One example in which this utilitarian argument pertains to civilian practice is the "duty to warn" someone whom a patient has identified they would want to harm (Tobriner 1976).

To add in another comparative factor to the same general case study, the patients—now Mr. Smith, Sergeant John Smith, and Police Officer Smith—have taken some time off to stabilize and now wish to return to work. They are no longer suicidal and no longer have active symptoms. In Mr. Smith's case, there is no indication that his job will re-traumatize him. However, for both the police officer and the service member, the job very well might—and for the service member, the timeline for this potential re-traumatization is likely to be much shorter than it would be for the police officer patient. Is it ethical to return either of them to their duties, knowing that there is a likelihood that the factors that precipitated their initial clinical scenario are potentially going to be reexperienced and thus may re-traumatize the patients?

This chapter explores how, in such difficult scenarios, the utility of informed consent and transparency is of the utmost importance when engaging patients in an ethically sound manner. Being transparent with service member patients about the potential risks and benefits of both returning to duty and not returning to duty invites an honest discussion.

Most people who serve in the military prefer to remain with their units, citing their sense of being a valued member of the team, and their desire to not let their comrades down, as more important than the risk of being re-traumatized. Additionally, they have the sense that they would be leaving their comrades to be traumatized, while they themselves escape further exposure. Other patients may realize their limits and not have the motivation to remain on duty, despite knowing that there are also risks to not remaining. Many military psychiatrists have had the experience of either removing people in the latter category from the combat zone or, at a minimum, working with their commands to find them a job in the combat zone that minimizes the risk of repeated exposure. National Guard units often have additional flexibility to keep a service member in their guard unit, as the National Guard includes duties such as stateside disaster assistance that the active component of the military does not include. Once an active military service member is removed from a combat zone for a psychiatric disability, they are more frequently than not separated from the military either by a medical retirement or by an administrative separation.

Confidentiality and Dual Agency

The American Psychiatric Association's (APA) 2013 "Principles of Medical Ethics with Annotations" make the following comment regarding a psychiatrist's commitment to confidentiality and transparency:

> The psychiatrist should diligently guard against exploiting information furnished by the patient and should not use the unique position of power afforded him/her by the psychotherapeutic situation to influence the patient in any way not directly relevant to the treatment goals. (American Psychiatric Association 2013)

There are instances in which a military psychiatrist may be required by law or regulation to report information to military commanders for reasons other than the furtherance of treatment goals (Department of Defense 2011). These communications and privacy breaches take several forms and include, for example, a "fitness for duty" determination, which leads to a decision of whether to medically retire a service member. It is not always obvious that sharing this information is directly relevant to treatment goals. Some areas of civilian psychiatric practice also experience tension when dealing with this principle, specifically in the practice of forensic psychiatry and in child and adolescent psychiatry. In both of these psychiatric subspecialties, information obtained from a patient could be used for purposes other than those directly relevant to treatment goals. Forensic psychiatrists solve this conundrum by making it explicit "up-front" that when they conduct evaluations they are not engaging in treatment. They do so by providing a statement of non-confidentiality, warning the patient that they are not collecting information to treat the patient's psychiatric problem, but rather are gathering information to answer a third party's specific questions about this subject's psychiatric issues. This is an example of using transparency to inform the patient that the ethical principle of beneficence is being potentially "transgressed." This allows the patient more autonomy to decide what information they may decide to share.

A child and adolescent psychiatrist must balance the treatment goals of the patient with the parent's right to know information about their child. Again, in these situations, being transparent and "up-front" about what information will and will not be shared is key to managing the boundaries of confidentiality. Similarly, psychiatrists who work in correctional facilities, and psychiatrists who work for law enforcement or other government agencies like the Department of State, the CIA, or other elements of national security, encounter such tensions with an espoused principle. Civilian psychiatrists in these settings are contractually bound to the institution for which they work, much as are military psychiatrists.

This section will examine how military psychiatrists can also manage these conundrums in the context of the APA's 2013 "Principles of Medical Ethics with Annotations" as they relate to confidentiality, listed as follows:

> Psychiatric records, including even the identification of a person as a patient, must be protected with extreme care. Confidentiality is essential to psychiatric treatment. This is based in part on the special nature of psychiatric therapy as well as on the traditional ethical relationship between physician and patient. Because of the sensitive and private nature of the information with which the psychiatrist deals, he or she must be circumspect in the information that he or she chooses to disclose to others about a patient. The welfare of the patient must be a continuing consideration. (American Psychiatric Association 2013)

This ethical requirement of confidentiality may seem daunting for the military psychiatrist, as there are requirements to report certain information to a patient's commander and/or to decide if a service member continues to meet the military's requirements for employment in specific positions, such as maintaining a security clearance or working in sensitive classified positions or such as being on a presidential detail or working in an environment that involves strategic warfare assets like the country's nuclear missile arsenal. Civilian psychiatrists working for other federal agencies, such as the State Department, the CIA, or other law enforcement agencies, may also encounter tensions with fully adhering to this guideline in all instances.

The APA expands on this tension inherent to the principle of confidentiality in dual agency roles:

> A psychiatrist may release confidential information only with the authorization of the patient or under proper legal compulsion. The continuing duty of the psychiatrist to protect the patient includes fully apprising him/her of the connotations of waiving the privilege of privacy. This may become an issue when the patient is being investigated by a government agency, is applying for a position, or is involved in legal action. The same principles apply to the release of information concerning treatment to medical departments of government agencies, business organizations, labor unions, and insurance companies. (American Psychiatric Association 2013)

Psychiatrists are often asked to examine individuals for security purposes, to determine suitability for various jobs, and to determine legal competence. The psychiatrist must fully describe the nature, purpose, and lack of confidentiality of the examination to the examinee at the beginning of the examination (American Psychiatric Association 2013).

The key to managing the dual agency issue in any organization, including the military, is to aspire to always obtain patient authorization and also to know the proper "legal compulsion," which in the case of the military may involve military policies or regulations set forth to inform the psychiatrist how to manage the tension. In these instances, maintaining transparency about the requirements, and how a patient's information may be used, is paramount to maintaining one's obligation to the patient in as faithful manner as possible.

According to the Department of Defense, confidential information may be revealed in specific circumstances: "When, in the clinical judgment of the treating psychiatrist, the risk of danger is deemed to be significant, the psychiatrist may reveal confidential information disclosed by the patient" (Department of Defense 2011). This statement, although agreed upon in both civilian and military settings, potentially has more "at stake" when performed in a military setting, as the outcome may have implications for the ability of the service member to maintain their position. While this principle is supported and agreed upon in all settings, the decision may appear to be more difficult for the military psychiatrist.

The APA upholds the importance of a stable working relationship between a patient and physician and states that physicians, in some instances, may decide to refuse service to patients:

> Physicians generally agree that the doctor-patient relationship is such a vital factor in effective treatment of the patient that preservation of optimal conditions for development of a sound working relationship between a doctor and his or her patient should take precedence over all other considerations. An ethical psychiatrist may refuse to provide psychiatric treatment to a person who, in the psychiatrist's opinion, cannot be diagnosed as having a mental illness amenable to psychiatric treatment. (American Psychiatric Association 2013)

With regard to this principle, military psychiatrists may find themselves in settings where there are no other options for care if they are deployed to a remote environment. Service members are not allowed to be referred out of the military health system, and, as such, military providers are at times unable to recuse themselves from providing care. Additionally, sometimes commanders will put pressure on the provider to "fix" situations where these issues may be in play, thereby putting pressure on the psychiatrist to engage in care they may not believe to be in adherence with this principle.

On occasion, psychiatrists are asked for an opinion about an individual who is in the light of public attention or who has disclosed information about himself/herself through public media. In such circumstances, a psychiatrist may share with the public his or her expertise about psychiatric issues in general. However, it is unethical for a psychiatrist to offer a professional opinion unless he or she has conducted an examination and has been granted proper authorization for such a statement (American Psychiatric Association 1973). This ethical guideline has become known as the "Goldwater Rule," as it pertains to the commentary of the fitness of Senator Barry Goldwater as a political candidate for office. The Goldwater Rule is operationalized frequently in the military when psychiatrists are in the role of a command consultant. Military psychiatrists must always be vigilant of the boundaries espoused in this principle when performing in these roles.

The APA makes the following annotation to the principle regarding the psychiatrist's role in "contributing to the improvement of the community":

> The psychiatrist may permit his or her certification to be used for the involuntary treatment of any person only following his or her personal examination of that person. To do so, he or she must find that the person, because of mental illness, cannot form a judgment as to what is in his/her own best interests and that, without such treatment, substantial impairment is likely to occur to the person or others. (American Psychiatric Association 2013)

A set of circumstances that can be compared and contrasted between military and civilian psychiatric practice is the management of the patient who may be a danger to themselves or others. All states have some version of a law that allows for citizens to be temporarily detained and evaluated if they are considered to be at risk to harm themselves or others and then to be held against their will if they remain a danger. The military has a similar process in place. The initial evaluation piece of this process is accomplished through the command-directed mental health evaluation (Department of Defense 1998). This process has been revised on occasion, and, in its most current form, the process has become more streamlined to allow commanders and supervisors to more easily refer service members for whose safety or ability to function they are concerned. Previously, the process was divided into emergency and routine processes. The emergency process required that the supervisor feel the safety concern was imminent and encouraged a consultation with a behavioral health provider. The routine process required written notification to the service member; provided them 72 h to contact an attorney, the inspector general, or a chaplain; and required consultation with a behavioral health provider who had to concur that this was a reasonable request (Lauretano 1998). In light of the increasing problems with suicides in the military during the period from 2005 to 2014, commanders felt that this was too restrictive; the due process requirements for the routine process were thus done away with, and first-line supervisors were also allowed to refer, no longer just the commander. The reason for the initial set of due process requirements was that these policies (and the policy known as the Boxer amendment, which directs the process for holding service members against their will for inpatient psychiatric treatment) grew out of the Whistleblower Protection Act (Boxer 1988). At the time of their creation, it was believed that commanders at times inappropriately utilized mental health referrals as forced hospitalizations in order to punish service members, thus going beyond reasonable command authority in those situations. More recently, however, the reason for a more permissive revision is due to the fact that leaders have felt they were hampered in obtaining care for their service members. This cultural shift came about as a result of senior military leadership making commanders evaluate every suicide and suicide attempt for lessons learned and breakdowns in processes. Some commanders were relieved from duty or chastised if it was believed that they were negligent in facilitating care for service members.

The other end of this process, in which clinicians can actually hold a service member against their will, will now be discussed. The Department of Defense Whistleblower Protection Act, frequently referred to as the Boxer Act for its author, came into existence in 1988. Amendments in 1990 and 1992 specifically addressed the command-directed mental health evaluations already discussed. The Department of Defense Directive that governs command-directed mental health evaluations, and the current process for involuntary hospitalization as written in the directive, is provided in Appendix 1. This discussion serves as a reminder that in real-world situations, the application and balancing of ethical principles often depends on the facts at hand and the practices of the system within which the care is given.

A new hypothetical case study will allow for the review of clinical and ethical decision-making issues that can arise in the process of enacting these directives.

Case Study 2

A command psychiatrist, Anna Minassian (pseudonym), is called into the commander's office to consult on a situation that has arisen regarding two soldiers in training status. David Adelman (pseudonym), a male soldier, has been accused of stalking Claudia Shin (pseudonym), a female soldier: Adelman has shown up at Shin's quarters and remained outside, causing her to hide in her closet and act as if she were not there. Adelman believes the two to be involved in a relationship, but Shin has denied this, indicating that they have gone out once and have interacted on occasion in a friendly manner. Shin also notes that Adelman has become increasingly more convinced that the relationship has progressed, despite her telling him that this is not the case. When the training director confronted Adelman about this behavior and told him to leave Shin alone, not only did he not follow these directions, but he also acted in a manner that made the training director feel threatened. The commander has consulted command psychiatrist Minassian for input on how to handle this situation. At this point, Adelman has not directly threatened others verbally, but is exhibiting a behavioral pattern that has caused people to feel very uncomfortable and to consider him to be a potential threat.

Minassian finds that the commander is within his rights to order Adelman to have a command-directed mental health evaluation. This recommendation is akin to a civilian employer requesting an evaluation for an employee, but the evaluation is far easier for a military commander to conduct than it is in the civilian world. A civilian would have to engage law enforcement or another legal authority to make an evaluation happen immediately, and the evaluation would normally be conducted under the laws of whichever state they were in and in an emergency department where the employee would be evaluated by clinicians. In the military, the person ordered to evaluation has more limited choice. As such, military psychiatrists who assist commanders in these decisions have much more authority—and, therefore, responsibility—to perform due diligence and ensure that the rationale for the referral is reasonably connected to a potential psychiatric issue that could put others in harm's way.

Case Study 2 demonstrates the balancing act between the ethical principle of autonomy and the military physician's duty to others. Although some may criticize the requirements of a military psychiatrist's dual agency as working against a larger cultural shift toward patient autonomy as the main guiding ethical principle, perhaps a psychiatrist trained in applying balance is best suited to handle situations that require a balancing act between the principle of autonomy and other organizational principles and duties. In this particular case, the consulted psychiatrist may have felt the patient was manic or paranoid and, coupled with more than one person saying they were uncomfortable with his behavior, could have been justified in advising the command to make the referral for command-directed mental health evaluation.

In this scenario, it may also be preferable to have a different clinician, other than the command's psychiatrist, perform the evaluation if possible. This decision would also be an attempt to balance patient autonomy with duty to others. In some instances, this alternative will not be logistically possible, and the psychiatrist must then be acutely aware of their dual agency role and how it may be affecting their decision-making process. Psychiatrists in this situation are advised to consult a colleague by phone, if possible, in order to ensure that they are not being blind to some unintended bias that has crept into the decision-making process and that might unduly infringe on the soldier's autonomy.

In this scenario, the clinician has to make a number of determinations once the patient is evaluated. Is the patient an acute danger to themselves or others? If they are, is hospitalization indicated, or can they be managed at a lower level of care? Is there a Tarasoff duty (Tobriner 1976)—a duty shared by all providers, military, and civilian—to warn any intended victim at the time of the evaluation? The Tarasoff duty presents another example of a "dual agency" issue, as it balances patient autonomy with a duty to warn. Moreover, should the clinician advise the command to make changes in the physical conditions that currently exist? For example, commands can order service members into government quarters, and they can make this order for the person being evaluated or for the service member who may be in danger and who is being warned. Further, the clinician must determine whether treatment is warranted and whether the soldier is willing to agree to the treatment recommendations.

In a military situation like this one, another issue that may arise involves where to hospitalize a service member—a decision that can account for the patient's own right to privacy (as there may be people involved with his training, this particular incident, or his chain command). In this scenario, the soldier was convinced that he had no medical issues, that the situation was not as it had been described, and that people were blowing the situation out of proportion. He maintained this stance even when confronted by some of the facts of the situation. Ultimately, due to lack of insight and corroborating evidence that the patient did not seem to manipulate in a completely reasonable manner, it was decided he should be hospitalized against his will. Due to at least one of these privacy issues, and the fact that people felt unsafe around this soldier, it was decided that he be hospitalized at a different base in a different state.

Inherent Conflicts in Military Psychiatry: Boundaries and Privacy Issues in the Military Context

Military psychiatrists live and work in the communities where they practice. While this may also be true in civilian practice, the military psychiatrist is an integrated member of the military community, a ranking officer, a member of the command structure, and a neighbor to potential patients, including fellow officers with whom he/she must serve. As such, the military psychiatrist is forced to interact with his/her patient population by the very nature of military communities. In this context, the psychiatrist will almost certainly work with, live with, and observe past, present, and future patients outside of the context and protections of the boundaries of the clinical relationship.

This blurring of boundaries creates tensions, experienced by both the psychiatrist and the patient, about the management of privacy and transparencies. While these potential boundary breaches could be handled by a referral to another colleague in a civilian setting, it is often the case that the military psychiatrist is the sole mental health practitioner for a community. In this case, the military psychiatrist may not have the luxury of being allowed the option to select or decline a referral.

The dual or triple relationship for the psychiatrist and patient must be discussed and negotiated as part of the therapeutic contract. For example, the doctor and patient should discuss how they will refer to each other in military community settings. They should negotiate if they will even acknowledge a therapeutic relationship or perhaps only acknowledge that they are familiar through their command relationship or some other context. As military communities are very close-knit, there is a high potential for spouses or families to develop relationships with the psychiatrist, and this possibility should be discussed as well. These instances all employ the principle of autonomy and are scenarios that providers who live in small civilian communities also encounter, as an example.

While on deployment, the potential for dual relationships intensifies. Service members must work together within the context of the mission with members of their commands. It is often not possible to refer a patient to a colleague at a distant location across the theater of combat. The psychiatrist must remain mindful of his/her role in this context, both as a consultant to commanders on combat stress control and as a direct-care clinician caring for members of the command to whom he/she serves as a consultant. This dual relationship often calls into question the boundaries around privacy and confidentiality. The service member seeking care can rightly ask the question "Whom is this psychiatrist working for—the commander or the patient?" It is imperative that this issue be addressed up front in the clinical evaluation through a discussion of the limits of confidentiality, in which the psychiatrist is obliged to breach confidentiality for any life-threatening ideation or behavior, any criminal conduct, or when any deployment-limiting condition is identified. Under these conditions, the provision of care can remain confidential, with the exception that the commander must maintain the accountability of the service member at all times and has a right to know if the service member is seeking medical care to the extent that he needs to know the location of his service members at all times.

Apart from the boundaries associated with the clinical encounters, the deployed psychiatrist lives, eats, and bathes with all the service members in the command. There is no anonymity or privacy for the psychiatrist—or the patients for that matter. The psychiatrist must maintain a professional posture in all of these settings, paying special attention to maintaining discretion and confidentiality while eating a meal at a dining hall, going to the latrine, or using recreational facilities. There are many situations in which a psychiatrist may be approached by potential patients, from informal consultations to clinical crises. The psychiatrist must work to safeguard the patient's privacy in all of these settings and either divert the encounter to a strict clinical setting or find a discrete area to meet with the potential patient.

Military members are generally concerned about the stigma of seeking mental health care (Acosta et al. 2014). It is a military psychiatrist's duty to minimize the stigma by enhancing privacy and confidentiality and, at the same time, to normalize help seeking and to make care accessible. One strategy frequently employed by combat stress control (CSC) units is to offer general health services like smoking cessation, relaxation training, or other morale building activities to destigmatize the mental health clinic or combat stress control unit. These strategies allow an apprehensive person a face-saving, normalized reason for coming to a clinic and engaging in care. On one of the author's deployments, the combat stress control unit procured golf equipment from the Army Navy Country Club and set up a driving range on a small base that served as a logistical hub for surrounding units. Service members could come by to hit a few balls and speak informally to behavioral health specialists and perhaps engage in care. Strategies such as these maintain the privacy and dignity of service members and break down barriers to care in order to optimize the health of the deployed troops.

Ethical Considerations in the Psychiatrist's Use of a Position of Power

Fitness for Duty

Military psychiatrists are required, during the course of evaluating service members, to continually determine whether the service member meets current standards of fitness to serve in the armed forces or if they will require a medical discharge because they are no longer medically fit. For example, the United States Army regulations list the requirement for entry into the Army and for retention on active duty (Department of the Army 2011). Usually the retention standards provide somewhat more latitude except for severe or recurrent psychiatric issues. Additionally, there may be more specialized directions and stricter requirements for service members with special skills or duties, such as pilots in any service, service members with high-level security clearances, and service members in specialized units, such as the presidential detail, the nuclear weapons program, or Special Forces units. As a result, psychiatrists are often put in the situation of making a diagnosis that potentially could result in the patient being medically retired and removed from active duty, which often is at odds with the service member's desire.

Another case study can help delineate the ethical considerations that may arise in such a situation. A common scenario in which patients are frequently relieved from duty and are medically retired is when a patient is diagnosed with a psychotic disorder. The Army lists the psychiatric diagnoses that provide cause for referral to a Medical Evaluation Board (MEB). The relevant excerpts applicable to this case study include:

> 3–31. Disorders with psychotic features
> a. Diagnosed psychiatric conditions that fail to respond to treatment or restore the soldier to full function within 1 year of onset of treatment.
> b. Mental disorders not secondary to intoxication, infections, toxic, or other organic causes, with gross impairment in reality testing, resulting in interference with social adjustment or with duty performance. (Department of the Army 2011)

The Medical Evaluation Board is the medical assessment that becomes the basis of the Human Resources division's determination of whether a service member meets the provisions for retention in the service. Historically, the provider was both the person who treated the patient and the person who was primarily responsible for writing and presenting the Medical Evaluation Board to the Human Resources staff. Starting in 2007, overseas engagements in Afghanistan and Iraq made the occurrence of medical boards much more frequent, especially for combat-related issues such as post-traumatic stress disorder (PTSD). Clinicians became more acutely aware of the dual agency conflict of interest of trying to both treat a patient and determine medical fitness, which would either return a patient to duty or require a medical separation process. As a result, these clinical and administrative processes have been uncoupled, and there is now a distinction between the psychiatrists who treat a patient and who belong to the clinical service and psychiatrists who work for the "board" and process these evaluations who do not directly treat the patient. The change in this process provides a helpful example of military psychiatrists being attuned to the inherent ethical dilemma of treating their patient and complying with government regulations. Civilian colleagues in many other federal and law enforcement agencies also face these types of ethical conundrums. In order for the clinician to remain true to the tenets of patient autonomy and informed consent, it is necessary to provide documents that state how the information collected may be used and to provide verbal formal consent. With these changes, the clinician can now feel more like an advocate for the patient rather than a person determining their future in the military.

A third case study can provide further insight into the ethical questions that arise when utilizing a Medical Evaluation Board to determine fitness of duty.

Case Study 3

Leila Khan (pseudonym), a Navy Petty Officer Corpsman, began acting strangely at her workplace. She became easily confused, started voicing odd beliefs, and was unable to follow the protocols required to do her duties in a primary care clinic due to her inability to keep her thoughts organized. The command referred Khan for evaluation. It was determined that the patient was psychotic, and a trial of treatment was recommended. Khan had little insight into her condition and did not agree with the treatment and was, therefore, frequently nonadherent with the treatment. As a result, the symptoms persisted and Khan ended up meeting the criteria for referral to a Medical Evaluation Board (MEB). She never required hospitalization, and never was a danger to herself or others, but was taken out of a care environment and given minimal administrative duties, such as delivering mail or answering phones. She would frequently forget the mail route and had difficulty communicating messages received over the phone. As such, she was referred to the MEB for determination of fitness for duty. Khan disagreed with this determination and filed an Inspector General complaint against her doctor for alleged "fraud, waste, and abuse" by saying that she should be eligible for medical benefits and disability retirement pay for the rest of her life. This complaint was dismissed, and Khan was ultimately medically discharged from military health service as 100 % disabled, which provides a monthly retirement benefit and access to healthcare from the military health system and the Veterans Affairs (VA) healthcare system.

In this case study, the patient met all administrative criteria for being medically retired. She was ill for a protracted time and was unable to perform her duties. Another criterion that must be considered is if the service member is worldwide deployable. This determination requires understanding the level of care typically available in remote theaters of operation where access to a full formulary or to labs required to monitor some medications is not available.

All of these issues require the clinician to maintain the highest level of transparency and provide constant reminders of the risks and benefits of moving forward with care. In this case, this requirement involved continually reminding the patient that her noncompliance with treatment meant that she was less likely to have resolution of symptoms and would ultimately be removed from active duty via a medical board despite her desire not to be removed and her belief that she was not ill. This example illustrates the provider attempting to balance the principles of autonomy and beneficence with a duty to others.

In another example, a patient with bipolar II disorder requires a mood stabilizer. Some mood stabilizers would be acceptable on a worldwide deployment and others would not. Therefore, a clinician must be up-front and explain the risks and benefits for both treatment and the patient's career when determining what medication to prescribe. To not do so, and to either purposefully undertreat to please the patient by prescribing a medication that allows for worldwide deployment or treat with a preferred medication but one that requires referral to a Medical Evaluation Board, would put a clinician in an ethically unfavorable situation with regard to their patient.

Medical Evacuation v. Return to Duty

One unique aspect of military psychiatry is the fact that psychiatrists deploy to theaters of combat with the soldiers they treat. This fact is frequently depicted in many movies and television shows such as *M*A*S*H* and *The Hurt Locker* and in the series about World War II called *The Pacific*, the companion to *Band of Brothers*. The rationale for having psychiatrists in or near the theater of combat is to provide triage and care close to combat in order to determine who needs to be evacuated for care and who can be returned to duty. In some cases this is a fairly easy determination and there is no blurring of ethical considerations. In other instances, the decision is much more nuanced and fraught with the potential for biases that may conflict with pure ethical decision-making. An example of the former is a patient who is clearly psychotic from a primary psychotic process. This patient would almost always be evacuated, especially if their psychotic symptoms included paranoia and delusions, which potentially could compromise the safety of the ill service member or the unit. On the other end of the spectrum, a patient who had a few days of intense combat and had not slept, and who had some acute change in mental state related to extreme lack of sleep but who responded to 2 or 3 days' rest with complete return to baseline, presents an instance where returning the patient to duty would be a fairly simple choice as well.

In between these two extremes, much gray area exists. The most common gray-area question that arises when considering fitness of duty regards "correct" decision-making for a patient who has PTSD and who may potentially be reexposed to trauma that could worsen the condition. This scenario was presented in this chapter's initial case study. Some would argue that it is unethical to make a decision that would potentially reexpose the patient to situations that could worsen their condition. They might say that, in this instance, or in any other where the patient might get worse or have a recurrence of symptoms (e.g., panic and depression), it is an unethical clinical decision to return the patient to duty. This decision would be based on the principles of beneficence and non-maleficence. Others might say that perhaps the rules are different for military service members in a time of war, especially when the service member has volunteered for service, has been trained to expect these conditions and exposures, and has access to treatment to help control any symptomatic reactions to further exposure. Commanders may worry that if psychiatrists start allowing anyone who might be at risk for reexposure to be evacuated, an "evacuation syndrome"—in which droves of soldiers would attempt to leave the combat zone—might occur and seriously diminish the capability of units to effectively fight. This could lead to even more service members being wounded or exposed to extreme circumstances. The ability to maintain a fighting force with the proper level of capability is an important aspect of a unit's readiness to engage the enemy in a manner that statistically puts them in the position to succeed in their mission. Every member of the team contributes to this capacity, so commanders prefer that their soldiers be returned to duty if at all possible.

In this scenario, one's "duty to others" presents a stark contrast to the other ethical principles. While there are no randomized studies to guide decision-making on this issue, service members who are evacuated from theater for a psychiatric condition, suicidal ideation, or inability to adapt to the mission tend to reintegrate poorly, and are at risk for chronic mental health problems. A service member returning "early" from their deployment will have to rationalize and perhaps explain to their families why they did not complete their tour of duty. A mental health reason for early evacuation is highly stigmatizing in and of itself. In addition, the service member may be perceived as a malingerer by unit members and their homefront community. All of these biases and attitudes create obstacles to a welcoming homecoming and supportive reintegration into the community.

On the other hand, service members who are able to receive treatment, and successfully complete their mission despite a mental health concern, receive all of the prestige associated with the successful mission. The service member can also feel pride for completing their mission, being true to their combat brothers, and not "getting off easy" when others were forced to stay. There is also the potential benefit to the service member of developing resilience through succeeding despite the odds—a source of pride that troops who are evacuated from theater do not experience. Psychiatrists work with the service member to make these decisions and help delineate who might have the capacity to succeed and who might not. One division that deployed to Iraq during Operation Iraqi Freedom followed all of its soldiers from start to finish and identified those at risk every step of the way, from predeployment through the end of deployment (Warner et al. 2011).

The proper balancing act for making the determination of whether to evacuate or return service members to duty requires having a transparent discussion with the service member and the command regarding the risks and benefits of the soldier being treated, or being followed closely in theater, or being evacuated back to the States. This discussion needs to consider numerous variables, such as the motivation of the service member to finish their tour and stay in the military, the ability to keep the service member and others safe, the level of symptoms being displayed, the response of those symptoms to interventions available in theater and the rapidity by which the symptoms resolve, the ability to monitor the service member's progress in theater, and the type of work or exposures the service member will be required to endure if they remain in theater. Once an honest discussion of all these factors has occurred, and the clinician and patient are able to come to a determination of what appears to be in the patient's best immediate interest, they can then monitor together over time to determine if the risk/benefit ratio is actually allowing for the patient to benefit or if the patient remains at risk and there needs to be a final decision to evacuate. This decision should be nuanced, informed, transparent, and ongoing rather than black and white or quickly decided based on limited data or interaction. It is only when a military clinician makes a true attempt to balance their dual agency roles of prioritizing the patient's needs and wishes (autonomy and beneficence) while still attempting to preserve fighting strength (duty to others) that one could say the test of ethical balancing is being met.

Disability Determination

Not only does the psychiatric condition of the service member create the potential for service-limiting disability, but it also creates incentives for long-term compensation in the form of medical retirement and disability pension. The Departments of Defense (DoD) and Veterans Affairs (VA) coordinate their efforts to determine what service-connected conditions qualify for a disability rating and potential benefits through the Integrated Disability Evaluation System (IDES). When a service member develops a health condition and seeks treatment, the treating clinicians first aggressively treat the condition to restore the service member's fitness for duty and worldwide deployability. If the service member cannot be restored to health within a reasonable period of time (defined in regulations as 1 year), then the service member is referred to the IDES, which has several phases.

The first phase is the Medical Evaluation Board (MEB), described above and conducted by the Department of Defense. During the evaluation, Department of Defense physicians establish all relevant diagnoses and identify any conditions incompatible with further military service. The MEB is also charged with determining whether any conditions may have existed prior to service in the military and were not caused by military service. For any conditions not directly attributable to military service, or incurred while on active duty service, the MEB comments whether that condition may have been aggravated by military service and therefore be eligible for disability recognition.

Inherent to this process are competing demands to treat an illness to restore health, to identify disqualifying conditions, and to refer the service member for disability benefits. These competing demands lead to potential ethical conflict regarding whether to maximize the restoration of health aligned with the values of a physician, to minimize the impact of illness and return the service member to active service aligned with the values of a military officer, or to ensure that only those members who are truly fit for duty are retained and those who are not are transitioned to civilian life.

There are many forces at play in the MEB process. The service member may be motivated by his/her warrior ethos to minimize any illness in an attempt to remain on active duty and continue to serve. Alternatively, the service member might be seeking separation from the military and long-term disability. The physician conducting the MEB must be aware of the dynamic forces at play and the potential for malingering and other secondary gain issues. The physician attempts to remain objective, but can be influenced by personal biases, military cultural influences, and the patient's interests. In this case, the patient's interests and those of the military may be in conflict, and the physician's role is that of a neutral arbitrator making objective findings and recommendations.

At the completion of the MEB, the service member is found to be either medically fit or unfit for duty. The service member has the opportunity to request consideration of transfer to a different military occupational specialty if the condition's limitations can be accommodated in a different type of military work. For example, if a service member has an amputation and can no longer perform light infantry patrols with a full combat load, he may transfer to a specialty that does not require such rigorous walking, running, or marching. If the service member requires a medication for a mood disorder that necessitates lab monitoring, he may be unable to be deployed, but he may be reassigned to permanent stateside duty if the mood disorder is stable. These requests are heavily weighted in the interest of the service and are granted to service members with unique or in-demand skills.

If the MEB concludes that the service member's medical condition is incompatible with further military service, the case is then referred to the Integrated Disability Evaluation System (IDES), which formally determines if the service member is fit for continued military service and determines his/her subsequent eligibility for disability compensation. If the service member's disability rating indicates minimal disability (20 % or less), then they are administratively separated with a severance package. If the disability is rated as moderate or above (30 % or more), then they will receive military retirement at that percentage of their base pay for life. This disability determination process represents a great deal of value for the service member and, therefore, can present untold pressures on the physician trying to balance his duties to the military and to the service member to maintain the integrity of the disability determination process.

Interface Between the Departments of Defense (DoD) and Veterans Affairs (VA)

Once the service member is retired from the military with any disability, he/she is automatically referred to the Department of Veterans Affairs for enrollment. This referral ensures that the service member/veteran becomes eligible for all applicable benefits. These benefits include access to healthcare for the service-connected disability and a host of financial benefits and disability compensation. The Department of Defense and Department of Veterans Affairs have forged a highly interoperable system of referral that includes access to each other's electronic medical record to seamlessly coordinate care between these complex systems. The veteran, now enrolled in the VA to receive the benefits he has earned, continues to be eligible for a lifetime entitlement to ongoing healthcare. In addition, all combat veterans from the wars in Iraq and Afghanistan receive a carte blanche 5-year benefit of access to VA healthcare regardless of any identified service-connected disability on the presumption that a health condition may emerge after a period of active service.

Psychiatrists' Involvement as Command Consultants: Torture and Enhanced Interrogation

"Psychiatrists shall not participate in torture." In 2006, the American Psychiatric Association adopted a position paper on the psychiatrist's role in so-called "enhanced interrogations". This paper, entitled "Position Statement on Psychiatric Participation in Interrogation of Detainees" (American Psychiatric Association 2006), was reaffirmed in 2014 and is provided for review in Appendix 2. While this position paper states that no provider may engage directly in interrogations of persons held in custody, it also states that psychiatrists may provide training to military or civilian investigative or law enforcement personnel on recognizing and responding to persons with mental illnesses and on the possible medical and psychological effects of particular techniques and conditions of interrogation.

The Department of Defense has also codified the roles for treatment in comparison with those for consultation in its directive entitled "DoD Intelligence Interrogations, Detainee Debriefings, and Tactical Questioning" (Department of Defense 2012). Applicable excerpts are provided in Appendix 3. This directive specifically defines the role of Behavioral Science Consultants:

> 14. BEHAVIORAL SCIENCE CONSULTANTS. Behavioral science consultants are authorized to make psychological assessments of the character, personality, social interactions, and other behavioral characteristics of interrogation subjects and to advise authorized personnel performing lawful interrogations regarding such assessments in accordance with Reference (r). During assignments in which a health care provider delivers behavioral science consultant services, the provider may not supply medical care for detainees except in an emergency when no other health care providers can respond adequately. Behavioral science consultants may not be used to determine detainee phobias for the purpose of exploitation during the interrogation process. In totality, these position papers and regulations provide the clinician with a framework for approaching the possibility that they may be tasked to engage in activities such as supporting interrogation operations. In this scenario, it is clear that the ethical principles of non-

maleficence and the principle of patient autonomy override the potential dual agency conflict of the psychiatrist feeling they have a duty to protect the greater good by assisting in interrogations which may lead to the prevention of acts of war or terrorism. (Department of Defense 2012)

Conclusion

In a report summarizing a workshop entitled "Military Medical Ethics: Issues Regarding Dual Loyalties" and convened by the Institute of Medicine (IOM), IOM President Harvey Fineberg acknowledges that "moments of tension" arise and states the belief that "these difficult issues do not benefit from being ignored or secretly managed or considered to be implicit." During the workshop, one of the consensus principles that emerged was the concept of transparency. As stated by participant Myron C. Harrison, "an act that deceives someone, whether the individual or the employer, probably is unethical. If no one—employee, manager, or labor union—is being deceived, then the matter probably is being handled transparently and on an ethical track." The other major principles in effect for making ethical decisions are autonomy, beneficence, and non-maleficence (Weisfeld et al. 2008).

As this chapter has described, the practice of military psychiatry may present a higher number of instances in which the ethics of patient care conflict with the dual agency role of a military psychiatrist. As such, all psychiatrists who practice in the military need to be aware of the types of situations in which these conflicts may arise. The clinician can aim to take an ethical stance that favors transparency over deception and can use informed consent of the potential inherent risks and benefits of each potential decision as the framework for ensuring the ethical management of the balancing act inherent in any dual agency situation.

Key Concepts

1. A military psychiatrist must be aware of the types of situations that give rise to potential ethical dilemmas.
2. Dual agency requirements may lead to ethical dilemmas that either do not exist in the civilian practice of psychiatry or are very similar to certain civilian practices (e.g., law enforcement).
3. Balancing ethical principles with dual agency requires a dynamic, rather than static, decision-making process, depending on changes in the circumstances and the facts of the case.
4. Utilizing transparency and informed consent in order to be up-front with and to educate patients of potential conflicts is paramount to maintaining an ethical practice while still maintaining dual agency requirements.

Appendix 1: Department of Defense Instruction (DoDI) 6490.04 (March 4, 2013)

Hospitalization for Psychiatric Evaluation and Treatment

(a) Pursuant to a referral, only a psychiatrist, or, when a psychiatrist is not available, a physician or another MHP [mental health-care provider] with admitting privileges may admit a service member for an inpatient MHE [mental health evaluation].

(b) The evaluation will be conducted in the most appropriate clinical setting, in accordance with the least restrictive alternative principle.

(c) Voluntary inpatient admission is appropriate when a psychiatrist, or, when a psychiatrist is not available, a physician or another MHP with admitting privileges, determines that admission is clinically indicated and the service member has the capacity to provide and does provide informed consent regarding treatment and admission.

(d) An involuntary inpatient admission to an MTF [military treatment facility] is appropriate only when a psychiatrist, or, when a psychiatrist is not available, a physician or another MHP with admitting privileges, makes an evaluation that the service member has, or likely has, a severe mental disorder or poses imminent or potential danger to self or others. Guidelines include:

1. Level of Care. Placement in a less restrictive level of care would result in inadequate medical care.
2. Admission Criteria. Admission is consistent with applicable clinical practice guidelines.
3. Reevaluation Following Admission. The service member will be reevaluated, under the purview of the admitting facility, within 72 h of admission by an independent privileged psychiatrist or other medical officer if a psychiatrist is not available:
   (a) The independent medical reviewer will notify the service member of the purpose and nature of the review and of the member's right to have legal representation during the review by a judge advocate or by an attorney of the member's choosing at the member's own expense if reasonably available within the required time period for the review.
   (b) The independent medical reviewer will determine and document in the inpatient medical record whether, based on clear and convincing evidence, continued involuntary hospitalization is clinically appropriate. If so, the reviewer will document the clinical conditions requiring continued involuntary hospitalization and the circumstances required for discharge from the hospital and schedule another review within five business days.
   (c) The independent medical reviewer will notify the service member of the results of each review.
4. Medical Record Documentation. Documentation of the evaluation encounter, findings, and disposition must be consistent with applicable standards of care and will additionally:
   (a) Document information pertaining to the inpatient admission in the service member's MTF electronic health record including at a minimum communication of the assessment of risk for dangerousness, treatment plan, medications, progress of treatment, discharge assessment, and recommendations to commanders or supervisors regarding continued fitness for duty and actions the MHP recommends be taken to assist with the continued treatment plan.
   (b) Upon discharge, MHPs will provide, consistent with Reference (l), memorandums or copies of consultation reports to the commander or supervisor with sufficient clinical information and recommendations to allow the commander or supervisor to understand the service member's condition and make reasoned decisions about the service member's safety, duties, and medical care requirements.
5. Additional Patient Rights. The service member has the right to contact a relative, friend, chaplain, attorney, any office of Inspector General (IG), and anyone else the member chooses, as soon as the service member's condition permits, after admission to the hospital.

(e) When a physician who is not an MHP admits a service member pursuant to the referral for an MHE to be conducted on an inpatient basis, the physician will:
   1. Make reasonable attempts to consult with an MHP with admitting privileges prior to and during the admission (e.g., by telecommunications).
   2. Arrange for transfer to an MHP with admitting privileges as soon as practicable.

(f) In the case of referral for an involuntary inpatient admission to a civilian facility, guidelines in Reference (n) will be considered, and the process established under the law of the State where the facility is located will be followed. If in a foreign country, the applicable laws of the host nation will be followed.

Appendix 2: "Position Statement on Psychiatric Participation in Interrogation of Detainees" (American Psychiatric Association 2006)

The American Psychiatric Association reiterates its position that psychiatrists should not participate in, or otherwise assist or facilitate, the commission of torture of any person. Psychiatrists who become aware that torture has occurred, is occurring, or has been planned must report it promptly to a person or persons in a position to take corrective action.

Furthermore, no psychiatrist should participate directly in the interrogation of persons held in custody by military or civilian investigative or law enforcement authorities, whether in the United States or elsewhere. Direct participation includes being present in the interrogation room, asking or suggesting questions, or advising authorities on the use of specific techniques of interrogation with particular detainees. However, psychiatrists may provide training to military or civilian investigative or law enforcement personnel on recognizing and responding to persons with mental illnesses, on the possible medical and psychological effects of particular techniques and conditions of interrogation, and on other areas within their professional expertise.

Appendix 3: Department of Defense Directive, "DoD Intelligence Interrogations, Detainee Debriefings, and Tactical Questioning" (Department of Defense 2012)

4.1. Basic Principles. Healthcare personnel (particularly physicians) perform their duties consistent with the following principles.

- 4.1.1. Healthcare personnel have a duty in all matters affecting the physical and mental health of detainees to perform, encourage, and support, directly and indirectly, actions to uphold the humane treatment of detainees and to ensure that no individual in the custody or under the physical control of the Department of Defense, regardless of nationality or physical location, shall be subject to cruel, inhuman, or degrading treatment or punishment, in accordance with and as defined in US law.
- 4.1.2. Healthcare personnel charged with the medical care of detainees have a duty to protect detainees' physical and mental health and provide appropriate treatment for disease. To the extent practicable, treatment of detainees should be guided by professional judgments and standards similar to those applied to personnel of the US Armed Forces.
- 4.1.3. Healthcare person23.443 ptnel shall not be involved in any professional provider-patient treatment relationship with detainees, the purpose of which is not solely to evaluate, protect, or improve their physical and mental health.
- 4.1.4. Healthcare personnel, whether or not in a professional provider-patient treatment relationship, shall not apply their knowledge and skills in a manner that is not in accordance with applicable law or the standards set forth in Reference (c).
- 4.1.5. Healthcare personnel shall not certify, or participate in the certification of, the fitness of detainees for any form of treatment or punishment that is not in accordance with applicable law or participate in any way in the administration of any such treatment or punishment.
- 4.1.6. Healthcare personnel shall not participate in any procedure for applying physical restraints to the person of a detainee unless such a procedure is determined to be necessary for the protection of the physical or mental

health or the safety of the detainee or necessary for the protection of other detainees or those treating, guarding, or otherwise interacting with them. Such restraints, if used, shall be applied in a safe and professional manner.

4.2. Medical Records. Accurate and complete medical records on all detainees shall be created and maintained. Medical records must be maintained for all medical encounters, whether in fixed facilities or through medical personnel in the field.

4.3. Treatment Purpose. Healthcare personnel engaged in a professional provider-patient treatment relationship with detainees shall not participate in detainee-related activities for purposes other than healthcare. Such healthcare personnel shall not actively solicit information from detainees for other than healthcare purposes. Healthcare personnel engaged in non-treatment activities, such as forensic psychology, behavioral science consultation, forensic pathology, or similar disciplines, shall not engage in any professional provider-patient treatment relationship with detainees (except in emergency circumstances in which no other healthcare providers can respond adequately to save life or prevent permanent impairment).

4.4. Medical Information. Healthcare personnel shall safeguard patient confidences and privacy within the constraints of the law. Under US and international law and applicable medical practice standards, there is no absolute confidentiality of medical information for any person. Detainees shall not be given cause to have incorrect expectations of privacy or confidentiality regarding their medical records and communications. However, whenever patient-specific medical information concerning detainees is disclosed for purposes other than treatment, healthcare personnel shall record the details of such disclosure, including the specific information disclosed, the person to whom it was disclosed, the purpose of the disclosure, and the name of the medical unit commander (or other designated senior medical activity officer) approving the disclosure. Similar to legal standards applicable to US citizens, permissible purposes include preventing harm to any person, maintaining public health and order in detention facilities, and any lawful law enforcement, intelligence, or national security-related activity.

4.4.1. When the medical unit commander (or other designated senior medical activity officer) suspects the medical information to be disclosed may be misused, or if there is a disagreement between such medical activity officer and a senior officer requesting disclosure, the medical activity officer shall seek a senior command determination on the propriety of the disclosure, or actions to ensure the use of the information will be consistent with applicable standards.

4.4.2. Consistent with applicable command procedures, International Committee of the Red Cross physicians shall be given access to review medical records of detainees during visits to detention facilities.

4.5. Reportable Incident Requirements. Any healthcare personnel who in the course of a treatment relationship or in any other way observes or suspects a possible violation of applicable standards, including those prescribed in References (b), (c), and (e), for the protection of detainees shall report those circumstances to the chain of command. Healthcare personnel who believe such a report has not been acted upon properly should also report the circumstances to the medical program leadership, including the Command Surgeon or Military Department specialty consultant. Officials in the medical program leadership may inform the Joint Staff Surgeon or Surgeon

General concerned, who then may seek senior command review of the circumstances presented. Other reporting mechanisms, such as the Inspector General, criminal investigation organizations, or Judge Advocates, also may be used.

4.5.1. Healthcare personnel involved in clinical practice activities shall make a written record of all reports of suspected or alleged violations in a reportable incident log maintained by the medical unit commander or other designated senior medical activity officer.

4.5.2 Healthcare personnel carrying out BSC [behavioral science consultant] functions under Enclosure 2 shall also comply fully with the reportable incident requirements of paragraph 4.5. They shall make a written record of all reports of suspected or alleged violations in a reportable incident log maintained by the detention facility commander or other designated senior officer.

4.6. Training. The Secretaries of the Military Departments and, as appropriate, Combatant Commanders shall ensure healthcare personnel involved in the treatment of detainees or other detainee matters receive appropriate training on applicable policies and procedures regarding the care and treatment of detainees. This training shall include at least the following elements:

4.6.1. A basic level of training for all military healthcare personnel who may be deployed in support of military operations and whose duties may involve support of detainee operations or contact with detainees. The overall purpose of this training is to ensure a working knowledge and understanding of the requirements and standards for dealing with healthcare of detainees.

4.6.2. Periodic provision of refresher training consistent with the basic level of training.

4.6.3. Additional training for healthcare personnel assigned to support detainee operations, commensurate with their duties.

4.7. Consent for Medical Treatment or Intervention. In general, healthcare will be provided with the consent of the detainee. To the extent practicable, standards and procedures for obtaining consent will be consistent with those applicable to consent from other patients. Standard exceptions for lifesaving emergency medical care provided to a patient incapable of providing consent or for care necessary to protect public health, such as to prevent the spread of communicable diseases, shall apply.

4.7.1. In the case of a hunger strike, attempted suicide, or other attempted serious self-harm, medical treatment or intervention may be directed without the consent of the detainee to prevent death or serious harm. Such action must be based on a medical determination that immediate treatment or intervention is necessary to prevent death or serious harm and, in addition, must be approved by the commanding officer of the detention facility or other designated senior officer responsible for detainee operations.

4.7.2. Involuntary treatment or intervention under subparagraph 4.7.1. in a detention facility must be preceded by a thorough medical and mental health evaluation of the detainee and counseling concerning the risks of refusing consent. Such treatment or intervention shall be carried out in a medically appropriate manner, under standards similar to those applied to personnel of the US Armed Forces.

4.7.3. Detention facility procedures for dealing with cases in which involuntary treatment may be necessary to prevent death or serious harm shall be developed with consideration of procedures established by Title 28, Code of Federal Regulations, Part 549 (Reference (g)).

4.8. Role of the Armed Forces Medical Examiner (AFME) in Death Investigations. As required by the Secretary of Defense Memorandum dated June 9, 2004 (Reference (h)), if a detainee dies, the commander of the facility (or if the death did not occur in a facility, the commander of the unit that exercised control over the individual) shall immediately report the death to the cognizant Military Criminal Investigation Organization (MCIO). The MCIO shall contact the Office of the AFME, which shall, consistent with Reference (h), Section 1471 of Title 10, United States Code, and DoD Instruction 5154.30 (References (i) and (j)), determine whether an autopsy will be performed. The body will be handled as directed by the Office of the AFME. The determination of the cause and manner of death will be the sole responsibility of the AFME or other physician designated by the AFME.

4.9. Health Care Personnel Management. As a matter of personnel management policy, except as provided in this paragraph, healthcare personnel's support of detainee operations is limited only to providing healthcare services in a professional provider-patient treatment relationship in approved clinical settings, conducting disease prevention and other approved public health activities, advising proper command authorities regarding the health status of detainees, and providing direct support for these activities. Medical personnel shall not be used to supervise, conduct, or direct interrogations. Healthcare personnel assigned as, or providing direct support to, BSCs, consistent with Enclosure 2, or AFME personnel, are the only authorized exceptions to this paragraph. The Assistant Secretary of Defense for Health Affairs (ASD(HA)), or designee, must approve any other exceptions to this paragraph.

4.10. BSCs. Standards and procedures for BSCs are established in Enclosure 2.

4.11. Effect on Legal Obligations. Nothing in this Instruction may be construed to alter any legal obligations of healthcare personnel under applicable law.

References

Acosta J, Amariah B, Cerully JL, Fisher MP, Martin LT, Vardavas R, Slaughter ME, Schell TL (2014) Mental health stigma in the military. Rand Corporation, Santa Monica

American Psychiatric Association (1973) The principles of medical ethics with annotations especially applicable to psychiatry. American Psychiatric Association, Arlington

American Psychiatric Association (2006) Position statement on psychiatric participation in interrogation of detainees. American Psychiatric Association, Arlington

American Psychiatric Association (2013) The principles of medical ethics with annotations especially applicable to psychiatry. APA, Arlington

Boxer B (1988) Military whistleblower protection Act, United States Code 10, Section 1034. US Congress, Washington, DC

Department of Defense (1998) DODD 6490.1 – command-directed mental health evaluations. Department of Defense, Washington, DC

Department of Defense (2011) Department of Defense Instruction 6490.08 – the military command exception and disclosing PHI of armed forces personnel. Department of Defense, Washington, DC

Department of Defense (2012) DoD intelligence interrogations, detainee debriefings, and tactical questioning. Department of Defense, Washington, DC

Department of the Army (2011) Army regulation 40–501, standards of medical fitness. Department of the Army, Washington, DC

Department of Veterans Affairs & Department of Defense (2013) VA/DoD clinical practice guideline for the assessment and management of patients at risk for suicide. Department of Veterans Affairs & Department of Defense, Washington, DC

Lauretano DA (1998) The military whistleblower protection act and the military mental health evaluation protection act. Department of the Army, Washington, DC

Payne SE, Hill JV, Johnson DE (2008) The use of unit watch or command interest profile in the management of suicide and homicide risk: rationale and guidelines for the military mental health professional. Mil Med 173(1):25–35

Tobriner M (1976) Tarasoff v. Regents of the University of California, 17 Cal. 3d 425, 551 P.2d 334, 131 Cal. Rptr. 14. California Supreme Court, San Francisco

Warner CH, Appenzeller GN, Parker JR, Warner CM, Hoge CW (2011) Effectiveness of mental health screening and coordination of in-theater care prior to deployment to Iraq: a cohort study. Am J Psychiatr 168(4):378–385

Weisfeld NE, Weisfeld VD, Liverman CT (2008) Military medical ethics: issues regarding dual loyalties. The National Academies Press, Washington, DC

Part II

Systems of Care for Mental Health Needs of Military and Veteran Populations

Veterans Affairs and Department of Defense Integrated Systems of Mental Health Care

7

Samuel L. Preston

Introduction and Scope

The Global War on Terror (GWOT) and associated campaigns (Operation Enduring Freedom, Operation Iraqi Freedom, and Operation New Dawn) resulted in an immediate need for veterans medical and mental health services. Since fiscal year 2002, nearly two million veterans became eligible for Department of Veterans Affairs (VA) care. Of that total, 1,185,160 (61%) were former active duty, while 754,799 (39%) were either National Guard or Reserve component (US Department of Veterans Affairs 2015a). Of this cohort, 685,540 (57.6%) carry a mental health diagnosis with 378,993 diagnosed with post-traumatic stress disorder (PTSD), making this diagnosis the most common mental health disorder evaluated at VA facilities for this population (US Department of Veterans Affairs 2015a). Furthermore, the National Center for Veterans Analysis and Statistics anticipates the number of VA-eligible post-9/11 veterans to expand to nearly 3.4 million by 2018. The bolus of incoming GWOT veterans increased utilization of VA outpatient services from 46.5 million visits in 2002 to 83.6 million visits in 2012 (Department of Veterans Affairs 2011). However, GWOT veterans only represent 33% of the total veteran population, roughly the same total number as Vietnam-era veterans (Department of Veterans Affairs 2014). Though the veteran population composition will shift toward GWOT veterans over time, this illuminates the resource impact of post-9/11 veterans on VA medical services in combination with veterans from previous eras already seeking medical care within VA facilities. The National Center for Veterans Analysis and Statistics reports that, of the over nine million veterans enrolled in the VA system of care, four million carry a service-connected disability, accounting for nearly $50 billion in cash payments annually. This speaks to the personal sacrifices performed by many veterans associated with their military services and to the American people's willingness to financially support veterans with service-connected disability.

Furthermore, the demographic composition of the veteran populations is changing over time. By 2030, the percentage of female veterans is projected to nearly double, while nonwhite minorities will continue to steadily increase to approximately 34% of the total veteran population (Department of Veterans Affairs 2011). The shift of veteran composition requires flexibility and enhanced services to ensure cultural, gender, and socioeconomic sensitivities and capabilities within the continuum of care for the next generations of veterans.

To meet the needs of the expanding, dynamic composition of the eligible veteran population with mental health treatment needs, the Department

S.L. Preston (✉)
US Army, Regional Health Command-Atlantic,
Washington, DC 20001, USA
e-mail: Samuel.l.preston@mail.mil

L.W. Roberts, C.H. Warner (eds.), *Military and Veteran Mental Health*,
https://doi.org/10.1007/978-1-4939-7438-2_7

of Defense (DoD) and Department of Veterans Affairs (VA) developed an integrated model of mental health services. The continuum of mental health services begins with service-specific mental health resources consisting of established military treatment facilities, programs, and partnerships, continuing through established programs developed for the transition of in-need service members to the VA behavioral health system of care. Though the primary focus of this chapter is the Department of Veterans Affairs continuum of mental health care, the importance of the transition of medical and mental health services from military treatment facilities to the VA system of care cannot be overstated. Providing streamlined, seamless continuity of mental health services to the veteran population is a national priority (Commission on Care 2016).

With the highest national visibility placed on veteran care services, it is important to underscore that entry into the DoD-VA mental health continuum of care is as diverse as the population served, with some enrollees first seeking treatment while on active duty and others beginning services upon discharge from service (Mental Health Advisory Team 2007). Accessible services and multiple entry points available for veterans continue to evolve with the veteran population served. This chapter provides a general outline of expected and available mental health services within the DoD-VA continuum of mental health care and includes resources within the DoD-VA community in support of veterans with mental health care needs.

Case Study

Staff Sergeant (SSG) (ret.) Julius Mericido (pseudonym) is a combat veteran with 15 years of service with the Guam Army National Guard, an organization he deployed with three times in support of the Global War on Terror (GWOT). Upon return from his third deployment, SSG Mericido began isolating from his friends and family. During the first drill weekend after the unit returned, it was obvious to SSG Mericido's company something was wrong: SSG Mericido looked exhausted and his breath smelled of alcohol from the night before. When his platoon sergeant discussed the odor, SSG Mericido broke down into tears; he was not sleeping due to severe combat-related nightmares and alcohol seemed to help. He knew he was losing control of his alcohol use. The platoon sergeant escorted him to the unit behavioral health officer who conducted an interview. The behavioral health officer determined SSG Mericido suffered from depression, alcohol use disorder, and post-traumatic stress disorder (PTSD). The behavioral health officer recommended movement to Naval Hospital Guam for immediate assessment.

SSG Mericido received medical treatment at Naval Hospital Guam to assist with his withdrawal from alcohol. Upon discharge, he was enrolled in the Regional Health Command-Pacific telemental health service, where he connected with a psychologist at Tripler Army Medical Center for therapy. However, SSG Mericido needed a higher level of care than what was available in Guam for his severe PTSD symptoms. As a result, he was attached to the Warrior Transition Unit at Schofield Barracks, HI, and enrolled in the Honolulu VA's residential PTSD treatment program. While in this program, SSG Mericido received residential, focused treatment for his PTSD.

Upon completion of the program, his behavioral health providers agreed the best disposition for SSG Mericido was through the integrated disability evaluation system (IDES). SSG Mericido remained at Schofield Barracks on active duty status through his medical board completion, a process that took approximately 4 months. While at Schofield completing the IDES process, SSG Mericido concurrently received outpatient mental health and medical services from Schofield Army Health Clinic, including Schofield's trauma resolution intensive outpatient program (TR-IOP). Upon completion of the IDES process, SSG

Mericido was enrolled in the *inTransition* program by his Warrior Transition Unit case manager, which linked him with VA services in Guam and ensured that his transitional care plan was seamless. Currently, SSG Mericido is engaged in services through the Guam VA medical clinic. His PTSD symptoms continue to improve with outpatient interventions.

Military Treatment Facility (MTF) Mental Health Services

Each branch and service component possesses mental health capabilities supporting the medical readiness of service-specific missions in accordance with respective, service-specific medical retention, and disposition policies (Department of Defense 2015a). The composition, capacity, and population served by military treatment facility (MTF) providers vary based on multiple influences including geographic location, available conjoint civilian capabilities, treatment facility size, installation mission, available resourcing, and military service affiliation. For instance, some military installations house large medical centers with every level of inpatient and outpatient mental health service treating service members, dependents, and veterans; still, other installations are supported by a small clinic capable of supporting only active duty outpatient beneficiaries, leveraging non-DoD-affiliated mental health providers within the community TRICARE network for inpatient and family member services. Though access to care timelines and in-house services vary between installations due to available mental health capabilities, the process of engaging mental health care at military treatment facility is consistent across the Department of Defense (2015a).

Service members engage mental health services through five general ways: voluntary treatment by self-referral (including emergent treatment); through a medical referral by primary care or other medical professionals; by administrative assessment for a position of trust, advanced training, or due to mission; within the context of established mental health assessment and treatment after domestic violence or substance use disorder incidents; or via a command-directed mental health referral due to concerns for safety or ability to complete mission (Department of Defense 2013a).

At a minimum, every service member completes an annual periodic health assessment with a primary care provider, including general mental health and suicide screens along with a physical exam and medical review (Department of Defense 2016). Deploying service members receive mental health evaluations preceding and after completing the mission assessing fitness for and potential mental health issues resulting from deployment, respectively (Department of Defense 2013b). Additionally, all service members completing their time in service and most service members separating for administrative reasons complete a final screen and assessment of service-connected diagnoses. Upon separation, eligible veterans are able to engage in Department of Veterans Affairs care for identified conditions (Department of Defense 2014b).

Recurrent, mandated medical and mental health screening affords service members opportunities to identify medical and mental health needs resulting in referral to appropriate services. Though periodic assessments are conducted within the primary care, non-specialty clinics, there is a body of evidence supporting both screening and treatment of behavioral health conditions, including post-traumatic stress disorder (PTSD), within primary clinics. When utilized to maximum evidence-based scope, military treatment facility primary care behavioral health service efficiently provides behavioral health care, especially when geographic barriers or specialty behavioral health service unavailability are considered (Cigrang et al. 2015).

Once enrolled in mental health services, regardless of service affiliation, military beneficiaries are assessed and treated in accordance with professional clinical practice guidelines. The American Psychiatric Association's

Diagnostic Statistical Manual (*DSM*) is the standard classification and nomenclature for mental health diagnoses mandated for all military treatment facility mental health providers (Assistant Secretary of Defense for Health Affairs 2013). Further providing consistency across the care continuum, the Department of Defense and Department of Veterans Affairs continue collaborative clinical strides through standardizing practice guidelines, ensuring consistent, evidence-based, quality mental health treatment. DoD-VA clinical practice guidelines, including for post-traumatic stress disorder, substance use disorders, depression, concussion, and bipolar disorders, provide clinical consistency across the vast DoD-VA system of care while setting mental health clinical benchmarks for thousands of mental health providers treating military and veteran beneficiaries (Department of Veterans Affairs and Department of Defense 2012). In addition to assessing and treating mental health diagnoses, military treatment facility providers, independent of affiliated branch, assess the capability for continued military service at every appointment. Military treatment facility providers must continually balance the clinical needs of the service member with the needs of the military (Ritchie 2014).

Each service possesses specific medical and mental health policies contoured to ensure readiness for unique branch-specific missions. For instance, the Air Force's policies for medical retention and disposition of airmen are relatively more specific regarding flight status considerations, while the Navy's retention policies are relatively more specific regarding considerations for nuclear submarine missions and marine warfare. These necessary service-specific medical retention variances may result in inconsistencies across service branches, including a provider's medical retention determination timeline, length or type of treatment trial influenced by mission, and variability between services regarding disqualifying treatments and diagnoses. In effect, service members with similar diagnoses and clinical presentations may receive different service retention dispositions by their mental health provider based upon branch policy, the service member's assigned mission, and unique branch needs.

As a general unifying rule, if a service member is engaged in medical or behavioral services requiring limitations for duty or deployment for over 12 months or if the treated diagnosis will not sufficiently improve to meet mission within 12 months, the service member is referred to a medical board for medical disposition from the military (Department of Defense 2014a). Once a provider determines that a service member does not meet service-specific retention standards based on specific retention policies, the service member is referred to the integrated disability evaluation system (IDES). During the IDES process, a determination will be made if the diagnosis is service connected, meaning the diagnosis was caused by or exacerbated by military service. The National Center for Veterans Analysis and Statistics reports a 60% increase of service-connected disabilities among veterans between 1990 and 2014, accounting for nearly 4 million of the 22 million veterans carrying a service-connected disability (Department of Veterans Affairs 2014). The increase of service-connected behavioral health casualties resulted in an immediate and critical shortage in military behavioral health capabilities.

Expanding Military Behavioral Health Requirements After Protracted Combat Operations

With the eclipse of combat operations in Iraq and Afghanistan, a relatively paradoxical increase of behavioral health requirements by the active duty force developed despite a reduction in force since 2012 (Table 7.1). Though the active duty force has decreased 13.6% from 2005 to 2015, the population diagnosed with a behavioral health diagnosis has increased by 9%. In 2015, 20.7% of the active duty force (307,633 service members) carried a behavioral health diagnosis, with the Army representing over 50% of all diagnosed members, and 28% of active duty land forces carrying a behavioral health

Table 7.1 Active Duty Service Member (ADSM) population diagnosed with a mental health disorder by military service, fiscal years 2005–2015 by fiscal year (DoD Deployment Health Clinical Center, April 2016)

Military service	Prevalence	2005	2006	2007	2008	2009	2010	2011	2012	2013	2014	2015
All	Mental health cases	203,319	227,755	263,217	318,450	328,968	343,889	360,244	366,613	351,402	327,852	307,633
	ADSM pop	1,719,753	1,632,373	1,623,462	1,646,538	1,686,521	1,708,575	1,678,487	1,636,693	1,591,669	1,552,467	1,486,438
	Percent diagnosed	11.8%	14%	16.2%	19.3%	19.5%	20.1%	21.5%	22.4%	22.1%	21.1%	20.7%
Army	Mental health cases	98,856	115,728	140,393	176,820	183,081	193,444	195,254	200,029	189,751	176,421	163,428
	ADSM pop	715,833	659,116	673,253	711,960	741,327	755,924	735,698	708,356	674,998	640,996	601,939
	Percent diagnosed	13.8%	17.6%	20.9%	24.8%	24.7%	25.6%	26.5%	28.2%	28.1%	27.5%	27.2%
Air Force	Mental health cases	48,029	51,651	56,857	67,467	66,916	66,645	69,003	67,490	65,009	61,693	57,893
	ADSM pop	409,765	394,562	384,338	369,867	372,252	380,260	377,459	375,841	374,405	367,602	349,144
	Percent diagnosed	11.7%	13.1%	14.8%	18.2%	18%	17.5%	18.3%	18%	17.4%	16.8%	16.6%
Marine Corps	Mental health cases	16,565	18,736	21,766	26,246	29,980	33,260	38,687	41,124	39,190	34,780	32,443
	ADSM pop	201,331	195,961	195,385	205,135	215,552	218,169	213,638	209,961	204,099	200,217	191,613
	Percent diagnosed	8.2%	9.6%	11.1%	12.8%	13.9%	15.2%	18.1%	19.6%	19.2%	17.4%	16.9%
Navy	Mental health cases	39,869	41,640	44,201	47,917	48,991	50,540	57,300	57,970	57,452	54,958	53,869
	ADSM pop	392,824	382,733	370,486	359,586	357,390	354,222	351,683	342,535	338,167	343,661	343,742
	Percent diagnosed	10.1%	10.9%	11.9%	13.3%	13.7%	14.3%	16.3%	16.9%	17%	16%	15.7%

diagnosis (DoD Deployment Health Clinical Center 2016a). The total number of direct care mental health-related outpatient visits among Active Duty Service Members (ADSMs) increased by 263% from fiscal year 2005 (935,608) through fiscal year 2012 (2,460,552), and subsequently decreased through fiscal year 2015 (2,288,219). The mean number of mental health-related outpatient visits among Active Duty Service Members with at least one mental health-related outpatient visit steadily rose from fiscal year 2005 (5.07) through fiscal year 2015 (8.14). However, the median number of mental health-related outpatient visits only increased slightly, from two in fiscal year 2005 to three in fiscal year 2015. The discrepancy between mean and median suggests a small subset of Active Duty Service Members utilize a disproportionately high number of mental health-related outpatient services compared to the remainder of the Active Duty Service Member population seeking mental health care (DoD Deployment Health Clinical Center 2016b). Additionally, the total number of direct care mental health-related inpatient stays rose from 8,958 in fiscal year 2005 to 12,663 in fiscal year 2011, declining to 11,816 in fiscal year 2015 (DoD Deployment Health Clinical Center 2016b).

The military behavioral health system, maximally extended from years of supporting protracted combat operations and inundated with the associated behavioral health casualties of these operations, had to evolve. While the acute and emergent medical service requirements of direct combat diminished, the hidden behavioral health wounds of many service members festered, becoming late casualties. This paradoxical phenomenon of shrinking forces but increased behavioral health requirements forced the services, specifically the Army in scope, to completely change its process of identifying, assessing, treating, and dispositioning service members with behavioral health needs. Without doing so, and with dwindling resources in the wake of combat operations, the behavioral health mission was unsustainable.

Department of Defense Example of Behavioral Health Evolution: Army Behavioral Health System of Care

Though military service provides differing levels of behavioral health support, they are required to supply a general framework for behavioral health services, including imbedded behavioral health providers in primary care clinics (Department of Defense 2013c). In 2012, the Army, facing the brunt of readiness issues associated with behavioral health casualty during early Operation Iraqi Freedom/Operation Enduring Freedom conflicts, aggressively developed sweeping modifications to its Behavioral Health System of Care (BHSOC) in an effort to curb critical readiness issues associated with behavioral health-related illnesses (Headquarters, US Army Medical Command 2010).

To capstone its rapid behavioral health (BH) evolution, Army Medical Command initiated the Behavioral Health Service Line (BHSL), a standardized system of care designed to identify, prevent, treat, and track behavioral health issues affecting soldiers and other beneficiaries (United States Army Medical Command 2013). Consistent with an Operating Company Model (OCM), the BHSL enhances behavioral health care through an enterprise-wide approach to the delivery of existing and emerging behavioral health programs. In effect, the Army ensured that commanders, soldiers, and beneficiaries, regardless of location, were offered standardized, readiness-oriented services with the same clinical nomenclature. This franchised approach simplifies and streamlines behavioral health services for beneficiaries and commanders with limited resources during a highly kinetic and turbulent time (Department of Defense 2015b).

The Army Behavioral Health Service Line includes 12 integrated behavioral health enterprise programs within the Behavioral Health System of Care (Fig. 7.1). The Army BHSOC operates as a single behavioral health system supporting the readiness of the force by promoting health, identifying behavioral health issues early in the course of the illness, delivering evidence-based treatment, fully leveraging other members of the Army community, and monitoring efficiency and

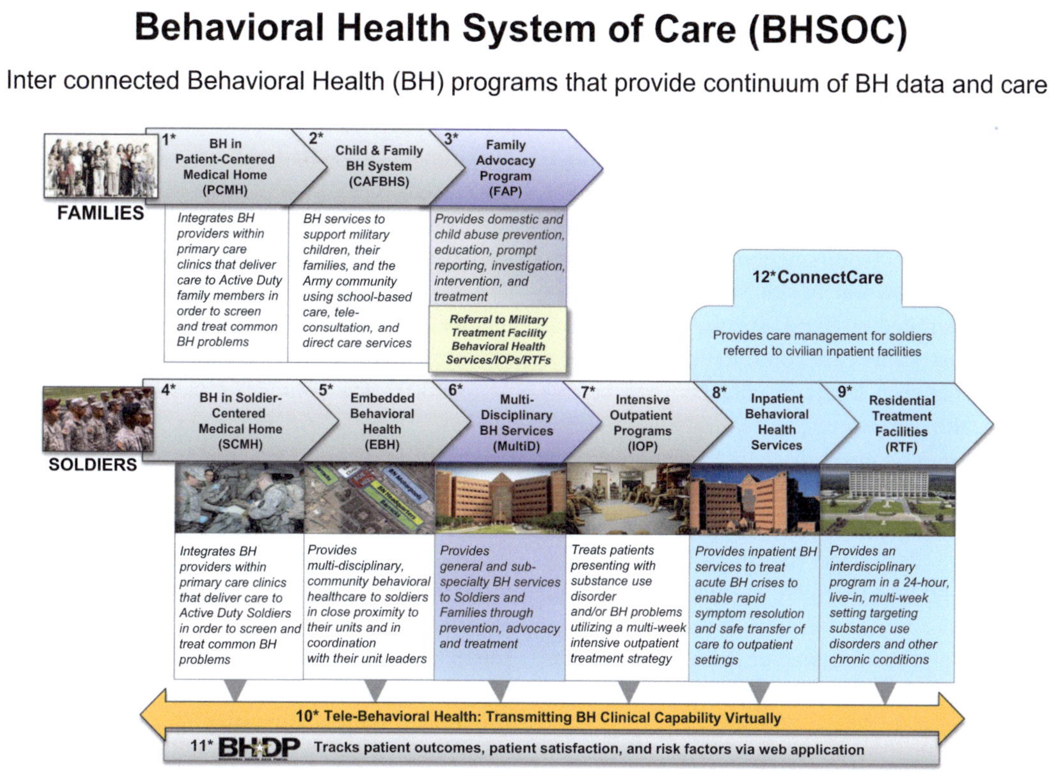

Fig. 7.1 US Army Behavioral Health Service Line (BHSL) structure (Office of the US Army Surgeon General, Behavioral Health Division 2017)

effectiveness through standardized metrics (United States Army Medical Command 2013). This multi-access system is incremental, providing basic psychoeducation, screening, and routine treatment in primary care settings to the most advanced residential and treatment modalities available at tertiary centers. Through the Embedded Behavioral Health (EBH) program, the Army BHSL is nested in the operational framework providing both direct care and community health assessment to best enable a ready force (Department of the Army 2012). By integrating key aspects of behavioral health, including inpatient, outpatient, substance use disorder, domestic violence, and community partners under one command and control mechanism, the Army BHSL essentially constructed a unique, truly comprehensive system of communicating behavioral health capabilities surrounding the soldier and his or her family, maximizing limited resources, and promoting a maximally ready force.

With more soldiers receiving care in the outpatient setting, behavioral health conditions are managed earlier, before crises occur. Soldiers required 67,000 fewer inpatient bed days for all types of behavioral health conditions in 2016, as compared to 2012 (approx. 41% decrease), due in part to improvements in outpatient services, intensive outpatient services, and case management (Office of the US Army Surgeon General, Behavioral Health Division 2017).

However, as discussed previously, behavioral health capabilities at each Army installation vary based on the population served and the installation's associated missions, among other factors. Because most installations do not possess all levels of the Behavioral Health System of Care, collaboration within Army installations, sister services, the VA, and community partners is paramount for the wide-range of treatment requirement needs from military beneficiaries. This is especially evident with higher levels of care including intensive outpatient, inpatient, and residential modalities. In 2014 alone, there were over \$117 M worth of nonmilitary treatment facility (MTF) purchased inpatient behavioral health care for all Army beneficiaries (soldiers and families), speaking to the scope of Army-private sector behavioral health utilization. Because of the collaborative care requirement for providing full-spectrum behavioral health services, the Army BHSL instituted at BHSL-specific *connect care* program to ensure care coordination, formalize a conduit between levels of care between behavioral health care sectors, and solidify warm hand-off through active discharge planning and outpatient follow-up (Headquarters, US Army Medical Command 2014).

Though developed in 2012, the US Army BHSL continues to evolve as new requirements, limitations, and best practices develop. The Army BHSL is a prime example of the military's focus and investment in behavioral health services for its beneficiaries.

Transition of Mental Health Care from Military Treatment Facility to VA

Though not all-inclusive, service members separating from the military generally do so through three main categories: End Time of Service or ETS (either through completion of their service contract or retirement), Judicial (Uniform Code of Military Justice, UCMJ) or Nonjudicial (administrative) separations, and medical separations through the integrated disability evaluation system (IDES) process. This section discusses the advancement in programs assisting eligible service members moving from military treatment facility (MTF) behavioral health services to VA services.

As a result of increased service-connected medical separations due to prolonged conflict, the process of connecting medically separating service members to VA services became a clear necessity. Previous legacy, disability evaluation systems implemented by the Department of Defense were self-contained, with limited VA involvement. Without VA involvement during the medical fitness and disposition process, effective, timely access for needed VA medical and mental health services were potentially delayed, disrupted, or discontinued due to fractured medical services between the Department of Defense and Department of Veterans Affairs systems. Prior to the current IDES system, case management and care continuum synchronization between the military treatment facility and the VA were not codified, resulting in some medically retired service members being left to navigate complex medical systems to ensure their care was not disrupted.

In 2007, *The Report of the Department of Defense (DoD) Task Force on Mental Health* called for improved Department of Defense programs designed to secure continuity of behavioral health care services during periods of transition for service members engaged in behavioral health services. These transition periods (between installations, geographic location, or separation from service) were associated with a higher risk for treatment disengagement or deterioration of their health status. In response to the report, the Department of Defense instituted the *inTransition* program, mandating and standardizing continuity of behavioral services for eligible service members (Assistant Secretary of Defense for Health Affairs 2010).

As a result of continued VA/DoD behavioral health care delivery evolution, once a service member is enrolled in the IDES process by a military treatment facility behavioral health provider due to assessed inability to meet mission requirements, the service member is assigned a physical evaluation board liaison officer (PEBLO) charged with assisting with the evaluation process, including transition to VA services. The IDES process is standardized across services via Department of Defense Instruction (DoDI) 1332.18 and provides a vital conduit for VA assessment and engagement early in the medical disposition of the service member.

Currently, military treatment facility behavioral health providers are required to refer all service members meeting established criteria (Table 7.2) to the *inTransition* program (Assistant Secretary of Defense for Health Affairs 2010). Eligible service members can opt out after a provider enrolls the service member, but the referral is mandatory.

Table 7.2 *InTransition* eligibility (Assistant Secretary of Defense for Health Affairs 2010)

Eligible service members for the *inTransition* program
Those currently or recently engaged in behavioral health care scheduled for permanent change of duty station or an extended temporary duty station
Wounded, ill, and injured service members receiving behavioral health services returning to home station following rehabilitative care at a military treatment facility, Warrior Transition Unit, or Department of Veterans Affairs facility
Those currently or recently engaged in behavioral health care separating from active duty and transitioning to Department of Veterans Affairs or TRICARE network for continued services
Reserve Component service members being activated currently or recently engaged in behavioral health care and must transfer Department of Veterans Affairs care to a military treatment facility or TRICARE network
Service members transitioning to one location to another, including deployment, who are/have been receiving behavioral health care and who do not fall into one of the above categories

Once enrolled, the service member is assigned a transition coach responsible for delivering instruction in life skills such as stress management, problem solving, rest, nutrition, and exercise. The transition coach also provides guidance in obtaining assistance and resources in the service member's immediate area while providing expert information on behavioral health treatment options and techniques and on existing support networks and benefits. The transition coach makes recurrent contact with the enrolled service member until the service member establishes care with a behavioral health provider or until the service member requests to discontinue services. Though the *inTransition* program is not a crisis or suicide hotline, transition coaches can refer enrolled service members to emergency services when indicated (Assistant Secretary of Defense for Health Affairs 2010).

The *inTransition* program, when leveraged, maximizes available support for eligible service members with behavioral health conditions ensuring continuity of care regardless of location, service affiliation, or type of military separation and is a powerful tool for Department of Defense providers in support of beneficiaries during periods at elevated risk for treatment disruption and general health deterioration (Assistant Secretary of Defense for Health Affairs 2010). Additionally, this process provides service members separating from the military a defined conduit into continuity VA mental health services. The Department of Defense acknowledges the importance of mitigating risks associated with life transitions and established a program to supporting eligible beneficiaries' continuation of behavioral health care to the VA.

Military Treatment Facility Conclusion

Military treatment facility behavioral health sections are developing to meet the needs of the next generation of beneficiaries. Each military service focuses available, limited resources to meet the mission requirements of their respective services. With standardized, programmed, and recurrent behavioral health screening within primary care, combat movements, and upon transition between stations, the services afford service members multiple opportunities to engage in behavioral health care. Once a service member is engaged, all services provide evidence-based care in accordance with DoD/VA treatment guidelines and utilize the same diagnostic criteria to best ensure consistency within the highly dynamic behavior health medical service. Treatment is available through multiple avenues including local military treatment facilities, distant military treatment facilities, VAs, and in coordination with community behavioral health partners.

Ultimately, the intent of military behavioral health is to adequately treat and return service members to premorbid functioning. With that said, each of the services' behavioral health providers must make a readiness determination based upon the unique mission requirements of the service members seeking care. If a full return to duty is not possible due to one or several behavioral health conditions and per service regulation, military behavioral health providers make the sometimes difficult determination to refer the service member to the IDES process. Once in the IDES process, the service member continues treatment with his or her provider until final determination is made whether he or she is fit to remain in service by clinicians outside of the direct care team. This decision-making process minimizes the dualistic role of the military provider, allowing the provider to concentrate on the health and well-being of the patient and not the determination of disability.

The military behavioral health process, in general terms, requires interfaces between command, family members, unit members, and care team members on and off post while maintaining fidelity to both the service member and the operational mission. The recent explosion of behavioral health requirements, both anticipated and paradoxical, forced the services on differing levels to reevaluate, refine, and evolve behavioral health services in rapid sequence. In the broadest refinement of behavioral health operations, the Army provides one example of redesigned structure and care delivery through integration of primary care and specialty services within a behavioral health continuum to meet this need. Further military behavioral health service developments and refinement are inevitable with emboldened behavioral health focus by social, political, and military leadership.

The VA Integrated System of Mental Health Care

Up to this point, this chapter has focused on military treatment facility identification and disposition of service members with mental health diagnoses with an emphasis on the critical transition of care services from military treatment facility to the VA.[1] However, it is important to also emphasize the population of VA-eligible veterans needing mental health services who were minimally or never engaged in mental health services while in the military. Unlike military treatment facilities requiring service members to participate in recurrent screening for mental disorders, VA facilities rely on veterans' willingness and ability to access mental health services. The VA invests heavily in expanding mental health resources and accessibility for veterans with mental health needs, understanding that distance to VA specialty mental health care is a known barrier in some areas. The remainder of this chapter will focus on the current VA system of mental health care, describing expanded services to previously geographically isolated locations. The section's primary source of information is the Veterans Health Administration (VHA) Handbook 1160.01, *Uniform Mental Health Services in VA Medical Centers and Clinics*. This section primarily digests the handbook through the lens of integrated mental health services.

VA Organization

The VA is geographically organized into Veterans Integrated Service Networks (VISNs) (Fig. 7.2). Each VISN contains at least two medical centers (i.e., tertiary centers or specialty care centers). The medical centers contain outpatient clinics on-site, and there are community-based outpatient clinics (CBOCs) throughout the VISN. Community-based outpatient clinics are classified according to number of individual veterans treated per year. Very large CBOCs treat more than 10,000 individual veterans per year. Large CBOCs treat 5,000–10,000 individual veterans per year. Mid-sized CBOCs treat 1,500–5,000 individual veterans per year, and small CBOCs treat fewer than 1,500 individual veterans per year. As will be discussed later, the CBOC classification is associated with respective mental health services.

In terms of scope, there are 1,211 CBOCs aligned with 144 VA hospitals providing care to roughly nine million VA-eligible beneficiaries (Department of Veterans Affairs 2016). Because veterans typically seek routine care at the location closest to their homes with referral to a larger clinic or medical center as needed, this medical system configuration is designed to provide a

[1] To this point, the medical section associated with the treatment of mental health illness has been referred to as "behavioral health" services. This nomenclature is military specific and, for all intents and purposes of this chapter, is interchangeable with "mental health" services, the VA's preferred nomenclature.

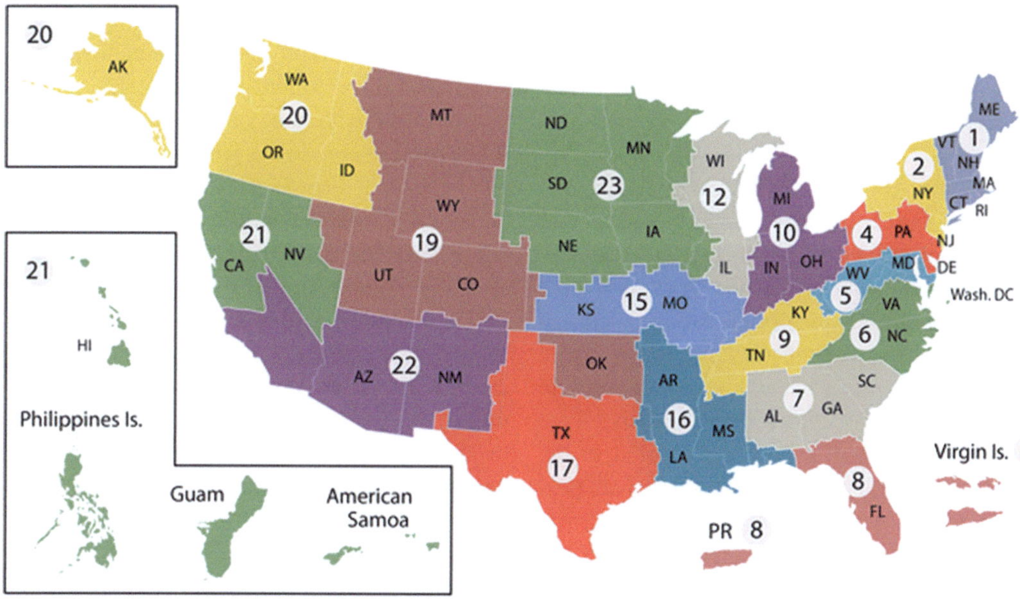

Fig. 7.2 Graphic Depiction of VA Veterans Integrated Service Network (VISN) organization and service areas (US Department of Veterans Affairs 2015b)

wheel-and-spoke model, maximizing limited medical and behavioral health services.

On the seventh year anniversary of the terrorist attacks on 9/11, the Department of Veterans Affairs introduced Veterans Health Administration (VHA) Handbook 1160.01, *Uniform Mental Health Services in VA Medical Centers and Clinics*, specifying the mental health services that VA hospitals and clinics are required to offer to veterans and their families, depending on the size and type of VA hospital or clinic. This manual essentially standardized mental health resources across the VA mental health continuum and provided guiding principles for VISN leadership focusing on mental health capability outreach and access to geographically isolated veterans.

Structure of VA Mental Health Services Under Veterans Health Administration (VHA) Handbook 1160.01

VHA Handbook 1160.01 integrated mental health within the VISN leadership structure by requiring a mental health professional in each VISN's primary decision-making body. Additionally, each VA medical center was required to establish and maintain a Mental Health Executive Council responsible for proposing strategies to improve care and consulting with management to improve treatment programs, coordinating communication among and between various departments and specialty mental health programs, and reviewing the mental health impact of facility-wide policies. The VA's intent is that mental health professional presence within VA clinical management structures will ensure mental health consideration and integration within medical service planning, implementation, and delivery.

Community outreach is also a focus of the VA mental health reorganization. Each VISN and VA medical center appoints a mental health staff member as a liaison with state, county, and local mental health systems ensuring coordination of VA activities with those of other public mental health and mental health systems. This requirement prioritizes mental health outreach and education and provides an avenue toward community understanding of available resources in support of veteran mental health.

Clinically, VHA Handbook 1160.01 integrates behavioral health within primary care and interdisciplinary medical and mental health settings. VA primary care clinics use Patient Aligned Care Teams (PACTs) to provide the veteran's health care. Patient Aligned Care Teams are led by the Patient Aligned primary care provider and include a mental health provider as a consultant to the primary care team. Mental health providers on primary care teams offer guidance to primary care providers, expanding available mental health resources for veterans in the primary care setting. However, if more complex or intensive care beyond the scope of available resources in the primary care setting is needed, primary care providers refer veterans to a specialized mental health program for further treatment.

Veterans receiving care in specialty mental health clinics will still have their primary care closely coordinated with the Patient Aligned Care Team. Once referred to specialty mental health care, a veteran will have a Mental Health Treatment Coordinator (MHTC) assigned. The Mental Health Treatment Coordinator ensures continuity for veterans though their mental health care and life transitions and is responsible for the overall mental health care coordination for the veteran. Mental Health Treatment Coordinators ensure each veteran has a stable, lasting relationship with a mental health care team member who serves as a point of contact, especially during times of care transitions.

Veterans referred to specialty mental health may receive same-day assessment or make an appointment for a later date, depending on services available at the treatment location. However, mental health consultation and comprehensive assessment must occur within 14 days by policy. This policy is more readily met in some areas; however, underserved areas require support and ingenuity to meet this assessment benchmark.

To better meet the needs of remote or underserved areas, community-based outpatient clinics offer tele-behavioral health services as an option, providing timely specialty mental health consultation. Tele-behavioral health allows mental health providers located at larger VA medical centers to evaluate and provide treatment for veterans at smaller community-based VA clinics through closed-circuit video. Telemedicine provides routine outpatient mental health services for veterans who are stable enough for this modality and who do not have a cognitive, mental, or physical disorder preventing adequate participation through this service. Expansion of tele-behavioral health will provide mental health specialty services to areas previously underserved and allow access to mental health care in otherwise remote or unsupported regions of the country. In the example presented at the beginning of this chapter, SSG Mericido, who was located in the remote island territory of Guam, used telemedicine services to ensure timely specialty assessment and treatment.

The VA provides 24 h a day, 7 days a week (24/7) mental health care access as a portion of its mental health care delivery system. Emergency mental health care by an independently licensed mental health professional is available 24/7 at VA medical centers. If the VA in an area does not have a 24-h emergency room, it must provide these services through a local, non-VA hospital. Additionally, all VA medical center telephonic triage services are equipped with mental health capabilities able to direct and respond to veteran mental health concerns. VA telephonic triage services are also able to facilitate access to the National Suicide Prevention Hotline when appropriate. This ensures systemic vigilance for veterans seeking mental health services, regardless of time or location.

Similar to the Army Behavioral Health Service Line example, the structure of mental health treatment settings available for veterans based on clinical presentation provides an incremental system of mental health care delivery. The underlying intent of the system is to provide veterans with readily available and least restrictive levels of care delivery while ensuring safe, quality, evidence-based treatment.

VA Mental Health Specialty Services

As with the military, VA mental health providers are required to follow DoD/VA practice guidelines for evidence-based treatment of specific mental health disorders. The continuum of specialty behavioral health services within the VA looks similar to the US Army example, in terms of general services provided, incremental care, and primary care and treatment team collaboration (Fig. 7.3). However, due to the relatively decentralized patient population base when compared to military beneficiaries surrounding installations, the VA emphasizes outreach and expanded services providing remote mental health care. Where the military requires touch points for mental health assessment, the VA largely depends on veteran participation and independent care-seeking behavior. This is a key consideration when conceptualizing the VA mental health care continuum and why the VA invests largely in outreach programs, bringing the services as close to the veteran as possible.

One method of providing far-forward outreach to communities with high numbers of veterans is through *Vet Centers*. Currently, the VA operates 300 community-based counseling Vet Centers offering readjustment counseling services. Vet Centers provide readjustment counseling and outreach services to all veterans who served in any combat zone. Additionally, military sexual trauma counseling and bereavement counseling are also provided at Vet Centers. Services are available for family members for military-related issues, and bereavement counseling is offered for parents, spouses, and children of Armed Forces, National Guard, and Reserves personnel who died in the service of their country.

Similar to the military, the VA recognizes the importance of integration of mental health specialists within the VA mental health continuum of care. VA *Mental Health within Primary Care/Ambulatory Care* addresses routine, outpatient mental and behavioral problems within the primary care setting by leveraging mental health experts working as part of the Patient Aligned Care Team. General mental health services within this program include assessment and treatment of general mental health conditions as well as patient education, family education, and referrals as needed to inpatient and residential care programs.

VA *Outpatient Specialty Mental Health Care*, which may include telemedicine services, provides evidence-based psychiatric and psychotherapy interventions to address mental disorders or to support veterans through phase-of-life stresses. In addition to the general mental health services provided at ambulatory clinics, specialty mental health within VA medical centers provides mental health case management, psychosocial rehabilitative services (including

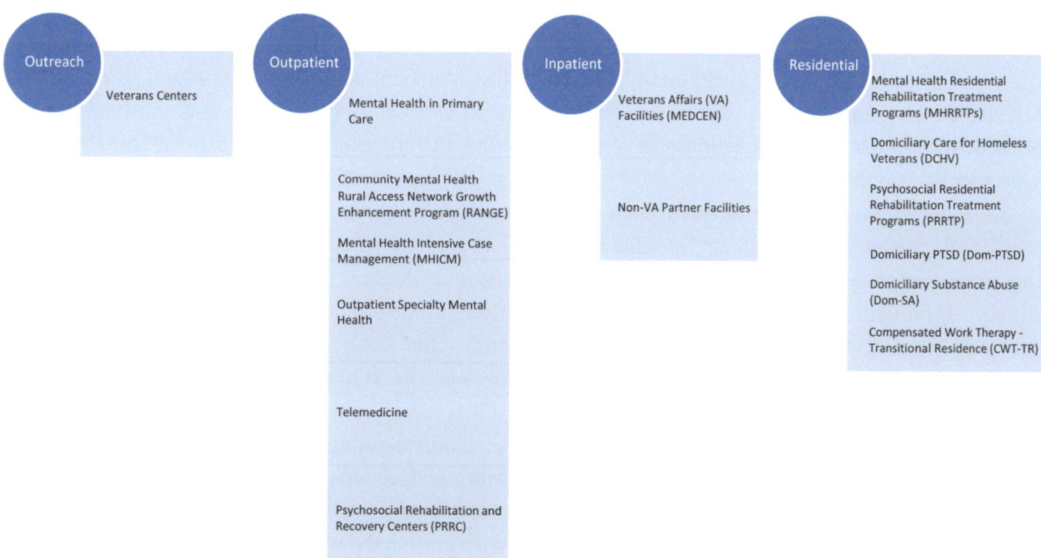

Fig. 7.3 VA mental health programs within the continuum of care

Psychosocial Rehabilitation and Recovery Centers, family psychoeducation, skills training, peer support, and supported employment), PTSD teams or specialists, military sexual trauma special clinics, homeless veteran outreach programs, and specialty substance abuse treatment services.

Community-Based Mental Health Services are provided to support the most seriously ill veterans through "on-the-street" veteran assessment and support through outreach efforts. Examples of community-based VA mental health programs include *Mental Health Intensive Case Management* (MHICM) and the *Rural Access Network Growth Enhancement Program* (RANGE). Mental Health Intensive Case Management consists of a team of mental health physicians, psychologists, nurses, and social workers who treat patients in their homes and in their community. The intent of MHICM is to reduce the need for recurrent hospitalization for veterans experiencing severe mental illness by meeting the veteran where they are and providing outpatient mental health services. While most MHICM programs are located in urban areas, Rural Access Network Growth Enhancement Program teams are of a similar composition but are primarily in rural locations with a lower concentration of veterans and veteran resources. These teams also support and assist veterans who are homeless or at risk for homelessness who may not have access to transportation to VA mental health resources. Both of these services attempt to address the most vulnerable veterans with mental health concerns.

Short-term, Inpatient Units provide a structured, safe therapeutic milieu for veterans suffering from very severe or life-threatening mental illness. Inpatient treatment typically includes medication and individual and group counseling. For veterans who receive inpatient and residential mental health treatment, VA staff or case managers will check on the veteran's progress within 1 week after hospital discharge. This evaluation might be by telephone or, possibly, in person, to ensure the veteran is safe and integrating into the outpatient setting. VA facilities will also ask the veteran to come back for a follow-up appointment no later than 2 weeks after discharge from the hospital to further promote treatment plan adherence and safety.

VA *Residential Rehabilitation Treatment Programs (RRTP)* are treatment settings for veterans with a wide range of mental health problems and/or rehabilitative care needs who would benefit from treatment in a structured environment for a period of time. Residential treatment programs include domiciliary programs. Specifically, *Mental Health Residential Rehabilitation Treatment Programs (MH RRTP)* provide a therapeutic, residential setting for veterans with a wide range of problems, illnesses, or rehabilitative care needs that can include mental health, substance use disorder, and co-occurring medical concerns. Veterans may also be homeless or unemployed or have other psychosocial needs. Residential Rehabilitation Treatment Programs help veterans work on improving their quality of life, maintaining their health, and participating in their communities. They also offer evidence-based treatment for mental illness, including PTSD and substance use disorders. There are several types of Mental Health Residential Rehabilitation Treatment Programs that can be standalone programs or larger domiciliary programs (DOM) where several programs are located in one location (Table 7.3).

Psychosocial Rehabilitation and Recovery Centers (*PRRC*) are a specialized component of the VA mental health continuum for veterans with serious mental illness and significant problems in functioning. Psychosocial Rehabilitation and Recovery Centers are outpatient programs assisting veterans with serious mental illness to learn to more fully participate in and integrate into their communities. Psychosocial Rehabilitation and Recovery Centers treat veterans with severe mental illnesses, like major depression, schizophrenia, bipolar disorder, and schizoaffective disorder.

Understanding the importance of financial stability and occupation, the VA provides *Supported Work Settings (SWS)* programs assisting veterans with joining the workforce and improving function within their community. Though not a specific mental health treatment modality, occupational

Table 7.3 Mental Health Residential Rehabilitation Treatment Programs (MH RRTP)

MH RRTP program	Program description
Domiciliary Care for Homeless Veterans (DCHV)	Provides a 24/7 structured and supportive residential treatment environment for veterans who are homeless
General Domiciliary (General Dom) or Psychosocial Residential Rehabilitation Treatment Programs (PRRTP)	Provide residential care for the general veteran population, treating medical and psychiatric problems, substance use disorders, PTSD, and homelessness. General Doms and PRRTPs provide a 24/7 structured and supportive residential environment as a part of treatment
Domiciliary PTSD (Dom PTSD) or Post-traumatic Stress Disorder Residential Rehabilitation Treatment Program (PTSD-RRTP)	Provide residential care for veterans with PTSD including Military Sexual Trauma (MST). Both Dom PTSD and PTSD-RRTPs provide a 24/7 structured and supportive residential environment with evidence-based treatment for PTSD
Domiciliary Substance Abuse (Dom SA) or Substance Abuse Residential Rehabilitation Treatment Program (SARRTP)	Provide residential care to veterans with substance use disorders. Dom SA and SARRTPs provide a 24/7 structured and supportive residential environment as a part of specialized substance use disorder treatment
Compensated Work Therapy-Transitional Residence (CWT-TR)	Offers therapeutic work-based residential rehabilitation services designed to help veterans return to their communities. Veterans participating in CWT-TR live in transitional residences and are enrolled in compensated work therapy working directly on employment goals

and community return to functioning is a cornerstone of effective mental health treatment. VA Supported Work Settings services provided in the community, rather than in mental health treatment or rehabilitation settings, include *Transitional Work Experience*, which offers assignments in businesses helping veterans to function in the work environment and to reintegrate into the community, and *Supported Employment*, which provides veterans with job-support services to help them obtain and maintain a job.

However, *incentive therapy*, a pre-vocational program for veterans to perform work at some VA Medical Centers, provides a more structured vocational experience for occupational rehabilitation. Incentive therapy provides veterans the ability to improve occupational skills in a controlled, therapeutic environment designed to construct a bridge from unemployment to employability.

As discussed earlier in this section, the VA mental health service delivery construct is a wheel-and-spoke model, with full-spectrum services available at medical centers and contoured services available at the community-based outpatient clinics. Per VHA Handbook 1160.01, each echelon of care is required to maintain a minimal amount of mental health services, with larger facilities responsible for a wider array of mental health services. Though smaller community-based outpatient clinics are not required to carry the full spectrum of mental health outpatient services on-site, it is important to note that the VA requires the mental health capabilities either through telemedicine or by community partnerships (Table 7.4).

In addition to providing a general structure for the VA continuum of care settings, VHA Handbook 1160.01 also outlines considerations for special subpopulations through services for families and couples, elderly and geriatric services, gender and cultural sensitive services, and services supporting those affected by military sexual trauma. The VA system of care incorporates residential and inpatient programs that provide treatment to women only or that have separate tracks for men and women. Each Veterans Integrated Service Network must have residential care programs able to meet the needs of women veterans. However, the need for some types of sub-specialty care (e.g., women with PTSD) is limited, and women veterans who need these services may be referred to regional or national resources. Additionally, the VA has available resources to treat conditions associated with military sexual trauma (MST). VA medical centers are required to provide MST-specific outpatient, inpatient, and residential services to

Table 7.4 Minimal mental health services provided by VA facilities per VHA handbook 1160.01 (U.S. Department of Veterans Affairs 2012)

Mental health problem	Medical center	Very large community-based outpatient clinic (CBOC) (more than 10,000 veterans per year)	Large CBOC (5,000–10,000 veterans per year)	Mid-sized CBOC (1,500–5,000 veterans per year)	Small CBOC (fewer than 1,500 veterans per year)
Post-traumatic stress disorder (PTSD)	Specialized outpatient programs; evidence-based talk therapies; medications on-site	Specialized outpatient programs; evidence-based talk therapies; medications on-site	Evidence-based talk therapies; medications on-site or through telemedicine	Evidence-based talk therapies; medications on-site or through telemedicine	General and specialty services on-site or via telemedicine [referral to residential treatment program, VA medical center, or community services]
Schizophrenia, schizoaffective disorder, bipolar disorder, depression anxiety	General and specialty services; family services; skills training; peer support; evidence-based therapies for depression/ anxiety; larger facilities may have psychosocial rehabilitation and recovery centers (PRRCs) or Mental Health Intensive Case Management (MHICM) programs on-site	General and specialty services; family services; skills training; peer support; evidence-based therapies for depression/ anxiety [MHICM, PRRC] on-site	Majority of general and specialty services on-site or via telemedicine; evidence-based therapies for depression/ anxiety on-site or through telemedicine [referrals to VA medical center or community services]	General and specialty services on-site or via telemedicine; referral to residential treatment program, VA medical center, or community services; evidence-based therapies for depression/ anxiety, on-site or through telemedicine	General and specialty services on-site or via telemedicine; referral to residential treatment program, VA medical center, or community services
Substance use disorders (alcohol, drugs, prescription medications, tobacco)	General and evidence-based specialty services; inpatient or outpatient detoxification; opioid treatment programs providing methadone at some medical centers	Specialized outpatient treatment programs with evidence-based therapies and medication management on-site	Specialized outpatient programs; evidence-based therapies on-site or through telemedicine	Specialized outpatient programs; evidence-based therapies on-site or through telemedicine	General and specialty services on-site or via telemedicine; referral to residential treatment program, VA medical center, or community services
Homelessness	Emergency or transitional housing with support services; homelessness outreach specialist and community links	Emergency or transitional housing with support services; homelessness outreach specialist and community links	Referrals to community providers for emergency or transitional housing, and/or basic emergency services	Referrals to community providers for emergency or transitional housing, and/or basic emergency services	Referrals to community providers for emergency or transitional housing, and/or basic emergency services

support veterans. The VA ensures these veteran subpopulations, as well as others, receive the best possible services and attention to the unique experience or needs associated with their population.

Alternative Access to VA Mental Health Services

Though many veterans may receive mental health consultation via a referral by primary care or other medical services, the VA developed several other methods designed for ready availability, routing in-need veterans toward mental health services. These programs further improve mental health treatment and support access for veterans. To meet the needs of veterans with metal health concerns, many of whom may be in acute crisis and remote, the VA implemented and maintains active mechanisms ensuring medical vigilance (Table 7.5).

Conclusion

The Department of Defense and the Department of Veterans Affairs continue to evolve to meet the mental needs of the next generation of service members and veterans. As an example, the VA announced further support for expanding partnerships with community mental health organizations and providers, further enhancing access to services for in-need beneficiaries. Integration of mental health resources at every level of the care continuum, coupled with advancements in telemedicine and alternative mental health access points, provide improved access to mental health services for service members and veterans who previously may not have engaged in services due to stigma or mental health service unavailability at their locations. Investment in mental health case management, with specific attention to periods of transition and to those with serious mental illness or significant psychosocial challenges, provides service members and veterans warm

Table 7.5 VA mental health crisis and alternative resources within the continuum of care

Mental health resource	Description	Access
Veterans crisis line	Connects veterans in crisis and their families and friends with Department of Veterans Affairs responders through a confidential toll-free hotline	The service is available through phone call at 1-800-273-8255, on the internet at www.Veteranscrisisline.et, or via text at 838255
		This crisis line is available 24 h a day, 7 days a week, 365 days a year
Coaching into care resources	Free and confidential telephone coaching service designed to support family members and loved ones who are supporting veterans potentially suffering from mental illness. It helps callers develop ways to talk with the veteran about their concerns and about treatment options	Callers can reach the service at (888) 823-7458 or at www.mirecc.va.gov/coaching
VA general information hotline	For those veterans who believe that they may have a mental health condition or concern, and have previously not been engaged in mental health services, this hotline can assist them in determining which clinic or VA center is best situated to support the identified need	The hotline number is 1-800-827-1000 and VA clinic location services are also available at the VA website www.va.gov

hand-offs between treatment locations. In turn, this continuum reduces care disruption for at-risk populations, improving the continuity of treatment for veterans. Continued expansion of intranet and smart phone technology will bring more mental health resources to beneficiaries and their families, providing patients access to mental health-related educational applications and treatment options in the convenience of their homes.

The enhancement of mental health services through technology is causing tremendous strides in mental health accessibility, and technological expansion is already supporting veterans and their care teams, especially in areas with limited resources. This enhancement represents a new frontier in military and veteran mental health treatment that the continuum of care is only beginning to tap.

Vigilance between Department of Defense and Department of Veterans Affairs mental health leaders will allow continued expansion and development of efficient, contoured, and seamless mental health care delivery systems in a dynamic and vast population with varying and unique needs. A collaborative approach between departments, with sharing of information and resources, will continue the positive trajectory of this comprehensive, patient-centered system of mental health care.

Key Concepts

1. The Department of Defense/Department of Veterans Affairs (DoD/VA) continuum of care begins with prevention and outreach services intended to identify mental health needs early, reducing illness impact and improving clinical outcomes.
2. Department of Defense and VA providers practice evidence-based medicine by prioritizing clinical practice guidelines and ensuring beneficiaries receive safe, quality mental health services.
3. Transitions from service to the VA system of care are a known vulnerability with the potential of in-need beneficiaries falling through the cracks. The Department of Defense and VA provide multiple resources designed to bridge active duty and VA mental health services.
4. VA Mental Health resources are integrated in Patient Aligned Care Teams (PACTs) within primary care, while telemedicine provides mental health services in remote VA locations.
5. The Department of Defense and VA continue to adapt services to meet the needs of service members, veterans, and their families with development of internal and community partnerships as new opportunities expanding services.

References

Assistant Secretary of Defense for Health Affairs (2010) ASD(HA) memo: the Department of Defense in Transition Program

Assistant Secretary of Defense for Health Affairs (2013) ASD(HA) memo: transitioning to the fifth edition of the diagnostic and statistical manual of mental disorders

Cigrang J, Rauch S, Mintz J, Brundige A, Avila L, Bryan C et al (2015) Treatment of active duty military with PTSD in primary care: a follow-up report. J Anxiety Disord 36:110–114

Commission on Care (2016) Final report on the commission on care. Commission on Care, Washington, DC

Department of Defense (2013a) DoDI 6490.04: mental health evaluations of members of the military services

Department of Defense (2013b) DoDI 6490.12: mental health assessments for service members deployed in connection with a contingency operation

Department of Defense (2013c) DoDI 6490.15: integration of Behavioral Health Personnel (BHP) services into Patient-Centered Medical Home (PCMH) primary care and other primary care service settings

Department of Defense (2014a) DoDI 1332.18: Disability Evaluation System (DES)

Department of Defense (2014b) DoDI 6490.10: transferring Family Advocacy Program (FAP) and behavioral healthcare during Permanent Change of Station (PCS) and Expiration of Time in Service (ETS)

Department of Defense (2015a) DoDI 1304.26: qualification standards for enlistment, appointment, and induction

Department of Defense (2015b) DoD/VA Report to the Congress in Response to Senate Report 113–44, pg. 133, Accompanying S. 1197, the National Defense Authorization Act for Fiscal Year 2014: mental health counselors for service members, Veterans, and their families. Under Secretary of the Army for Personnel and Readiness

Department of Defense (2016) DoDI 6200.06: periodic health evaluations

Department of Defense Deployment Health Clinical Center (2016a) Mental health care utilization among active duty service members. http://www.pdhealth.mil/clinical/psychological-health-numbers/mental-health-care-utilization-among-active-duty-service/outpatient-visits-2689. Accessed 4 Oct 2016

Department of Defense Deployment Health Clinical Center (2016b). Mental health disorder prevalence among active duty service members. http://www.pdhealth.mil/clinical/psychological-health-numbers/mental-health-disorder-prevalence-among-active-duty-service. Accessed 4 Oct 2016

Department of the Army (2012) HQDA EXORD 236–12: army implementation of Behavioral Health System of Care (BHSOC) Embedded Behavioral Health (EBH). Pentagon Telecommunications Center, Washington, DC

Department of Veterans Affairs (2011) Veteran Population Projection Model – VetPop2011. Washington, DC

Department of Veterans Affairs (2012) Guide to VA mental health services. Veterans Health Administration, Office of Patient Care Services, Mental Health Services, Washington, DC

Department of Veterans Affairs (2014) Veteran population projection model – VetPop2014. Department of Veterans Affairs, Washington, DC

Department of Veterans Affairs (2015a) Office of Public Health Highlights report. Department of Veterans Affairs, Washington, DC

Department of Veterans Affairs (2015b) Veterans health administration locations. http://www.va.gov/directory/guide/division.asp?dnum=1. Accessed 4 Oct 2016

Department of Veterans Affairs (2016) VA pocket card, 4th Quarter FY16. http://www.va.gov/vetdata/docs/pocketcards/fy2016q4.pdf. Accessed 4 Oct 2016

Department of Veterans Affairs and Department of Defense (2012) Department of Veterans Affairs and Department of Defense Joint Executive Committee Joint Strategic Plan Fiscal Years 2013–2015

Headquarters, US Army Medical Command (2010) Operations order 10–70: USAMEDCOM comprehensive behavioral health system of care campaign plan. Office of the Surgeon General US Army Medical Command, Ft. Sam Houston

Headquarters, US Army Medical Command (2014) MEDCOM/OTSG policy 14–058: absent and sick accountability and management of soldiers receiving inpatient care outside of military treatment facilities. Office of the Surgeon General, US Army Medical Command, Washington DC

Mental Health Advisory Team (2007) Mental health advisory team IV: operation Iraqi Freedom. Office of the Surgeon General, US Army Medical Command, Washington, DC

Office of the US Army Surgeon General, Behavioral Health Division (2017) Behavioral Health Service Line Home page. https://bhsl.army.mil. Accessed 27 February 2017

Ritchie E (ed) (2014) Forensic and ethical issues in military behavioral health. Borden Institute, Office of the Surgeon General & AMEDD Center and School, Fort Sam Houston

United States Army Medical Command (2013) MEDCOM policy 13–059: behavioral health service line policy (BHSL), consolidated behavioral health (BH). Office of the Surgeon General, US Army Medical Command, Fort Sam Houston

Screening for Mental Health Disorders in the Military

8

Daniel J. Lee, Christopher H. Warner, and Charles W. Hoge

History

The first recorded instances of mental health screening occurred in the Napoleonic French Army when French physicians began screening their soldiers to identify "nostalgia" (Rosen 1975). The first major military psychological screening efforts for the United States began during World War I when mental health professionals instituted a testing and interview process to identify those mentally suitable for military and to estimate intellectual functioning for selecting particular military duties (McGuire 1994). Of note, these initial efforts were based on a belief that psychiatric symptoms and illnesses reflected a "weak personality" and that individuals with psychoneurotic illness were not normal and not capable of marshaling defenses needed to serve during war. Some of these perspectives may still influence stigma toward mental health conditions in the military today (McGuire 1994). While these early screening methods are viewed as failures, they did create a belief that psychological screening could be effective in predicting military performance potential, leading to many other screening efforts (Page 1996).

During the early stages of World War II, Harry Stack Sullivan was appointed as a psychiatric consultant to create a comprehensive screening system. His initial efforts were viewed as successful; however, as the war continued and there remained a demand for an increasing number of troops, attitudes about the effectiveness of the screening methods changed. By late in World War II, Sullivan's methods were viewed as ineffective in accurately predicting the resilience of individuals to withstand the risks of war and believed to result in a substantial and excessive loss of suitable soldiers. During post-World War II, mental health screening methods were modified to what remains the present-day method of identifying and disqualifying only gross psychiatric disorders (Glass et al.1966). Debate remains focused on which pre-existing conditions contribute to combat zone attrition (Warner et al. 2008). The exception to this method involves certain highly specialized duties such as special forces, nuclear material handlers, and high-level security clearance positions in which mental health providers are asked to determine the psychological fitness for these specific tasks as part of extensive vetting and training processes (Stokes and Jones 1995).

D.J. Lee (✉)
Division of Psychiatry Products, Center for Drug Evaluation and Research, U.S. Food and Drug Administration, Silver Spring, MD, USA
e-mail: Daniel.Lee2@fda.hhs.gov

C.H. Warner
US Army Medical Department Activity – Fort Stewart, Fort Stewart, GA, USA

C.W. Hoge
Center for Psychiatry and Neuroscience, Walter Reed Army Institute of Research, Silver Spring, MD, USA

L.W. Roberts, C.H. Warner (eds.), *Military and Veteran Mental Health*,
https://doi.org/10.1007/978-1-4939-7438-2_8

In more recent years, attention has focused on mental health and medical screening in relation to a specific deployment. This focus began in the wake of the Persian Gulf War after US service members who deployed to the Arabian Peninsula began complaining of a number of medically unexplained symptoms that became known as Gulf War Syndrome (Hyams et al. 2002). By the late 1990s, congressional requirements mandated post-deployment screening for medical conditions and environmental exposures, and the initial standardized instruments were developed. Over the course of the next decade, the screening tools and administration timelines were modified significantly based on lessons learned from the US peacekeeping efforts in the Balkans and subsequently the wars in Iraq and Afghanistan. Today, deployment assessments are aimed at identifying service members with post-traumatic stress disorder (PTSD), depression, generalized anxiety, and substance use disorders. They are provided both before and after deployment and utilize screening tools validated largely in primary care settings. There are ongoing efforts to increase and refine screening methods throughout the system of care.

Case Study: Part 1

Juan Jiménez (pseudonym) grew up in one of the roughest areas of Los Angeles, CA. By age 13, he had directly witnessed the deaths of two friends from gang violence. Symptoms of depression and PTSD began in the aftermath of their deaths. His school referred him for evaluation when his academic performance fell significantly. Juan was seen for weekly counseling sessions and took an antidepressant for roughly 9 months before dropping out of treatment abruptly. His mother worked two jobs to support the family and was not around for the majority of his childhood. Juan fell in with a gang from age 14 to 16 but turned his life around after a number of his friends were arrested and he realized that he was likely to end up in more serious trouble in the future. Upon finishing high school, he decided to join the military. At his accession physical, he reported no behavioral health treatment history based on his desire to leave Los Angeles and his recruiter's casual suggestion that he might want to leave mention of his prior behavioral health treatment off the application. Juan had too much to lose to report honestly and was concerned that, had he reported honestly, he would likely have been blocked from joining the military.

Disqualifying Medical Conditions and Incentives to Conceal Disqualifying Conditions

While the Army, Navy, Air Force, and Marine Corps each have different regulations governing disqualifying medical conditions, they each originate from an overarching Department of Defense (DoD) policy (DoD Directive 6130.4). The goal is to ensure that individuals are not accessed into the military who have a condition that would make them unqualified for deployment to a remote or austere environment where medication access and specialty care might be limited (e.g., epilepsy or bipolar disorder). However, there are many exclusions that do not necessarily involve chronic conditions or conditions with poor prognoses. For example, exclusion because of a history of an uncomplicated concussion is likely to lead to exclusions of well-qualified applicants who may have received concussions during high school sports. The regulations are generally written to ensure clarity about minimum standards for health (usually referred to as *fitness* in military language) for all recruits in a way that promotes efficiency in moving individuals through the standardized process. When there are questions about potentially unfitting conditions, a waiver process provides a second set of eyes on a particular recruit before entry into the military is granted.

Although new recruits sign documents indicating that the military may obtain medical records and prosecute them for dishonest answers, the system ultimately depends on the willingness of recruits to report their prior medical history honestly and thoroughly. As seen in this chapter's case study, the incentives to join the military, coupled with the concern about potential exclusion, may lead to less-than-honest reporting during accession. Furthermore, there are sometimes incentives at the level of the military recruiter to achieve recruitment goals. Incentives and desires for joining the military are myriad, including career goals, funding for college, escaping a challenging home situation, traveling the world, gaining friends or a new family, making oneself a better person, increasing social status, continuing a family tradition, gaining financial stability, providing health care to a sick spouse or child, improving health, increasing self-esteem, and/or being a part of something larger than oneself. A point that cannot be stressed more strongly is that the military represents far more than a job to most service members. It is a unique culture, a series of values and ideals, and a family. As such, there is often a high level of concern about stigma from one's peers or supervisors, among other reasons to not report a condition. Unless a condition is reported, screening clinicians have no clear way to seek out civilian treatment records. This process is further complicated by the fact that the consequences for not reporting prior mental health conditions are largely unenforceable. It is difficult to incentivize honest reporting of medical conditions without the uniform availability of corresponding medical records.

An understanding of military accession standards is important for all mental health providers who work with teenage or young adult populations, as many of these youths may be interested in including military service in their life plans. Having awareness and understanding of what is and is not feasible allow for realistic expectation setting and management. As these standards continue to develop and change, based on our medical understanding, evolving treatments, and political directives, it is important that providers know where to find out if a condition is conducive to military service. Tables 8.1and 8.2 highlight the applicable regulations and the current guidance on key mental health conditions.

Case Study: Part 2

Juan married his high school sweetheart 6 months after joining the Army and thrived in the military, making several close friends, performing well at work, and being regarded as a good solider by his command. Soon after the honeymoon, he was notified that his unit would be deploying within the next 3–6 months. The tempo of work increased dramatically as his unit began sending soldiers to deployment health and readiness clinics as part of the deployment preparation. Screenings involved questionnaires for current depression, PTSD, anxiety, and substance use, as well as prior behavioral health treatment. Juan felt a duty to his friends and did not want to let them down by not going on the deployment. He again answered every single question negatively and was rapidly cleared for deployment. A small number of his peers were blocked from deployment following the screening. They were labeled "dirtbags" and/or "broken" by other soldiers in the unit, although several of them were later able to join the deployment after some treatment.

The deployment itself was difficult, as the unit was tasked with clearing and ensuring route security of several key roads in a highly volatile and dangerous combat sector. They were involved in several major firefights that fortunately resulted in only a few minor injuries. The true danger of this assignment came from the improvised explosive devices (IEDs) that were regularly placed in and around the operationally necessary routes. Juan experienced several concussions from explosions in and around the up-armored vehicle. The worst blast, to which he would later refer as "the day I got blown up," occurred 9 months into his 15-month deployment and after he dismounted his vehicle to pull security for another vehicle that had been disabled by an IED. After this blast, he experienced several minutes of lost consciousness, followed by feeling dazed and experiencing loud tinnitus for hours afterward, in addition to the effects of a shattered eardrum. While the standard protocol involves traumatic brain injury (TBI) screening with the military acute concussion evaluation (MACE), the mission did not allow for this screening to occur, and no written account of the blast was entered into his medical record. From that time on, he was noted by peers to be continuously irritable, jumpy, paranoid, and isolative. His sleep became increasingly disrupted, and he was often seen awake during times when his team was supposed to be resting.

Upon return from deployment, Juan again answered negatively to all of the screening questions due to fear of being delayed from returning to his wife and family. However, over the next several months, he began to experience problems with hypervigilance, anger, depressed mood, sleep disturbance, fatigue, decline in work performance, and strain in his relationship with his wife. His wife began to urge him to seek treatment, which he initially refused. However, when he completed his next round of post-deployment screening at 90–180 days upon return, he reluctantly answered the depression and PTSD questions honestly, leading to specialty mental health-care referral. The treatment ultimately led to improved health and work performance, and he was able to successfully complete his enlistment contract.

Pre- and Post-deployment Screening

The need for deployment-related military mental health screening became apparent when a high percentage of service members returning from Desert Shield/Desert Storm began complaining of vague illnesses and somatic symptoms months to years after the conflict. Large-scale epidemiological studies and specialized clinics were developed to attempt to understand and mitigate these health concerns, but these analyses were hindered in part by lack of available deployment and post-deployment surveillance data. This ultimately led to the formation of the Department of Defense Deployment Health Clinical, Research, and Surveillance Centers and numerous efforts by the Department of Defense (DoD), the Department of Veteran's Affairs (VA), and the Institute of Medicine to focus on guidelines for post-deployment monitoring and management.

As a result, a prototype of the Post-Deployment Health Assessment (PDHA) was introduced in 1998. The Post-Deployment Health Assessment differed from earlier screening instruments because it included both a survey and a face-to-face interview and evaluation with a primary care provider (Hyams et al. 2002). This early Post-Deployment Health Assessment contained a total of six questions with only one focused on mental health ("During this deployment have you sought, or intend to seek, counseling or care for your mental health?") (PDHA 1999). However, research continued with expanded screening instruments in personnel deploying to the Balkans (Wright et al. 2002), and in 2003, in association with the first deployment to Iraq, the Post-Deployment Health Assessment was modified to include screening tools for depression (Patient Health Questionnaire-2) and PTSD (Primary Care PTSD) (Wright et al. 2005). This Post-Deployment Health Assessment stood as the only mandatory screen for deploying service members until 2005 when the Post-Deployment Health Re-assessment (PDHRA) was instituted 3–6 months post-deployment.

Introduced as part of the 2005 National Defense Authorization Act, the Post-Deployment Health Assessment was required for all service members 90–180 days following return from deployment (NDAA 2005). The additional

Table 8.1 Summary of behavioral health enlistment medical standards (standards of medical fitness)

	Pertinent regulation	Mood disorders	Adjustment disorder	Anxiety disorders	Psychotic disorders	Substance disorders	ADHD, learning disorders	Eating disorders	Somatoform disorders	Personality disorders	Enuresis, encopresis, sleepwalking	Dissociative disorders	Paraphilias
Department of Defense (DoD)	DoD Instruction 6130.4	Any mood disorder requiring >6 months of outpatient treatment or inpatient hospitalization or residential treatment or causes recurrent impairment is disqualified	Waiverable if recruit has been symptom-free for 3+ months	Disqualified	Disqualified	Disqualified	Waiverable if recruit can demonstrate passing academic performance without accommodation and is off all medications for 12 months	Disqualified if symptoms present after a recruit's 13th birthday and last >3 months	Disqualified	Disqualified	Disqualified if symptoms present after a recruit's 13th birthday	Disqualified	Disqualified
US Army	Army Regulation (AR) 40–501, Chap. 2												
US Navy and Marine Corps	Navy Manual of the Medical Department (NAVMED P-117), Chap. 15, section 3												
US Air Force	Air Force Instruction 48-123, Section 1A												

Table 8.2 Summary of neuropsychiatric enlistment medical standards (standards of medical fitness)

	Pertinent regulation	Mild Traumatic Brain Injury (TBI)	Moderate Traumatic Brain Injury (TBI)	Severe Traumatic Brain Injury (TBI)	Cerebrovascular incidents	Meningeal disorders	Neurodegenerative disorders	Recurrent headaches	Narcolepsy and cataplexy	Tourette's and tic disorders	Epilepsy	Other chronic conditions
Department of Defense (DoD)	DoD Instruction 6130.4	Waiverable 1 month after injury	Waiverable 2 years after injury	Disqualified	Disqualified	Disqualified	Disqualified	Disqualified if it has interfered with function in last 3 years or requires medication to manage	Disqualified	Disqualified	Disqualified unless recruit has been seizure-free for 5+ years without medications and has a normal EEG	Disqualified
US Army	Army Regulation (AR) 40–501, Chap. 2											
US Navy and Marine Corps	Navy Manual of the Medical Department (NAVMED P-117), Chap. 15, section 3											
US Air Force	Air Force Instruction 48–123, section 1A											

screening was added based on initial studies in Afghanistan and Iraq veterans, which showed that rates of service members with symptoms of PTSD increased 90 days following deployment (Bliese et al. 2004; Hoge et al. 2006; Milliken et al. 2007). These studies also identified various barriers to care, such as stigma about behavioral health conditions and seeking behavioral health care, which further influenced other behavioral health initiatives throughout the military and VA system.

During this time, multiple other initiatives and changes to the screening process were considered. Proposals included having all returning service members complete a face-to-face evaluation with a mental health provider or undergo a full mental health intake evaluation, but a 2008 study found that potential benefits of this process were outweighed by the risks, including drawing the limited number of mental health personnel away from where they were most needed in treating identified patients (Warner et al. 2008). Thus, the general process of completing the initial questionnaire and reviewing it with a primary care provider has remained intact. However, most post-deployment screening stations did add the presence of on-site or tele-available behavioral health providers to allow for immediate evaluation of behavioral health referrals, when indicated, though this was not a Department of Defense requirement (Warner et al. 2007).

Iraq and Afghanistan represented the first prolonged wartime deployment of an all-volunteer force, and the multiple deployments for many service members resulted in new challenges. As service members repeatedly deployed, media reports began asserting that military mental health and medical providers were sending mentally unfit service members into the combat zone (Chedekel and Kauffman 2006; Rogers 2006). This led to the creation of minimum mental health standards for deployment (Warner et al. 2011a). Specifically, these standards (outlined in Table 8.3) required at least 90 days of treatment (usually medication) stabilization before deployment and specified medications that precluded deployment regardless of duration of treatment (e.g., lithium, antipsychotics, and tricyclic antidepressants). One study found that when coupled with a coordination of care process, these standards were shown to be effective in reducing the incidence of mental health complications (Warner et al. 2011a).

Even with the screening timing changes as well as the addition of questions on drug/alcohol abuse and family violence, concerns remained that current efforts were insufficient, prompting Congress to require additional screening. In the 2012 National Defense Authorization Act (NDAA), lawmakers increased the frequency of screening again to the current schedule of 120 days before deployment, upon return from deployment, 90–180 days after deployment, 180–365 days after deployment, and 18–30 months after deployment (NDAA 2012). Additional screenings are also conducted on entry into the VA health-care system and prior to separation from the military.

In one study, pre-deployment behavioral health screening has been shown to be effective in its current form, provided that there is coordination of care in-theater for service members who have a stable behavioral health condition. In contrast, the effectiveness of post-deployment screening is unknown. It is not likely to be effective immediately post-deployment, based on research that has shown that service members tend to conceal behavioral health problems at that time, due to stigma, fears of not being able to go on leave after deployment, and other concerns (Hoge et al. 2006; Warner et al. 2011b). The willingness to report mental health concerns increases several months after coming home, though the effectiveness of post-deployment screening during this time period in preventing or mitigating negative health outcomes is unknown. Anecdotally, many senior noncommissioned officers and officers delay seeking treatment until retirement or separation from the military is approaching.

Primary Care Screening and Outcome Management

As noted in the previous section, post-deployment mental health screening failed to identify a large number of those service members who would benefit from mental health treatment. For example, one study showed that less than 40% of those

Table 8.3 Disqualifying health conditions with behavioral health applications and rationale for disqualification

Diagnoses, problems, or medications	Rationale for disqualification
Service members taking antipsychotics	Close follow-up unavailable; possibility of serious side effects; most conditions treated with antipsychotics disqualified from deployment; withdrawal could be temporarily disabling
Service members taking lithium	Close follow-up unavailable; possibility of serious side effects; most conditions treated with lithium disqualified from deployment; dehydration in hot climates could be fatal; proper hydration cannot be ensured in a deployed environment; withdrawal could be temporarily disabling or potentially fatal
Service members taking anticonvulsants, tricyclic antidepressants, or MAO-Is	Close follow-up unavailable; possibility of serious side effects; most conditions treated with anticonvulsants disqualified from deployment; withdrawal could be temporarily disabling or potentially fatal
Service members at significant risk of deterioration in a deployed environment	Deterioration could lead to service member becoming disabled or a risk to self and others; air evacuation not always available; deterioration could lead to multiple other service members becoming unavailable due to need to monitor disabled individual; high-stress environment, sleep disruption, and lack of control over home environment raises risk of deterioration
Service members with chronic or residual psychiatric symptoms	Risk of relapse is high; service member likely to have difficulty coping with deployed environment; service member will likely not be fully effective even with optimal monitoring and support
Service members without at least 3 months of psychiatric symptom and medication stability prior to deployment	Close follow-up unavailable; possibility of side effects or medication becoming non-effective; air evacuation not always available; risk of relapse is high; service member likely to have difficulty coping with deployed environment; service member may not be fully effective even with optimal monitoring and support; deterioration could lead to service member becoming disabled or a risk to self and others
Services members with current or a history of psychotic episodes	High-stress environment, sleep disruption, and lack of control over home environment raises risk of deterioration; consequences of a psychotic episode in a fully armed service member could be dire; air evacuation not always available
Service members with current or history of bipolar I or II disorder	High-stress environment, sleep disruption, and lack of control over home environment raises risk of deterioration; consequences of a psychotic/manic episode in a fully armed service member could be dire; air evacuation not always available
Service members with current or a history of seizures or psychosomatic conditions	High-stress environment, sleep disruption, and lack of control over home environment raises risk of sudden incapacitation; withdrawal from antiepileptics could result in sudden incapacitation; air evacuation not always available
Service members requiring durable medical equipment such as a CPAP	Electricity, equipment servicing, and equipment maintenance cannot be ensured; lack of equipment may result in incapacitation
Service members with pain disorders or phobias which prevent proper wear of helmets and body armor	Service member becomes a liability to self and rest of team
Service members with current or a history of self-mutilation, suicidal ideation, or suicide attempts	High-stress environment, sleep disruption, and lack of control over home environment raises risk of deterioration; consequences of recurrence in a fully armed service member could be dire; air evacuation not always available
Service members with current or a history of inappropriate violence, reckless behavior, or impulsiveness	Service member becomes a liability to self and rest of team
Service members currently abusing alcohol or other substances	Withdrawal may result in incapacitation or potentially be fatal; addiction may compromise judgment and reaction time

being screened honestly reported their mental health symptoms due to ongoing stigma (Warner et al. 2011b). To address this stigma, the US military began screening service members for depression, PTSD, and alcohol misuse during all primary care encounters. This initiative, which began at Fort Bragg, NC, in 2006 was initially called Re-Engineering Systems of Primary Care for PTSD and Depression in the Military or RESPECT-Mil (Engel et al. 2008).

Under the RESPECT-Mil program, service members who screened positive for symptoms of depression, PTSD, or alcohol misuse then had the issue addressed by their primary care physician and were invited to participate in the RESPECT-Mil program, which assigned them a nurse case manager and resulted in a psychiatrist conducting provider-to-provider consultation with the primary care physician. Over time, this program transitioned to having an embedded licensed mental health professional in the primary care clinic to provide supportive counseling needs and brief cognitive-behavioral interventions and to assist in care coordination. The effectiveness of this program is unknown, but a large randomized trial is currently assessing the effectiveness of additional care management enhancements, stepped treatment (including web and phone options), and more intensive outcomes management compared with usual care (Engel et al. 2014).

Another change the military has instituted is the introduction of the Behavioral Health Data Portal (BHDP). This automated system contains multiple screening instruments such as the PTSD checklist (PCL-5) and PHQ-9 depression screen, which service members complete when attending mental health appointments. This portal allows a clinician to view the historical record of symptom scores and provides a standardized mechanism for monitoring treatment progress and assessing outcomes across the large military health-care network. Data acquired through widespread use of this program may enable the development of better instruments capable of being validated for repeated administration over time (Hoge et al. 2015). Unfortunately, despite all of these increases in screening efforts, many service members who develop symptoms of psychiatric disorders leave after one to two tours and do not access, delay to access, or fail to complete an adequate course of treatment while on active duty (Tanielian and Jaycox 2008; Hoge et al. 2014).

Future Screening Initiatives and Improvements

As noted with each of these current screening mechanisms, the major limitation is that each relies on the service member to honestly report symptoms. While there will continue to be efforts to decrease stigma toward mental health care and to increase self-reporting, there is a growing level of interest in identifying biomarkers to diagnose PTSD. However, as noted in a recent comprehensive review, it is increasingly unlikely that a single biomarker for PTSD will be identified; although there is some evidence that future efforts will identify biomarkers associated with one or more clinically significant PTSD symptom (Lehmer and Yehuda 2014), there is low likelihood of a biomarker in the near future that could be useful for screening or diagnostic purposes.

In summary, screening for mental health problems has become routine in military and VA settings, and there is much greater attention on mental health issues now than in prior generations. While prior efforts focused on premilitary identification, more recent efforts have focused on using screening tools for early identification of underlying mental health conditions (military or nonmilitary related), routine screening in primary care, incorporating mental health providers into primary care, and educating service members to reduce stigma. Unfortunately, despite these efforts, a high percentage of service members with symptoms of depression, PTSD, or other mental health problems never seek treatment within the military system, and many also fail to access adequate services after leaving military service. Improving engagement and retention in treatment is a high priority.

Key Concepts

1. Pre-enlistment behavioral health screening has unknown effectiveness in its current form. Incentives for recruits to hide disqualifying conditions are high, given the benefits of being selected for a military occupation. Consequences for recruits hiding disqualifying conditions are largely unenforceable.
2. Pre-deployment behavioral health screening has been shown to be effective in its current form in one study, provided that there is coordination of care in-theater for service members who have a stable behavioral health condition. This method is not effective for service members who are receiving or have received mental health treatment outside the military system and choose to conceal it.
3. The effectiveness of post-deployment screening is unknown. It is not likely to be effective immediately post-deployment, based on research that has shown that service members tend to conceal behavioral health problems at that time, due to stigma, fears of not being able to go on leave after deployment, and other concerns. The willingness to report mental health concerns increases several months after coming home, though the effectiveness of post-deployment screening during this time period in preventing or mitigating negative health outcomes is unknown.
4. Despite dramatic increases in screening, many individuals with symptoms of PTSD leave the military never having sought treatment. Service members remain reluctant to report behavioral health symptoms due to perceived stigma, fear of damage to career, concerns for security clearances, and other reasons. As a result, the majority of new PTSD diagnoses in veterans are made by community or VA clinicians.

References

Bliese PD, Wright KM, Adler AB, Thomas JL (2004) Validation of the 90 to 120 day post-deployment psychological short screen: research report 2004–002. US Army Medical Research Unit-Europe and Walter Reed Army Institute of Research, Heidelberg. Available at: http://usamru-e.amedd.army.mil/assets/docs/publications/bliese_et_al_2004_report_2004-002_short_screen_development_and_validation.pdf

Chedekel L, Kauffman M (2006) Mentally unfit, forced to fight. Hartford Courant 14 May 2006. Accessed at http://www.courant.com/news/special-reports/hc-mentallyunfit-sg,0,4649032.storygallery on 25 Apr 2017

Engel CC, Oxman T, Yamamoto C, Gould D, Barry S, Stewart P, Kroenke K, Williams JW, Dietrich AJ (2008) RESPECT-Mil: feasibility of a systems-level collaborative care approach to depression and post-traumatic stress disorder in military primary care. Mil Med 173:935–940

Engel CC, Bray RM, Jaycox LH, Fred MC, Zatzick D, Lane ME, Brambilla D, Rae Olmsted K, Vandermaas-Peeler R, Litz B, Tanielian T, Belsher BE, Evatt DP, Novak LA, Unutzer J, Katon WJ (2014) Implementing collaborative primary care for depression and post-traumatic stress disorder: design and sample for a randomized trial in the U.S. military health system. Contemp Clin Trials 39:310–319

Glass AJ, Bernucci RJ, Anderson RS (1966) Neuropsychiatry in world war II. Office of the Surgeon General, Washington, DC, pp 153–191

Hoge C, Auchterlonie J, Milliken C (2006) Mental health problems, use of mental health services, and attrition from military service after returning from deployment to Iraq or Afghanistan. JAMA 295:1023–1032

Hoge CW, Grossman SH, Auchterlonie JL, Riviere LA, Miliken CS, Wilk JE. (2014). PTSD treatment for soldiers after combat deployment: low utilization of mental health care. Psychiatry Services. 65(8): 997–1004

Hoge CW, Ivany CG, Brusher EA, Brown III MD, Shero JC, Adler AB, Warner CH, Orman DT (2015). Transformation of mental health care for US soldiers and families during the Iraq and Afghanistan wars: where science and politics intersect. American journal of psychiatry. Nov 10;173(4):334–343

Hyams K, Riddle J, Trump D, Wallace M (2002) Protecting the Health of US Military forces in Afghanistan: applying lessons learned since the Gulf War. Clin Infect Dis 34(Suppl 5):S208–S214

Lehmer A, Yehuda R (2014) Biomarkers of PTSD: military applications and considerations. Eur J Psychotraumatol 5. https://doi.org/10.3402/ejpt.v5.23797

McGuire F (1994) Army alpha and beta tests of intelligence. In: Sternberg RJ (ed) Encyclopedia of intelligence volume I. Macmillan, New York, pp 125–129

Milliken C, Auchterlonie J, Hoge C (2007) Longitudinal assessment of mental health problems among active and reserve component soldiers returning from the Iraq war. JAMA 298(18):2141–2148

National Defense Authorization Act (NDAA) FY 2005 (2005) H.R. 4200, section 723

National Defense Authorization Act (NDAA) FY 2012 (2012) H.R. 4310, sections 582 and 1212

Page GD (1996) Clinical psychology in the military: developments and issues. Clin Psychol Rev 16:383–396

Post Deployment Health Assessment, DD Form 2796 (1999) Available at http://www.dtic.mil/whs/directives/forms/eforms/dd2796.pdf. Accessed 25 Apr 2017

Rogers R (2006) Some troops headed back to Iraq are mentally ill. San Diego Tribune. 18 March 2006 Available at http://legacy.signonsandiego.com/news/military/20060319-9999-n19mental.html. Accessed on 25 Apr 2017

Rosen G (1975) Nostalgia: a "forgotten" psychological disorder. Psychol Med 5:340–354

Stokes JW, Jones FD (1995) Combat stress control. In: Jones FD, Sparacino LR, Wilcox VL, Rothberg JM, Stokes JW (eds) Joint operations in war psychiatry. Office of the Surgeon General – Borden Institute, Washington, DC, pp 243–270

Tanielian T, Jaycox L (2008) Invisible wounds of war: psychological and cognitive injuries, their consequences, and services to assist recovery. RAND Corporation, Santa Monica

Warner C, Breitbach J, Appenzeller G, Yates V, Grieger T, Webster W (2007) Division mental health: its role in the new brigade combat team structure part II: re-deployment and post-deployment. Mil Med 172:912–917

Warner CH, Appenzeller GN, Mullen K, Carolynn M. Warner CM, & Grieger T (2008). Soldier Attitudes toward Mental Health Screening and Seeking Care upon Return from Combat. Military Medicine, 173(6), 563–569

Warner C, Appenzeller G, Parker J, Warner C, Hoge C (2011a) Effectiveness of mental health screening and coordination of in-theater care prior to deployment to Iraq: a cohort study. Am J Psychiatry 168:378–385

Warner CH, Appenzeller GN, Grieger TA, Belenkiy S, Breitbach JE, Parker JR, Warner CM, Hoge CW (2011b) Importance of anonymity to encourage honest reporting in mental health screening after combat deployment. Arch Gen Psychiatry 68(10):1065–1071

Wright K, Huffman A, Adler A, Castro C (2002) Psychological screening program overview. Mil Med 167:853–861

Wright K, Thomas J, Adler A, Ness J, Hoge C, Castro C (2005) Psychological screening procedures for deploying US forces. Mil Med 170:555–562

9 Mental Health Command Consultation

Rebecca I. Porter and Danielle K. Clauss

History of Command Consultation

Command consultation in the military refers to the practice of subject matter experts providing information and advisement to a commander within their area of expertise. With regard to mental health command consultation, a behavioral health professional provides subject matter expertise in the area of mental health to support the commander's responsibility for the health and welfare of the individual, the unit, and the command. The use of the term "behavioral health professional" in the military may refer to a uniformed or civilian employee of the Department of Defense (DoD) and includes psychiatrists, psychologists, psychiatric nurse practitioners, social workers, and technicians. When requesting mental health consultation, the commander is seeking information regarding the psychological health of the individual, the unit, and/or the command as it relates to mission readiness. It may be helpful to conceptualize this type of consultation as sharing features with employment evaluations, which assess an individual's psychological functioning as it relates to work suitability or performance, but with a broader focus within the military given the commander's responsibility for the overall health and functioning of the individual and the unit. The behavioral health professional essentially has two clients: the individual and the organization, represented by the commander. To provide context for this framework, a brief review of the history of mental health command consultation is provided.

Screening

The history of mental health command consultation in the military is well documented (e.g., Camp 2015; McCarroll et al. 1994; Warner et al. 2011). There is evidence that this type of command consultation occurred at least as early as the nineteenth century during the Napoleonic and Crimean Wars (Jones 1995). The initial focus of this consultation was the screening and identification of psychiatric dysfunction and determination of fitness for military duty. The need for mass screening to facilitate the selection and assignment of recruits in the USA during World War I led to the creation of the first group intelligence tests, the Army Alpha and Beta tests. These instruments were designed to assess the intellectual functioning of recruits and represented a formalized system of mental health

R.I. Porter
United States Army Medical Command,
San Antonio, TX, USA

D.K. Clauss (✉)
Philadelphia College of Osteopathic Medicine,
Philadelphia, PA, USA
e-mail: Danielle.clauss@gmail.com

L.W. Roberts, C.H. Warner (eds.), *Military and Veteran Mental Health*,
https://doi.org/10.1007/978-1-4939-7438-2_9

command consultation within the US military. As the effectiveness of this type of screening process was questioned (e.g., Warner et al. 2011), the role of the behavioral health professional in the US military shifted from one of personnel selection and placement to one of prevention, conservation, and treatment during World War II.

Prevention

The shift to prevention, conservation, and treatment by behavioral health professionals occurred as there was increased recognition that mental health dysfunction negatively impacts mission readiness, particularly in times of war, and that a focus on preventing and treating these conditions could prevent the loss of valuable manpower. As evidence of this shift, Brigadier General William C. Menninger, Psychiatric Consultant to the Surgeon General of the Army during World War II, stated that the "most important functions of military psychiatry are primarily preventive," highlighting the role of the psychiatrist to "give counsel and advice" to the commander (Camp 2015, p. 375; Menninger 1948). Borrowing from the preventive psychiatry models used in the civilian sector, military behavioral health professionals focused on primary, secondary, and tertiary prevention of psychiatric conditions (Camp 2015; Caplan 1964; Warner et al. 2011). This three-tiered prevention model continues to be used by behavioral health professionals within the military environment.

Primary prevention refers to decreasing psychiatric morbidity by reducing risk at the group or unit level. Education is the main tool of primary prevention and tends to take the form of unit-level trainings (Warner et al. 2011). Secondary prevention occurs at the individual level and involves intervening to prevent further disability. The goal within the military is to treat the individual promptly and within the unit environment to increase the likelihood of the individual returning to duty with minimal disruption to the mission (e.g., Salmon 1917; Camp 2015; Warner et al. 2011). Tertiary prevention refers to the practice of treating the individual outside of the unit environment, for example, in a medical treatment facility, with the goal of preventing permanent disability (Camp 2015).

With this prevention model in place, behavioral health professionals were increasingly likely to engage in consultation activities related to the prevention of psychiatric casualties, with a much broader focus than treating individual cases of pathology. Further evidence of this paradigm shift is seen in the formalization of the consultant role for behavioral health professionals in military regulations, for example, in Army Regulation (AR) 40-216, *Medical Service: Neuropsychiatry* (US Department of the Army 1959), which states as a primary task "advising the commander in matters pertaining to the morale of troops and the impact of current policies upon the psychological effectiveness of troops" (Camp 2015, p. 374). The consultant role further evolved during the Korean and Vietnam War eras as commanders witnessed the impact of low morale on the psychological functioning of troops. Consistent with the community psychiatric movement in the civilian sector at that time (e.g., Community Mental Health Act of 1963), behavioral health professionals were expected to provide consultation on factors such as morale, motivation, discipline, and substance abuse as they related to decreased psychological functioning and increased psychological morbidity (Camp 2015).

Advances in Consultation Since the Wars in Afghanistan and Iraq

Command consultation has evolved over the years. According to the Office of Medical History in the Office of the (Army) Surgeon General, psychiatric command consultation was routinely used by the US military during World War II (Appel 1966) and was known as Mental Hygiene Consultation Services. With this model, mental health services were provided in closer proximity to service members' units and away from the camp hospital. Such an arrangement afforded mental health practitioners (the psychiatrists, psychologists, and psychiatric social workers who staffed the consultation services) an opportunity to witness the combat events a unit was facing and therefore a better understanding of the challenges and conditions they were confronted with on a daily basis. Additionally, service members in the unit became accustomed to mental health providers and were more likely to seek out their services.

Taking a page from this wartime history, behavioral health professionals have been embedded with military units to varying degrees over the years. Beginning in World War II, behavioral health assets were consolidated at the division level (two-star general headquarters) and provided command consultation from a centralized position, across the entire division of approximately 10,000–15,000 soldiers (Rock et al. 1995). More recently, the military began to embed behavioral health professionals at even lower levels in military units. With the advent of the wars in Afghanistan and Iraq, behavioral health officers and technicians were assigned to brigades, and they trained and deployed with their units (Warner et al. 2007). These "organic" behavioral health assets were instated in addition to Combat and Operational Stress Control units.

Also during the wars in Afghanistan and Iraq, the Army deployed Mental Health Advisory Teams (MHATs) into theaters of combat. Chartered by the Army Surgeon General and the Army's Deputy Chief of Staff for Personnel, the MHATs first went into Iraq and later Afghanistan with the mission of determining the effects the wars were having on soldiers' mental health and well-being (and later with the Joint-MHATs, Marines as well). These teams assessed mental health services in theater, reviewed processes for evacuating mental health casualties, and examined suicide prevention programs (US Department of the Army 2003). Several iterations of the teams deployed, gathering valuable data that has informed commanders, Congress, policymakers, and mental health practitioners for more than a decade.

In January 2012, the Vice Chief of Staff of the Army directed the formal expansion of a program to locate behavioral health teams (often composed predominantly of civilian psychologists and social workers) near the brigades they support in garrison (i.e., at their stateside post) (US Army 2012). These Embedded Behavioral Health teams (EBH teams) currently support approximately 31 Brigade Combat Teams and 142 other battalion-sized (500–800 personnel) and brigade-sized (1,500–4,000 personnel) units (Army Medicine 2016). Aligning behavioral health professionals with specific units has the advantage of facilitating habitual relationships among commanders, providers, and soldiers and has been correlated with decreased acute psychiatric hospitalizations, increased command satisfaction, and improved mission readiness (Army Medicine 2016). This approach, which is designed for early identification and intervention when soldiers experience difficulties, is consistent with the military's recent emphasis on resiliency.

An important aspect of the Embedded Behavioral Health teams is that their location in or near brigade areas helps to increase the likelihood that a soldier will utilize services. The providers develop a relationship with the unit and with command, maintaining visibility on upcoming missions and specific stressors for the organization. Although not assigned to the organization, they interface regularly with leadership; reinforce trust and an understanding of the limits of confidentiality among leaders, soldiers, and the care team; and note that the stigma of seeking mental health care is eroded (Army Medicine 2016).

Service members have historically reported stigma surrounding mental health care, fearing that seeking treatment will jeopardize their career or that they will be seen as weak (Miggantz n.d.). Programs such as the Embedded Behavioral Health teams and the Department of Defense "Real Warriors" campaign (www.realwarriors.net) encourage service members to seek help when needed and educate leaders on how they can decrease the stigma associated with seeking mental health care.

Case Study

The command psychologist, LTC Renee Sanchez (pseudonym), was summoned to Brigadier General (BG) Arthur Smith's (pseudonym) office to discuss an urgent matter. One of the company commanders in the organization, CPT Joshua Trimble (pseudonym), was being accused of fraternization with a soldier, an offense that is punishable by court martial. CPT Trimble was considered a talented young officer and had been selected to be the general's next aide-de-camp (personal assistant). Since being informed that he was under investigation, CPT Trimble had been texting a friend that his situation was hopeless, and he had decided to stop taking his insulin for type 1 diabetes. The friend reported the texts to the officer's chain of command and escorted CPT Trimble to the health clinic where a suicide assessment was conducted. CPT Trimble was deemed not to be at imminent risk of suicide, which was reported through the chain of command to BG Smith. BG Smith was concerned for CPT Trimble's safety and questioned the veracity of the information provided by the young officer during the assessment. BG Smith called LTC Sanchez to his office to be apprised of the situation. He directed LTC Sanchez to conduct another assessment because he was convinced that the captain was a risk to himself. In fact, the general wanted the captain to be assessed every day. LTC Sanchez explained that she was prohibited from conducting "serial evaluations" of the captain if his situation had not changed. Such a practice could be perceived as punitive and was in violation of Department of Defense Instruction (DoDI) 6490.4 (Department of Defense 2013b). BG Smith (who was in LTC Sanchez's chain of command) again directed LTC Sanchez to conduct the evaluation, at which time she reiterated that another assessment could not be completed unless something in CPT Trimble's situation changed to suggest his risk of suicide might increase. In discussing this aspect of the Department of Defense guidance, BG Smith came to the realization that a second evaluation might be more appropriate after court martial charges were filed, and so he coordinated with LTC Sanchez to make preparations for the evaluation following charges being filed.

Types of Command Consultation

Command consultation may take many forms, ranging from informal requests to assess the morale of a unit to a formal request to assess the fitness for duty of a particular service member. Given the range of possible consultation requests, and given that all requests relate in some form to mission readiness, the first step in the consultative process is to clarify and understand the nature of the request. This is particularly important as certain consultation tasks must adhere to Department of Defense policy and specific military branch regulations.

In both civilian and military environments, it is imperative that the consultant be viewed as credible, knowledgeable, and effective. When working within a military environment, behavioral health professionals should possess an awareness of the unique challenges that may be associated with providing mental health consultation. For example, a commander may have the view that behavioral health professionals "take his soldiers out of the fight" or service members may believe that talking with a behavioral health professional has a negative effect on one's military career. The behavioral health professional can build credibility and engender trust by having regular contact with command and unit members during their regular operations, not only at times of crisis or conflict. Maintaining regular contact provides the opportunity to observe command and the unit in their naturalistic environment, as well as to establish working relationships with members of the organization such that the professional is able to generate recommendations that are practical and demonstrate an understanding of the organization. For example, a behavioral health professional may take part in a physical training exercise with a unit, a particularly effective way to build credibility within the military. A successful consultation outcome has the potential to increase acceptance of behavioral health services in general and may make it more likely that command will seek consultation in the future. If the request for consultation falls outside the behavioral health professional's area of expertise, the professional should serve as a liaison to connect command with a professional who is able to address the consultation request. Whenever possible, the behavioral health professional should maintain contact with command to ensure that the initial consultation request is adequately addressed. This topic is reviewed in greater detail accompanied with specific recommendations in the "Facilitating/Creating an Effective Consultation Process" section of this chapter.

Problem-Oriented Consultation

This type of consultation involves a commander seeking a behavioral health professional's expertise regarding a problem that may impact mission readiness. The broad term "problem" may refer to such diverse issues as an accident, natural disaster, death of a unit member, conflict or lack of cohesion within a unit, or unit performance problems. The consultation may involve assessing an entire unit or a group of individuals or may be focused on a specific individual. The consultation may be ongoing or may be limited to a one-time assessment. Additionally, the consultation may be performed by one behavioral health professional or by a team of professionals, individuals who may or may not be endogenous to the unit. The overarching goal of this type of consultation is for the behavioral health professional to provide specific, practical recommendations that assist command in addressing the problem so as to maximize mission readiness.

Command-Directed Mental Health Evaluations

A command-directed mental health evaluation consists of a formal assessment of a specific service member initiated by a commander to evaluate safety concerns, including risk of harm to self or others, significant changes in performance, or behavior changes that suggest a mental status change or psychological disorder. The requirements and procedures for initiating and completing a command-directed mental health evaluation are outlined in Department of Defense Directive (DoDD) 6490.1 and Instruction (DoDI) 6490.4 (DoD 2013a, b). The behavioral health professional performs the evaluation and is expected to provide written feedback to the commander within 24 h of the evaluation. The feedback at a minimum addresses the concerns outlined in the request for the evaluation, provides a summary of the psychological functioning of the individual, specifies any duty limitations or safety concerns, provides a treatment plan, and outlines any specific recommendations to maintain the health and welfare of the individual (e.g., restricting access to alcohol). Given the complexities associated with navigating the issues that necessitate the evaluation, and the need to systematically adhere to and execute the steps outlined in DoDI 6490.4 (DoD 2013b), the behavioral health professional plays a key role as a consultant. For example, the commander may consult with the behavioral health professional prior to initiating the request for the evaluation to ensure that it is an appropriate request and that the commander has exhausted all self-referral options. The behavioral health professional may also educate the commander regarding the nature and type of information that can be expected from the evaluation, provide guidance as to how the commander may use this information, and review recommendations that are in the best interest of command and the service member.

As highlighted in the case vignette included in this chapter, when conducting the evaluation, the psychologist has the responsibility of both assessing the service member for risk of suicide and educating the commander that his insistence on serial evaluations without a change in situation violates DoDI 6490.4 (DoD 2013b). By educating the leadership, the behavioral health professional protects command, ensures that the rights of the service member are not violated, and facilitates an effective working relationship for the future.

Fitness for Duty Evaluations

A fitness for duty evaluation is designed to address whether a service member is able to perform the tasks and responsibilities of his position from a psychological functioning perspective. The behavioral health professional considers the service member's specific duty position as well as the greater military environment when performing the assessment. Because of the expectation within the military that a service member is prepared to serve the needs of the organization at any time, the behavioral health professional considers such factors as the chronicity and severity of psychiatric impairment, the level of treatment required (e.g., hospitalization), the anticipated effect of varying and changing environmental conditions (e.g., 24 h duty assignment, remote geographical assignment), the impact on judgment and reality testing, and the likelihood of persistent inability to perform work tasks. The unique demands and features of the military environment may necessitate evaluation of factors beyond what is typical for fitness for duty evaluations in nonmilitary environments. To effectively perform this evaluation, the behavioral health professional must have a thorough understanding of the service member's position and functional responsibilities as well as military regulations governing the retention standards for specific positions.

The findings from a fitness for duty evaluation may lead to the determination that a service member is not fit for military duty. Depending on the reason for the finding, the service member may be referred for a medical evaluation board or administratively separated from the military. The distinction between a medical evaluation board and an administrative separation is an important one, as they each lead to significantly different outcomes. A medical evaluation board is initiated when a medical professional, including a behavioral health professional, identifies a condition that is believed will permanently impede a service member's ability to perform the duties of his position. The service member may be returned to service if it is determined that the individual is able to meet the demands of the position or may be medically retired if the disability causes permanent functional impairment. A service member who is medically retired is assigned a disability rating which may provide health benefits and financial compensation. An administrative separation is an involuntary separation of a service member from the military initiated by command.

Behavioral health professionals are involved with administrative separations when there is a presumed diagnosis of a personality disorder or other disorder that does not result in complete disability but impairs one's ability to successfully perform the duties of a given position (e.g., claustrophobia, enuresis, sleepwalking) (Warner et al. 2011). Of particular importance is that an administrative separation due to a personality disorder presumes that the personality disorder was a pre-existing condition and does not result in health benefits or financial compensation. It is imperative that the behavioral health professional consider the possibility that the service member's impairment is not better accounted for by another diagnosis, for example, post-traumatic stress disorder, particularly when assessing a service member who has had a history of successful functioning in the military prior to the current period of impairment. Given the presumption that the personality disorder is an inherent part of the individual's characterological structure, a thorough history taking regarding the service member's premilitary functioning and collection of collateral data, when possible, will assist the behavioral health professional in understanding the timeline and nature of the service member's impairment. The behavioral health professional has a pivotal role as a consultant in educating and assisting command during this process to ensure that the administrative separation action is the appropriate course of action.

Preventive Consultation

Preventive mental health consultation involves behavioral health professionals providing subject matter expertise to command in order to prevent or decrease the risk for adverse psychological outcomes at the group and individual level. These activities are commonly discussed in terms of primary, secondary, and tertiary prevention (Camp 2015; Caplan 1964) and have been explored in detail in the context of the military environment in other texts (e.g., Warner et al. 2011).

A behavioral health professional may provide subject matter expertise to command regarding a matter that has the potential to negatively impact the functioning of the unit. Typically, command has identified general risks to mission readiness (e.g., low morale, sleep deprivation, substance abuse) and is seeking guidance to address these risk factors. The focus is on the unit rather than the individual, and the emphasis is preventing problematic outcomes through risk reduction. As education is the primary tool of this type of consultation, the behavioral health professional will typically lead a unit-level training on a topic related to the consultation request, such as sleep hygiene training. While unit-level briefings may be the preferred method of delivery for this type of preventive consultation, the behavioral health professional may also provide tailored recommendations for specific consultation requests. For example, a commander may request recommendations for maintaining morale and effectiveness when a deployment requires service members to be separated from their families for a sustained period of time. As another example, the professional may advise command about sleep hygiene principles to facilitate structuring training schedules to ensure adequate sleep for service members.

Behavioral health professionals may also assist in the identification of service members who are at increased risk for developing a mental health condition through screening measures, with the idea being that early intervention may prevent disability. As discussed by Warner et al. (2011), this screening may take the form of post-deployment assessments, which seek to identify service members who are potentially experiencing mental health issues following a deployment. A significant challenge associated with this type of screening is the possibility that service members are reluctant to disclose difficulties they are experiencing out of concern that doing so will negatively impact their career and delay their return to their families. This challenge reinforces the benefit of having a behavioral health professional who is trusted by service members available to address and discuss these common concerns related to the stigma associated with seeking mental health care. Because command may share similar beliefs, the behavioral health professional may intervene at the command level by educating command about the screening process, outcomes, and the potential benefits of identification, such as the ability to intervene early and prevent or decrease disability. In this way, the behavioral health professional demonstrates to command that behavioral health intervention can be a force multiplier, or a means of enhancing the mission capabilities of the unit, rather than an approach that decreases mission readiness.

Preventive consultation may also occur after a service member has developed a mental health condition. This type of consultation may take the form of the behavioral health professional recommending an increased level of treatment to prevent chronic disability or a recommendation for specific duty limitations. With this type of consultation, it is important to convey the rationale for these recommendations and to assist command in viewing them as relevant to maintaining the health and welfare of the individual service member and the larger organization. This type of consultation is akin to a medical professional recommending that a coach temporarily remove a player from the game after the player sustains a concussion. These recommendations may initially be viewed as decreasing the organization's effectiveness, and it is therefore critical that the professional advises the leadership about the immediate and long-term consequences of the recommendations. For example, a behavioral health professional may increase acceptance of a recommendation to temporarily remove a service member from overnight guard duty if the professional educates command and the service member about sleep hygiene principles and the relationship between sufficient sleep and mood, decision-making ability, and global functioning.

Unique Aspects of Seeking Mental Health Care in the Military

In general, behavioral health professionals have many roles within the field and provide a myriad of services to the populations they serve. Within the military environment, behavioral health professionals assume many of the same roles as their civilian counterparts; however, the unique context of providing services to a military population necessitates an understanding of the broader military culture and the unique aspects associated with seeking and receiving mental health care within this environment. Arguably, the most important factor to understand is the extent to which a service member's personal and professional lives are intertwined. Given the expectation that service members are mission ready at all times and that commanders are responsible for ensuring that service members are fit to perform the duties and responsibilities of their positions, command generally has a greater level of access to personal information than the typical employer, which may alter the limits of confidentiality in mental health care. Additionally, the notion of stigma related to seeking and receiving mental health care within the military environment has the potential to affect the utilization of these services by service members and command.

Limits of Confidentiality

Because command bears the ultimate responsibility to ensure that service members are able to safely and effectively perform the duties of their positions, a commander may seek information pertaining to any area of the service member's life that impacts mission readiness—including the commonly cited areas of physical and psychological health but also extending to domains such as financial and family well-being. Behavioral health professionals working in a military environment must balance the need to keep commanders informed with the ethical responsibility to protect service members' privacy. These dual professional requirements require that behavioral health professionals be familiar with the broader limits to confidentiality that may exist in the military environment and able to effectively communicate and discuss these limits with the service member and command as appropriate. For example, in certain circumstances, a behavioral health professional may disclose information if it is deemed essential to the accomplishment of a military mission, a limit to confidentiality uncommon in most civilian outpatient settings. Viewed within the context of a multiple relationship, a behavioral health professional should clarify who the client is (e.g., organization vs. service member) depending on the nature of services being provided (e.g., fitness for duty evaluation, personnel selection evaluation, psychotherapy), communicate this information to the service member and command, and explicitly review the limits to confidentiality prior to obtaining information. This approach allows for clear communication and provides the opportunity to build collaborative relationships with the service member and command.

In the case vignette presented at the beginning of this chapter, CPT Trimble, the service member, was assessed by LTC Sanchez, the psychologist, due to command's concerns for imminent risk of suicide. LTC Sanchez was required to provide feedback to the command and did so under the established limits of confidentiality. LTC Sanchez appropriately educated BG Smith of the potential of violating Department of Defense policy by conducting serial evaluations that could be viewed as punitive, protecting both command and the rights of the service member. In this situation, LTC Sanchez was able to effectively serve as a command consultant, building credibility by providing subject matter expertise in a collaborative manner that ensured the welfare of both the organization and the service member. If CPT Trimble were to subsequently initiate psychotherapy with LTC Sanchez, this would require a review of the limits of confidentiality, particularly as the nature of services changes from assessment of risk to treatment. Ideally, LTC Sanchez would review the limits of confidentiality with CPT Trimble and command prior to the initiation of psychotherapy services, with a specific discussion of how these limits may be impacted by the filing of court martial charges and potential future outcomes (e.g., having another psychologist conduct the risk assessment while LTC Sanchez continues as the treating provider).

Another unique aspect of seeking mental health care in the military environment relates to the personnel who provide care and the location where treatment occurs. Behavioral health professionals are often military personnel, Department of Defense personnel, or civilian providers located on the military installation. In a sense, service members are seeking mental health care at the workplace, and this arrangement may appear to increase limits to privacy, whether or not this is actually the case. As highlighted in the case vignette, the decision by CPT Trimble to stop taking his insulin for type 1 diabetes was communicated to his command, effectively his "boss," and CPT Trimble was subsequently assessed at the health clinic at his "workplace," by another service member, effectively another "employee," within the same chain of command. While the expectation is that behavioral health professionals are familiar with and adhere to privacy rules and regulations, the service member and command may not have the same familiarity with and understanding of this information. This discrepancy, in combination with the co-location of services, may serve as a potential barrier to seeking mental health care. Again, clear communication with the service member at the beginning of treatment regarding the limits to confidentiality has the potential to address specific concerns, establish rapport, and build a collaborative relationship. Whenever possible, and ideally prior to a crisis situation, behavioral health professionals should seek opportunities to educate command about potential privacy and confidentiality issues related to the delivery of mental health care. In particular, behavioral health professionals should highlight the ways in which these policies facilitate a therapeutic relationship and enhance treatment outcomes, rather than constitute a convention that prevents command from receiving information. At all opportunities, behavioral health professionals should educate command regarding the ways in which mental health care can serve as a force multiplier and maintain the health and well-being of the larger organization.

Stigma Associated with Seeking Mental Health Care

There is a well-documented perception among service members that receiving mental health care has negative professional consequences. This perception includes the belief that other individuals will view them as weak, superiors will blame them for unit problems, they will be treated differently in general, they will lose their security clearance, and it will harm or end their military careers (e.g., Acosta et al. 2014; Britt et al. 2008; Hoge et al. 2004). Given findings that combat exposure increases risk for mental health problems (e.g., Britt et al. 2008; Hoge et al. 2004), and the fact that the United States was engaged in the longest sustained combat operations since Vietnam during the wars in Afghanistan and Iraq, there is increased recognition that addressing the stigma associated with receiving mental health care is critical to sustaining the health and well-being of service members and ensuring mission readiness. As evidence of this awareness, the Department of Defense issued a mandate in 2011 to all branches of service to "foster a culture of support" for seeking and receiving mental health care (DoD 2011, p. 2).

In their roles as command consultants and service providers, behavioral health professionals have the opportunity to educate both command and service members regarding the "myths" and "realities" of receiving mental health care. Perhaps the most important message to convey is that not being able to perform one's duties will almost certainly have a negative impact on a service member's career, while seeking mental health care provides the opportunity to address the issue before it has a detrimental effect on that career. For example, in a 2006 study of Air Force personnel receiving mental health care, service members who were command-directed for mental health care were 13 times more likely to have a negative career outcome (defined as a change in duty or discharge) than service members who self-referred for treatment (Rowan and Campise 2006). Moreover, in this same study, less than 1% of service members who sought mental health care had a change in their duty status (defined as a change to security clearance, flight, or weapons bearing status). These findings highlight that impairment in functioning harms service members' careers rather than receiving mental health care. Said another way, service members are far more likely to experience negative career outcomes when they are unable to perform the duties and responsibilities of their job due to unaddressed mental health problems. Behavioral health professionals have the opportunity to challenge the belief that seeking mental health care is detrimental to a military career by sharing such research findings with command and service members.

Another commonly cited belief held by service members is that seeking mental health care will result in the loss of one's security clearance. In the role of command consultant, a behavioral health professional should challenge this belief with data whenever possible. For example, a review of the adjudicative history of the US Army Central Personnel Security Clearance Facility, the agency responsible for making personnel security decisions for the Army, found that "99.8% of cases with psychological concerns obtained or retained their security clearance eligibility" (Haire 2009). As both a command consultant and provider, a behavioral health professional has the opportunity to challenge the stigma associated with receiving mental health care by sharing data with command and service members and discussing their concerns. Building credibility with both command and service members greatly increases the acceptance of this type of information and subsequent use of mental health care services.

Special Populations

Each of the military branches includes occupations that are deemed to require exceptional reliability, perception, and judgment. Military guidelines and instructions require personnel in such positions as nuclear material handlers, explosive ordinance drivers, pilots, or submariners, for example, to maintain an excellent level of mental health. Because an in-depth review of the applicable rules and regulations would become quickly outdated, practitioners are encouraged to refer to the most current publications of service-specific guidance (see Table 8.1 for examples).

Generally, individuals who work in areas that require exceptionally clear cognition, prolonged independent work, and unquestionable judgment and reliability must be free of current or poorly managed mental health conditions. Adjustment disorders are typically acceptable, as is bereavement or a history of mood disorder that was resolved more than 6 months in the past. The services and occupations vary in the permissibility

Table 8.1 Military guidance for special populations

Branch of service	Basic applicable guidelines
Department of Defense	Department of Defense Instruction, 6490.4, Mental Health Evaluations of Members of the Military Services
US Army	Army Regulation (AR) 40-501, Standards of Medical Fitness
US Navy	Manual of the Medical Department (MANMED), Chap. 15, Article 15-103, Nuclear Field Duty and Article 15-106, Submarine Duty; US Navy Aeromedical Reference and Waiver Guide
US Air Force	Air Force Instruction (AFI) 48-123, Medical Examinations and Standards
US Marine Corps	US Marine Corps receive medical care in accordance with the US Navy MANMED, above
US Coast Guard	Coast Guard Aviation Medicine Manual, COMMANDANT INSTRUCTION M6410.3A
Veterans	Veterans seeking special occupation must meet requirements of the military or civilian (e.g., Federal Aviation Administration) agency

of the use of psychotropic medications for managing depression or anxiety. Psychosis, controlled or otherwise, is disqualifying from these occupations. Behavioral health professionals may be asked to provide an assessment of the individual's reliability, judgment, or other suitability for employment in a given role. It is always permissible, and prudent, to seek guidance from military medicine authorities regarding the most current relevant instructions or regulations.

Controversies Related to Behavioral Health Role

Military behavioral health professionals have long balanced the challenge of serving at least two masters (Hines et al. 1998; Staal and King 2000; Warner et al. 2009). The question of whether their first responsibility is to the service member, or to the military command, is perpetual. More recently, military behavioral health professionals have had to be more mindful of the impact of their diagnostic impressions, particularly as they pertain to separation from military service. At times a consultant may feel at risk of inadvertently disadvantaging the service member or of damaging his or her own career if his or her findings and recommendation are somehow controversial. Such feats of balance and differentiation must often be accomplished in the context of what could be likened to a rural community: a small, closed military base. It is not uncommon for a consultant to be at odds with someone for whom they work—for example, their commander, who is also the commander of an individual service member being evaluated. For example, in the case vignette, LTC Sanchez, the psychologist, and CPT Trimble, the service member being evaluated, both worked for BG Smith. LTC Sanchez made a recommendation that was in the best interest of the service member and command; however, the recommendation did not comply with BG Smith's request, essentially placing the psychologist in a position of conflict with her "boss." Finally, consultants may find the requirements of their military mission in conflict with the ethical guidelines of their professions—for example, in the case of military psychologists and psychiatrists advising interrogators or a behavioral health professional beginning to have concerns about a service member's potential as a security risk.

The training programs for military behavioral health professionals typically spend significant time addressing the particulars of more common ethical dilemmas and strongly encourage consultation. Consultation can take place with a colleague who works in the same organization, on the same installation, or even—remotely through technology—halfway around the world.

Consultants may also find themselves facing scrutiny if their diagnoses have implications for a service member's continuing service. For example, if a consultant diagnoses a service member with a personality disorder, and the service member had combat experience, the system may require additional screening for PTSD and/or traumatic brain injury (TBI) to ensure that the behaviors that contributed to a personality disorder diagnosis (and possible separation from service without benefits) are not in fact due to PTSD or head trauma. A service member may not necessarily be separated because of a PTSD diagnosis, but if he is, there are medical and disability benefits associated with it. Consultants may feel that their clinical skills are being second-guessed by administrative behavioral health professionals, when oftentimes it is simply a matter of ensuring that the clinician's documentation adequately supports the diagnosis.

Facilitating/Creating an Effective Consultation Process

As with so many situations, the relationship can make or break the effectiveness of a partnership. This is definitely the case in a behavioral health consultation. The command consultant should assume responsibility for developing and securing the relationship with command. He or she must establish credibility with command and highlight how his or her role can be a "force multiplier" or a means to enhance the mission capabilities of the unit. The relationship should become collaborative, and the consultant can take steps to ensure this is the case.

Leadership in an organization and service members alike experience the stigma and lack of understanding surrounding interaction with a behavioral health professional. Developing a relationship with the leadership is an important step that consultants can take to counter such stigma. Ideally, this relationship will be developed long before a commander has the need to consult with a behavioral health professional or before the behavioral health professional needs to convey important information to the commander. Upon being designated as the consultant to a given unit, behavioral health professionals should schedule an office call with the unit's commander and other key leadership (e.g., First Sergeant (Army), Squadron Commander (Air Force), or Command Master Chief (Navy)).

A consultant should aim to be seen frequently around the organization, whether it is at training exercises, social functions, or sporting events. It is important to foster trust with the leadership, communicating an understanding and respect for the demands they face. For example, in this chapter's case study in which the psychologist, LTC Sanchez, was advising BG Smith against repeated assessments of CPT Trimble that might be misinterpreted as punitive, BG Smith may have more readily accepted LTC Sanchez's recommendations if Smith and Sanchez had an existing professional relationship through which Sanchez had established her competence and sound judgment. The situation would have gone much differently if Sanchez had suggested to Smith that "fraternization" is a minor offense and would hardly be cause for suicidal ideation or intent.

Similarly, had Sanchez not been able to communicate confidently in the vernacular of the Army, with a clear understanding of the regulations and nuances of the situation, Smith would have likely sought out other counsel or inadvertently badgered Trimble about whether he was a suicide risk. Commanders (like BG Smith in this case) bear ultimate responsibility for their troops, and they are unlikely to accept counsel from someone who equivocates or seems disconnected from the military culture. Engendering the commander's trust is paramount.

Role of Civilian Providers in the Consult System

Civilian providers have a critical role in providing health care to service members and veterans. With the United States engaged in sustained combat operations for over 13 years during the wars in Afghanistan and Iraq, and with the simultaneous aging of Vietnam-era veterans, the number of service members and veterans seeking mental health care currently exceeds the capacity of the Military Health System (MHS) and the Veterans Health Administration (VHA), the two agencies responsible for providing health care to these populations. As evidence of this increased need for mental health care, over 10,000 civilian mental health providers were hired by the Department of Defense and Department of Veterans Affairs between 2007 and 2010 to provide mental health care to service members and veterans (Westphal and Convoy 2015). As the number of civilians providing mental health care to service members and veterans continues to increase, civilian providers need to be familiar with and understand the military and veteran cultures.

Facilitating an effective relationship with service members, command, and veterans starts with civilian providers being knowledgeable about the population being served. This awareness begins with understanding the potential differences in needs and expectations of active duty service members and veteran populations. For example, an active duty service member may be concerned that a civilian provider will make recommendations that negatively impact her career and therefore may omit important information, while a veteran may believe that a civilian provider's assessment will adversely affect his disability rating and decrease financial compensation.

Moreover, the policies and procedures of the Military Health System and Veterans

Health Administration differ, which may impact the acceptance of services. Whenever possible, civilian providers should establish relationships with the organization, build credibility, and clarify expectations. For example, if a civilian provider regularly provides mental health care to active duty service members via Tricare, the government-provided insurance plan for service members, a commander may be concerned that command will not be kept appraised of information relating to the safety and well-being of service members. Ideally, in this case, the provider should establish a relationship with command prior to the initiation of services and demonstrate an understanding of the unique aspects of treating an active duty service member outside the military medical system. A collaborative relationship with command can allow a civilian provider to better serve service members.

A model for this type of collaborative relationship comes from the Embedded Behavioral Health (EBH) program established by the Army. As discussed earlier, this program places primarily civilian behavioral health professionals and administrative support personnel within a brigade combat team to serve as both providers and consultants to command. The placement of the behavioral health team within the unit fosters regular contact between the providers and command, provides the opportunity for the team to give feedback to command regarding potential barriers to mental health care, and facilitates continuity of care for service members because the team is endogenous to the unit. In order to be viewed as an asset, behavioral health professionals should communicate information in a way that is understandable and useful to command, always keeping in mind command's responsibility for the health and welfare of the individual service member, the unit, and mission readiness. As an example, providers should avoid diagnostic jargon and explain the impact and manifestations of a particular disorder in terms that are specific to the service member's role, functional responsibilities, and behavior. If, for example, a service member is diagnosed with PTSD, the provider may communicate to command that the service member's tendency to constantly scan the environment (i.e., hypervigilance) and drive defensively may be beneficial in Iraq when the service member is driving a combat vehicle, but problematic when the service member drives on the shoulder of a highway in northern Virginia to avoid stopping in traffic. In this way, the behavioral health professional can use salient examples to build the case for treatment, increasing command's and the service member's acceptance of mental health care.

Conclusion

The case of LTC Sanchez's command-directed mental health evaluation of CPT Trimble exemplifies several important aspects of command consultation within the military. The psychologist (or other professional), LTC Sanchez, bore much of the responsibility to ensure that proper procedures were followed in accordance with Department of Defense Instruction (DoDI) 6490.4 and that the service member's rights were protected while at the same time ensuring that command (BG Smith) received the important information needed to maintain the service member's welfare and ability to safely and reliably execute the organization's mission.

Mental health command consultants have the opportunity to increase acceptance and use of mental health care services by command and service members, particularly if the consultant is viewed as credible, competent, and knowledgeable of military culture and regulations. When the consultant is unfamiliar with the job requirements of the service member being evaluated or another aspect of the consultation request, consultation with other behavioral health professionals is permissible and encouraged. Despite efforts of the Departments of Defense and Veterans Affairs, service members will necessarily be seen in a civilian setting. In these instances, consultation and reference to governing instructions and guidance is especially useful and appropriate.

Key Concepts

1. Building an effective relationship as a mental health command consultant requires the behavioral health professional to be perceived as credible, competent, and knowledgeable of military culture and regulations.
2. Mental health command consultants have the opportunity to increase acceptance and use of mental health care services by command and service members.
3. Military commanders are entitled to an assessment of the mental health of their troops, within the standards set out in Department of Defense Instruction (DoDI) 6490.4, Mental Health Evaluations of Members of the Armed Forces.
4. Service members may have concerns or fears about seeking mental health care or disclosing critical information during an interview or therapeutic session. Practitioners can mitigate these concerns with an open discussion of what may or may not be shared under specific circumstances.
5. Command consultants may advise commanders on psychological trends in their unit, the stressors of a training or wartime environment, or concerns related to specific individuals with proper release of information and informed consent.

References

Acosta J, Becker A, Cerully J et al (2014) Mental health stigma in the military. RAND Corporation, Santa Monica. Available at: http://www.rand.org/pubs/research_reports/RR426.html. Accessed 1 Oct 2016

Appel J (1966) Preventive psychiatry. In: Heaton L, Anderson R, Glass A et al (eds) Neuropsychiatry in World War II. Office of the Surgeon General Department of the Army, Fort Sam

Army Medicine (2016) Embedded Behavioral Health (EBH) (n.d.). Available at: http://armymedicine.mil/Pages/EBH.aspx. Accessed 2 Nov 2016

Britt T, Greene-Shortridge T, Brink S, Nguyen Q, Rath J, Cox A, Hoge C, Castro C (2008) Perceived stigma and barriers to care for psychological treatment: implications for reactions to stressors in different contexts. J Soc Clin Psychol 27(4):317–335

Camp N (2015) Preventive social psychiatry and command consultation: who is the patient-the soldier or his military unit. In: US Army psychiatry in the Vietnam war: new challenges in extended counterinsurgency warfare. Office of the Surgeon General, Fort Sam Houston, p 373–392

Caplan G (1964) Principles of preventive psychiatry. Basic Books, New York

Community Mental Health Act (1963) (Pub. Law 88–164)

Department of Defense (2011) Department of Defense instruction 6490.08. Command notification requirements to dispel stigma in providing mental health care to service members. Office of the Secretary of Defense, Washington, DC

Department of Defense (2013a) Department of Defense directive 6490.1, mental health evaluations of members of the Armed Forces. Office of the Secretary of Defense, Washington, DC

Department of Defense (2013b) Department of Defense instruction 6490.4, requirements for mental health evaluations of members of the Armed Forces. Office of the Secretary of Defense, Washington, DC

Haire T (2009) Financial problems or PTSD need not affect security clearance. [online] USarmy.mil. Available at: https://www.army.mil/article/24053/financial-problemsor-ptsd-need-not-affect-security-clearance. Accessed 2 Nov 2016

Hines A, Ader D, Chang A, Rundell J (1998) Dual agency, dual relationships, boundary crossings, and associated boundary violations: a survey of military and civilian psychiatrists. Mil Med 163(12):826–833

Hoge C, Castro C, Messer S et al (2004) Combat duty in Iraq and Afghanistan, mental health problems, and barriers to care. N Engl J Med 351(1):13–22

Jones F (1995) Psychiatric lessons of war. In: Jones F, Sparacino L, Wilcox V et al (eds) War psychiatry. Office of the Surgeon General, US Department of the Army, Falls Church

McCarroll J, Jaccard J, Radke A (1994) Psychiatric consultation to command. In: Jones F, Sparacino L, Wilcox V, Rothberg J (eds) Military psychiatry: preparing in peace for war. Office of the Surgeon General, US Department of the Army, Falls Church, pp 151–170

Menninger W (1948) Psychiatry in a troubled world. MacMillan, New York

Miggantz E (n.d.) Stigma of mental health care in the military. [online] Naval Center for Combat & Operational Stress Control. Navy Bureau of Medicine and Surgery (BUMED). Available at: http://www.med.navy.mil/sites/nmcsd/nccosc/healthProfessionalsV2/reports/Documents/Stigma% 20White% 20Paper.pdf. Accessed 2 Nov 2016

Rock N, Stokes J, Koshes R et al (1995) US Army combat psychiatry. In: Jones F, Sparacino L, Wilcox V et al (eds) War psychiatry. Office of the Surgeon General Borden Institute, Falls Church

Rowan A, Campise R (2006) A multisite study of Air Force outpatient behavioral health treatment-seeking patterns and career impact. Mil Med 171(11):1123–1127

Salmon T (1917) The care and treatment of mental disease and war neuroses ("shell shock") in the British army. Ment Hyg 1:509–547

Staal M, King R (2000) Managing a multiple relationship environment: the ethics of military psychology. Prof Psychol: Res Pract 31(6):698–705

US Department of the Army (1959) Army regulation 40–216, neuropsychiatry and mental health. Department of the Army, Washington, DC

US Department of the Army (2003) Operation Iraqi freedom (OIF) mental health advisory team (MHAT) report. Department of the Army, Washington, DC

US Department of the Army (2012) HQDA EXORD 236–12, army-wide implementation of embedded behavioral health teams. Department of the Army, Washington, DC

Warner C, Breitbach J, Appenzeller G et al (2007) Division mental health in the new brigade combat team structure: part I. Predeployment and deployment. Mil Med 172(9):907–911

Warner C, Appenzeller G, Grieger T et al (2009) Ethical considerations in military psychiatry. Psychiatr Clin North Am 32(2):271–281

Warner C, Appenzeller G, Breitbach J et al (2011) Psychiatric consultation to command. In: Ritchie E (ed) Combat and operational behavioral health. Office of The Surgeon General US Army, Falls Church, pp 171–188

Westphal R, Convoy S (2015) Military culture implications for mental health and nursing care. OJIN: Online J Issues Nurs [online] 20(1), Manuscript 4. Available at: http://www.nursingworld.org/MainMenuCategories/ANAMarketplace/ANAPeriodicals/OJIN/TableofContents/Vol-20-2015/No1-Jan-2015/Military-Culture-Implications.html. Accessed 1 Oct 2016

The Perpetrator Hypothesis: Victimization Involving LGBT Service Members

10

Carl Andrew Castro and Jeremy Goldbach

Minority Stress Theory and LGBT Service Members

It has been well established that minority status confers a substantial risk to health. When compared to their majority peers, health disparities have been found among women (Weber and Parra-Medina 2003), ethnic and racial minorities (Cervantes et al. 2011; Kessler 1979; McLeod and Kessler 1990), and lesbian, gay, bisexual, and transgender (LGBT) people (Goldbach et al. 2014; Thoits 1991). Various stress theories have been developed to account for these minority-related health disparities, generally rooted in the stress-illness paradigm (Lazarus and Folkman 1984). For the health disparities observed amongst LGBT people, minority stress theory has received considerable attention and support (see, e.g., Dentato et al. 2013; Hatzenbuehler 2009; Meyer 2003).

At its core, minority stress theory postulates that prejudice and stigma directed toward LGBT people results in unique stressors that cause adverse health outcomes, especially mental health disorders. For example, a number of studies find that LGBT people are more likely to experience victimization in social environments such as school/work, the home, and in religious communities. These experiences have been shown to impact mental health patterns including suicidal risk in both youth and adults (Goldbach and Gibbs 2015). Empirical support for several minority stress theory constructs has been established in prospective studies as well as meta-analyses (Goldbach et al. 2014; Marshal et al. 2011; Mustanski et al. 2010).

While there is strong empirical evidence that LGBT people experience minority-related stressors at higher rates than non-LGBT people and report disproportionate mental health concerns (Meyer 2003; Rosario et al. 2002), scholars have also argued that experiences common to both LGBT and non-LGBT people should be considered (for example, see Cole et al. 1996; Hatzenbuehler 2009). Indeed, when controlling for differences in levels of discrimination (e.g., Mays and Cochran 2001) or sexual assaults (Lucas et al. under review) between LGBT and non-LGBT people, the observed mental health disparities are explained, at least in part, by differences in the *likelihood of experiencing* the stressor rather than whether the stressor itself is unique to LGBT individuals. Thus, external factors that may be present (regardless of sexual identity) and that are common across minority populations should also be considered within the

C.A. Castro (✉) • J. Goldbach
Suzanne Dvorak Peck School of Social Work, University of Southern California, Los Angeles, CA, USA
e-mail: carl.castro@usc.edu; jermy.goldbach@usc.edu

L.W. Roberts, C.H. Warner (eds.), *Military and Veteran Mental Health*, https://doi.org/10.1007/978-1-4939-7438-2_10

context of minority stress, including (a) the targeting of minority people, (b) the role of organizational policies and support, and (c) social support and individual factors. The present chapter provides an additional heuristic when considering disparities among LGBT individuals: the Perpetrator Hypothesis. To demonstrate the potential utility of this approach, this chapter presents the Perpetrator Hypothesis in the context of LGBT personnel serving in the military.

Case Study

Specialist Maria Stone (pseudonym) is a female Army veteran in her late 30s who left the military approximately 2 years ago. She reported that she was raped by her squad leader while on active duty. She also reported that fellow male soldiers constantly asked her out on dates, but that she always turned them down since she identifies as a lesbian. On one occasion, after turning down a date, she was asked if she was a lesbian; since she enlisted in the Army during the "Don't Ask, Don't Tell" policy era, she wanted to keep her sexual identity private. Thus, in an attempt to "fit in" and dispel rumors about her sexual orientation, she agreed to go out with a group of male soldiers from her unit, thinking it would be "safe" since there would be others present. After being out drinking all night, she accepted an offer by her squad leader to escort her back to her room since she trusted him. Upon arriving to her barracks room, her squad leader forced his way into her room and raped her. The rape was not reported, though at the time of the rape, the "Don't Ask, Don't Tell" policy had been recently rescinded. The veteran reported that she became depressed, her performance deteriorated, and she left the military just over a year after the rape occurred. She has been in treatment for the past year to help her deal with the assault.

Distinction Between Sexual Orientation and Gender Identity

Before presenting the Perpetrator Hypothesis, it is important to distinguish between "sexual orientation" and "gender identity," as not all readers may appreciate the difference between these terms. Individuals engaging in same-sex sexual behaviors or reporting same-sex attractions have been documented across a wide range of historical periods and cultural experiences (Blackwood 1986). In the early 1900s, sexual orientation was described in terms of psychology and behavior (Sell 1997). As early as 1905, Freud began to publish on sexuality, identifying the defining characteristic of sexual orientation as the sex an individual is, compared with the sex of an individual to whom the individual is attracted.

Also during this time, researchers began to recognize that gender roles, expression, and sexual behaviors were not parts of the same construct but rather multiple aspects of one's identity. Many regard the work of Alfred Kinsey (Kinsey et al. 1948, 1953) as the first attempt to describe sexuality as a multidimensional construct rather than as a binary one; that is, being only either heterosexual or homosexual. This early work of Kinsey and his colleagues helped us to understand that sexual behavior and identity is an ongoing process that can change over time.

More recently, the sophistication in defining sexual orientation has advanced beyond behavior alone to include dimensions of attraction (Janssen et al. 2000), romantic beliefs (Diamond 2003a, b, 2005), and identity (Kauth and Kalichman 1995). Given this complexity, a number of definitions have emerged. In the early 1990s, sexual orientation was defined as "the direction of sexual feelings or behaviors toward individuals of the opposite sex, same sex, or combination of the two" (LeVay 1993; Sell 1997). According to the American Psychological Association (2011), sexual orientation is defined as "the sex of those to whom one is sexually and romantically attracted." Still others have tried to embrace all of these constructs, asserting that sexual orientation is "an enduring emotional, romantic, sexual or affection, attraction or non-attraction to other people; sexual orientation is fluid and people use a variety of labels to describe their sexual orientation" (UC Davis 2015).

Gender is another concept that is an important element of identity. Gender and sex can be related but are not synonymous. Gender can be defined as "a socially constructed system of classification that ascribes qualities of masculinity and femininity to people" (UC Davis 2015). Gender is a socially constructed, emotional, expressed, and internal experience of masculinity and/or femininity along the spectrum that can be inclusive or exclusive of both male and female. Toomey et al. (2010) state that gender-nonconforming individuals, such as boys who are more feminine than other boys, or girls who are more masculine than other girls, can be described as transgressing social gender norms. These social norms include both the way a person feels as well as how they behave or express themselves. However, these social gender norms change over time. For example, 20 years ago when a woman cut her hair short, this was considered a transgression of gender norms, and, indeed, this act was often associated with feminism and lesbian identity. Today, however, this social norm has shifted, and many women choose to wear their hair short without the automatic, socially constructed assumption that the woman is lesbian.

On the other hand, sex is not a socially constructed concept. Rather, sex is "a medical term designating a certain combination of gonads, chromosomes, external gender organs, secondary sex characteristics and hormonal balances" (UC Davis 2015.). Sex, then, is a biological definition, describing physiological aspects of the body only. Often, gender has been used to describe the sex of an individual at birth (i.e., "it's a girl!"). Gender, however, is a socially constructed and personal experience. Thus, it is more accurate to refer to the sex of a baby as opposed to the gender of a baby, as a baby is incapable of having awareness of their gender at such a young age.

By preschool, most children have a strong concept of gender and are able to label their own and others' gender (Toomey et al. 2010). Those who conform to socially constructed gender norms are often reinforced to maintain those roles by society, whereas those who do not conform may face criticism within various community and family settings. Egan and Perry (2001) suggest that "by middle childhood, a strong concept has developed regarding the degree to which [children] typify their gender category; degree of connection with gender assignment; whether they are free to explore cross-sex options or are compelled to conform to gender stereotypes; and whether their own sex is superior to another" (p. 459). Pressure to conform and shaming by family members and other members of society often create oppressive environments for many youths who are gender nonconforming, who are exploring their gender identity, or whose gender identity is not consistent with their biologically determined sex.

Gender nonconformity is defined as "not conforming to society's expectations of gender expression based on the gender binary expectations of masculinity and femininity, or how they should identify their gender" (UC Davis 2015). Transgender, on the other hand, can be defined as a psychological self (i.e., gender identity) differing from the social expectations for the physical sex a person was born with, a gender identity that does not fit within dominant-group social constructs of assigned sex and gender, or having no gender or multiple genders. It is important to emphasize that gender identity and sexual identity are usually related, but are not always. A transgender individual who is attracted to a male individual, for example, may identify as heterosexual, gay/lesbian, queer, or any other sexual identity.

Most estimates suggest that lesbian, gay, and bisexual (LGB) persons represent approximately 3%–5% of the general population in the United States (Gallup 2012; Marshal et al. 2008), yet new estimates indicate perhaps as many as 10% of young people identify as something "other than exclusively heterosexual" (Marshal et al. 2011). It is also quite possible that fewer youth identify as LGB because of uncertainty in how they will identify later in life (Savin-Williams 2001). When offered a range of reporting choices about sexuality, approximately 25% of 12-year-olds report they are "unsure" of their sexual orientation. This rate decreases significantly by age 18, where only about 5% report uncertainty (Remafedi et al. 1992; Robinson 1994).

It has been estimated that LGB service members comprise nearly 3% (71,000) of the total force, including National Guard and reserves, with 15,000 transgender service members serving. In fact, 21% of all transgender adults in the United States have served in the military compared to 10% for the general population (Zarembo 2015). Surprisingly, given the military's long history of discriminating against LGBT service members (see Goldbach and Castro 2016), it has been suggested that many LGBT people, especially transgender people, who are struggling with their sexual orientation or identity join the military as a means to help them resolve this uncertainty (Brown 1988; Moradi 2009).

The Perpetrator Hypothesis

A schematic of the Perpetrator Hypothesis is shown in Fig. 10.1. At its core, the Perpetrator Hypothesis contends that the poorer health status, attitudes and beliefs, and job performance indicators occur as a result of deliberate and malicious perpetrator behaviors that target LGBT people. The responsibility for LGBT victimization lies with the perpetrator and organizational climate, policies, programs, and culture that enable such victimization to occur. Each component of the model is described below.

Violent and Non-violent Behaviors

LGBT service members experience a wide range of violent experiences that exceed those of their peers (e.g., Friedman et al. 2011). LGBT service members experience higher of rates stigma, harassment, discrimination, bullying, and sexual assaults than do non-LGBT service members (Goldbach et al. 2014; Friedman et al. 2011). The Perpetrator Hypothesis postulates that the three primary types of violence likely to be experienced by LGBT service members are sexual assaults, hazing, and bullying. All of these behaviors undermine the espoused military values of dignity and respect (see US Army 2014). Further, all three are crimes in the military, punishable under the Uniform Code of Military Justice. Despite these behaviors being crimes, seldom do such behaviors result in military convictions or other forms of military punishment (see Castro et al. 2015).

Sexual Assault Sexual assault has been defined by the Department of Defense as, "Intentional sexual contact characterized by use of force, threats, intimidation, or abuse of authority or when the victim does not or cannot consent. The term includes a broad category of sexual offenses consisting of the following offenses: rape, sexual assault, aggravated sexual contact, abusive sexual contact, nonconsensual sodomy (forced oral or anal sex), or attempts to commit these acts" (Department of Defense 2015). Acts of sexual assault can therefore range from unwanted sexual contact to rape. To obtain a conviction for sexual assault, two things must be proven: the behavior or action must be shown to have occurred, and the behavior must be shown to have occurred without consent. Not surprisingly, it is this latter aspect of sexual assault that has been shown to be difficult to prove in both military and civilian courts, with conviction rates in the military of 10% or less (see Castro et al. 2015).

LGB individuals experience higher rates of sexual assault not only within the general population but also within the veteran population. LGB veterans have been found to have significantly higher rates of sexual assault in their life (Ray-Sannerud et al. 2015). In one study of LGB veterans, 8% of the LGB veterans reported experiencing sexual assault while in the military, known as military sexual assault (MSA), due to their sexual orientation

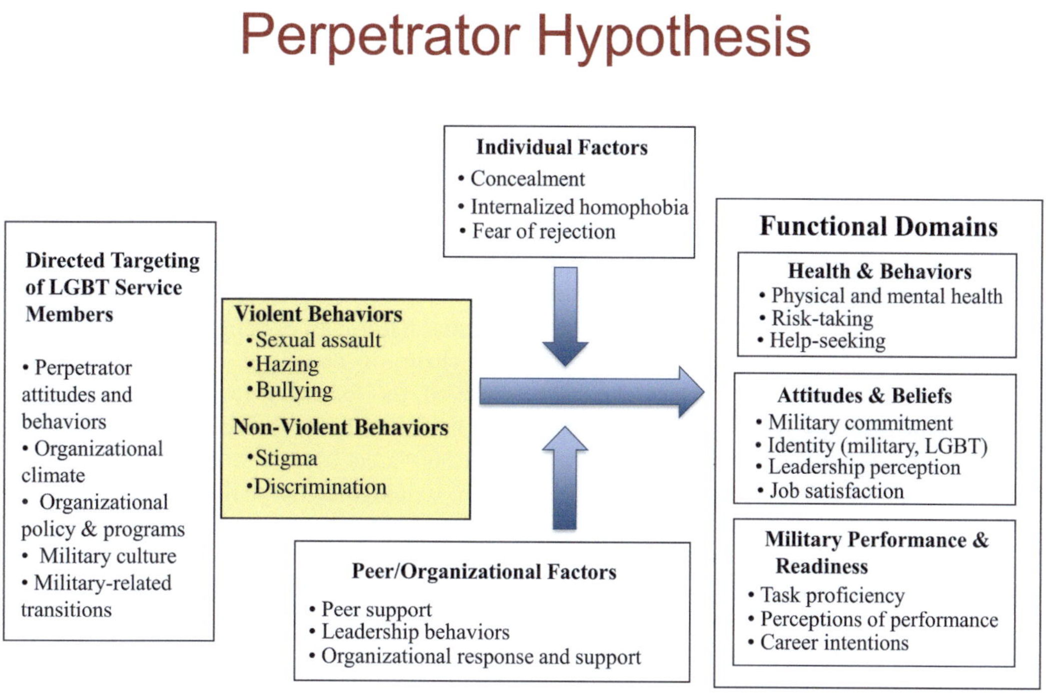

Fig. 10.1 Perpetrator hypothesis

(American Psychological Association – Joint Task Force on Sexual Orientation and Military Service 2009). One recent study found that LGB veterans reported more than twice the rate of military sexual assault when compared with their heterosexual peers (33%–14%, respectively; Lucas et al. under review).

Bullying The US military defines bullying as "any conduct whereby a service member or members, regardless of service, rank, or position, intends to exclude or reject another service member through cruel, abusive, humiliating, oppressive, demeaning, or harmful behavior, which results in diminishing the other service member's dignity, position, or status" (US Army, AR 600-20). Bullying may include an abuse of authority. Bullying tactics include, but are not limited to, making threats, spreading rumors, social isolation, and attacking someone physically, verbally, or through the use of electronic media (known as cyberbullying). Bullying behaviors usually happen more than once, and, absent outside intervention, bullying will typically continue without any identifiable endpoint. Within the military, bullying will continue until either the bully or the service member being bullied moves to another duty location, yet even then, cyberbullying may occur. It is important to appreciate that there is very little research on this topic in the US military, although it is thought to impact upwards of one-third to half of all military personnel. By comparison, the incidence of civilian workplace bullying has been estimated at 27%, where bullying was defined as having experienced one of the following types of repeated mistreatment: abusive conduct that is threatening, intimidating, humiliating; work sabotage; or verbal abuse (Namie et al. 2014).

Hazing The military defines hazing as "any conduct whereby a service member or members regardless of service, rank, or position, and without proper authority, recklessly or intentionally causes a service member to suffer or be exposed to any activity that is cruel, abusive, humiliating, oppressive, demeaning, or harmful. Soliciting or coercing another to participate in any such activity is also considered hazing. Hazing need not involve physical contact among or between military members or employees; it can be verbal or psychological in nature. Likewise, it need not be committed in the physical presence of the victim; it may be accomplished through written or phone messages, text messages, email, social media, or any other virtual or electronic medium. Actual or implied consent to acts of hazing does not eliminate the culpability of the perpetrator. Without outside intervention, hazing conduct typically stops at an identified endpoint" (US Army 2014, pp. 29).

While hazing and bullying can include both physical and nonphysical interactions, there are important differences between the two. Hazing typically involves conduct directed at new members of an organization or individuals who have recently achieved a career milestone. Hazing may occur during graduation or promotion ceremonies or similar military "rites of passage." However, it may also happen in military settings, such as in small units, to initiate or "welcome" a new member to the unit. That is, hazing is typically limited to key transition points within the military. It may result from any form of initiation, "rite of passage," or congratulatory act that includes unauthorized conduct such as physically striking a service member while intending to cause, or causing, the infliction of pain or other physical marks such as bruises, swelling, broken bones, and internal injuries; piercing another's skin in any manner; forcing or requiring the consumption of excessive amounts of food, alcohol, drugs, or other substances; or encouraging another to engage in illegal, harmful, demeaning, or unauthorized dangerous acts.

Unlike hazing, bullying often, but not always, takes the form of excessive corrective measures that, like hazing, involve the infliction of physical or psychological pain and go beyond what is required for authorized corrective training. Hazing and bullying are not limited to superior-subordinate relationships. They may occur between peers or, under certain circumstances, may involve actions directed toward senior personnel by those who are junior in rank, grade, or position. Bullying often appears as excessive correction of, or punishment for, perceived performance deficiencies. Hazing and bullying are prohibited in all cases, including off-duty or "unofficial" celebrations or unit functions, on or off post.

There are actions that may appear to be bullying or hazing that in fact are not. For instance, the obligation of necessary or proper duties and the requirement of their performance do not constitute bullying even though the duties may be arduous, hazardous, or both. When authorized by the chain of command and/or operationally required, the following activities do not constitute hazing or bullying: the physical and mental hardships associated with operations or operational training; lawful punishment imposed pursuant to the Uniform Code of Military Justice; administrative corrective measures, including verbal reprimands and command-authorized physical exercises; and extra military instruction or corrective training, including physical training, that is a valid exercise of military authority needed to correct a soldier's deficient performance.

Functional Domains

The effects of perpetration on the functioning of the victims can be profound. In nearly all cases of perpetration—whether the perpetration involves hazing, bullying, or sexual assault—physical and mental health, job attitudes, and work performance are adversely affected (Aquino et al. 1999; Turner et al. 2006). In the case of LGBT service members, however, how perpetration affects these functional domains is effectively unknown Burrelli (2010). In large part, this lack of knowledge is due to the "Don't Ask, Don't Tell" policy in which LGBT service members were not allowed to openly serve, and thus this important topic did not receive attention Cochran (2013). Since the repeal of the "Don't Ask, Don't Tell" policy, the Department of Defense has funded several efforts to begin filling this research gap. The following discussion draws heavily from the findings in the LGBT civilian and military veteran literature.

Health and Behavioral Disparities The Perpetrator Hypothesis predicts that the increased violent behaviors experienced by LGBT service members will lead to health and behavioral disparities between LGBT service members and non-LGBT service members. LGBT service members will suffer from both poorer physical and mental health, as well as increased risk-taking behaviors.

In addition, LGBT service members are less likely than their non-LGBT counterparts to engage in help-seeking behaviors, such as health care and other forms of social support. Given the limitations of physician-patient privacy in the military, it is not surprising that LGBT service members were reluctant to discuss their medical and psychosocial needs with doctors prior to the repeal of "Don't Ask, Don't Tell." Smith (2008) found in a small sample of 11 gay male service members that all of them reported fear of seeing their military doctor because of the repercussions of possible disclosure of their sexual orientation. Even after the repeal of "Don't Ask, Don't Tell," LGBT service members may remain less likely to access medical care. Poor access to health-care services leads to delays in seeking care and forgone preventative care (Renshaw et al. 2010; Conley and Heerwig 2011) including mental health services (Jones et al. 2012), resulting in degraded readiness for the individual and the unit as a whole. Fear of disclosure prior to "Don't Ask, Don't Tell" and continued fears about "coming out" mean that little is known about the specific needs among LGBT service members.

Attitudinal and Belief Differences The Perpetrator Hypothesis suggests that, as a result of being victimized, LGBT service members will have lower military commitment and be more likely to hold negative views of their leaders. LGBT service members who have been victims of violence will also have weaker military identity than non-LGBT service members. Further, LGBT service members will also have lower job satisfaction, morale, and unit cohesion than non-LGBT service members.

Given the importance of leadership and unit support and cohesion in the military (Griffith 1988; Manning 1991; Siebold 1999), victimizing experiences such as hazing and assault may be particularly relevant not only to the mental health outcomes of this population but also to the health and well-being of the unit. Leadership and cohesion within the military have been shown to influence health and performance in combat and in garrison (Bliese and Castro 2000; Castro and McGurk 2007; Wong et al. 2003). In a study conducted in garrison among soldiers with a high workload, soldiers in units with higher cohesion displayed fewer mental health symptoms associated with depression and anxiety than did soldiers where cohesion was lower (Bliese and Castro 2000). In a conceptually similar study conducted in Iraq where combat operations were ongoing, constructive and positive leadership behaviors were shown to attenuate the adverse effects of combat (Castro and McGurk 2007). Subordinates whose leaders displayed positive leader behaviors were less likely to screen positive for probable posttraumatic stress disorder (PTSD) and depression following combat experiences than leaders who displayed negative leader behaviors. Viewed in the context of minority stress theory, it is expected that LGBT service members who report supportive leadership and higher unit cohesion will report fewer health concerns than LGBT service members who report unsupportive or negative leadership and lower unit cohesion (Kaplan and Rosenmann 2012).

Reduced Military Performance and Readiness The Perpetrator Hypothesis predicts that LGBT service members who have been victims of violence display lower military performance and readiness compared to non-LGBT service members. As a result of experiencing violent behaviors targeted at them, LGBT service members will suffer a drop in task proficiency. Further, leaders' perceptions of LGBT service members who have experienced violent behaviors will be lower than non-LGBT service members, as self-confidence and resilience of LGBT service members who have experienced violent behavior will be lower than non-LGBT service members. LGBT service members who have suffered victimization will also show lower career intentions; that is to say, they will be less likely to make the military a career.

Combating Victimization of LGBT Service Members

The Perpetrator Hypothesis identifies numerous points where interventions can be employed to combat victimization of LGBT service members.

Directed/Targeting of LGBT Service Members A critical component of the Perpetrator Hypothesis is that LGBT service members are specifically targeted by perpetrators for violent aggressive attacks because they are known to be or perceived to be LGBT individuals. Thus, the attacks are thoughtful, deliberate, and premeditated and are typically not opportunistic attacks. Further, perpetrators are likely to be other service members. The reasons perpetrators target LGBT service members are numerous.

First, perpetrators often target those who they perceive as weak and unable to marshal resources to protect themselves (Murray 2000). Thus, perpetrators may target LGBT service members because they believe LGBT service members are less likely to report the perpetrating behaviors than non-LGBT service members. In fact, during the "Don't Ask, Don't Tell" policy era, service members would be discharged from the military if their sexual orientation or identity was revealed. Burks (2011) also presents a compelling conceptual framework that suggests "Don't Ask, Don't Tell" may have uniquely "served to increase LGBT victimization, decrease victim reports and help-seeking, and prevent sexual orientation military research" (p. 604). The Perpetrator Hypothesis incorporates this aspect of increased victimization as well. Even after the repeal of the "Don't Ask, Don't Tell" policy, perpetrators continue to target LGBT service members because many LGBT service members still wish to keep their sexual orientation and/or identity private. Reporting acts of abuse, even when the acts involved sexual assaults, would likely reveal the sexual orientation or identity of the victim.

Second, unit climate and organizational variables might exist that enable perpetration against LGBT service members. For instance, unit leaders might make disparaging comments about homosexual behavior being incompatible with military service, thereby signaling that bullying and hazing behaviors, and even sexual assaults, are acceptable treatment of LGBT service members. Even leaders using or tolerating the use of words such as "fag," "queer," or "pretty lady" can convey the message to other unit members that LGBT service members are less desirable or are unwanted in the military. Such behaviors by unit leaders may embolden perpetrators to believe that, even if LGBT service members report victimization, no action will be taken by leaders in the unit.

The important organizational factors that allow perpetrators to victimize LGBT service members are policies that prohibit LGBT service members from serving in the military or the lack of enforcement of policies and regulations governing victimization. As previously mentioned, the "Don't Ask, Don't Tell" policy likely placed LGBT service members at increased risk for all types of victimization. And even after the repeal of "Don't Ask, Don't Tell," LGBT service members are still at increased risk of victimizing behaviors, especially if rules and laws prohibiting such victimization are not rigorously enforced.

Finally, there are many aspects of military culture that could unintentionally facilitate LGBT service member victimization. The hypermasculine social norms that are fostered within the military (Moradi 2009) can lead to more acceptable sexual aggression, bullying, and hazing. In the case of hazing or bullying, gay and transgender male service members may be at increased risk for these types of physically victimizing behaviors. The numerous job changes that involve moving service members from one location to another can also place the LGBT service member at increased risk for victimization.

Reducing the Impact of Victimization of LGBT Service Members

The Perpetrator Hypothesis makes important assertions about how numerous individual, peer, leadership, and organizational factors can have an impact upon the effects of targeted victimization of LGBT service members and the subsequent impact of these violent behaviors on the functioning of LGBT service members. Understanding these factors is especially important since they point to possible means for ameliorating or attenuating the adverse effects of violent behaviors targeted at LGBT service members.

Individual Factors Associated with LGBT Service Members There are several individual or personal factors that can moderate the adverse effects of LGBT service member victimization. These individual factors include concealment, internalized homophobia, and fear of rejection (Meyer 2003; Rosario et al. 2002, 1996). Within the Perpetrator Hypothesis framework, these individual factors do not link directly to the functional domains (i.e., the outcomes); rather, they serve as moderators or mediators that can attenuate or eliminate the adverse effects of the experienced violent behaviors.

Many LGBT service members may not wish to have their sexual orientation or identity known, or they may limit whom they tell about their sexual orientation or identity. The reasons for not wanting to be open about one's sexual orientation or identity are numerous, ranging from fear of rejection or losing relationships to concerns over discrimination in promotion or other career-enhancing opportunities. These concerns may limit the reporting of victimization, as doing so may result in one's sexual orientation or identity being revealed. LGBT service members may also harbor internalized homonegativity, which could also cause LGBT service members who have been victims of sexual assault or bullying to similarly not report. The Perpetrator Hypothesis predicts that concealment of sexual orientation or identity and internalized homophobia are related to the impact that victimization has on the functional domains. When either is highly present, adverse outcomes associated with victimization will be exacerbated. Conversely, when concealment and/or internalized homophobia are low, the adverse effects of victimization will be lessened or attenuated.

Peer and Organizational Factors In addition to individual factors that can moderate the adverse impact of victimization, the Perpetrator Hypothesis postulates that there are also peer and organizational factors that can lessen or attenuate the adverse effects produced by victimization. First, support received from fellow service members is especially important when reporting victimization. LGBT service members who have been victimized need to know that they will be believed and supported by other unit members and that appropriate actions will be taken. LGBT service members need to feel confident that they will not be blamed for the victimization, nor will they suffer from retaliation for reporting the victimization. Support for LGBT service members who have been victimized needs to come from both non-LGBT service members and from other LGBT service members. For instance, internalized homophobia might impede the support that fellow LGBT service members provide to those who report victimization, as they might blame victims for "being too gay" or "being too butch."

Leader behaviors following a report of LGBT victimization are equally critical. Leaders need to take all reports of LGBT victimization seriously. Leaders must openly support LGBT service members who report being victimized and ensure that retaliation against them does not occur. In particular, leaders need to ensure that LGBT victims receive all necessary health care, as well as the support and time needed to recover from acts of violence.

Finally, how the organization responds to and supports LGBT service members who report victimization is essential. The military must be committed to ensuring that the needs of the LGBT service member take priority. Military agencies outside the unit, such as criminal investigation, legal, and medical agencies, among others, must also be equally supportive.

Often, due to the unique culture of these organizations, such as criminal investigation, there is a tendency to initially challenge claims of victimization, which can be perceived by the victim as not believing the claim of victimization or blaming the victim.

Implications of the Perpetrator Hypothesis

The Perpetrator Hypothesis provides a conceptual framework for understanding the impact of acts of violence committed by perpetrators on the health and well-being of LGBT service members by building upon the minority stress theory (Meyer 2003). The Perpetrator Hypothesis presented here focuses on the causes and the consequences of violent and non-violent behaviors directed at LGBT service members. Importantly, the Perpetrator Hypothesis identifies numerous approaches to how perpetration can be either reduced or eliminated or, when perpetration does occur, how the potential adverse impact of perpetration can be minimized or attenuated. Viewed within the perspective of the Perpetrator Hypothesis, numerous suggestions for improving acceptance and integration of LGBT service members in the military have been provided.

It should be appreciated that the Perpetrator Hypothesis has important implications for understanding perpetration among nonmilitary populations and communities. For most minority or marginalized groups, the Perpetrator Hypothesis has direct applicability, as marginalized groups are at greater risk for being targets of perpetration for the same fundamental reasons that LGBT service members are victimized. That is, existing laws, cultures, or beliefs create an atmosphere in which perpetration is either condoned or enabled by members of the community or society. Therefore, women, children, undocumented immigrants, sex workers, as well as certain ethnic and racial groups, among others, are all at increased risk for perpetration. The Perpetrator Hypothesis can be expanded to encompass all of these vulnerable groups. Such a conceptual framework is necessary if clinicians wish to achieve a holistic approach in addressing perpetration and the adverse impacts that perpetration causes.

Key Concepts

1. Minorities should never be viewed as the cause of or be blamed for their victimization by perpetrators.
2. Minorities, such as lesbian, gay, bisexual, and transgender (LGBT) service members, are targeted by perpetrators because of perceptions of their perceived vulnerability.
3. There are many cultural and organizational enablers that allow for perpetrators to target LGBT service members, such as the "Don't Ask, Don't Tell" policy.
4. The impact of experiencing violent and non-violent behaviors includes adverse health, poor job attitudes and beliefs, and a decrease in work performance and career intentions.
5. There are a wide variety of interventions that can be developed and employed to combat LGBT service member victimization.

References

American Psychological Association (2011) Practice guidelines for LGB clients: guidelines for psychological practice with lesbian, gay, and bisexual clients. American Psychological Association, Washington, DC

American Psychological Association – Joint Task Force on Sexual Orientation & Military Service (APAJTF) (2009) Final report. Society of military psychology (division 19) and society for psychological study of lesbian, gay, and bisexual issues (division 44). Retrieved from: https://www.apa.org/pi/lgbt/resources/19-44-taskforce-report.pdf

Aquino K, Grover S, Bradfield M, Allen DG (1999) The effects of negative affectivity: hierarchical status and self-determination on workplace victimization. Acad Manag J 42:260–272

Blackwood E (1986) Breaking the mirror: the construction of lesbianism and the anthropological discussion of homosexuality. In: Blackwood E (ed) The many faces of homosexuality: anthropological approaches of homosexual behavior. Harrington Park, New York, pp 1–17

Bliese PD, Castro CA (2000) Role clarity, work overload and organizational support: multilevel evidence of the importance of support. Work Stress 14:65–73
Brown LS (1988) Feminist therapy with lesbians and gay men. In: Dutton-Douglas MA, Walker LEA (eds) Feminist psychotherapies: integration of therapeutic and feminist systems. Ablex, Norwood, p 206227
Burks DJ (2011) Lesbian, gay, and bisexual victimization in the military: an unintended consequence of "Don't Ask, Don't Tell"? Am Psychol 66(7):604–613
Burrelli DF (2010) "Don't ask, Don't Tell": the law and military policy on same-sex behavior (CRS report 40782). Congressional Research Service, Washington, DC
Castro CA, McGurk D (2007) The intensity of combat and behavioral health status. Traumatology 13:6–23
Castro CA, Kintzle S, Schuyler AC, Lucas CL, Warner CH (2015) Sexual assault in the military. Curr Psychiatry Rep 17:54–xx. https://doi.org/10.1007/s11920-015-0596-7
Cervantes RC, Fisher DG, Cordova D, Napper LE (2011) The Hispanic stress inventory-adolescent version: a culturally informed psychosocial assessment. Psychol Assess 24(1):187–196. https://doi.org/10.1037/a0025280
Cervantes R, Padilla A, KJip L, Goldbach J (2013) Acculturation-related stress among three generations of Hispanic adolescents. Hisp J Behav Sci 35:451–468. https://doi.org/10.1177/0739986313500924
Cochran BN, Balsam K, Flentje A, Malte CA, Simpson T (2013) Mental health characteristics of sexual minority veterans. J Homosex 60:419–435
Cole SW, Kemeny ME, Taylor SE, Visscher BR (1996) Elevated physical health risk among gay men who conceal their homosexual identity. Health Psychol 15(4):243–251
Conley D, Heerwig J (2011) The war at home: effects of Vietnam-era military service on postwar household stability. Am Econ Rev 101:350–354. https://doi.org/10.3386/w16671
Davis UC (2015) LGBTQ+ Glossary. Retrieved from: https://www.ucdrnc.ucdavis.edu/diversity-inclusion/LGBTQI/LGBTQ-Plus.html
Dentato MP, Halklitis PN, Orwat J (2013) Minority stress theory: an examination of factors surrounding sexual risk behavior among gay and bisexual men who use club drugs. J Gay Lesbian Sch Serv 24:509–525. https://doi.org/10.1080/10538720.2013.829395
Department of Defense (2015) Sexual assault prevention and response (SAPR) program. Directive Number 6495.01
Diamond LM (2003a) Love matters: romantic relationships among sexual-minority adolescents. In: Florsheim P (ed) Adolescent romantic relations and sexual behavior: theory, research, and practical implications. Lawrence Erlbaum, Mahwah, pp 85–107
Diamond LM (2003b) What does sexual orientation orient? A biobehavioral model distinguishing romantic love and sexual desire. Psychol Rev 110:173–192
Diamond LM (2005) From the heart or the gut? Sexual-minority women's experiences of desire for same-sex and other-sex partners. Fem Psychol 15:10–14
Egan SK, Perry DG (2001) Gender identity: a multidimensional analysis with implications for psychosocial adjustment. Dev Psychol 37:451–463
Fisher CM (2012) Assessing developmental trajectories of sexual minority youth: discrepant findings from a life history calendar and a self-administered survey. J LGBT Youth 9:114–135. https://doi.org/10.1080/19361653.2012.649643
Friedman MS, Marshal MP, Guadamuz TE, Wei C, Wong CF, Saewyc EM, Stall R (2011) A meta-analysis of disparities in childhood sexual abuse, parental physical abuse, and peer victimization among sexual minority and sexual nonminority individuals. Am J Public Health 101:1481–1494. https://doi.org/10.2105/AJPH.2009.190009
Gallup. (2012). Special report: 3.4% of U.S. adults identify as LGBT: inaugural gallup findings based on more than 120,000 interviews. Gallup politics. Retrieved from http://www.gallup.com/poll/158066/special-report-adults-identify-lgbt.aspx
Gibbs J, Goldbach JT (2015) Religious conflict, sexual identity, and suicidal behaviors among sexual minority youth. Arch Suicide Res 19(4):472–488. https://doi.org/10.1080/13811118.2015.1004476
Goldbach JT, Castro CA (2016) Lesbian, gay, bisexual and transgender (LGBT) service members. Curr Psychiatry Rep 18:1–7. https://doi.org/10.1007/s11920-016-0695-0
Goldbach JT, Tanner-Smith EE, Bagwell M, Dunlap S (2014) Minority stress and substance use in sexual minority adolescents: a meta-analysis. Prev Sci 15:350–363. https://doi.org/10.1007/s11121-013-0393-7
Goldbach JT, Gibbs J (2015) Strategies employed by sexual minority adolescents to cope with minority stress. Psychol Sex Orientation Gend Divers 2:297–306
Griffith J (1988) Measurement of group cohesion in U.S. army units. Basic Appl Soc Psychol 9:149–171
Hatzenbuehler ML (2009) How does sexual minority stigma "Get Under the Skin"? A psychological mediation framework. Psychol Bull 135(5):707–730. https://doi.org/10.1037/a0016441
Janssen E, Everaerd W, Spiering M, Janssen J (2000) Automatic processes and the appraisal of sexual stimuli: toward an information processing model of sexual arousal. J Sex Res 37:8–23. https://doi.org/10.1080/00224490009552016
Jones L, Bellis MA, Wood S, Hughes K, McCoy E, Eckley L, Bates G, Mikton C, Shakespeare T, Office A (2012) Prevalence and risk of violence against children with disabilities: a systematic review and meta-analysis of observational studies. Lancet 380(9845):899–907
Kaplan D, Rosenmann A (2012) Unit social cohesion in the Israeli military as a case study of "Don't Ask, Don't Tell". Polit Psychol 33:419–436. https://doi.org/10.1111/j.1467-9221.2012.00914.xView/save
Kauth MR, & Kalichrnan SC (1995) Sexual orientation and development: An interactive approach. *The psychology of sexual orientation, behavior, and identity*, 81–103

Kerrigan MF (2012) Transgender discrimination in the military: the new don't ask don't tell. Psychol Public Policy Law 18(3):500–518
Kessler RC (1979) Stress, social status, and psychological distress. J Health Soc Behav 20:259–272
Kinsey AC, Pomeroy WB, Martin CE (1948) Sexual behavior in the human male. WB Saunders, Philadelphia
Kinsey AC, Pomeroy WB, Martin CE (1953) Sexual behavior in the human female. WB Saunders, Philadelphia
Lazarus RS, Folkman S (1984) Stress, appraisal and coping. Springer, New York
LeVay S (1993) The sexual brain. MIT Press, Cambridge
Manning FS (1991) Morale, cohesion, and esprit de corps. In: Gal R, Mangelsdorff DA (eds) The handbook of military psychology. Wiley, Chichester, pp 453–470
Marshal MP, Dietz LJ, Friedman MS, Stall R, Smith HA, McGinley J, Brent DA (2011) Suicidality and depression disparities between sexual minority and heterosexual youth: a meta-analytic review. J Adolesc Health 49:115–123. https://doi.org/10.1016/j.jadohealth.2011.02.005
Marshal MP, Friedman MS, Stall R, King KM, Miles J, Gold MA et al (2008) Sexual orientation and adolescent substance use: a meta-analysis and methodological review. Addiction 103:546–556. https://doi.org/10.1111/j .1360-0443.2008.02149.x
Mays VM, Cochran SD (2001) Mental health correlates of perceived discrimination among lesbian, gay, and bisexual adults in the United States. Am J Public Health 91:1869–1876
McLeod JD, Kessler RC (1990) Socioeconomic status differences in vulnerability to life events. J Health Soc Behav 31:162–172. https://doi.org/10.2307/2137170
Meyer IH (2003) Prejudice, social stress, and mental health in lesbian, gay, and bisexual populations: conceptual issues and research evidence. Psychol Bull 129:674–697
Moradi B (2009) Sexual orientation disclosure, concealment, harassment, and military cohesion: perceptions of LGBT military veterans. Mil Psychol 21:513–533. https://doi.org/10.1080/08995600903206453
Murray JB (2000) Psychological profile of pedophiles and child molesters. J Psychol 134:211–224. https://doi.org/10.1080/00223980009600863
Mustanski BS, Garofalo R, Emerson EM (2010) Mental health disorders, psychological distress, and suicidality in a diverse sample of lesbian, gay, bisexual, and transgender youths. Am J Public Health 100:2426–2432. https://doi.org/10.2105/AJPH.2009.178319
Namie G, Christensen D Phillips D (2014) WBI U.S. Workplace bullying survey. Workplace bullying institute. Retrieved from the workplacebullying.org
Ray-Sannerud BN, Bryan CJ, Perry NS, Bryan AO (2015) High levels of emotional distress, trauma exposure, and self-injurious thoughts and behaviors among military personnel and veterans with a history of same sex behavior. Psychol Sex Orientation Gend Divers 2(2):130–137
Remafedi G, Resnick M, Blum R, Harris L (1992) Demography of sexual orientation in adolescents. Pediatrics 89:714–721
Renshaw KD, Rodebaugh TL, Rodrigues CS (2010) Psychological and marital distress in spouses of Vietnam veterans: importance of spouses' perceptions. Anxiety Disord 24:743–750. https://doi.org/10.1016/j.janxdis.2010.05.007
Robinson KE (1994) Addressing the needs of gay and lesbian students: the school counselor's role. Sch Couns 41:326–332
Rosario M, Rotheram-Borus MJ, Reid HM (1996) Gay-related stress and its correlates among gay and bisexual male adolescents of predominantly black and Hispanic background. J Community Psychol 24: 136–159
Rosario M, Schrimshaw EW, Hunter J, Gwadz M (2002) Gay-related stress and emotional distress among gay, lesbian and bisexual youths: a longitudinal examination. J Consult Clin Psychol 70:967–975
Savin-Williams RC (2001) Mom, dad, I'm gay: how families negotiate coming out. American Psychological Association, Washington, DC
Sell RL (1997) Defining and measuring sexual orientation: a review. Arch Sex Behav 26(6):643–657
Siebold GL (1999) The evolution of the measurement of cohesion. Mil Psychol 11(1):5–26
Smith DM (2008) Active duty military personnel presenting for care at a gay men's health clinic. J Homosex 54:277–279. https://doi.org/10.1080/00918360801982173
Thoits PA (1991) On merging identity theory and stress research. Soc Psychol Q 54(2):101–112
Toomey RB, Ryan C, Diaz RM, Card NA, Russell ST (2010) Gender-nonconforming lesbian, gay, bisexual, and transgender youth: school victimization and young adult psychosocial adjustment. Dev Psychol 46:1580–1589. https://doi.org/10.1037/a0020705
Turner HA, Finkelhor D, Ormrod RK (2006) The effect of lifetime victimization on the mental health of children and adolescents. Soc Sci Med 62(1):13–27
US Army (2014) Army regulation 600–20: army command policy. Headquarters Department of the Army, Washington, DC
Weber L, Parra-Medina D (2003) Intersectionality and women's health: charting a path to eliminating health disparities. In: Segal MT, Demos V, Kronenfeld JJ (eds) Gender perspectives on health and medicine, Advances in Gender Research, vol 7. Emerald Group Publishing Limited, Bingley, pp 181–230
Wong L, Kolditz TA, Millen RA, Potter TM (2003) Why they fight: combat motivation in the Iraq war. Strategic Studies Institute, U.S. Army War College, Carlisle
Zarembo A (2015) Why do transgender people join the military in such high numbers? Los Angeles Times, Sept 4. http://www.latimes.com/nation/la-na-transgender-military-20150904-story.html

The Military Mental Health Disability System

11

Jeffrey Guina, Randon S. Welton,
Pamela J. Broderick, and Ryan P. Peirson

Overview of the Mental Health Disability System

The system for determining mental health disability and compensation for service members is termed the Integrated Disability Evaluation System (IDES), combining Department of Defense and Veterans Affairs (VA) processes. The IDES process can vary between service branches but always includes treatment, Medical Evaluation Board (MEB), Physical Evaluation Board (PEB), and, potentially, transitioning out of the military. This process is resource intensive as well as a significant source of stress for service members, in part because it typically takes 6 months or longer. However, that period of time is spent in service, which is the reason the IDES was created (i.e., to address concerns about disabled veterans being separated but then being delayed for long periods of time before receiving VA benefits). For veterans who are no longer serving, disability claims are filed with the Veterans Benefits Administration, which may directly initiate a Separation-Compensation and Pension examination (Worthen and Moering 2011).

The process begins with identification of service members with potentially disqualifying mental health conditions that render them unfit for duty. Fitness for duty is determined by mental health providers evaluating the impact of a condition on occupational functioning (e.g., the ability to deploy overseas). In general, disqualifying conditions are determined by the *Diagnostic and Statistical Manual of Mental Disorders* (*DSM*) as required by Title 38 of the US Code (38 U.S.C. 4.125). While the *DSM* was not initially intended for determining occupational fitness for duty or disability eligibility, this has become standard in the military, which has led many clinicians to worry about how it will affect access to care and who gets financial benefits (Guina et al. 2016; McFarlane 2014). Some mental disorders are considered unfitting for military duty and can result in medical discharge with disability benefits, while others are considered unsuiting for military duty and can result in administrative separation without benefits or require a waiver to return to certain military duties (AFI 48-123 2014). What is disqualifying may vary between

J. Guina (✉) • P.J. Broderick
Wright-Patterson Medical Center, Wright-Patterson Air Force Base, Dayton, OH, USA

Wright State University Boonshoft School of Medicine, Dayton, OH, USA
e-mail: jeffrey.guina@us.af.mil

R.S. Welton
Wright State University Boonshoft School of Medicine, Dayton, OH, USA

R.P. Peirson
U.S. Air Force School of Aerospace Medicine, Wright-Patterson Air Force Base, Dayton, OH, USA

Wright State University Boonshoft School of Medicine, Dayton, OH, USA

L.W. Roberts, C.H. Warner (eds.), *Military and Veteran Mental Health*,
https://doi.org/10.1007/978-1-4939-7438-2_11

service branches and between job duties (e.g., pilots have stricter standards than others). Table 11.1 provides examples of potentially disqualifying conditions based on US Air Force standards (US Air Force 2016). Most disorders are not automatically disqualifying, with disqualification typically depending on impact on functioning, treatment requirements, and risk of recurrence. For example, the US Air Force considers the following unfitting: mental disorders causing impairment beyond 1 year, requiring continuing mental health treatment (e.g., weekly psychotherapy) beyond 1 year in order to perform military duty, requiring psychoactive medications managed by a licensed mental health provider beyond 1 year, requiring mood stabilizers (i.e., lithium, anticonvulsants, antipsychotics), and requiring recurrent psychiatric hospitalizations (US Air Force 2016). Similarly, the US Air Force only considers neurodevelopmental disorders (e.g., learning, communication, attention deficit/hyperactive) disqualifying if they have "ever compromised military duty or training, required treatment, or required special accommodations for job or academic performance" (US Air Force 2016).

Table 11.1 Mental health conditions that are potentially unsuiting or unfitting for military service

Potentially unsuiting conditions	Potentially unfitting conditions
Neurodevelopmental disorders	Schizophrenia
Disruptive, impulse control, and conduct disorders	Bipolar and related disorders
Substance-related and addictive disorders	Depressive disorders
Personality disorders	Anxiety disorders
History of suicide or suicidal behavior	Obsessive-compulsive and related disorders
Nonrecurrent adjustment disorder <60 days	Chronic trauma- and stressor-related disorders
Specific phobia to flying	Dissociative disorders
Schizophrenia in both parents	Somatic symptom and related disorders
Bipolar disorder in both parents	Feeding and eating and elimination disorders
Maladaptive personality traits[a]	Neurocognitive disorders
A pattern of maladaptive behavior[a]	Sexual disorders[b]

[a]Potentially unsuiting for flyers only and only when significantly interfering with safety or mission

[b]Gender nonconforming or transgender is not disqualifying from continued service if there is no duty impact

Service members may be referred to the IDES for a number of reasons, by both commanders and clinicians. Members may be referred for several reasons including, but not limited to, having an automatically disqualifying diagnosis (e.g., psychotic and bipolar disorders), showing continued impairment after receiving optimal medical benefit (i.e., after an adequate trial of treatment), having an unfavorable prognosis, following a suicide attempt, following cancelation of a deployment due to a mental health condition, or requiring significant time away from work or on duty restrictions (e.g., no firearms, no deployments). Once referred, a Medical Evaluation Board (MEB) provider or panel of medical personnel determines if a MEB is required.

If a MEB is deemed appropriate, it requires a mental health evaluation. Service members undergoing MEBs and veterans filing disability claims are evaluated in Separation-Compensation and Pension examinations (Worthen and Moering 2011). These evaluations can be completed by a VA mental health provider or by a trained, private mental health provider. If a service-connected mental health disorder is diagnosed, a rating is assigned. The rating represents the percentage of impairment of the veteran's average earning capacity. The current VA Schedule for Rating Disability is based on a standardized rating for disability that was developed in 1945 (IOM 2007). Veteran disability requires that examiners consider the frequency, severity, and duration of psychiatric symptoms and the veteran's capacity for readjustment during periods of remission (38 U.S.C. 4.125). The examiner must consider the veteran's degree of social and occupational functioning based on all existing evidence and not just the veteran's self-report (38 U.S.C. 4.126). The General Rating Formula for Mental Disorders is based on a 0–100 scale with specific descriptions for ratings of 0%, 10%, 30%, 50%, 70%, and 100% (38 U.S.C. 4.130). For active duty members, a Department of Defense mental health provider also completes a report including a thorough mental health history, diagnosis, impairment assessment, prognosis, and recommendations and outlines if the condition existed prior to service.

These reports go to the MEB, which must include "at least one psychiatrist or psychologist with a doctorate in psychology"—military or civilian employees—with at least one having "detailed knowledge of the standards pertaining to medical fitness, the disposition of patients, and disability separation processing" (DoDI 1332.18 2014). If requested by the service member, an impartial physician independent of the MEB will review the MEB findings and advise the service member. Service members are permitted to at least one rebuttal of the MEB findings. If the MEB determines that service members cannot perform their duties based on all the required examinations and reports, it refers the case to a Physical Evaluation Board (PEB). The PEB consists of a president who is a military O-6 (i.e., the pay grade of a colonel in the US Army, Air Force, and Marines or a captain in the Navy and Coast Guard) or the civilian equivalent, a medical officer who cannot be the service member's clinician and cannot have served on the service member's MEB examination, and a line officer familiar with duty assignments. PEBs determine fitness for duty and the reason an unfitting condition is or is not compensable (the amount of which is based on the percentage rating of a disability determined by the VA). Determinations may include a medical retirement with compensation, a return to duty with no restrictions, a return to duty with restrictions (e.g., no deployments, must be assigned to bases with mental health providers), a separation with or without severance pay, or a Temporary Disability Retired List (TDRL). A Temporary Disability Retired List provides members temporary retirement including continuing medical benefits for up to 5 years, during which they are reevaluated every 12–24 months by a military mental health provider, and after 5 years or earlier, a permanent determination is made. Whatever the MEB determination, once the rating is assigned, the findings are forwarded to the service member who can choose to accept the determination or appeal. If separation from the military is initiated, the member has a 90–120-day transition period.

Case Study

John Peralta (pseudonym), a 40-year-old male US Air Force Technical Sergeant with a history of post-traumatic stress disorder (PTSD), was referred by his commander for a Medical Evaluation Board (MEB) to determine fitness for duty and medical disability eligibility. He denied any psychiatry history until experiencing combat-related traumas in Afghanistan. He received mental health treatment for the 3 years preceding the MEB, including supportive psychotherapy, sertraline 50 mg daily for mood/anxiety, and hydroxyzine 50 mg daily as needed for anxiety. He had no treatment history other than failing brief trials of trazodone and prazosin. With only minimal improvements from treatment, he continued to have occupational dysfunction, largely due to poor concentration, excessive startle, re-experiencing instances, and irritability. Because he had not received adequate treatment for PTSD, the active duty psychiatrist that evaluated him recommended that he receive a full course of evidence-based trauma-focused psychotherapy and that his sertraline be titrated to a therapeutic dose or changed to another agent if he continued to not respond. His prognosis was deemed to be fair with respect to military service if he received adequate treatment, and it was recommended that he be reassessed in 1 year. An independent VA psychiatric examination concurred with the diagnosis and recommendations. The military placed him on the Temporary Disability Retirement List, medically separating him from the military and awarding him 50% service-connected medical disability for PTSD. Six months later, he started cognitive processing therapy at the VA but dropped out of treatment before completion. One year after the MEB, his sertraline 50 mg was increased to 100 mg. A different active duty psychiatrist reassessed him 18 months after the MEB and determined there had been little change in symptoms or functioning and repeated the same recommendations for a full course of psychotherapy, maximizing medications and reassessing in 1 year.

Common Concerns

While pensions were given to disabled veterans since the formation of the US, the focus had historically been on physical injuries and diseases like tuberculosis. Although mental health professionals had long recognized the connection between combat and mental health pathology, the *DSM* did not recognize PTSD until 1980—in large part due to lobbying by veterans (Herman 2015). This recognition was partially responsible for the VA increasing resources for the treatment and research of mental disorders since the 1980s (VA 2016). With increased recognition of how combat can impact mental health and increased survival rates from catastrophic injuries—largely due to improved body armor and medical advances—in recent wars (Dunbar 2015; Goldberg 2014), veteran disability compensation for mental health conditions has become more prevalent. In fact, PTSD has become the third most common VA disability, behind tinnitus and hearing loss (McNally and Frueh 2013). The number of veterans receiving PTSD-related disability benefits increased 80% from 1999 to 2004 (Frueh et al. 2007). Among veterans receiving compensation for mental disorders, 58% are for PTSD, and, among Operation Enduring Freedom/Operation Iraqi Freedom (OEF/OIF) veterans, the number rises to 75% (McNally and Frueh 2013). In 2010, the VA implemented the Disability Benefits Questionnaire, a shorter version than previous examination templates to handle the increased load of disability claims following Operation Enduring Freedom/Operation Iraqi Freedom (Worthen and Moering 2011). Beginning in 2011, private mental health providers (in addition to VA providers) were eligible to conduct Separation-Compensation and Pension examinations. Although both changes were intended to streamline the compensation process, concerns regarding accuracy and completeness of the assessments have arisen.

Both over- and underdiagnosis of mental health conditions are fraught with potential occupational/financial consequences for veterans. Since diagnoses can result in service members being limited in their duties or even losing their job—by medical discharge with disability compensation and healthcare benefits, administrative separation without benefits, or dishonorable discharge due to problematic behaviors—proper diagnosis is important for service members' finances, the military's manning, and the VA's budget. Veterans often experience psychological distress and dysfunction but do not meet *DSM* criteria and may be denied VA healthcare services or disability compensation. Conversely, some veterans receive benefits for feigned or exaggerated symptoms or have a true mental health condition but receive benefits despite never attempting or completing treatment. Besides fiscal reasons, accurate diagnosis and proper treatment are important because veterans with service-connected disabilities have lower suicide rates than those without (VA/DoD 2010). Unfortunately, policies such as 50% disability for combat-related mental health conditions have led many to suggest that the military is financially incentivizing individuals to be or remain ill.

Overreporting and Malingering

Detecting malingering is important not only for legal and financial reasons but also clinical and ethical ones. While malingering PTSD for legal and financial gain is common in the civilian setting (Guriel and Fremouw 2003; Kunst et al. 2011), these rates may be even higher in the military, with 37–75% of veterans that report PTSD exaggerating or malingering (McNally 2007; Smith and Frueh 1996). However, these high rates are controversial, and the military has been criticized for overemphasizing malingering, resulting in increased standardization of disability evaluations (Vergun 2012). Nevertheless, overreporting does occur in the military disability

Table 11.2 Possible reasons for over- and underreporting symptoms in military populations

	Overreporting	Underreporting
Help-seeking incentives/deterrents	Desire for care/pity	Stigma
	Decrease legal responsibility/liability	Lack of mental health knowledge
	Benzodiazepines	Denial of mental health problems
Cultural attitudes	Belonging to a group of sufferers	Overvaluing self-reliance
	Desire to be distinct/important	Stoicism/masculinity
		Perceive mental disorders as weakness
Contextual factors in military	Seeking disability payments	Issues of confidentiality
	Avoid service/deployment	Negative career impacts
		Perceive clinician conflict of interest
Common issues with trauma	Fear of not being believed/understood	Avoidance of trauma discussion
	Excessive blame of military/government	Embarrassment or shame
	Excessive self-blame	Normalization of trauma
	Blaming all life problems on trauma	Belief that nothing can help

From Guina et al. (2016)

system and is important for recommending and monitoring treatment and assuring access to limited treatment resources.

Numerous factors complicate detecting overreporting. With high comorbidity rates among mental disorders, the most scrupulous patients may have difficulty separating trauma-related problems and those from other conditions. Structured interviews found 53% of Vietnam veterans had "clear exaggeration" of PTSD symptoms, but 70% of these had major depressive disorder and 58% alcohol dependence (McNally 2007). Among Vietnam veterans applying for PTSD-related disability in one study, 52% had no documented combat exposure, and 5% either had never been in the military or never deployed (Frueh et al. 2005). Clinicians are generally left with the dilemma of diagnosing mental disorders or malingering without supporting documentation. An alternative to this dichotomous schema is delineating a true mental disorder, "pure malingering," "partial malingering," and "feigning symptoms" (Resnick 1999; Wooley and Rogers 2015). Pure malingering involves fabricating symptoms (and, possibly, trauma). Partial malingering involves exaggerating symptoms (e.g., from an actual trauma). Feigning involves ascribing symptoms to a condition which actually emanate from another source (e.g., ascribing alcohol-induced anxiety to PTSD).

The spectrum of overreporting hints at several causes (Table 11.2), including both primary and secondary gain. Some individuals' desires for disability arise from a sense they are owed recompense, viewing their suffering as the responsibility of a person or system. For others, trauma becomes the single dominant event that precipitated their future distress; all subsequent problems with relationships, substances, and career are blamed on trauma regardless of the real cause (Frueh et al. 2000). For many, overreporting is more like factitious disorder than true malingering. A label like "PTSD" makes them distinct, important, and the object of concern and serves primary gain: receiving care, pity, or the psychosocial benefits of belonging to a self-identified group of sufferers (Ali et al. 2015). Clinicians should consider all of these potentially contributing factors before assuming malingering.

In general, clinicians tend to take everything patients say at face value, but in forensic and occupational settings where motives may exist beyond the desire for treatment, further efforts, tools, and techniques become necessary. Asking open-ended questions, having patients spontaneously report symptoms, inquiring into specific examples of personal manifestations of a condition, and focusing on evidence of dysfunction rather than symptom self-report are all preferable to allowing patients to recite memorized criteria or affirming symptoms proffered by interviewers. The development of objective measures and screening tools, the standardized evaluation methodology, and the military pushing for more research into biomarkers for PTSD have attempted to improve this, but clinician judgment will always be the most important factor in disability evaluations. However, considering that many veterans seek help from civilian clinicians who are not culturally competent with military patients and policies, there is still a potential for overdiagnosis. Inconsistencies should be explored thoroughly, including within self-report, between what is reported and observed (e.g., inattention, agitation, excessive startle), between self-report and collateral information (e.g., military, police and medical records, and interviews with significant others), and between individual and typical presentations (Ali et al. 2015). Unfortunately, clinicians often do not have access to all military records, or frequently, veterans delay reporting about mental health symptoms or a trauma until years later. The current system is designed to give the benefit of the doubt, as compared to a workman's compensation model requiring the claimant to prove their disability (Worthen and Moering 2011). Diagnosis is improved with structured interviewing techniques such as the Structured Clinical Interview for *DSM* and Clinician-Assessed PTSD Scale (Morgan et al. 2005). Several psychometric tests include subscales for exaggeration: the Minnesota Multiphasic Personality Inventory-2 (MMPI), the Structured Interview of Reported Symptoms, the Miller Forensic Assessment of Symptoms Test (which can be taken and scored in 15 min), and the Traumatic Stress subscale of the Anxiety-Related Disorders Scale of the Personality Assessment Inventory (Smith and Frueh 1996; Freeman et al. 2008). Distinguishing between those who are honestly reporting and inflating symptoms/distress is important for patients, clinicians, the military, and taxpayers.

Underreporting and Reverse Malingering

There are many tangible reasons to underreport (Table 11.2), and minimizing symptoms may be more common in the military than the general population. Service members are probably more likely to "fake good," which is verifiable by the Minnesota Multiphasic Personality Inventory-2 (MMPI) (Elhai et al. 2000), or avoid treatment altogether. A military culture of stoicism and hypermasculinity can lead to underreporting and avoiding and rejecting help (Lollis et al. 2009; Tolin and Foa 2008). Among those with PTSD, it is common to normalize their symptoms or trauma, to feel ashamed about a trauma, or to perceive their symptoms as a failure to cope as well as others they served with, which can further impede help seeking (Nazarov et al. 2015). It is important that military leaders avoid perpetuating mental health stigma, actively support their troops who are suffering (rather than waiting for members to come to leadership for help), and publicly discuss general mental health concerns.

While malingering receives significant attention because of the costs of fraudulent disability compensation (Zarembo 2014), reverse malingering is understudied. Reverse malingering is the intentional underreporting of symptoms or distress (Lurati 2013). Some try to avoid the legal, disciplinary, and social consequences that may result from the revelation of unhealthy behaviors. Others fear negative career impacts, including being prevented from changing to more attractive duty stations, being limited in duties (e.g., leadership, aircrew, medical, police, presidential assignments), and even losing one's career (Lollis et al. 2009). Contrary to popular belief, most service members—unlike Sergeant Klinger from *M*A*S*H*—want to keep their job (including salary and benefits, especially for those nearing 20 years of active duty service when retirement benefits become available), and many want to deploy (whether out of a sense of duty or honor or because it may help their careers). Reverse malingering is most commonly associated with considering work a part of self-worth (military service is accompanied by a deep sense of purpose and identity) and considering work as therapy or a distraction for problems, having many responsibilities, and income (Lurati 2015). Clinicians have a responsibility to determine with reasonable certainty fitness for duty because failure to recognize limitations in unfit service members can increase their risk to themselves, others, and even national security. For these reasons, the military needs to be careful about over-incentivizing or disincentivizing self-disclosure of mental health concerns.

Stigmatizing and over-punishing mental health problems can be a major deterrent for service members seeking mental health care. Because there are more exceptions for confidentiality in military than civilian medicine, including being deemed unfit for duty to perform a mission, violation of military standards and laws, and substance use (DoDI 6025.18-R 2003), concerns about clinician conflicts of interest can be particularly off-putting. Even if members are comfortable seeking mental health treatment, they are often concerned how leadership will respond. It is important that military leaders find a balance between lenient (even those with a mental health condition should be held responsible for their criminal or insubordinate behaviors) and punitive actions (which can exacerbate mental health conditions and deter honest self-disclosure of problems), because both ignoring and castigating mental health problems are harmful.

Disability Without Adequate Treatment

Veterans seeking compensation for mental disorders without completing treatment (i.e., being deemed permanently disabled without knowing if recovery is possible) is a pervasive problem for the military, complex in its causes, and an ethical and clinical conundrum for those evaluating disability. Most veterans receiving PTSD-related disability payments report increasing symptoms until given 100% disability ratings after which mental health visits precipitously decrease implying that compensation—not treatment—was the primary focus (Frueh et al. 2007). However, avoidance (of treatment and discussing problems) is common in many mental disorders—especially PTSD—and may partially explain why many receive disability compensation without adequate treatment.

Many clinicians and researchers implicate dropouts in the volume of veterans not receiving adequate treatment. A systematic review of psychotherapies for Operation Enduring Freedom/Operation Iraqi Freedom-related PTSD reported a 36% dropout rate (Goetter et al. 2015). Most dropouts occur within three sessions, prior to starting exposure (Najavits 2013), leading many to theorize that fears of revisiting trauma lead to dropouts. However, the most robust correlate of dropouts is younger age, with no significant correlations to exposure, symptom severity, comorbidity, or disability status (Goetter et al. 2015). Most studies define adequate treatment as attending 8 PTSD-related sessions within 12 months (Hoge et al. 2014), but most standard treatment courses are longer, such as cognitive processing therapy (CPT) (12 sessions) and prolonged exposure (PE) (8–15) (Najavits 2013). Despite this low bar, only one-third of Operation Enduring Freedom/Operation Iraqi Freedom veterans with PTSD obtain "adequate care" (Hoge et al. 2014), and that is likely an overestimate as number of visits provides little information about treatment quality and patient engagement.

Another concern is whether veterans receive evidence-based PTSD treatments, including cognitive processing therapy, prolonged exposure, eye movement desensitization and reprocessing (EMDR), cognitive restructuring therapy, trauma-focused cognitive behavioral therapy, brief eclectic psychotherapy, narrative therapy, stress inoculation training, and serotonergic antidepressants (Haagan et al. 2015; VA/DoD 2010). Although the VA and Department of Defense have invested substantially into training clinicians in prolonged exposure and cognitive processing therapy (Karlin et al. 2010; Eftekhari et al. 2013), less than 10% of veterans with PTSD have completed either cognitive processing therapy or prolonged exposure (Seal et al. 2010; Shiner et al. 2013; Mott et al. 2014), and supportive therapy continues to be the most common treatment (Najavits 2013). Clinician barriers include low confidence in effectiveness, fear of dropout or symptom exacerbation, and lack of training (Najavits 2013). Additionally, many clinicians modify treatment protocols, homework, and number or structure of sessions—changes which have unknown efficacy (Najavits 2013).

Of veterans who engage in treatment, recovery rates are 70–80% for evidence-based treatment completers but decrease to 40% after accounting for dropouts (Hoge et al. 2014). Some speculate that real-world conditions further limit effectiveness since studies often exclude suicidal, homicidal, substance-using, and cognitively impaired patients (Najavits 2013). Nevertheless, number of sessions and focus on traumatic content are most predictive of improvement (Haagan et al. 2015).

Treatment dropout and lack of evidence-based treatment commonly contribute to veterans making claims for mental health disabilities without adequate treatment. How should the VA/Department of Defense respond? Is it ethical to withhold or delay compensation until treatment is completed? Is it ethical to declare someone disabled without adequate treatment? Even with treatment, how often will secondary gain deter recovery? If veterans drop one treatment, it is reasonable to recommend further treatment with a different provider and/or modality. The system should work to incentivize getting healthy, but many argue the current system disincentivizes recovery. Increased training and consultation with senior clinicians to discuss cases may help address clinicians who opt for nonevidence-based approaches, alter treatment protocols, or are limited in the modalities they provide (e.g., only cognitive processing therapy or prolonged exposure for PTSD). Implementing these proposals is almost certainly cost-effective because if recovery rates improve, so will disability rates.

Implications for the Future

While most clinicians are trained to diagnose in clinical settings, many are unfamiliar with occupational and forensic settings (Morgan et al. 2005), where evaluees have motivations for dishonesty and under- and overreporting. Although it is easy to give examples when most clinicians are appropriately skeptical of a patient's intent (e.g., doctor shopping, efforts to obtain controlled substances, etc.), it could be argued that clinicians should take a trusting stance and accept the information given by patients. All the while assessing for historical reliability, some have argued that reciprocal trust is an important aspect of the healthcare relationship (Thorne and Robinson 1988). It has even been said that trusting patients is a "moral duty" (Rogers 2002). This notion has face validity—who wants to see a provider who does not believe him/her? Yet, clinicians have good reason to be skeptical of many subjective reports, especially those of behaviors related to eating, substance use, and medication adherence (Gadkari and McHorney 2012; Mertz 1984; Morgan et al. 2005; Palamar et al. 2015). Indeed, even in settings where malingering is more common, it can be difficult to stave cynicism and preserve empathy. A middle ground is possible, where individuals are trained to respect, empathize, and trust their patients but also are trained to be aware of possible secondary gain and the signs of malingering. As always, the differential diagnoses must be broad, and all possibilities must be systematically ruled in or ruled out. Clinicians need to be able to identify typical vs. atypical symptoms and should avoid leading, coaching, or suggesting. Administration must insist that professionals are thorough and a culture of immediate suspicion or dismissal of patients must not be tolerated. On the other hand, they must ensure that clinicians are provided with ongoing training and support about the issues of feigning and malingering. Support for obtaining an access to necessary sources of collateral data (e.g., VA *and* Department of Defense's medical *and* personnel records) is crucial, and clinicians should be more familiar with validated instruments and structured interviews.

The VA/Department of Defense (and others treating service members) should expand their treatment armamentarium (e.g., currently the military only provides cognitive processing therapy and prolonged exposure trainings for PTSD) and address the needs of those who do not respond to first-line treatments or do not fit in the current procrustean *DSM* bed. Treatment model fidelity and adherence to protocol are notoriously difficult to achieve, but efforts should be made to ensure members receive the correct treatment for the correct duration. Currently, disability benefits are not tied to treatment adherence. This begs the question: is it just to provide benefits for individuals who never attempt a valid course of treatment? Perhaps this is an uncomfortable question, but clinicians should not shy away from discussions about the need for evidence-based treatment and efforts to ensure veterans and service members have the opportunities to receive the treatment they deserve. As assessments and biomarkers become available, they should be utilized as appropriate. Clearer policies for treatment requirements may improve outcomes and retention. The disability system must not be structured to discourage individuals from improving their health.

While clearer policies for fitness requirements can make evaluations easier for clinicians (especially civilians), they may also make feigning symptoms easier. Clinical judgment and case-by-case determinations are essential as absolutist policies can be exploited for secondary gain. The structure of the disability system must be carefully designed as not to over-incentivize or disincentivize fitness/compensation evaluations.

Finally, in keeping with the Institute of Medicine's recommendation that healthcare workers have better education in social determinants of health, it would be wise to ensure the healthcare workforce understands social determinants as risk factors for future mental illness and other health burdens (Institute of Medicine 2016). This is a component of resiliency training but should be considered as practitioners assess individuals with symptoms. Better knowledge of these factors may help leadership target preventative interventions, help clinicians focus treatment, and may help with selection and retention.

Conclusions

Treating active duty and veteran military personnel can involve complex clinical and occupational decisions. It can be difficult to determine when what is reported is true (or feigned, overreported, or minimized), when adequate levels and the right types of treatment have been utilized, and when there is sufficient distress/dysfunction to warrant changes in diagnosis, treatment, and occupational status. More research is needed to best understand and care for service members with psychiatric disorders, both their mental health and their careers.

Key Concepts

1. The Integrated Disability Evaluation System may vary between service branches but always includes treatment, occupational evaluations, and Department of Defense/Veterans Affairs' determinations of fitness for duty, medical disability eligibility, and compensation.
2. The military disability process is time and resource intensive and can be stressful for service members.
3. Some mental health conditions are considered potentially unfitting and may result in medical retirement with disability compensation, while others are considered potentially unsuiting and may result in administrative separation without benefits.
4. Overreporting, misattribution of symptoms, and malingering can result in overdiagnosis and misappropriation of limited resources (e.g., compensation, treatment).
5. Minimization and reverse malingering can result in underdiagnosis and are common in the military, where a culture of stoicism and self-reliance, and fear of negative career impacts, often deters forthrightness.
6. Thorough reviews of records and collateral information, structured interviews, psychometric testing, and training evaluators in occu-

pational/forensic issues can help ensure the validity of diagnoses, though the current system is designed to give the benefit of the doubt to service members and veterans.

7. Symptomatic avoidance, stigma, treatment dropouts, and limited evidence-based treatment resources often lead to service members qualifying for medical disability without adequate treatment (i.e., deeming someone is permanently disabled without determining if recovery is possible with treatment).
8. Expanding and providing regular evidence-based treatment trainings and ensuring veterans are not disincentivized from recovering may improve outcomes, increase rates of returning service members to duty, and make available limited resources.

References

AFI 48-123 (2014) Department of the Air Force instruction on medical examinations and standards

Ali S, Jabeen S, Alam F (2015) Multimodal approach to identifying malingered posttraumatic stress disorder: a review. Innov Clin Neurosci 12(1–2):12–20

DoDI 1332.18 (2014) Department of Defense instruction on disability evaluation system

DoDI 6025.18-R (2003) Department of Defense instruction on health information privacy regulation

Dunbar VL (2015) Trauma registry yields significant increase in traumatic injury survival rates. Army News Service http://www.army.mil/article/150990/Trauma_registry_yields_significant_increase_in_traumatic_injury_survival_rates. Accessed 7 Feb 2016

Eftekhari A, Ruzek JI, Crowley JJ, Rosen CS, Greenbaum MA, Karlin BE (2013) Effectiveness of national implementation of prolonged exposure therapy in Veterans Affairs care. JAMA Psychiatr 70(9):949–955

Elhai JD, Gold PB, Rue BC, Gold SN (2000) Cross-validation of the MMPI-2 in detecting malingered posttraumatic stress disorder. J Pers Assess 75(3):449–463

Freeman T, Powell M, Kimbrell T (2008) Measuring symptom exaggeration in veterans with chronic posttraumatic stress disorder. Psychiatry Res 158(3):374–380

Frueh BC, Hamner MB, Cahill SP, Gold PB, Hamlin KL (2000) Apparent symptom overreporting in combat veterans evaluated for PTSD. Clin Psychol Rev 20(7):853–885

Frueh BC, Elhai JD, Grubaugh AL, Monnier J, Kashdan TB, Sauvageot JA, Hamner MB, Burkett BG, Arana GW (2005) Documented combat exposure of US veterans seeking treatment for combat-related post-traumatic stress disorder. Br J Psychiatry 186:467–4755

Frueh BC, Grubaugh AL, Elhai JD, Buckley TC (2007) US Department of Veterans Affairs disability policies for posttraumatic stress disorder: administrative trends and implications for treatment, rehabilitation, and research. Am J Public Health 97(12):2143–2145

Gadkari AS, McHorney CA (2012) Unintentional non-adherence to chronic prescription medications: how unintentional is it really? BMC Health Serv Res 12:98

Goetter EM, Ojserkis RA, Zakarian RJ (2015) A systematic review of dropout from psychotherapy for posttraumatic stress disorder among Iraq and Afghanistan combat veterans. J Trauma Stress 28:401–409

Goldberg MS (2014) Updated death and injury rates of U.S. military personnel during the conflicts in Iraq and Afghanistan. Congressional Budget Office https://www.cbo.gov/sites/default/files/113th-congress-2013-2014/workingpaper/49837-Casualties_WorkingPaper-2014-08_1.pdf. Accessed 7 Feb 2016

Guina J, Welton RS, Broderick PJ, Correll TL, Peirson RP (2016) DSM-5 criteria and its implications for diagnosing PTSD in military service members and veterans. Curr Psychiatr Rep 18(5):43

Guriel J, Fremouw W (2003) Assessing malingered posttraumatic stress disorder: a critical review. Clin Psychol Rev 23(7):881–904

Haagan JF, Smid GE, Knipscheer JW (2015) The efficacy of recommended treatment for veterans with PTSD: a metaregression analysis. Clin Psychol Rev 40:184–194

Herman J (2015) Trauma and recovery: the aftermath of violence – from domestic abuse to political terror, 2nd edn. Basic Books, New York

Hoge CW, Grossman SA, Auchterlonie JL (2014) PTSD treatment for soldiers after combat deployment: low utilization for mental health care and reasons for dropout. Psychiatr Serv 65(8):997–1004

Institute of Medicine (2007) A 21st century system for evaluating veterans for disability benefits. The National Academies Press, Washington, DC

Institute of Medicine (2016) A framework for educating health professionals to address the social determinants of health. Retrieved from: http://www.nap.edu/catalog/21923/a-framework-for-educating-health-professionals-to-address-the-social-determinants-of-health

Karlin BE, Ruzek JI, Chard KM, Eftekhari A, Monson CM, Hembree EA, Foa EB (2010) Dissemination of evidence-based psychological treatments for posttraumatic stress disorder in the Veterans Health Administration. J Trauma Stress 23(6):663–673

Kunst M, Winkel FW, Bogaerts S (2011) Recalled peritraumatic reactions, self-reported PTSD, and the impact of malingering and fantasy proneness in victims of interpersonal violence who have applied for state compensation. J Interpers Violence 26(11):2186–2210

Lollis BD, Marsh RW, Sowin TW, Thompson WT (2009) Major depressive disorder in military aviators: a ret-

rospective study of prevalence. Aviat Space Environ Med 80(5):734–737
Lurati AR (2013) Reverse malingering-staying on the job at any cost. Work Health Saf 61(7):297–298
Lurati AR (2015) Identifying reverse malingering in the civilian occupational setting. Workplace Health Saf pii: 2165079915607484
McFarlane A (2014) PTSD and DSM-5: unintended consequences of change. Lancet Psychiatr 1(4):246–247
McNally RJ (2007) Can we solve the mysteries of the national Vietnam Veterans Readjustment Study? J Anxiety Disord 21(2):192–200
McNally RJ, Frueh BC (2013) Why are Iraq and Afghanistan War veterans seeking PTSD disability compensation at unprecedented rates? J Anxiety Disord 27(5):520–526
Mertz W (1984) Beltsville one-year dietary intake study. Am J Clin Nutr 40(6 suppl):1323–1403
Morgan CA, Feuerstein S, Fortunati F, Coric V, Temporini H, Southwick S (2005) Posttraumatic stress disorder within the forensic arena. Psychiatry 2(10):21–24
Mott JM, Hundt NE, Sansgiry S, Mignogna J, Cully JA (2014) Changes in psychotherapy use among veterans with depression, anxiety, and PTSD. Psychiatr Serv 65(1):106–112
Najavits LM (2013) The problem of dropout from "gold standard" PTSD therapies. F1000Prime Rep 7(43):7–43
Nazarov A, Jetly R, McNeely H, Kiang M, Lanius R, McKinnon MC (2015) Role of morality in the experience of guilt and shame within the armed forces. Acta Psychiatr Scand 132(1):4–19
Palamar JJ, Martins SS, Su MK, Ompad DC (2015) Self-reported use of novel psychoactive substances in a US nationally representative survey: Prevalence, correlates, and a call for new survey methods to prevent underreporting. Drug Alchol Depend 1:112–119
Resnick PJ (1999) Malingering of posttraumatic disorders. In: Rogers R (ed) Clinical assessment of malingering and deception, 2nd edn. Guilford Press, New York, pp 84–103
Rogers WA (2002) Is there a moral duty for doctors to trust patients? J Med Ethics 28(2):77–80
Seal KH, Maguen S, Cohen B, Gima KS, Metzler TJ, Ren L, Bertenthal D, Marmar CR (2010) VA mental health services utilization in Iraq and Afghanistan veterans in the first year of receiving new mental health diagnoses. J Trauma Stress 23(1):5–16
Shiner B, D'Avolio LW, Nguyen TM, Zayed MH, Young-Xu Y, Desai RA, Schnurr PP, Fiore LD, Watts BV (2013) Measuring use of evidence based psychotherapy for posttraumatic stress disorder. Admin Pol Ment Health 40(4):311–318
Smith DW, Frueh BC (1996) Compensation seeking, comorbidity, and apparent exaggeration of PTSD symptoms among Vietnam combat veterans. Psychol Assess 8(1):3–6
Thorne SE, Robinson SE (1988) Reciprocal trust in health care relationships. J Adv Nurs 13(6):782–789
Tolin DF, Foa EB (2008) Sex differences in trauma and posttraumatic stress disorder: a quantitative review of 25 years of research. Psychol Trauma S(1):37–85
US Air Force (2016) US Air Force Medical Standards Directory, approved by AF SG3/5P on 02 Feb 2016
VA (2016) VA history in brief. http://www.va.gov/opa/publications/archives/docs/history_in_brief.pdf. Accessed 8 Feb 2016
VA/DoD (2010) Veterans Affairs and Department of Defense clinical practice guideline for management of post-traumatic stress. http://www.healthquality.va.gov/guidelines/MH/ptsd/cpg_PTSD-FULL-201011612.pdf. Accessed 14 Jan 2016
Vergun D. (2012) Army standardizes PTSD diagnosis, treatment. Army News Service http://www.army.mil/article/84928. Accessed 4 Feb 2016
Wooley CN, Rogers R (2015) The effectiveness of the personality assessment inventory with feigned PTSD: an initial investigation of Resnick's model of malingering. Assessment 22(4):449–458
Worthen MD, Moering RG (2011) A practical guide to conducting VA compensation and pension exams for PTSD and other mental disorders. Psychol Inj Law 4:187–216
Zarembo A. (2014) As disability awards grow so do concerns with veracity of PTSD claims. LA Times http://www.latimes.com/local/la-me-ptsd-disability-20140804-story.html. Accessed 24 Dec 2015

12 Vocational Rehabilitation

Charles Drebing, Lisa Mueller, Christopher Waltrous, and Walter Penk

Employment as a Clinical Concern

Vocational problems are common in adults with mental illness and can often respond well to clinical interventions designed specifically for adults with mental health treatment needs who are seeking to achieve an employment goal. Vocational problems come in many different forms, including (1) unemployment, (2) underemployed (being employed in day labor, temporary work, or work that requires substantially lower skill levels than prior work successfully engaged in), or (3) being employed at an appropriate level but functioning poorly at work secondary to mental health problems. While unemployment is the most commonly recognized and treated, other needs are important to recognize and to treat. As in the case of Maria, underemployment and poor functioning at work are often a part of the pathway to unemployment and all of its associated problems.

C. Drebing (✉) • L. Mueller • C. Waltrous • W. Penk
Bedford VA Medical Center, Bedford, MA 01730, USA
e-mail: Charles.drebing@va.gov; Lisa.Mueller@VA.gov; Christopher.Waltrous@VA.gov; WEPenk@att.net

Case Study

Sergeant (Sgt.) Maria Alvarez (pseudonym) served two tours in Iraq as a military police officer in the Army. When she was discharged, there were no openings for police officers in her area, but she had friends going back to school to become emergency medical technicians. She signed up for training, and as soon as she started, she felt convinced that this type of work was a perfect match for her.

She was very successful during the first 5 years working for a private ambulance company. She performed well and was respected by co-workers and supervisors. On at least two occasions, she received awards for excellent work in dangerous situations. In one particularly difficult situation, she was fired upon and almost killed while saving an attempted murder victim.

Surprisingly, Alvarez's work performance declined over the next 12 months, and she left that job unexpectedly. She then took an evening job as an emergency medical technician for a competing firm. Her work for that company did not go as well. She used a lot of sick leave and felt less enthusiastic about her work. She had more conflict from her supervisor and left the job within 6 months. She then left another

L.W. Roberts, C.H. Warner (eds.), *Military and Veteran Mental Health*,
https://doi.org/10.1007/978-1-4939-7438-2_12

emergency medical technician job only 4 months after starting and was then unemployed for 8 months.

It was during this time that she was referred for specialty mental health care by her primary care doctor for symptoms of posttraumatic stress disorder (PTSD). She was having recurring nightmares related to combat experiences in Iraq, as well as experiences from her first emergency medical technician job. On closer evaluation, it was clear that she was suffering from combat-related PTSD. Her symptoms were initially manageable when she started as an emergency medical technician but became worse over time. Eventually, she would feel anxious whenever she heard a radio call. She was particularly anxious when she had to drive in the neighborhood in which she was nearly shot. While working, she often felt like the prior incidents were just about to happen again. Unfortunately, she did not feel comfortable talking about her anxiety with her supervisor, feeling embarrassed for needing help and worried that she would lose her job. She used sick leave and substance use as a means of coping with her anxiety. Her loss of three jobs left her demoralized and thinking that she was not "smart enough" to do this type of work. She was concerned that she would never go back to work at all and was starting to feel that she had no future.

Employment and Recovery

There are a number of reasons for viewing employment or re-employment as central to mental health treatment and rehabilitation outcomes. Deterioration in functioning in employment is a central element in the definition and measurement of disability (see the World Health Organization's International Classification of Functioning, Disability and Health and VA compensation determination process) and of many of the most common health conditions (see *DSM-V* diagnostic criteria). The notion of recovery and community integration as the ultimate goal of rehabilitation, described in foundational documents such as the President's New Freedom Commission ("President's New Freedom Commission on Mental Health," 2003) and the Americans with Disabilities Act, emphasizes the primacy of helping participants resume valued roles like employment. In this framework, clinical care, and specifically those clinical efforts designed primarily to reduce clinical symptoms, is seen as part of the overall approach to helping adults to move toward or to maintain full integration in their communities.

Similarly, the current philosophical emphasis on client-centered approaches to healthcare (Stewart et al. 2000) emphasizes the need for all clinical services to serve the goals of clients. A growing body of evidence indicates that most adults with disabilities want to be employed in their community (McQuilken et al. 2003). Finally, there is growing support for the longstanding view of many vocational service providers and researchers that "Work is Therapy" (Kukla and Bond 2009; Siu et al. 2010). Participating in employment has important clinical benefits that rival the benefits of many common clinical interventions. These benefits are wide-ranging and, while not achieved by every participant, are generally experienced by most participants across most work settings. They include the benefits of social contact and engagement; learning and cognitive activity; physical activity; enhanced opportunities to play valued social roles, including a valued family role as "provider" and a valued societal role as a "worker"; a broader sense of purpose and meaning; opportunities to use and develop skills; opportunities for distraction from clinical symptoms such as anxiety; as well as the indirect benefits of earning income, such as paid leisure time and employer-supported healthcare benefits (Kukla and Bond 2009; Siu et al. 2010).

Unfortunately, unemployment is all too common among disabled adults and among veterans in particular (Zivin et al. 2011). The employment rate for individuals with disabilities aged 16–64 is only 36% compared to 75% for the non-disabled population ("Annual Disability Statistics

Compendium: 2009" 2009). This employment gap is present across disability types (45% for adults with sensory disabilities, 31% for physical disabilities, and 28% for mental disabilities) with the poorest employment rates found for the largest disability subgroups, particularly those with disabilities secondary to mental illnesses. When disabled adults do acquire employment, on average they earn 33% less than their non-disabled peers. The result is higher rates of poverty, with disabled adults facing a 25% poverty rate compared to 10% for non-disabled adults (22% for adults with sensory disabilities, 26% for physical disabilities, 31% for mental disabilities). Similar patterns are noted for veterans, with higher unemployment rates found among veterans with mental health conditions (Zivin et al. 2011), and particularly elevated risks of unemployment for recently returning female veterans (Kleykamp 2013).

Some form of vocational problems will be part of the experience of most adults and most veterans, but when they are secondary to mental health conditions, they tend to develop in predictable patterns (Penk et al. 2002). In a recent study, examining naturalistic data documenting the pathways-to-care to vocational services, the authors of the present chapter interviewed 155 veterans who were receiving some form of Veterans Health Administration (VHA) mental health care and had a vocational need but were not currently enrolled in vocational services (Drebing 2011; Drebing et al. 2012b). The median length of the participants' vocational need was more than 4.2 years. The vocational problems typically occurred after the mental health problem was present, and showed a clear progression in severity over time, often starting with performance or interpersonal problems at work and eventually resulting in multiple job losses and sustained unemployment. As with most mental health conditions, adults with vocational problems are slow to pursue treatment. Delays associated with recognition, help-seeking, and treatment entry all contribute to the overall delay in entering appropriate care. Factors associated with slower recognition, seeking help, and receiving services included diagnosis, level of disability, type of vocational need, and support from primary providers, family and friends. These results suggest that without proactive efforts by clinical providers to identify vocational problems and to actively refer veterans for vocational services, many will suffer vocational problems for years, with the accompanying difficulties for their family, the employment market, and society as a whole.

Models of Vocational Services

To address vocational problems among veterans and broader populations, governmental agencies, including the US Department of Veterans Affairs (VA), have invested heavily in vocational services. They are administered by a wide variety of organizations, using a range of different intervention models, most of which have resulted in relatively modest success rates (Bond et al. 2008; Resnick et al. 2006). Over the past 25 years, research efforts to systematically evaluate and improve these services have grown steadily both in number and in quality, with a fairly dramatic increase in the number of clinical trials and in overall methodological rigor (Drebing et al. 2012a). These research efforts have been the driving force behind relatively rapid changes in the broader field of vocational services and in vocational services targeted specifically for veterans with mental health concerns. For example, 10 years ago, the Veterans Health Administration vocational services programming consisted primarily of transitional employment, which has been found to have poor competitive employment outcomes (Penk et al. 2010a), and sheltered workshops, which have been found to have undesirable rehabilitation outcomes. Based on research findings inside and outside the VA (Bond 2004; Rosenheck and Mares 2007), Veterans Health Administration now provides Supported Employment (SE) services in each of its medical centers (Resnick et al. 2006). Individual Placement and Support Supported Employment (IPS SE) is an evidence-based model of vocational services for adults with mental health concerns, with significantly better employment outcomes noted in over 15 clinical trials (Bond et al. 2008). The Veterans Health Administration has dramatically reduced sheltered workshop services and has stopped the expansion of transitional employment, shifting funding to the expansion of Supported Employment capacity. Veterans Health Administration vocational services are now serving more veterans, including veterans with a broader range of disabilities, and using more effective models of care that are resulting in more participants acquiring community-based jobs (Resnick et al. 2009). Common and emerging models of care either within or outside the Veterans Health Administration include the following.

Simple Job Placement Services (JPS)

Job placement is the primary service offered by most state vocational rehabilitation programs to any citizen with a vocational need. Job placement services consist almost exclusively of the provision of job search skills training, coaching, and support, including access to public and agency job listings, computer access to Internet job listings and job search tools, and support and resources for resume creation and interview preparation. The focus is entirely on competitive employment and services are provided only during the process of an active job search. Job placement services are widely available to adults through state offices, which are often funded at least in part by the US Department of Labor. Unlike many vocational services, these services are available regardless of whether applicants have clinical problems and typically involve little or no additional support for adults with clinical needs. This lack of support for clinical population may be the primary reason for the very modest efficacy suggested in the limited outcome data on JPS in mental health populations (Penk et al. 2010b). In general, job placement services participation is very flexible and typically managed by the participant. There is no standard for the number of sessions for job placement services.

Individual Placement and Support Supported Employment (IPS SE)

Supported Employment, as conceptualized and evaluated by Robert Drake and Deborah Becker (Becker and Drake 1993), refers to a service model developed specifically to help adults with psychiatric disabilities find and maintain competitive employment. This approach has been carefully defined and boasts widely used treatment fidelity measures for use with Supported Employment. The key principles of Supported Employment include:

(a) Focus on competitive employment as the primary outcome.
(b) Open access: consumer desire for participation is the only inclusion/exclusion criteria.
(c) Job search activities begin at the earliest possible time, determined by the consumer's willingness to start.
(d) Integration of Supported Employment services with psychiatric care.
(e) Individualization of treatment.
(f) Ongoing support: there is no limit to the duration of support received by the participant; services may continue after job acquisition in order to support ongoing employment.

The Individual Placement and Support Supported Employment (IPS SE) model has been studied in at least 15+ randomized controlled trials using a variety of alternative vocational rehabilitation models as comparison conditions (Becker et al. 1996; Bond et al. 1995; Chandler et al. 1997; Drake et al. 1999; Gervey and Kowal 1994; Gold et al. in submission; Lehman et al. 2002; McFarlane et al. 2000; Mueser et al. 2004). In one review of IPS SE trials, Gary Bond (Bond 2004) notes that, in every case, the SE condition resulted in higher employment rates than the comparison condition. In one review, mean competitive employment rates for Supported Employment participants ranged from 28% to 78%, with an average rate of 56%. The comparison conditions, which included sheltered workshops, rehabilitation programs, and partial Supported Employment services, resulted in employment rates between 6% and 40%, with a mean of 19%. It has been found to be effective in adults from various age groups (Bond et al. 2012; Twamley et al. 2012), different diagnostic groups, and those with disability income (Frey et al. 2011). Within veteran populations, the efficacy of Supported Employment has been documented in populations of veterans with PTSD (Davis et al. 2012), with co-occurring mental illness and substance use disorders (Mueser et al. 2011), and with spinal cord injury (Ottomanelli et al. 2012). In fact, the authors are not aware of any clinical population in which SE has not been found to be more efficacious than other established models of vocational services.

Customized Employment (CE) Described by some authors as "the natural evolution of Supported Employment" (Griffin et al. 2008), Customized Employment is an emerging intervention that is beginning to develop a base of empirical support. The model emphasizes an extensive job development process to meet individualized job goals that reflect the unique needs of the employment seeker. Small caseloads reflect the effort to spend more time in understanding emerging participant interests and goals as well as a key focus on employment facilitated by additional funding and support resources. The limited data from empirical evaluations show promise (Griffin et al. 2008; Magura et al. 2007).

Diversified Placement Approach (DPA) and Transitional Work Experience With the publication of fidelity guidelines for services (Koop et al. 2004), a group of services commonly provided for adults with mental health and vocational concerns are likely to be increasingly studied. The Diversified Placement Approach (DPA) most closely describes vocational services common in clubhouse settings. They are also similar to Veterans Health Administration "Transitional Work Experience" services, which are also fairly common across the country (Penk et al. 2010a). Existing evidence suggests that these models have been relatively ineffective at helping participants obtain competitive employment. However, they are relatively effective at helping participants engage in "work activity." The value of "work activity" and its role in helping participants return to competitive employment is one aspect that needs further study. With 100 Veterans Health Administration vocational programs, including both DPA-type services alongside IPS SE, there is further need for investigation about how these services can most effectively interface both with other vocational services and with the broader range of clinical care.

A specialized Transitional Work Experience model called the "Veterans Construction Team" has been operating within the Veterans Health Administration vocational services program for approximately 20 years, providing focused rehabilitation for veterans seeking to enter or re-enter the construction trades (Schutt et al. 2003). This innovative enclave model of rehabilitation uses construction dollars from federal construction projects to simultaneously fund transitional work experiences in construction trades for veterans in need of that type of transitional experience.

Interventions to Enhance Employers' Involvement Major interventions to enhance employer's involvement include (1) liaison with employers soon after injury, (2) employer education, and (3) long-term employer support. In one study (Malec et al. 2000), while 80% of participants with brain injury returned to full- or part-time employment or education overall, almost 40% returned to their pre-injury employment, although not necessarily at the same level. Employer education has been identified as critical to vocational re-entry after brain injury (Malec 2005; Malec et al. 2000). Such education includes both general information dispelling employer myths about brain injury and specific information about the client's needs for physical and cognitive accommodations. Ongoing employer support (Malec 2005; Malec et al. 2000) has also been identified as critical. Such support begins with regular follow-up, which becomes increasingly less frequent as confidence in the durability of the placement increases.

Psychological Interventions to Enhance Vocational Outcomes There is preliminary research support for adding psychological interventions to vocational services to address relevant psychological processes that are known predictors of work performance and vocational outcomes. These interventions employ neurocognitive and social cognitive retraining (Bell et al.

2005, 2008; McGurk et al. 2005), cognitive behavior therapy that targets beliefs related to work (Lysaker et al. 2009), detailed work feedback and goal setting (Bell et al. 2003), or work-related social skills training (e.g., Workplace Fundamentals, Liberman 2008). These interventions, alone and in combination, may improve vocational outcomes. A curriculum-based psychoeducational intervention designed to reduce perceptions of disability among participants (Progressive Goal Attainment Program) is associated with higher return-to-work rates among those at risk for long-term disability and has now been piloted with veterans (Hossain et al. 2013).

Interventions to Enhance Individual Placement and Support Supported Employment (IPS SE) There have been a number of efforts to enhance the existing Individual Placement and Support Supported Employment (IPS SE) model in order to either improve outcomes or to adapt it to other populations. Supported Employment has been paired with a range of additional interventions including cognitive rehabilitation (Bell et al. 2008; McGurk et al. 2005), motivational interviewing (Drebing 1999; Drebing et al. 2008b), social skills training (Chan et al. 2009), and supported education (Rudnick and Gover 2009). This trend will hopefully continue in an effort to improve upon the outcomes and broaden the application of this well-established model.

It is important to recognize that the IPS SE model has some important limitations, most notably limited efficacy in terms of job retention outcomes (Drake and Bond 2008). This is a serious limitation, as any benefits of job acquisition are minimized by job tenures of less than 3 months, which are not uncommonly noted in randomized controlled trials of IPS SE. For some participants, job acquisition followed by rapid job loss may have an untoward effect in terms of reduced self-efficacy and eroded motivation to pursue employment. To address this key limitation in the IPS model, the Boston University Center for Psychiatric Rehabilitation undertook the initiative to enhance the employment outcomes of recipients of vocational services through an add-on intervention that fosters participants' capacity to manage their mental illness in the context of work and to improve their work functioning and vocational self-management once they are employed. This promising new intervention, entitled the Vocational Illness Management and Recovery program, is an innovative modification of the original Illness Management and Recovery program, which has been established as the evidence-based practice targeting both capacity to manage one's own mental illness and functional outcomes (Gingerich and Mueser 2005).

Contingency Management Integrated with Vocational Services Contingency management has primarily been used to enhance substance abuse treatments, but there have been at least two randomized controlled trials that document its efficacy at enhancing the outcomes of transitional employment (Drebing et al. 2005, 2008a). Both acquisition and maintenance goals were rewarded, with the result that participants were more active in job search and moved to competitive employment more quickly and at higher rates. The "therapeutic workplace" is a unique variation on this theme, using employment and a structured therapeutic work setting to reinforce abstinence among unemployed adults with substance use disorders (Wong and Silverman 2007). Though substantial empirical data support its efficacy at establishing abstinence, the model has not been applied widely (Silverman et al. 2007; Wong et al. 2004).

Self-Employment Interventions Self-employment and microenterprise development interventions have a number of advantages over interventions that result in placements in traditional jobs for veterans with mental health concerns. Self-employment typically focuses on jobs that more closely reflect the personal interests and skills of the individual. Self-employment also offers a greater degree of autonomy and flexibility. Adults who work for themselves have a greater ability to shift their work activities and schedules to address their other needs, including their needs to attend clinical appointments.

Criminal records can represent a significant barrier to being employed in many companies, and thus some adults seek self-employment as a more viable means of work. Finally, self-employment also offers the potential for higher pay rates for those who are successful in some types of businesses. In these ways, self-employment can be a means of raising the value of being employed for some people and so may lead to enhanced tenure. It does pose some risks as well, including the potential of less job stability and reliable pay, and greater stress, and greater range of skill requirements. Clearly, interventions that promote or support self-employment are not the ideal service for everyone but rather are a valuable option for a significant fraction of VR participants. Supported Self-Employment services are available at some Veterans Health Administration centers and are likely to grow in availability over time.

Resource Facilitation (RF) (Connors 2001) Developed in the field of brain injury rehabilitation, Resource Facilitation (RF) involves a coordinator providing assistance and advocacy to "break down barriers, increase access, and facilitate timely, coordinated management of resources" to return the individual with brain injury to full participation in family and community life (Trexler et al. 2010). Resource Facilitation seeks to increase access to community services and supports. A primary goal of Resource Facilitation is to develop a service support network that not only directly supports return to work (e.g., job search, placement, Supported Employment, transportation to work) but also provides a network of social support for work while giving work meaning. The Resource Facilitation coordinator is an advocate who assists the participant in developing a self-directed plan for community re-entry, identifying needed services and supports, and developing a sustainable network of these services and supports.

Paid Co-workers as Trainers This model involves the selection of a well-established senior lead or journey-level worker to mentor the vocational services participant. Mentorship involves training, observation, self-management concerns, and advocacy. Co-workers are paid on an hourly basis for their training activity (e.g., pre-work, over lunch, on break, end of day) and receive 2–4 h of training to gain access to training tools for both themselves and the participant. The model was developed by Curl and colleagues (Curl and Chisholm 1993; Curl et al. 1996) and has been used with adults with learning and behavioral disorders, developmental disabilities, and traumatic brain injury.

"Work Trials" With or Without Pay Work trials are time-limited job placements to assess the client's ability to succeed at a specific job and in a specific work environment. Work trials may be paid or unpaid and typically include elements of Supported Employment (Curl and Chisholm 1993; Curl et al. 1996). Work trials provide a means of assessing the client's ability to manage many aspects of the employment, such as the specific work skills required by the job, time demands and other expectations for performance, and the interpersonal and physical environment of the workplace. These latter aspects of work that are not directly related to job skills are often the most challenging for individuals with brain injury. Since the early 1990s, it has been recognized that such on-the-job assessments are of greater value in assessing the ability of the client with brain injury to succeed on the job than standardized job skill or interest assessments (Corthell 1990; Thomas and Menz 1993).

Supported Education (SEd) Education is a key activity in career development, and given the number of veterans who use their GI Bill benefits to attend college, interventions that reduce the risk of academic failure are of particular interest for those working with veterans. Supported Education (SEd) shares many of the basic principles and practices of Supported Employment. Among these practices are as follows: goals are achieved in natural community settings (community colleges, adult education programs); support is time unlimited and can ebb and flow according to the needs of the person; clinical and vocational services are integrated; and goals are driven by the person's choice. Supported Employment also uses the place/train philosophy, emphasizing the importance of placing a person directly into the target setting and providing wraparound support to facilitate success (Corrigan and McCracken 2005). The place/train model has demonstrated better outcomes within education and employment settings when compared with train/place models of service, such as sheltered workshops, transitional employment, and self-contained classrooms.

Ellison and colleagues (Ellison et al. 2012) conducted focus groups of Operation Iraqi Freedom/Operation Enduring Freedom veterans with self-reported PTSD regarding their needs for education supports. Participants reported barriers to entry or return to school, including meeting academic requirements; lack of information about financial aid and the GI Bill; symptoms of PTSD, depression, and substance abuse; lack of social support; and difficulties with the transition from military to civilian life. Results were consistent with findings from a previous study of the same population (Glover-Graf et al. 2010). In addition to services that would address the barriers they already reported, there were a number of common recommendations across the focus groups: interventions should include peer support, veteran-driven service intensity, integration of vocational and clinical teams, and greater connection between the VA and educational institutions. Ellison and colleagues (Ellison et al. 2012) then created a manual based on the focus group data and participatory action research team consisting of veterans, peer providers, clinicians, college administrators and professors, and community education providers. Another randomized, controlled trial of SEd (Smith-Osborne 2012) found that those randomized to the control group of this intervention showed a decrease in social and personal resilience and an increase in PTSD symptoms during their time in the study when compared to the experimental group.

Supported Volunteerism (SV) Supported Volunteerism is an emerging model of care that, like Supported Education, is modeled after Supported Employment. Using similar principles of care, Supported Volunteerism helps participants find meaningful volunteer opportunities in their communities that match their interests and abilities. While some Supported Employment providers have expressed concern that Supported Volunteerism can be an undesirable alternative that competes with Supported Employment, others have found the Supported Volunteerism can function as a stepping stone to employment for those adults who are initially not interested in returning to employment. After a period of time as a volunteer, many may find that their interest in returning to work, and their confidence that they can successfully maintain a job, has helped them decide to enter Supported Employment or another vocational service. Clearly, Supported Volunteerism needs more study and has to be used cautiously to avoid any negative impact on final vocational outcomes.

Family and Clinical Provider Interventions The growing evidence documenting the key role of stakeholders such as family, friends, and healthcare providers in vocational services outcomes has begun to spawn a range of new interventions designed to influence these stakeholders to support return-to-work efforts. Motivational interviewing interventions designed specifically to enhance support from family and friends for Individual Placement and Support Supported Employment (IPS SE) have been developed (Mueller and Rose 2008) and are being evaluated. Contingency management approaches that reward support for employment outcomes among vocational and nonvocational healthcare providers have been developed (Noone 2005) and may well be found to have a powerful effect on employment outcomes.

Clinical Strategies for Approaching Vocational Problems

In the case example at the beginning of this chapter, Maria found her way to specialty mental health care, but how should her clinicians work to address her vocational problems? Many mental health practitioners have little or no experience referring adults to vocational services. This is unfortunate, given the frequency of vocational problems among adults with mental illness and the availability of a wide range of services. The following recommendations are made for the broader range of mental health practitioners:

1. Routinely screen adults with mental health conditions for vocational problems. These problems are common and often respond well to vocational services. Without active screening and referral by providers, many adults will wait for years before seeking treatment (Drebing 2011).
2. Talk with clients about the functional impact of their mental illness on their work life. Adults frequently fail to recognize the links between their illness and their work problems and will benefit in a number of ways by seeing how these connect.
3. When exploring vocational problems, help the client examine the potential impacts of mental illness in terms of lost income and benefits, lost social status in their family and community, lost structure of their time, lost participation in valued work, and lost confidence in their ability to work. Explore how their family has reorganized around their vocational problem and any resistances that may have developed to their returning to work. For some, this may involve a "grieving process" for the losses that they have suffered (Drebing 2011). A full recognition of these losses is often critical to establishing solid motivation for change.
4. Become familiar with vocational services available to clients. Vocational services are available from a range of providers and in a range of formats and vary by location. Different clients will prefer different models and some will only tolerate some types of care (Penk 2000). Mental health providers who have relationships with vocational service providers will have the greatest ability to pick the best services for their clients.
5. Do not underestimate the ambivalence most clients will have about returning to work. Most adults are ambivalent about work, but those who have had job failures due to mental health problems are often very anxious about moving back toward employment, fearing that they may fail again (Drebing 2011).
6. Look for resistance among family members, friends, and even other clinical providers. While social support is a key resource for those seeking to return to work, family and friends are often cited as trying to discourage clients from returning to work (Drebing et al. 2012b). They are often concerned about whether returning to work will negatively impact the mental health of their relative, friend, or client.
7. Be aware of the role of disability income on feelings of ambivalence. Programs like Social Security Disability Income and VA disability pensions provide financial income to adults with disabilities. Participation in these programs is associated with poorer vocational outcomes and poorer participation in vocational services over and above the degree of disability (Drew et al. 2001). While most programs provide incentives for returning to work, there are still clear disincentives for some participants in terms of lost benefits. Clients often do not understand the incentives and so are even more concerned about lost benefits than they need to be.
8. Be cautious about referring clients to any services or programs that include significant time or programming "preparing" participants for employment. This may be preparation in the form of lengthy testing, or months of classes about returning to work, or intermediate employment activities before a real job is sought. Behavioral economics shows that the reward value of anything sought is discounted to the degree that one has to wait for it (Drebing et al. 2006). Supported Employment is very successful, in part, because it involves immediate efforts to obtain the job the client wants.
9. Continue to maintain a clinical focus on work after the client obtains employment. Obtaining a job is easier than keeping a job (Bond and Kukla 2011). If a client obtains a valued job that they quickly lose, their confidence in their ability to work may actually be further diminished. The challenges that arise as clients seek to maintain jobs are often cen-

tral to their vocational problems and provide valuable clinical material to work on.
10. Continue to maintain a clinical focus on work after the client establishes stability in employment. Most clients returning to work through vocational services start in jobs that are not their ideal work. Often these are jobs that they can get and so are not central to their occupational interests and do not offer the pay and benefits they want. Working with clients to continue their efforts to eventually reach the job that they truly want should be part of clinical follow-up in many situations in which vocational services have been used (Bond and Kukla 2011).

Implications for the Future

Growing Visibility of Employment as a Key Clinical Outcome Community reintegration is evolving as a key, if not the key, clinical outcome, and employment is central to community reintegration (Resnik et al. 2012). The growing focus on functional decline as part of the definition of clinical disorders, and the national and international focus on addressing "disability," will ensure that clinical care, and in particular mental health care, includes vocational interventions within clinical efforts. The growing focus on "evidence-based practice" and the fact that Supported Employment is one of the most well-established evidence-based practices across any mental health area will further strengthen the role and visibility of vocational services within clinical care.

Further Enhancement of Available Vocational Interventions The next decade is likely to produce research evaluating a number of adaptations of existing models, either for improvements in general outcomes or for improved services for target populations (Drebing et al. 2012a). Individual Placement and Support Supported Employment (IPS SE), which is the most effective model of care in terms of employment outcomes, still results in employment rates between 40% and 60%. Job tenure is a particular area of concern, as most vocational services participants who do obtain competitive jobs, including IPS SE participants, keep those jobs less than 16 weeks. While the evidence base for IPS SE supports its use with some clinical groups, there is a need to determine its efficacy with other common clinical populations.

New interventions and adaptations are being developed and disseminated (Drebing et al. 2012a) and will need to be evaluated for their effectiveness. Some of the most promising directions include (a) enhancements of existing models like IPS SE, Diversified Placement Approach (DPA), and Transitional Work Experience (TWE); (b) evaluation of new and emerging models of care like Supported Self-Employment, Customized Employment (CE), and Resource Facilitation (RF); (c) enhancing existing treatment models by adding psychological interventions like cognitive rehabilitation, cognitive behavior therapy, contingency management, detailed work feedback and goal setting, work-related social skills training, and motivation interventions to vocational services; (d) or developing entirely new types of services such as interventions targeting employers, clinical providers, family members, or co-workers.

Effective models of care are only valuable if they are widely available and utilized. Evidence from Veterans Health Administration vocational services suggests that available services are generally underutilized (Twamley et al. 2013). As VA and other systems of care increasingly include vocational rehabilitation as a central clinical resource, efforts to raise the rates and consistency of referral and utilization will ensure all veterans receive timely help returning to work.

Expansion of Vocational Services Targeting Veterans The Veterans Health Administration is reorganizing and reinvigorating the vocational programming available to veterans. There are new models of care being piloted and evaluated and more research funding available to those studying how to help veterans deal with vocational problems. All of these developments point to a larger trend in the expansion of services targeting veterans and the greater investment by the US Department of Veterans Affairs, by the Department of Labor, by state and local governments, and by the community to ensure that veterans who are facing employment challenges secondary to mental health concerns have available and effective services to help them meet their goals of returning to productive lives.

Key Concepts

1. Employment is often central to mental health treatment and rehabilitation outcomes and so should be a routine part of clinical evaluation and treatment planning.
2. Among the common models of vocational services available to potential participants, Individual Placement and Support Supported Employment (IPS SE) is one of the most well-researched and supported models of care, with consistent findings from over 15 randomized control trials finding that it results in better employment outcomes than a range of comparison conditions.
3. There are a growing number of interventions that appear to positively enhance employment outcomes, when they are added to interventions like Individual Placement and Support Supported Employment, including motivational interviewing, contingency management, cognitive rehabilitation, social skills training, and Supported Education.
4. Mental health providers should routinely screen for vocational problems and refer appropriate clients to the model of services that is most likely to meet their goals of obtaining employment, stabilizing employment, or improving their vocational situation.

References

Annual Disability Statistics Compendium: 2009 (2009) Retrieved 1 Sept 2010, 2010, from http://neweditions.net/statsrrtc/Compendium2009.pdf

Becker DR, Drake RE (1993) A working life: the individual placement and support (IPS) program. New Hampshire-Dartmouth Psychiatric Research Center, Concord

Becker D, Drake RE, Farabaugh A, Bond GR (1996) Job preferences among people with severe psychiatric disorders in supported employment programs. Psychiatr Serv 47:1223–1226

Bell MD, Bryson G, Greig TC, Fiszdon JM, Wexler BE (2005) Neurocognitive enhancement therapy with work therapy: productivity outcomes at 6-month and 12-month follow-up. J Rehabil Res Dev 42:829–838

Bell M, Lysaker PH, Bryson GA (2003) A behavioral intervention to improve work performance in schizophrenia: work behavior inventory feedback. J Vocat Rehabil 18:43–51

Bell MD, Zito W, Greig TC, Wexler BE (2008) Neurocognitive enhancement therapy with vocational services in schizophrenia: work outcomes at two year follow-up. Schizophr Res 105:18–29

Bond GR (2004) Supported employment: evidence for an evidence-based practice. Psychiatr Rehabil J 27(4):345–359

Bond GR, Dietzen LL, McGrew JH, Miller LD (1995) Accelerating entry into supported employment for persons with severe psychiatric disabilities. Rehabil Psychol 40:91–111

Bond GR, Drake RE, Becker DR (2008) An update on randomized controlled trials of evidence-based supported employment. Psychiatr Rehabil J 31(4):280–290

Bond GR, Drake RE, Becker DR (2012) Generalizability of the individual placement and support (IPS) model of supported employment outside the US. World Psychiatry 11(1):32–39

Bond GR, Kukla M (2011) Is job tenure brief in individual placement and support (IPS) employment programs? Psychiatr Serv 62(8):950–953. https://doi.org/10.1176/appi.ps.62.8.950

Chan AS, Tsang HW, Li SM (2009) Case report of integrated supported employment for a person with severe mental illness. Am J Occup Ther 63(3):238–244

Chandler D, Meisel J, Hu T, McGowen M, Madison K (1997) A capitated model for a cross-section of severely mentally ill clients: employment outcomes. Community Ment Health J 33:501–506

Connors SH (2001) Resource facilitation: a consensus of principles and best practices to guide program development and operation in brain injury. Brain Injury Association of America, McLean

Corrigan P, McCracken S (2005) Place first, then train: an alternative to the medical model of psychiatric rehabilitation. Soc Work 50(1):31–40

Corthell D (ed) (1990) Traumatic brain injury and vocational rehabilitation. University of Wisconsin – Stout, Menomonie

Curl RM, Chisholm LD (1993) Unlocking co-worker potential in competitive employment: keys to a cooperative approach. J Vocat Rehabil 3:72–84

Curl RM, Fraser RT, Cook RG, Clemmons DC (1996) Traumatic brain injury vocational rehabilitation: preliminary findings for the co-worker as trainer project. J Head Trauma Rehabil 11:75–85

Davis LL, Leon AC, Toscano R, Drebing CE, Ward LC, Parker PE, Kashner TM, Drake RE (2012) A randomized controlled trial of supported employment among veterans with posttraumatic stress disorder. Psychiatr Serv 63(5):464–470. https://doi.org/10.1176/appi.ps.201100340

Drake RE, Bond G (2008) The future of supported employment for people with severe mental illness. Psychiatr Rehabil J 31(4):367–376
Drake RE, McHugo GJ, Bebout RR, Becker DR, Harris M, Bond GR, Quimby E (1999) A randomized clinical trial of supported employment for inner-city patients with severe mental illness. Arch Gen Psychiatry 56:627–633
Drebing C (1999) Trends in the content and methodology of Alzheimer's caregiving research. Alzheimer Dis Related Disord *13*(S-1):S93–S100
Drebing C (2011) Pathways to vocational services: addressing barriers to rehabilitation. Paper presented at the mental health services research division meeting. Yale University School of Medicine, New Haven
Drebing CE, Bell M, Campinell EA, Fraser R, Malec J, Penk W, Pruitt-Stephens L (2012a) Vocational services research: recommendations for next stage of work. J Rehabil Res Dev 49(1):101–119
Drebing CE, Mueller L, Van Ormer EA, Duffy P, LePage J, Rosenheck R, Rose GS, King K, Penk W (2012b) Pathways to vocational services: factors affecting entry by veterans enrolled in veterans health administration mental health services. Psychol Serv 9(1):49–63. https://doi.org/10.1037/a0026662
Drebing C, Hebert M, Mueller L, Van Ormer EA, Herz L (2006) Vocational rehabilitation from a behavioral economics perspective. Psychol Serv 3(3):181–194
Drebing CE, Van Ormer EA, Krebs C, Rosenheck R, Rounsaville B, Herz L, Penk W (2005) The impact of enhanced incentives on vocational rehabilitation outcomes for dually diagnosed veterans. J Appl Behav Anal 38(3):359–372. https://doi.org/10.1901/jaba.2005.100-03
Drebing CE, Van Ormer EA, Mueller L, Hebert M, Penk W, Petry N, Rosenheck R, Rounsaville B (2008a) Adding a contingency management intervention to vocational rehabilitation: outcomes for dually diagnosed veterans. J Rehabil Res Dev 44(6):851–866
Drebing CE, Van Ormer EA, Mueller L, Rosenheck R, Drake RE, King K (2008b) Understanding and enhancing entry and completion of rehabilitation and recovery services: A pathways-to-care approach. Paper presented at the veterans administration conference on transforming mental health Care: Promoting Recovery and Integrated Care, Arlington, Virginia
Drew D, Drebing CE, Van Ormer EW, Losardo M, Krebs C, Penk W, Rosenheck.R. (2001) Effects of disability compensation on vocational rehabilitation participant and outcome. Psychiatr Serv 52(11):1479–1484
Ellison ML, Mueller L, Smelson D, Corrigan PW, Torres Stone RA, Bokhour BG, Najavits LM, Vessella JM, Drebing C (2012) Supporting the education goals of post-9/11 veterans with self-reported PTSD symptoms: a needs assessment. Psychiatr Rehabil J 35(3):209–217. https://doi.org/10.2975/35.3.2012.209.217
Frey WD, Drake RE, Bond GR, Lynde DW, Ganju VJ, Goldman HH (2011) Mental health treatment study: final report to social security administration. Westat, Rockville
Gervey R, Kowal H (1994) A description of a model for placing youth and young adults with psychiatric disabilities in competitive employment. Paper presented at the International Association of Psychosocial Rehabilitation Services, Albuquerque
Gingerich S, Mueser KT (2005) Illness management and recovery. Norton, New York
Glover-Graf NM, Miller E, Freeman S (2010) Accommodating veterans with posttraumatic stress Disorder symptoms in the academic setting. Rehabil Educ 24(1):43–56
Gold PB, Meisler N, Santos AB, Willians OH, Kelleher J, Carnemolla MA (n.d.) (in submission). A randomized clinical trial of integrated supported employment and assertive community treatment for rural Southern patients with severe mental illness
Griffin C, Hammis D, Geary T, Sullivan M (2008) Customized employment: where we are; where we're headed. J Vocat Rehabil 28:135–139
Hossain F, Baird P, Pardoe R (2013) Improving employment outcomes and community integration for veterans with disabilities
Kleykamp M (2013) Unemployment, earnings and enrollment among post 9/11 veterans. Soc Sci Res 42(3):836–851. https://doi.org/10.1016/j.ssresearch.2012.12.017
Koop JI, Rollins AL, Bond GR, Salyers MP, Dincin J, Kinley T, Shimon SM, Marcelle K (2004) Development of the DPA fidelity scale: using fidelity to define an existing vocational model. Psychiatr Rehabil J 28(1):16–24
Kukla M, Bond GR (2009) The working alliance and employment outcomes for people with severe mental illness enrolled in vocational programs. Rehabil Psychol 54(2):157–163
Lehman AF, Goldberg RW, Dixon LB, McNary S, Postrado L, Hackman A, McDonnell D (2002) Improving employment outcomes for persons with severe mental illness. Arch Gen Psychiatry 59:165–172
Liberman RP (2008) Recovery from disability. American Psychiatric Association Press, Washington, DC
Lysaker PH, Davis LW, Bryson GJ, Bell MD (2009) Effects of cognitive behavioral therapy on work outcomes in vocational rehabilitation for participants with schizophrenia spectrum disorders. Schizophr Res 107:186–191
Magura S, Blankertz L, Madison EM, Friedman E, Gomez A (2007) An innovative job placement model for unemployed methadone patients: a randomized clinical trial. Subst Use Misuse 42:811–828
Malec J (2005) Vocational rehabilitation. In: High WM, Sander AM, Struchen MA, Hart KA (eds) Rehabilitation for traumatic brain injury. New York. Oxford University Press
Malec JF, Buffington ALH, Moessner AM, Degiorgio L (2000) A medical/vocational case coordination system for persons with brain injury: an evaluation of employment outcomes. Arch Phys Med Rehabil 81:1007–1015
McFarlane WR, Dushay RA, Deakins SM, Stastny P, Lukens EP, Toran J, Link B (2000) Employment outcomes in family-aided assertive community treatment. Am J Orthop 70:203–214

McGurk SR, Mueser KT, Pascaris A (2005) Cognitive training and supported employment for persons with severe mental illness: one-year results from a randomized controlled trial. Schizophr Bull 31:898–909

McQuilken M, Zahniser JH, Novak J, Starks RD, Olmos A, Bond GR (2003) The work project survey: consumer perspectives on work. J Vocat Rehabil 18(1):59–68

Mueller L, Rose G (2008) Strategies for final success in rehabilitation services. Paper presented at the 117th Annual Meeting of the American Psychological Association, Boston

Mueser KT, Campbell BK, Drake RE (2011) The effectiveness of supported employment in people with dual disorders. J Dual Disord 7:90–102

Mueser KT, Clark RE, Haines M, Drake RE, McHugo GJ, Bond GR, Essock SM, Becker DR, Wolfe R, Swaine K (2004) The Hartford study of supported employment for persons with severe mental illness. J Consult Clin Psychol 72(3):479–490

New Freedom Commission on Mental Health: Achieving the Promise: Transforming Mental Health Care in America. Final Report. DHHS pub no SMA-03—3832. Rockville Md, Department of Health and Human Services, 2003. Available at www.mentalhealthcommission.gov/reports/finalreport/fullreport-02.htm

Noone W (2005) Federal Community Based Employment Services (CBES) program supported employment title VIc federal funding cost-benefit study. Massachusetts State Rehabilitation Commission, Boston

Ottomanelli L, Goetz LL, Suris A, MCGeough C, Sinnott P, Toscano R, Barnett SD, Cipher DJ, Lind LM, Dixon TM, Holmes SA, Kerrigan AJ, Thomas FP (2012) Effectiveness of supported employment for veterans with spinal cord injuries: results from a randomized multisite study. Arch Phys Med Rehabil 93:740–747

Penk W (2000) Designing work experiences for person with serious mental disorders. In: Frese FJ (ed) The role of organized psychology in treatment of the seriously mentally ill. Jossey-Bass, San Francisco, pp 17–26

Penk W, Drebing CE, Rosenheck R, Krebs C, Van Ormer EA, Mueller L (2010a) VHA transitional work experience vs. job placement in veterans with con-morbid substance use and non-psychotic psychiatric disorders. Psychiatr Rehabil J 33(4):392–407

Penk W, Drebing CE, Rosenheck RA, Krebs C, Van Ormer A, Mueller L (2010b) Veterans health administration transitional work experience vs. job placement in veterans with co-morbid substance use and non-psychotic psychiatric disorders. Psychiatr Rehabil J 33(4):297–307. https://doi.org/10.2975/33.4.2010.297.307

Penk W, Drebing C, Schutt R (2002) Posttraumatic stress disorder in the workplace. In: Thomas JC, Hersen M (eds) The handbook of mental health in the workplace. Sage Publications, Thousand Oaks, pp 215–249

Resnick SG, Kaczynski R, Sieffert D, Baldino R, Showalter D, Gray S et al (2009) Twelfth Progress Report on the Compensated Work Therapy (CWT) program: fiscal year 2008. Northeast Program Evaluation Center (NEPEC), West Haven

Resnick SG, Medak S, Baldino R, Corwel L, Rosenheck R (2006) Ninth progress report on the compensated work therapy (CWT)/veterans INdustries (VI) program. Northeast Program Evaluation Center, West Haven

Resnik L, Bradford DW, Glynn SM, Jette AM, Johnson Hernandez C, Wills S (2012) Issues in defining and measuring veteran community reintegration: proceedings of the working group on community reintegration, VA rehabilitation outcomes conference, Miami, Florida. J Rehabil Res Dev 49(1):87–100

Rosenheck R, Mares AS (2007) Implementation of supported employment for homeless veterans with psychiatric or addiction disorders: two-year outcomes. Psychiatr Serv 58(3):325–333

Rudnick A, Gover M (2009) Combining supported education with supported employment. Psychiatr Serv 10(12):1690

Schutt RK, Cournoyer B, Penk WE, Drebing CE, Van Ormer EA, Krebs C, Losardo MO (2003) Building the future: psychosocial rehabilitation with a veterans construction team. Psychiatr Rehabil J 27(2):186–189

Silverman K, Wong CJ, Needham M, Diemer KN, Kneeling T, Crone-Todd D, Fingerhood M, Nuzzo P, Kolodner K (2007) A randomized trial of employment-based reinforcement of cocaine abstinence in injection drug users. J Appl Behav Anal *40*(3):387–410

Siu PS, Tsang HW, Bond GR (2010) Nonvocational outcomes for clients with severe mental illness obtaining employment in Hong Kong. J Vocat Rehabil 32:15–24

Smith-Osborne AM (2012) Supporting resilience in the academic setting for student soldiers and veterans as an aspect of community reintegration: the design of the student veteran project study. Adv Soc Work 13(1):34–50

Stewart M, Brown JB, Doner A, McWhinney IR, Oates J, Weston WW, Jordan J (2000) The impact of patient-centered care on outcomes. J Fam Pract 49(9)

Thomas DF, Menz FE (1993) Development of a model of community-based employment for persons with traumatic brain injury. In: Thomas DF, Menz FE, McAlees DC (eds) Community-based employment following traumatic brain injury. University of Wisconsin-Stout, Menomonie

Trexler LE, Trexler LC, Malec JF, Klyce D, Parrott D (2010). Prospective randomized controlled trial of resource facilitation on community participation and vocational outcome following brain injury. J Head Trauma Rehabil 25(6): pp 440–446. https://doi.org/10.1097/HTR.0b013e3181d41139

Twamley EW, Baker DG, Norman SB, Pittman JO, Lohr JB, Resnick SG (2013) Veterans health administration vocational services for operation Iraqi freedom/operation enduring freedom veterans with mental health conditions. J Rehabil Res Dev 50(5):663–670

Twamley EW, Vella L, Burton CZ, Becker D, Bell MD, Jeste DV (2012) The efficacy of supported employment for middle-aged and older people with schizophrenia. Schizophr Res 135:100–104

Wong CJ, Dillon EM, Sylvest CE, Silverman K (2004) Contingency management of reliable attendance of chronically unemployed substance abusers in a therapeutic workplace. Exp Clin Psychopharmacol 12(1):39–46

Wong CJ, Silverman K (2007) Establishing and maintaining job skills and professional behaviors in chronically unemployed drug abusers. Subst Use Misuse 42:1127–1140

Zivin K, Bohnert AS, Mezuk B, Ilgen MA, Welsh D, Ratliff S, Miller EM, Valenstein M, Kilbourne AM (2011) Employment status of patients in the VA health system: implications for mental health services. Psychiatr Serv *62*(1):35–38. https://doi.org/10.1176/appi.ps.62.1.35

13 Risk Factors, Service Delivery, and Prevention of Veteran Homelessness

Jack Tsai and Robert A. Rosenheck

Introduction

Homelessness is a persistent problem in the USA and one that has been a public health concern among veterans for over three decades (Lewin 1987; US Department of Housing and Urban Development 2013). Homelessness among veterans was first documented after the US Civil War (Robertson 1987) and was widely recognized during the Great Depression (Dickson and Allen 2006). But it was not until the early 1980s after the Vietnam War, a period characterized by high inflation and two economic recessions, that veteran homelessness began to be recognized as an important social problem (Lewin 1987; Rosenheck et al. 1989; Wright 1988).

Homelessness can be defined as not having a "fixed, regular, and adequate nighttime residence" (McKinney-Vento Homeless Assistance Act, amended 2009) and includes moving frequently between different types of accommodations and staying in homeless shelters and places not meant for human habitation (e.g., vehicles, abandoned buildings). Some consider homelessness a violation of a basic human right—the right to have access to safe and secure housing (United Nations 1948). Homelessness is also a concern because it is associated with a host of other negative outcomes, including a wide range of serious medical problems (Hwang 2001; Schanzer et al. 2007), mental health and substance abuse problems (Fazel et al. 2008; Folsom et al. 2005), premature mortality (Hibbs et al. 1994; O'Connell 2005), frequent hospitalizations and excessive costs per hospital stay (Gladwell 2006; Rosenheck and Seibyl 1998; Salit et al. 1998), and incarceration (McGuire 2007; Tsai et al. 2014a, b, c).

Veterans constitute a unique segment of the US population due to their honored service to the country as reflected in their access to special federal and state government benefits such as Department of Veterans Affairs (VA) healthcare, disability and education benefits, and home-loan guarantees. Many regard the presence of veterans within the general US homeless population as a point of shame, and public concern for their health and well-being is strong (Donovan and Shinseki 2013). In 2009, Secretary Shinseki of the Department of Veterans Affairs pledged to end homelessness among veterans by the end of 2015 and has

J. Tsai, PhD (✉) • R.A. Rosenheck
Department of Psychiatry, VA New England MIRECC; Yale University School of Medicine, West Haven, CT 06516, USA
e-mail: Jack.Tsai@yale.edu; Robert.Rosenheck@yale.edu

L.W. Roberts, C.H. Warner (eds.), *Military and Veteran Mental Health*,
https://doi.org/10.1007/978-1-4939-7438-2_13

since poured millions of dollars into creating new VA homeless services and expanding existing ones (US Department of Veterans Affairs 2009). A growing component of those efforts is a focus on the prevention of homelessness.

Case Study

Lieutenant (ret.) Arnold Grisham (pseudonym) is a 60-year-old, male, Vietnam era veteran with an extensive history of substance abuse, depression, homelessness, and medical problems including hepatitis C and chronic pain. Lt. Grisham was staying at a homeless shelter when a Department of Veterans Affairs (VA) social outreach worker referred him to the VA's supported housing program. He was admitted to the VA's supported housing program and moved into his subsidized apartment about 4 months later. He remained connected to VA medical and substance abuse treatment services.

Soon after moving into supported housing, he was approved for social security disability and began to receive monthly disability income. With guidance from his case manager, he began to save money and build credit. He also found part-time work as a painter. Seven years after moving into supported housing, he bought his own home and successfully left the supported housing program. However, several years later, Lt. Grisham had a serious motorcycle accident and suffered substantial physical injuries. He was experiencing great pain and began to abuse drugs again. He was subsequently arrested for a drug-related offense and incarcerated for 1 year. During that time, his house went into foreclosure and he lost his house.

After being discharged from jail, Lt. Grisham reconnected with VA homeless program staff. For a period of time, Lt. Grisham lived in the woods and in homeless shelters before he was able to obtain an apartment in a Section 8 (non-VA affiliated) subsidized building. He now regularly sees his VA mental health and primary care providers. He reports that he diligently pays his bills on time and dreams of owning his own home again.

This chapter provides an overview of the problem of homelessness among US veterans. First, a case study of a homeless veteran illustrates a veteran's story of homelessness and the challenges encountered. Second, the rates of veteran homelessness are compared to the general population, and the significance of veteran homelessness is described. Third, the research on risk factors for veteran homelessness is reviewed. Fourth, some of the large existing programs for homeless veterans, along with empirical evidence of their effectiveness when available, are described. Fifth, current efforts to prevent homelessness and the implications of research on prevention are addressed. The chapter concludes by discussing future directions for research and practice and continued efforts to end veteran homelessness.

Scope of the Problem

Most recent estimates report that veterans constitute 12.3% of all homeless adults in the USA (US Department of Housing and Urban Development 2013) but only 9.7% of the total US population (US Department of Veterans Affairs 2013). The proportion of veterans among homeless adults appears to be on the decline when compared to data from the late 1980s (Rosenheck et al. 1994). Table 13.1 shows this breakdown by gender, which demonstrates several important points. The vast majority of homeless veterans are male, which is not surprising as they make up the majority of the general veteran population. However, female veterans are particularly overrepresented in the US homeless female population as compared to their representation in the general US population, while male veterans are not overrepresented in the US homeless male population. Most homeless veterans are sheltered veterans, i.e., they use emergency

Table 13.1 Descriptive statistics of homelessness among veterans

Homeless veterans (n = 57,849)	
Homeless male veterans	7.7%
Homeless female veterans	92.3%
Male veterans among all homeless male adults	0.9%
Female veterans among all homeless female adults	11.3%
Sheltered veterans	60.0%
Unsheltered veterans	40.0%

Estimates are based on the 2013 Annual Homeless Assessment Report (US Department of Housing and Urban Development 2013)

shelters or transitional housing facilities, although there are also substantial numbers of unsheltered veterans living on the streets and other places not meant for habitation.

Homelessness among veterans is of special concern because of their service to the country and the public's view that it is disgraceful and unpatriotic that veterans become homeless. At the same time, homelessness in the general US population has also been of widespread concern, and there have been various notable efforts to address this problem. For example, in 2000, the National Alliance to End Homelessness released a 10-year strategy to end homelessness in the USA, which was followed by a Bush administration initiative to end chronic homelessness in 10 years. The US Interagency Council on Homelessness then urged cities to create local plans to end homelessness, and over 200 of these plans have been completed across the country (National Alliance to End Homelessness 2014). In 2010, *Opening Doors* was released, which was the nation's first federal strategic plan to end homelessness and represents a joint action by the 19 member agencies of the US Interagency Council on Homelessness and local and state partners in the public and private sectors (US Interagency Council on Homelessness 2010).

In 2009 the Obama administration and Department of Veterans Affairs Secretary Shinseki announced a 5-year federal initiative to end homelessness specifically among veterans by 2015. This commitment to end veteran homelessness includes increased capital funding for supported housing units and housing vouchers, supportive services for low-income veterans and their families, increased employment opportunities for veterans, a national referral center to link veterans to local service providers, and various preventive measures like providing outreach to veterans involved in the criminal justice system, discharge planning for incarcerated veterans, and developing a homeless screener for all veterans. The National Center on Homelessness Among veterans was also created to address policy, research, and practice issues related to homeless veterans.

With the US involvement in the wars in Afghanistan (2001–present) and in Iraq (2003–2011), a large number of veterans serving in these conflicts are returning stateside with various medical and behavioral health problems (Hoge et al. 2004, 2006; Seal et al. 2007). Support for the nation's military during wartime has increased scrutiny on the healthcare of veterans and efforts to prevent problems like homelessness from occurring. There has been limited research specifically on homelessness among veterans who have served in Operation Enduring Freedom/Operation Iraqi Freedom (OEF/OIF). However, one study found that Operation Enduring Freedom/Operation Iraqi Freedom service appeared to be protective against homelessness when examined among all VA service users, even after adjusting for age (US Department of Veterans Affairs 2013). Another study found that OEF/OIF war zone service moderately increased the risk for homelessness when examined among only Iraq and Afghanistan era veterans (Metraux et al. 2013). Therefore, it seems that among veterans of all service eras, OEF/OIF service is not a current risk factor, but it is specifically among veterans who have served since September 11, 2001. Moreover, higher rates of combat exposure and PTSD have been found among homeless OEF/OIF veterans compared to previous cohorts of homeless veterans and nonveterans, with a recent estimate that 70% of homeless OEF/OIF male veterans and 53% of homeless female OEF/OIF veterans have been given a clinical diagnosis of PTSD at the time of initial assessment (Tsai et al. 2012).

Identified Risk Factors

Numerous studies have identified risk factors for homelessness among veterans. Most of these studies have found that identified risk factors for homelessness among veterans are not vastly different than those found among the general adult population. A comprehensive review of risk factors for homelessness in the general population (Susser et al. 1993) identified many of the same risk factors described in this section on veteran homelessness.

An unpublished review of veteran homelessness conducted by VA's Evidence-based Synthesis Program (ESP) Center aimed to address questions regarding the prevalence, incidence, and risk factors of homelessness among veterans. This review noted the high prevalence of psychiatric illness, substance abuse, and chronic mental illness among homeless veterans (Balshem et al. 2011). The review also identified that the risk factors strongly associated with homelessness in both veteran and nonveteran populations include difficulties in childhood (e.g., inadequate care by parents, experiencing foster care, running away from home), low income, low social support, and history of incarceration.

Some of these risk factors may become more salient over time as the veteran population and military era cohorts change. For example, more women are entering the military, and military sexual trauma may become an increasingly important risk factor to consider. Repeated tours of duty in the wars in Iraq and Afghanistan may put some veterans at increased risk due to the relationship between combat exposure and post-deployment mental health and functioning, indirectly increasing the risk for homelessness. Although the main risk factors for homelessness do not appear to differ between veteran and non-veteran population, homeless veterans tend to be older and better educated, show evidence of stronger family cohesion, and are more likely to have been married than homeless nonveterans.

A comprehensive and published review of risk factors for homelessness among veterans (Tsai and Rosenheck 2015) identified 31 studies that examined risk factors and correlates of homelessness among veterans. This review categorized seven studies as "more rigorous studies," nine studies as "less rigorous studies," and 15 studies as "comparative studies of homeless veterans and homeless nonveterans." More rigorous studies employed a cohort, case-control, or clearly formulated research design that provided support for causal factors, while less rigorous studies had weaker research designs or utilized smaller samples or a limited number of psychosocial and health measures. Comparative studies consisted of studies that compared veterans and nonveterans on homeless risk factors and characteristics.

Among the more rigorous studies, the most consistent risk factors for homelessness were substance abuse problems and mental illness. Substance abuse problems appeared to be the risk factor with the greatest magnitude of effect. Schizophrenia was also a major risk factor, and post-traumatic stress disorder was a risk factor but found to be of the same magnitude as other mental health disorders. Low-income and income-related variables, such as military pay grade and unemployment, were also consistently found to be risk factors for homelessness (Edens et al. 2011; Elbogen et al. 2013). A few studies also identified lack of social support, criminal history, and adverse childhood events as potential risk factors.

The less rigorous studies largely supported the findings of the more rigorous studies. Substance abuse and mental health problems were found to be related to veteran homelessness. Further evidence of the link between childhood problems and homelessness were provided by the less rigorous studies. Neurological deficits, problematic military discharges, weak social support, and history of incarceration were all also found to be related to veteran homelessness.

The comparative studies of homeless veterans and homeless nonveterans found that veterans have been at greater risk for homelessness than nonveterans across numerous time periods, although there are substantial differences between age strata representing different eras of military service (Gamache et al. 2001; Rosenheck et al. 1994). These studies further found particular subgroups of veterans who were at particularly greater risk than nonveterans. Male post-Vietnam era veterans, i.e., those who served in the early years of the All-Volunteer Force (1973–1983), appeared to be at particularly greater risk for homelessness than other male adults in the same age cohort possibly due to a "social selection" effect, in which men who volunteered to serve in the military during this time may have been escaping poor economic conditions and lacked family support. Two other case-control studies, conducted on data collected over a decade apart, both found that female veterans were particularly at greater risk than other women (Gamache et al. 2003; US Department of Housing and Urban Development and US Department of Veterans Affairs 2010). These findings suggest the substantial risk for homelessness among female veterans regardless of service era, perhaps because they have never been subject to a military draft and thus have always been volunteers susceptible to social selection effects (Gamache et al. 2003).

The other comparative studies found that there were consistent differences in sociodemographic characteristics between homeless veterans and nonveterans. Homeless veterans were older, better educated, and more likely to be male, to be or have been married, and to have health coverage. Earlier studies also found homeless veterans were more likely to be white than homeless nonveterans, but fewer racial/ethnic differences have been found in more recent studies as the veteran population has become more racially/ethnically diverse. A high prevalence of physical, mental health, and substance abuse problems was found among both homeless veterans and homeless nonveterans, but there were no consistent differences between veterans and nonveterans.

Table 13.2 summarizes the main risk factors that have been found from extant studies on veteran homelessness. As the table shows, a handful of factors have been found to be associated with homelessness among veterans, most of which are not unique to veterans. These factors may have implications for primary and secondary prevention efforts. And in fact, many programs have been developed for homeless veterans, which will be discussed in the next section.

Table 13.2 Main risk factors that have been identified for veteran homelessness

Risk factors
Adverse childhood experiences
Chronic medical problems
History of Incarceration
Neurological deficits
Poverty
Problematic military discharges
Severe mental illness
Social isolation
Substance abuse
Unemployment

Risk factors are those identified in previous reports and reviews (Balshem et al. 2011; Tsai and Rosenheck 2015)

Programs for Homeless Veterans

There are various VA and non-VA programs that have been developed for homeless veterans. This chapter cannot include a review of all of them but will describe several main programs worth noting. In the past decade, hundreds of millions of dollars have been spent on VA homeless services. Six of the VA's main homeless programs will be briefly described, and any research that has been conducted on their effectiveness will be mentioned in this section.

The US Department of Housing and Urban Development-Veterans Affairs Supportive Housing (HUD-VASH) program is the largest supported housing program for veterans in the nation and offers homeless veterans Housing and Urban Development Housing Choice vouchers to subsidize their rent and supportive case management from VA staff to help them acquire and retain permanent housing (US Department of Veterans Affairs 2010). A randomized controlled trial of HUD-VASH has shown it to be effective in improving housing outcomes compared to treatment as usual and intensive case management (Rosenheck et al. 2003). However, improvement in mental health, substance abuse, and quality of life outcomes (Cheng et al. 2007; Tsai et al. 2014a, b, c) was not different than in standard VA programs for homeless veterans. Additional programmatic efforts may be needed to improve the functioning of veterans in domains other than housing. This may include utilizing alternative case management models (Tsai and Rosenheck 2012b), leveraging peer support (Resnick et al. 2004), and citizenship type initiatives (Rowe et al. 2001).

The Grant and Per Diem (GPD) program funds community agencies to provide structured transitional housing for homeless veterans where they can stay for up to 2 years with the goal of helping them achieve residential stability, receive treatment for mental and addictive disorders, increase their skill levels and/or incomes, and obtain greater capacity for community reintegration. Many of these agencies require sobriety as an admission criterion for transitional housing, although one study of Grant and Per Diem and other VA transitional housing found that requiring sobriety at admission made little difference on housing outcomes after discharge from transitional housing (Tsai et al. 2012c, d).

The Veterans Justice Outreach (VJO) program, in contrast, serves veterans recently involved in the criminal justice system and seeks to rapidly link them with services to avoid incarceration entirely, when possible, and to otherwise minimize unnecessary criminalization of mental illness and extended incarceration by providing direct outreach, assessment, diversion, and case management services along with acting as a liaison with local courts, jails, and local justice system partners.

The Healthcare for Re-entry Veterans (HCRV) program assists incarcerated veterans soon to be reentering the community by connecting them to needed VA health services to prevent recidivism and homelessness through outreach, prerelease assessments, and post-release referrals and linkages to medical, psychiatric, and social services. Many veterans in the Healthcare for Re-entry Veterans program have histories of homelessness (Tsai et al. 2014), and many also have mental health and other psychosocial needs that would benefit from VA services (Tsai et al. 2014). Assisting recently incarcerated veterans at especially high risk of experiencing homelessness or re-incarceration to obtain adequate resources and services is an important component of VA efforts to prevent veteran homelessness.

The Domiciliary Care for Homeless Veterans (DCHV) program provides time-limited residential rehabilitation and treatment services on VA grounds, including medical, psychiatric, and substance abuse treatment and vocational rehabilitation (Seibyl et al. 2011).

The Supportive Services for Veteran Families (SSVF) program provides grants to community providers that offer services that provide rapid rehousing outreach, case management, temporary rental and financial assistance, and help with other psychosocial needs including civil legal problems to veterans and their families to help them stay in or acquire permanent housing. Analyses of the Supportive Services for Veteran Families program have shown that many homeless veterans, particularly female veterans, have benefitted from SSVF-provided funds (US Department of Veterans Affairs 2014), although a formal comparative evaluation has yet to be conducted.

Outside the VA system, many other federal, local, nonprofit, and private programs serve homeless veterans. The Department of Housing and Urban Development (HUD) alone offers many housing assistance programs available to homeless adults, including veterans, including emergency, transitional, and permanent housing programs. The Department of Labor Veterans' Employment and Training Service (DOL-VETS) offers employment assistance for homeless veterans, including the Homeless Veterans Reintegration Program which offers job counseling, resume preparation, job placement, and periodic follow-up, as well as essential supportive services for clothing, shelter, transportation, and mental health treatment. The National Health Care for the Homeless Council (HCH) is a national network of providers that work to improve the health of homeless people, including veterans. There are also various well-known nonprofit organizations such as the Salvation Army and Goodwill Industries, as well as various veteran service organizations like American Legion and the Disabled American Veterans, that offer service programs to support homeless veterans.

Many community programs have been implemented on the local and regional level that offer residential and transitional housing services to homeless veterans. An updated list of other non-VA resources available to homeless veterans is available online at http://www.va.gov/HOMELESS/NonVAResources.asp.

Primary and Secondary Prevention

Primary prevention by definition seeks to prevent the onset of conditions by altering behaviors or exposures (i.e., risk factors) that can lead to their development or by enhancing resistance to the effects of exposure before conditions have developed. Secondary prevention aims to treat and control the progression of conditions after they have developed, i.e., to prevent further exacerbation of identified problems such as reducing chronicity or relapse.

For primary and secondary homeless prevention, VA has implemented a universal, two-question screener for current homelessness and imminent risk called the Homelessness Screening Clinical Reminder (HSCR) that is being administered at all VA healthcare facilities (Montgomery et al. 2013). The Homelessness Screening Clinical Reminder comprises two questions: "In the past two months, have you been living in stable housing that you own, rent, or stay in as part of a household?" (a "no" response indicates veteran is positive for homelessness) and "Are you worried or concerned that in the next two months you may NOT have stable housing that you own, rent, or stay in as part of a household?" (a "yes" response indicates veteran is positive for risk). This screener is intended to target prevention interventions at those most vulnerable for homelessness. Preliminary analyses on more than 4.3 million unique veterans who responded to the Homelessness Screening Clinical Reminder in 2012–2013 found that 36,081 (0.8%) screened positive for current homelessness and 41,450 (0.9%) screened positive for imminent risk (Fargo et al. 2014). Of those who responded to a rescreen 6–12 months later, the vast majority (85%) was no longer homeless, suggesting many homeless veterans engaged in VA services are able to exit from homelessness.

The Supportive Services for Veteran Families (SSVF) program also focuses on both primary and secondary prevention. Created in 2012 to prevent veteran homelessness, the SSVF program rapidly rehouses homeless and at-risk veterans through time-limited case management, temporary financial assistance for moving expenses or rental fees, landlord mediation services, and other supportive services. In conjunction with the Homelessness Screening Clinical Reminder (HSCR), the Supportive Services for Veteran Families program has the potential to identify and directly target prevention interventions toward those most vulnerable. Other programs like the Healthcare for Re-entry Veterans (HCRV) and Veterans Justice Outreach (VJO) program offer primary prevention by connecting justice-involved veterans with VA health and social services to prevent homelessness.

VA services such as benefits outreach and supported employment can also be used to ameliorate poverty and other socioeconomic risk factors for veteran homelessness. Receipt of VA service-connected disability compensation has been found to be a protective factor against homelessness (Edens et al. 2011), and helping veterans obtain VA disability as well as social security income and other forms of disability benefits may help prevent or minimize the homeless risk or its chronicity.

Implementation of VA-supported employment for homeless veterans has shown to be associated with improved employment outcomes and more rapid housing placement (Rosenheck and Mares 2007). A randomized controlled trial of the VA's compensated work therapy program on homeless veterans with substance abuse problems showed that those who received work therapy were more likely to initiate outpatient substance abuse treatment, experienced fewer substance abuse problems, reported better physical health, and had fewer episodes of homelessness and incarceration than a control group (Kashner et al. 2002). Together, these studies suggest that employment supports should be offered, whenever possible, to homeless veterans in addition to the other psychosocial and housing services they are offered.

The Department of Housing and Urban Development-Veterans Affairs Supportive Housing (HUD-VASH) program is mainly designed to house veterans who are already homeless, so it can be characterized as focused on secondary prevention. The predominant model for permanent supported housing for homeless adults in the USA has become the model developed at Pathways to Housing, simply known as the Housing First model. The Housing First model has shown to be effective in improving housing outcomes better than treatment as usual in several randomized controlled trials in the USA and Canada (Hwang et al. 2012; Padgett et al. 2008; Patterson et al. 2013; Tsemberis et al. 2004). However, this model has not been formally evaluated in a randomized controlled trial. In 2013, the VA officially adopted the Housing First model in the HUD-VASH program although the implementation process has been gradual (Austin et al. 2014; Tsai 2014). The transition to the Housing First model in the VA also brings up questions about what role VA transitional and residential programs have, as the focus shifts to providing immediate, permanent housing instead of transitional types of housing. As for now, it appears the VA has taken the approach of maintaining a continuum of housing options with the recognition that "one size does not fit all."

Prevention interventions need to be individualized to address the unique needs of individual veterans. For example, homeless female veterans may have needs that are different from those of male veterans. Some studies have shown that homeless female veterans are more likely to have minor children with them, have experienced various types of trauma, may have more limited housing options, and have other special needs (Byrne et al. 2013; Hamilton et al. 2011; Tsai et al. 2012b, c; Tsai et al. 2014). Analysis of VA homeless program referral and admission patterns have shown that there are major gender differences in VA services that are offered or are available for male and female veterans (Tsai et al. 2014a, b, c; US Department of Veterans Affairs 2014). Beyond gender, homeless veterans may have other differences in their need profiles. Using latent class analysis of data from over 120,000 VA homeless service users from 142 sites, one study identified four need profiles, including a group with relatively few problems, a dual diagnosis group, a poverty-substance abuse-incarceration group, and a disabling medical problems group (Tsai et al. 2013). These different groups were referred and admitted to different VA homeless programs at different rates supporting the role of individualizing services for veterans with different patterns of need.

Future Directions

As Fig. 13.1 shows, recent governmental reports have reported declines in both adult homelessness in general and specifically veteran homelessness (US Department of Housing and Urban Development 2013). Although considerable progress has been made in research and practice on addressing homelessness among veterans, many programs for homeless veterans do not have substantial evidence of their effectiveness or cost-effectiveness. The authors have several suggestions for future directions and areas that need further development, research, and evaluation.

First, efforts are needed to devise demonstrably cost-effective primary prevention initiatives for veteran homelessness. The implementation of a homeless screener by the Veterans Health Administration is an important first step, but additional steps are needed to determine the most cost-effective ways of responding to veterans who screen positive for homelessness or are at risk for homelessness. As detailed in the previous two sections, there are many programs available to assist homeless veterans. However, there are no guidelines or treatment algorithms on which programs should be offered, to which veterans, and at what stage in their rehabilitation. The Supportive Services for Veteran Families (SSVF) program is particularly promising for primary prevention as it can offer many resources depending on the capabilities and resources of community grantees who receive the VA funds. But there is great variability in how these funds are used (e.g., legal services, moving expenses, rent, utilities, security deposits) and limited information on which approaches are most cost-effective. The Supportive Services for Veteran Families program is difficult to evaluate because it does not offer a clear set of alternative services than can be compared, and its active ingredients are not yet well defined. Thus, further evaluation research is needed to more optimally tailor prevention interventions to the needs of individual veterans, to identify "best practices," and to provide guidance to grantees and to clinicians on how to provide the most cost-effective care to homeless or "at-risk" veterans in VA's integrated healthcare system.

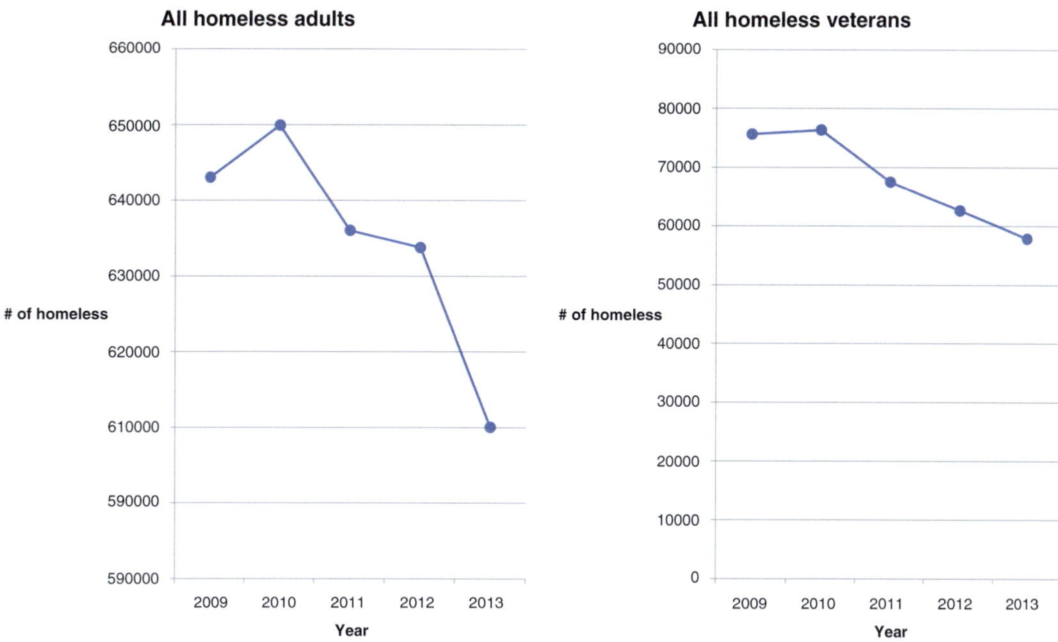

Fig. 13.1 Gradual decline in homelessness (Note: Estimates are based on the 2013 Annual Homeless Assessment Report (AHAR) to Congress (US Department of Housing and Urban Development 2013))

Second, with the Department of Housing and Urban Development-Veterans Affairs Supportive Housing (HUD-VASH) program now transitioning to the Housing First model, more attention is needed on developing methods for improving the lives of veterans after they obtain housing. In other words, if independent permanent housing is first, what comes next? Research on programs outside the VA has found that supported housing has little effect, by itself, on social and community integration (Tsai and Rosenheck 2012a). Obtaining housing per se, while a critical first step, does not automatically result in improvements in other psychosocial domains. Many adults with severe mental illness, including those who are formerly homeless, often report that they feel lonely, isolated, and without social support (Friedrich et al. 1999; Nelson et al. 1992; Siegel et al. 2006; Tsai et al. 2010). To prevent further homelessness and improve the lives of formerly homeless veterans, comprehensive recovery-oriented services may be needed to help veterans develop fully independent, fulfilling lives after housing is obtained.

Third, to prevent the problem of veteran homelessness, attention must be directed to the pathways by which veterans first fall into homelessness and why they continue to have multiple episodes of homelessness. The risk for homelessness may start as early as childhood. There is some evidence that adverse childhood events and experiences increase risk for homelessness in adulthood among veterans (Tsai and Rosenheck 2015). Moreover, veterans may be more likely to have had adverse childhood events than other adults (Blosnich et al. 2014), particularly veterans who have served since the advent of the All-Volunteer Force (i.e., after 1973). Better understanding of how the risks for veteran homelessness may accumulate or be mitigated over time is needed. Well-conducted population studies and longitudinal studies of homeless veterans after obtaining housing may shed light on the temporal sequence and factors that lead to first episode or multiple episodes of homelessness.

Many homeless veterans also have dependent children (Tsai et al. 2015), and there have been virtually no research or programs specifically addressing the needs of these children. We know from the homeless literature that these children may have many of the risk factors for experiencing homelessness in adulthood. To prevent the cycle of homelessness from recurring with the children of homeless veterans, services are needed to better support the parenting needs of homeless veterans and to help their children have lives with trajectories that lead away from homelessness.

Lastly, although VA has committed to ending homelessness among veterans, funding and efforts will need to be continued to maintain the progress that has been made. The federal initiative to end veteran homelessness by the end of 2015 has been superseded by the Mayors Challenge to End Veteran Homelessness (US Department of Veterans Affairs 2016). The Mayors Challenge to End Veteran Homelessness is an interagency initiative that calls on cities, counties, and states to commit to ending and preventing homelessness among veterans in their communities. To support these efforts, the Department of Housing and Development (HUD) has provided various resources including federal criteria and benchmarks review tools (US Department of Housing and Urban Development). However, local communities have to leverage their own funds to meet this challenge. Questions remain as to how resources can be most effectively allocated to garner public support and ultimately sustain long-term solutions to veteran homelessness in the future.

Conclusions

Veterans have a special status in US society because of their past military service, and intensive efforts to provide them with the health and social services they need have been marshaled in recent years to allow them to successfully reenter society after their service. Public concern about homelessness among veterans has led to a sizable body of research and the development and funding of a variety of Department of Veterans Affairs (VA) and non-VA homeless services. Some veteran cohorts are overrepresented among the general homeless population, although the proportion of veterans among homeless adults appears to be on the decline in recent years, which is encouraging. A body of studies has been conducted identifying certain risk factors for veteran homelessness, although more rigorous epidemiological studies may be needed. A variety of VA and non-VA homeless programs have been developed to provide primary and secondary prevention of homelessness among veterans. Some of these programs have been carefully evaluated and shown to be effective, while others lack empirical evidence and have not yet been adequately evaluated. There is considerable room for future program development and evaluation, for developing long-term solutions to ending veteran homelessness, and for identifying best practices for organizations to pool resources, collaborate, and deliver comprehensive services to address the needs of homeless veterans and to prevent its occurrence in the future.

Key Concepts

1. Veteran homelessness has been considered a public health problem for over three decades, and federal funds have been dedicated to addressing it.
2. The most consistent risk factors identified for veteran homelessness have been substance abuse problems and mental illness.
3. A range of Department of Veterans Affairs (VA) programs exist to help homeless and at-risk veterans with housing, medical and mental healthcare, employment, and criminal justice involvement.
4. Additional intervention research is needed on the health and social integration of veterans after obtaining housing.

References

Austin EL, Pollio DE, Holmes S, Schumacher J, White B, Lukas CV, Kertesz S (2014) VA's expansion of supportive housing: successes and challenges on the path toward Housing First. Psychiatr Serv 65(5):641–647

Balshem H, Christensen V, Tuepker A (2011) A critical review of the literature regarding homelessness among veterans. Department of Veterans Affairs Health Services Research & Development Service Evidence-based Synthesis Program, Washington, DC. VA-ESP Project #05–225

Blosnich JR, Dichter ME, Cerulli C, Batten SV, Bossarte RM (2014) Disparities in adverse childhood experiences among individuals with a history of military service. JAMA Psychiat. https://doi.org/10.1001/jamapsychiatry.2014.724

Byrne T, Montgomery AE, Dichter ME (2013) Homelessness among female veterans: a systematic review of the literature. Women Health 53(6):572–596

Cheng AL, Lin H, Kasprow WJ, Rosenheck RA (2007) Impact of supported housing on clinical outcomes: analysis of a randomized trial using multiple imputation technique. J Nerv Ment Dis 195(1):83–88

Dickson P, Allen TB (2006) The bonus army: an American epic. Walker & Company, New York

Donovan S, Shinseki EK (2013) Homelessness is a public health issue. Am J Public Health 103(S2):S180–S180

Edens EL, Kasprow W, Tsai J, Rosenheck RA (2011) Association of substance use and VA service-connected disability benefits with risk of homelessness among veterans. Am J Addict 20(5):412–419

Elbogen EB, Sullivan CP, Wolfe J, Wagner HR, Beckham JC (2013) Homelessness and money mismanagement in Iraq and Afghanistan veterans. Am J Public Health 103(Suppl 2):S248–S254

Fargo J, Byrne T, Montgomery AE, Roberts CB (2014) Universal screening for homelessness and risk among veterans: monitoring housing stability and exploring profiles of risk through repeated screening. National Center on Homelessness Among Veterans, Philadelphia

Fazel S, Kholsa V, Doll H, Geddes J (2008) The prevalence of mental disorders among the homeless in western countries: systematic review and meta-regression analysis. PLoS Med 5(12):e225

Folsom DP, Hawthorne W, Lindamer LA, Gilmer T, Bailey A, Golshan S, Unützer J, Hough R, Jeste D (2005) Prevalence and risk factors for homelessness and utilization of mental health services among 10,340 patients with serious mental illness in a large public mental health system. Am J Psychiatr 162(2):370–376

Friedrich RM, Hollingsworth B, Hradek E, Friedrich HB, Culp KR (1999) Family and client perspectives on alternative residential settings for persons with severe mental illness. Psychiatr Serv 50:509–514

Gamache G, Rosenheck RA, Tessler R (2001) The proportion of veterans among homeless men: a decade later. Soc Psychiatr Psychiatr Epidemiol 36(10):481–485

Gamache G, Rosenheck RA, Tessler R (2003) Overrepresentation of women veterans among homeless women. Am J Public Health 93(7):1132–1136

Gladwell M (2006) Million-dollar Murray. The New Yorker 13 Feb 2006:96

Hamilton AB, Poza I, Washington DL (2011) Homelessness and trauma go hand-in-hand: pathways to homelessness among women veterans. Womens Health Issues 21(4):S203–S209

Hibbs JR, Benner L, Klugman L, Spencer R, Macchia I, Mellinger A, Fife DK (1994) Mortality in a cohort of homeless adults in Philadelphia. N Engl J Med 331(5):304–309

Hoge CW, Castro CA, Messer SC, McGurk D, Cotting DI, Koffman RL (2004) Combat duty in Iraq and Afghanistan, mental health problems, and barriers to care. N Engl J Med 351(1):13–22

Hoge CW, Auchterlonie JL, Milliken CS (2006) Mental health problems, use of mental health services, and attrition from military services after returning from deployment to Iraq and Afghanistan. J Am Med Assoc 295(9):1023–1032

Hwang SW (2001) Homelessness and health. Can Med Assoc J 164(2):229–233

Hwang SW, Stergiopoulos V, O'Campo P, Gozdzik A (2012) Ending homelessness among people with mental illness: the at Home/Chez Soi randomized trial of a housing first intervention in Toronto. BMC Public Health 12(1):787

Kashner TM, Rosenheck R, Campinell AB, Suris A, Crandall R, Garfield NJ, Lapuc P, Pyrcz K, Soyka T, Wicker A (2002) Impact of work therapy on health status among homeless, substance-dependent veterans: a randomized controlled trial. Arch Gen Psychiatry 59(10):938–944

Lewin T (1987) Nation's homeless veterans battle a new foe: defeatism. The New York Times, p. A10

McGuire J (2007) Closing a front door to homelessness among veterans. J Prim Prev 28(3–4):389–400

McKinney-Vento Homeless Assistance Act as amended by S.896 (2009) The Homeless Emergency Assistance and Rapid Transition to Housing (HEARTH) Act of 2009 § 103, 42 USC 11302 General definition of homeless individual

Metraux S, Clegg LX, Daigh JD, Culhane DP, Kane V (2013) Risk factors for becoming homeless among a cohort of veterans who served in the era of the Iraq and Afghanistan conflicts. Am J Public Health 103(Suppl 2):S255–S261

Montgomery AE, Fargo JD, Byrne TH, Kane VR, Culhane DP (2013) Universal screening for homelessness and risk for homelessness in the Veterans Health Administration. Am J Public Health 103(S2):S210–S211

National Alliance to End Homelessness (2014) Ten year plan. http://www.endhomelessness.org/pages/ten-year-plan. Accessed 8 Jul 2014

Nelson G, Hall GB, Squire D, Walsh-Bower RT (1992) Social network transactions of psychiatric patients. Soc Sci Med 34:443–445

O'Connell JJ (2005) Premature mortality in homeless population: a review of the literature. National Health Care for the Homeless Council, Nashville

Padgett DK, Gulcur L, Tsemberis S (2008) Housing first services for people who are homeless with co-occurring serious mental illness and substance abuse. Res Soc Work Pract 16(1):74–83

Patterson M, Moniruzzaman A, Palepu A, Zabkiewicz D, Frankish CJ, Krausz M, Somers JM (2013) Housing first improves subjective quality of life among homeless adults with mental illness: 12-month findings from a randomized controlled trial in Vancouver, British Columbia. Soc Psychiatry Psychiatr Epidemiol 48(8):1245–1259

Resnick SG, Armstrong M, Sperrazza M, Harkness K, Rosenheck RA (2004) A model of consumer-

provider partnership: vet-to-vet. Psychiatr Rehabil J 28:185–187
Robertson MJ (1987) Homeless veterans: an emerging problem? In: Bingham RD, Green RE, White SB (eds) The homeless in contemporary society. Sage Publications, Newbury Park, pp 64–81
Rosenheck RA, Mares AS (2007) Implementation of supported employment for homeless veterans with psychiatric or addiction disorders: two-year outcomes. Psychiatr Serv 58:315–324
Rosenheck RA, Seibyl CL (1998) Homelessness: health service use and related costs. Med Care 36(8):1256–1264
Rosenheck RA, Leda C, Gallup P, Astrachan B, Milstein R, Leaf P, Thompson D, Errera P (1989) Initial assessment data from a 43-site program for homeless chronic mentally ill veterans. Hosp Community Psychiatr 40(9):937–942
Rosenheck RA, Frisman L, Chung A (1994) The proportion of veterans among homeless men. Am J Public Health 84(3):466–469
Rosenheck RA, Kasprow W, Frisman L, Liu-Mares W (2003) Cost-effectiveness of supported housing for homeless persons with mental illness. Arch Gen Psychiatry 60(9):940–951
Rowe M, Kloos B, Chinman M, Davidson L, Cross AB (2001) Homelessness, mental illness and citizenship. Soc Policy Adm 35(1):14–31
Salit SA, Kuhn EM, Hartz AJ, Vu JM, Mosso AL (1998) Hospitalization costs associated with homelessness in New York City. N Engl J Med 338(24):1734–1740
Schanzer B, Dominguez B, Shrout PE, Caton CL (2007) Homelessness, health status, and health care use. Am J Public Health 97(3):464–469
Seal KH, Bertenthal D, Miner CR, Sen S, Marmar C (2007) Bringing the war back home: mental health disorders among 103,788 US veterans returning from Iraq and Afghanistan seen at Department of Veterans Affairs Facilities. Arch Intern Med 167(5):476–482
Seibyl CL, Medak S, Baldino L, Desai RA (2011) The twenty-second progress report on the Department of Veterans Affairs (VA) domiciliary care for homeless veterans program: fiscal year (FY) 2010. Northeast Program Evaluation Center, West Haven
Siegel CE, Samuels J, Tang D, Berg I, Jones K, Hopper K (2006) Tenant outcomes in supported housing and community residences in New York City. Psychiatr Serv 57:982–991
Susser E, Moore R, Link B (1993) Risk factors for homelessness. Am J Epidemiol 15(2):546–556
Tsai J (2014) Timing and momentum in VA's path toward Housing First. Psychiatr Serv 65(6):836
Tsai, J., Rosenheck, R. A., & Kane, V. (2014). Homeless female US veterans in a national supported housing program: Comparison of individual characteristics and outcomes with male veterans. Psychological services, 11(3):309
Tsai J, Rosenheck RA (2012a) Does housing chronically homeless adults lead to social integration? Psychiatr Serv 63(5):427–434
Tsai J, Rosenheck RA (2012b) Outcomes of a group intensive peer-support model of case management for supported housing. Psychiatr Serv 63(12):1186–1194
Tsai J, Rosenheck RA (2015) Risk factors for homelessness among US veterans. Epidemiol Rev 37(1):177–195
Tsai J, Bond GR, Salyers MP, Godfrey JL, Davis KE (2010) Housing preferences and choices among adults with mental illness and substance use disorders: a qualitative study. Community Ment Health J 46:381–388
Tsai J, Pietrzak RH, Rosenheck RA (2012a) Homeless veterans who served in Iraq and Afghanistan: gender differences, combat exposure, and comparisons with previous cohorts of homeless veterans. Adm Policy Ment Health Ment Health Serv Res 40(5):400–405
Tsai J, Rosenheck RA, Decker SE, Desai RA, Harpaz-Rotem I (2012b) Trauma experience among homeless female veterans: correlates and impact on housing, clinical, and psychosocial outcomes. J Trauma Stress 25(6):624–632
Tsai J, Rosenheck RA, Kasprow WJ, McGuire JF (2012c) Sobriety as an admission criterion for transitional housing: a multi-site comparison of programs with a sobriety requirement to programs with no sobriety requirement. Drug Alcohol Depend 125(3):223–229
Tsai J, Rosenheck RA, McGuire JF (2012d) Comparison of outcomes of homeless female and male veterans in transitional housing. Community Ment Health J 48(6):705–710
Tsai J, Kasprow WJ, Rosenheck RA (2013) Latent homeless risk profiles of a national sample of homeless veterans and their relation to program referral and admission patterns. Am J Public Health 103(Suppl 2):S239–S247
Tsai J, Kasprow W, Kane V, Rosenheck RA (2014a) National comparison of literally homeless male and female VA service users: entry characteristics, clinical needs, and service patterns. Womens Health Issues 24(1):e29–e35
Tsai J, Kasprow WJ, Rosenheck RA (2014b) Alcohol and drug use disorders among homeless veterans: prevalence and association with supported housing outcomes. Addict Behav 39(2):455–460
Tsai J, Rosenheck RA, Kasprow WJ, McGuire JF (2014c) Homelessness in a national sample of incarcerated veterans in state and federal prisons. Adm Policy Ment Health Ment Health Serv Res 41(3):360–367
Tsai J, Rosenheck RA, Kasprow WJ, Kane V (2015) Characteristics and use of services among literally homeless and unstably housed US veterans with custody of minor children. Psychiatr Serv 66(10):1083–1090
Tsemberis S, Gulcur L, Nakae M (2004) Housing first, consumer choice, and harm reduction for homeless individuals with a dual diagnosis. Am J Public Health 94:651–656
Universal Declaration of Human Rights (1948) Article 25 (1)

US Department of Housing and Urban Development (2013) The 2013 annual homeless assessment report (AHAR) to congress: part 1, point-in-time estimates of homelessness. US Department of Housing and Urban Development, Washington, DC

US Department of Housing and Urban Development, US Department of Veterans Affairs (2010) Veteran homelessness: a supplemental report to the 2009 annual homeless assessment report to congress. US Department of Housing and Urban Development and the US Department of Veterans Affairs, Washington, DC

US Department of Veterans Affairs (2009) Secretary Shinseki details plans to end homelessness for veterans. http://www1.va.gov/opa/pressrel/pressrelease.cfm?id=1807

US Department of Veterans Affairs (2010) Department of Housing and Urban Development-Department of veterans affairs supported housing program (HUD-VASH). Northeast Program Evaluation Center, West Haven

US Department of Veterans Affairs (2013) Profile of veterans 2011. http://www.va.gov/VETDATA/docs/SpecialReports/Profile_of_Veterans_2011.pdf. Accessed 28 Jan 2014

US Department of Veterans Affairs (2014) Supportive Services for Veteran Families (SSVF) FY 2013 Annual Report. Washington, DC

US Department of Veterans Affairs (2016) Mayors challenge to end veteran homelessness. Interagency and cross-cutting initiatives to end and prevent veteran homelessness. http://www.va.gov/HOMELESS/Mayors_Challenge.asp. Accessed 2 Oct 2016

US Interagency Council on Homelessness (2010) Opening doors: federal strategic plan to prevent and end homelessness. United States Interagency Council on Homelessness, Washington, DC

Wright JD (1988) The worthy and unworthy homeless. Society 25(5):64–69

Part III

Clinical Care for Mental Health Needs of Military and Veteran Populations

Mood Disorders

14

Claudia B. Padula, Alicia B. Vanden Bussche, and Leanne M. Williams

Prevalence

Mood disorders are a group of diagnoses in which there is a disturbance in an individual's mood. Based on the current diagnostic classification system, disorders are classified as: major depression, dysthymia, and bipolar disorder. Major depression is one of the most common and debilitating mental health diagnoses in the United States. According to the World Health Organization (2010), major depression also causes the heaviest burden of disability among behavioral and mental health disorders (Kessler et al. 2003). Individuals who serve in the military may be prone to depression, at least partially as a result of exposure to combat, separation from family during deployment or training, and other traumatic factors (Hoge et al. 2006). For example, in 2011, The Army Study to Assess Risk and Resilience in service members (Army STARRS) described the 30-day prevalence of major depressive disorder (MDD) as 4.8% in service members compared to less than 1% among civilians (Kessler et al. 2014). A meta-analysis of 25 epidemiological studies estimated the prevalence of recent major depression at rates of 12.0% among currently deployed military service members, 13.1% among previously deployed, and 5.7% among those never deployed (Gadermann et al. 2012). However, the 25 studies from which these estimates are drawn described a wide range of prevalence depending on the screening or diagnostic instrument, population, and time period used. Being female, enlisted, 17–25 years old, unmarried, and having had less than a college education were reported risk factors for depression (Gadermann et al. 2012). In an analysis of current and former military personnel who were included in the Millennium Cohort Study, the risk of suicide increased in men and in those who were depressed (LeardMann et al. 2013).

In veterans, major depressive disorder (MDD), diagnosed by structured psychiatric interviews and specific diagnostic criteria, is present in 5–13% of patients seen by primary care physicians (Hofmann et al. 2003). Recent estimates suggest that 30% of veterans returning from Iraq and Afghanistan have a mental health condition requiring treatment (National Council of Behavioral Health 2012). This includes 5% prevalence of major depressive disorder in veterans. The prevalence of major depressive disorder in

C.B. Padula
Psychiatry and Behavioral Sciences, Stanford University School of Medicine and MIRECC VA Palo Alto Health Care System, Palo Alto, CA, USA

A.B. Vanden Bussche
Palo Alto University, Palo Alto, CA, USA

L.M. Williams (✉)
Psychiatry and Behavioral Sciences, Stanford University School of Medicine, Palo Alto, CA 94305-5717, USA
e-mail: leawilliams@stanford.edu

L.W. Roberts, C.H. Warner (eds.), *Military and Veteran Mental Health*,
https://doi.org/10.1007/978-1-4939-7438-2_14

the general population is approximately 3–5%. Major depressive disorder affects approximately 14.8 million American adults, or about 6.7% of the US population aged 18 and older, in a given year and is more common in women than in men (Takeuchi et al. 2014). In fiscal year 2015, among veterans served by the Veterans Health Administration (VHA), the documented prevalence of any depression (including depression not otherwise specified) was 19.8%, while the documented prevalence of major depressive disorder was 6.5% (VHA Mental Health Services 2015). According to the US Department of Veterans Affairs, 122,175 veterans were diagnosed with depressive disorders during 2002–2010. This number represents 20% of all patients seen and 31% of those being seen for mental health services. Of these service members and veterans who have depression, a small percentage of them experience a manic or hypomanic episode and become diagnosed with bipolar disorder. The lifetime prevalence of bipolar I disorder (depression and mania) is estimated at 0.8% of the adult population, with a range between 0.4% and 1.6%. Bipolar II disorder (depression and hypomania) affects approximately 0.5% or more of the population. Bipolar II disorder is more common in women, while bipolar I disorder appears to be evenly distributed between men and women (American Psychiatric Association 2000).

Case Study

Corporal Bella Davis (pseudonym) is a 48-year-old female veteran. She served in the Army for 5 years as a K9 drug detector handler specialist and was honorably discharged 20 years ago. Davis has always been bright and high achieving and has very high standards for herself. Since her separation from the Army, she has struggled with periods of significant feelings of worthlessness and shame. During these periods, she is unable to get out of bed, describes a fog that limits her ability to concentrate, and has increased urges to end her life. The episodes are so severe that she often ends up in the hospital. She struggles with substance use and is unable to maintain gainful employment. She describes her depression as "biochemical" and reports that there are no clear triggers for her deep sadness. She has had several trials of antidepressant medication and becomes frustrated when she finds them ineffective. She reports that she would like the "fog to be lifted" and is willing to try alternative treatments for her distressing experiences.

Symptoms

Symptoms of depressed mood can contribute to a spectrum of mood disorders including major depressive disorder and bipolar disorder. People with a depressive disorder may have experiences of depressed mood and extreme sadness, feelings of hopelessness, a profound loss of interest, problems getting motivated, loss of concentration, and/or changes in appetite and sleep. These experiences may continue for extended periods of time and also recur in episodes. For people experiencing bipolar disorder, periods of depression and feeling "down" may be interspersed with periods of feeling very "up" and energized. These "up" periods can be expressed as mania. Overall, mood disorders cause significant distress or impairment in an important area of functioning (e.g., social, occupational). Mood disorders can interfere with the usual activities of daily life, including social relationships and the capacity to work. These disorders cause pain and disability for the individual experiencing them as well as for those who care about them. Mood disorders have been associated with a greater prevalence in female individuals than in male individuals, with peak periods of onset in adolescence through early adulthood and then again in older age. As highlighted in the following section, these prevalence data are currently based on the general population, and research is needed to determine whether or not these patterns generalize to the veterans population.

Gender Differences in Depression

It is not yet known the extent to which the experience of depression may differ in men and women veterans. Right now, evidence is drawn from studies of the general population, and in these studies, depression is generally more prevalent in women than in men (Piccinello and Wilkinson 2000). In a small sample of Operation Enduring Freedom/Operation Iraqi Freedom (OEF/OIF) veterans, women were more likely to screen positive for depression in a primary care setting than their male counterparts (Haskell et al. 2010). Biological, life cycle, hormonal, and psychosocial factors that women experience may be linked to women's higher depression rate. Researchers have shown that hormones directly affect the brain chemistry that controls emotions and mood (McEwen 2005). Additionally, brain function, and specifically amygdala reactivity, appears to differ in men and women in response to affective stimuli, further suggesting a biological basis for difference in mood disorders between men and women (Williams et al. 2005).

Men, on the other hand, often experience depression differently than women (Padesky and Hammen 1981). Men are more likely to be very tired, irritable, lose interest in once-pleasurable activities, and have difficulty sleeping. Men may be more likely than women to turn to alcohol or drugs when they are depressed (Simbayi et al. 2007). They also may become frustrated, discouraged, irritable, angry, and sometimes abusive. Some men throw themselves into their work to avoid talking about their depression with family or friends or behave recklessly. Although more women attempt suicide, many more men die by suicide in the United States. In addition, veterans are twice as likely to die from suicide than non-veterans in the general population (Kaplan et al. 2007).

Older Veterans and Depression

Depression is not a normal part of aging. Studies show that most seniors feel satisfied with their lives, despite having more illnesses or physical problems (Ryan and Deci 2001). However, when older adults do have depression, it may be overlooked because seniors may show different, less obvious symptoms. They may be less likely to experience or admit to feelings of sadness or grief. Depression in older adults can also be associated with cognitive changes, like memory impairment, which is often confused with a neurodegenerative process like Alzheimer's disease. However, if late-life depression is properly treated, then the cognitive symptoms often subside (VA/DoD Clinical Practice Guideline for Management of Major Depressive Disorder 2009). Therefore, proper screening for depression in older veterans is of critical importance.

Older adults also may have more medical conditions such as heart disease, stroke, or cancer, which are associated with increased instances of depressive symptoms (Ariyo et al. 2000; Glenn et al. 2001; Deimling et al. 2005). Or, they may be taking medications with side effects that contribute to depression. Some older adults may experience what doctors call vascular depression, also called arteriosclerotic depression or subcortical ischemic depression. Vascular depression may result when blood vessels become less flexible and harden over time, becoming constricted. Such hardening of vessels prevents normal blood flow to the body's organs, including the brain. Those with vascular depression may have, or be at risk for, coexisting heart disease or stroke.

Older adults with depression improve when they receive treatment with an antidepressant, psychotherapy, or a combination of both (Depression Guideline Panel 1993). Research has shown that medication alone and combination treatment are both effective in reducing depression in older adults (Reynolds et al. 2006). Psychotherapy alone also can be effective in helping older adults stay free of depression, especially among those with minor depression (Williams et al. 2000), and can be a great option for older adults who are unable or unwilling to take medication.

Defining Mood Disorders

This chapter reviews the evidence for mood disorders relevant to veteran populations. These disorders have been defined by the following diagnostic criteria and symptoms by the *Diagnostic and Statistical Manual*, 5th Edition (*DSM-5*). The *DSM-5* is published by the American Psychiatric Association (APA) and offers a common language and criteria to classify mental disorders (American Psychiatric Association 2013). There is currently minimal information regarding prevalence rates of specific diagnosis in veterans beyond major depressive disorder and post-traumatic stress disorder (PTSD). For example, according to Bagalman (2013), the Veterans Health Administration does not separate prevalence figures for depression and bipolar disorder independently or combined but rather presents prevalence of:

- Affective psychosis at 14%, which includes a range of diagnoses that can include major depressive disorder and bipolar disorders, among others
- Depressive disorder not otherwise specified at 22%, which is a diagnosis assigned to individuals who report depressive symptoms but do not meet criteria for other depressive disorder

Thus, when veteran-specific data are unavailable, prevalence rates are extrapolated from the general population. It will be critically important for future studies to focus on specific diagnoses in order to ultimately tailor health care to specific veterans' needs.

Types of Mood Disorders

Major Depressive Disorder (MDD) Major depressive disorder is characterized by a constant sense of hopelessness and despair. Prevalence rates among veterans range from 5% to 13% (Hofmann et al. 2003), and the Millennium Cohort Study found that men and women deployed with combat exposures have the highest occurrence of new onset depression (5.7–15.7%), compared to non-deployed personnel (3.9–7.7%). Clinical depression is characterized by depression throughout the day and a loss of interest in normal activities and relationships, and symptoms persist most days for at least 2 weeks. *DSM-5* (APA 2013) specifies the following symptoms as indicators of major depressive disorder, with five required for diagnosis:

- Depressed mood
- Loss of interest or pleasure
- Significant weight loss or weight gain
- Insomnia or hypersomnia
- Psychomotor agitation or retardation
- Fatigue or loss of energy
- Feelings of worthlessness or guilt
- Diminished ability to concentrate, indecisiveness
- Recurring thoughts of death or suicide

Dysthymic disorder is similar in symptomatology to major depressive disorder but with reduced severity and longer duration of time.

Persistent Depressive Disorder (Dysthymic Disorder) Dysthymic disorder causes chronic, long-lasting sadness. Prevalence rates in the general population range from 3% to 7% (Sansone and Sansone 2009). Individuals who experience symptoms consistent with both major depressive disorder and dysthymic disorder for 2 years or longer may be diagnosed with both disorders simultaneously. Feelings of darkness invade life daily for 2 years or more. Common symptoms include:

- Poor appetite or eating too much
- Trouble sleeping or daytime sleepiness
- Fatigue or low energy
- Low self-esteem
- Trouble concentrating or making decisions
- Feelings of hopelessness or helplessness

Similar to major depressive disorder and dysthymic disorder, individuals with bipolar disorder and cyclothymic disorder can experience sadness and episodes of low mood.

Bipolar Disorder Bipolar disorder is a serious mental illness that is characterized by extreme changes in mood, from mania to depression. It can lead to risky behavior, damaged relationships and careers, and even suicidal tendencies if it is not treated. The National Comorbidity Study reported a lifetime prevalence of nearly 4% for bipolar disorder. Bipolar disorder results in medical separation from the military, but is often considered an existed-prior-to-service condition, and therefore it is not treated through the Department of Veterans Affairs (VA). There is a lack of bipolar disorder incidence data and temporal trends, specifically for diagnostic and demographic subgroups. One major longitudinal study (1997–2006) shows that there were 3,317 first-time hospitalizations for bipolar disorder with a mean of 1.2 hospitalizations per case. Bipolar in military members requires substantial medical, administrative, and financial resources and is among the leading causes of early discharge from the military. Bipolar disorder is diagnosed once an individual has experienced a manic episode. A manic episode is defined by *DSM-5* as three or more of the following symptoms:

- Inflated self-esteem or grandiosity
- Decreased need for sleep
- More talkative than usual or pressure to keep talking
- Flight of ideas or experience that thoughts are racing
- Distractibility
- Increase in goal-directed activity or psychomotor agitation
- Excessive involvement in pleasurable activities that have high potential for painful consequences

Cyclothymic Disorder In cyclothymic disorder, moods swing between short periods of depressed mood that does not meet criteria for a major depressive episode and periods of hypomanic symptoms that do not meet criteria for hypomanic episode. Lifetime prevalence is reported to be 0.4–1% in the general population (APA 2013). People with cyclothymic disorder have milder symptoms than occur in full-blown bipolar disorder. These symptoms last for at least 2 years.

Historical Overview of Mood Disorders

Mood disorders are a category of mental health diagnoses that include all subcategories of depression and anxiety disorders (American Psychiatric Association 2013). Included in their symptoms are sadness, fatigue, worry, tension, irritability, and rage. The World Health Organization estimates that depression was the leading cause of disability worldwide in the 15–44 years of age group, and bipolar disorder was the sixth leading cause (Murray, Lopez and World Health Organization 1996).

Symptoms of individuals suffering from mood disorders have been comparable for centuries; however, the label of specific criteria for diagnosis of these symptoms is relatively recent (American Psychiatric Association 2013). One of the earliest descriptions of mood disorders (Job's depression) is located in the Old Testament (Kruger 2005). There are countless other examples throughout history as well (e.g., the story of Egil; Ritschel et al. 2013), and there have been many well-known individuals and famous veterans who suffered from various mood disorders. For example, Elvis Presley (Hopkins 1986) and Clint Eastwood are both veterans of the military and suffered from depression throughout their lives.

Literature designates Hippocrates as the first physician to attempt to understand what is known today as depression and bipolar disorder (Goodwin and Jamison 2007). Centuries later, Adolf Meyer described psychosocial descriptions of depressive reactions to negative life experiences. He also expanded on psychodynamic descriptions of depression by Abraham and Freud (1911–1950; Ritschel et al. 2013). Mood disorders were not mentioned in the American Psychiatric Association's 1952 *Diagnostic and Statistical Manual* (*DSM-I*) (Grob 1991), and prior to the 1950s and 1960s, depression was considered a symptom of a variety of complaints (from neurasthenia to manic depressive psychosis; Ritschel et al. 2013). In the 1950s, before psychiatric medications, clinicians and researchers found that individuals experiencing symptoms of depression responded to electroconvulsive therapy (ECT), but individuals using ECT were not necessarily depressed (Beck and Alford 2009).

Around the 1970s, depression and mania became a widely discussed problem, even though they had only appeared in medical research less than two decades before. However, it was not granted the status of a diagnostic category until the third edition of the *Diagnostic and Statistical Manual* (*DSM-III*) in 1980. Throughout history, there have been many descriptions of melancholia; however, most of the literature suggests that the depression and mania that is known today is a twentieth-century phenomenon (Jackson 1986).

The VA recognizes and serves both active military and veteran personnel suffering from mood disorders, although the overwhelming majority of literature on veterans and VA care is focused on PTSD specifically. VA prevalence estimates indicate two differentiations of mood disorders: affective psychoses and depressive disorder not elsewhere classified (NEC). Affective psychoses are a range of diagnoses including major depressive disorder and bipolar disorder, among others (14%), and "not elsewhere classified" is a diagnosis assigned when a patient reports depressive symptoms that do not meet criteria for other depressive disorders (e.g., major depressive disorder; 22%; Bagalman 2013). Both categories of mood disorders receive service connection (financial assistance) within the current VA system if there is evidence of an incident in service that caused the mood disorder and medical evidence of causation between the current mood disorder diagnosis and the incident in service. However, mood disorders were not always viewed as debilitating conditions in need of such financial assistance like their counterpart PTSD, and because PTSD is the signature wound of war, VA resources have not allocated enough research and resources into mood disorders.

Per military health policy (Department of Defense 2013) both depression and, more so, bipolar disorder tend to be screened for prior to enrollment in the military. However, if symptoms develop during service, then the military has protocols in place to help treat its service members. A diagnosis of depression or bipolar disorder during one's service does not lead to automatic discharge from the military, but rather individuals who do not respond to treatment or whose symptoms interference with their duties are likely to be medically discharged. The Department of Defense (DoD) recently published a guidance memorandum that explains the armed forces' response to the deployment of individuals with psychiatric conditions. The stated goal is one of restoration, but if an individual's condition does not respond to treatment within 1 year, or is not anticipated to respond, then the person would be referred to a medical evaluation board for a possible medical discharge.

Individuals on particular medications (antipsychotics, lithium, and other mood stabilizers and benzodiazepines) may be disqualified from certain branch-specific jobs, such as flight pilot. Other issues surrounding medications, such as special storage, the need for blood work to monitor levels, and recently started psychiatric medications, might preclude an individual from being deployed or limit the positions in which she could be deployed. Specifically, the Department of Defense holds that "Personnel diagnosed with psychotic or bipolar spectrum disorders will be recommended for return to their home station,' and that "psychotic and Bipolar Disorders are considered disqualifying for deployment" (Department of Defense 2006).

By 2005, there were more than 200 Vet Centers providing various counseling services and treating PTSD (VA History in Brief). Mood disorders were still less understood and harder to receive assistance for because proving that they were caused during deployment or while in the field was difficult. The VA has greatly expanded its mental health staff, especially over the last 6 years. In 2005, the VA also had a staff of about 13,500 full-time individuals to deliver mental health care and other services. By 2011, that number had increased to over 21,000. Psychologists increased from 1,200 in 2005 to more than 2,500 in July 2011. Within the past few years, mood disorders have become more accepted and better understood (VA History in Brief).

Since 2014 the VA has outlined a vision for the future of mental health care that is patient-centered and driven by a holistic approach that integrates physical and emotional well-being (Fig. 14.1; US Department of Veterans Affairs 2014).

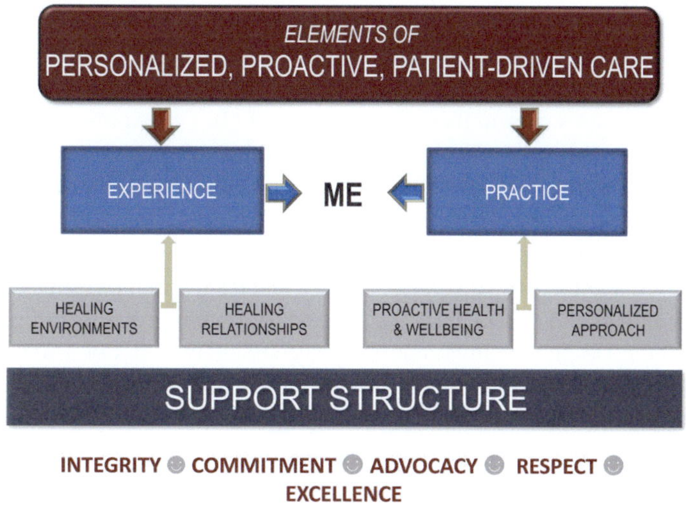

Fig. 14.1 An illustrative summary of the elements of personalized, patient-driven care within VA (Adapted from the VA BluePrint for Excellence, Strategy 6 (https://www.va.gov/patientcenteredcare/FY15AnnualNarrative/StaffFacing/OPC_Staff_Narrative_FY15-508.pdf)

History of the Treatment of Mood Disorders

Mood disorders can take on various forms, and treatment varies depending on the type of depression the person is experiencing (Drevets et al. 2008). The *DSM-5* separates mood disorders into two groups. Depressive disorders are those disorders that share a common feature of sad, empty, or irritable mood, accompanied by somatic/physical and cognitive changes that impair daily functioning. Bipolar and related disorders are those in which the person experiences both depressive periods and manic or hypomanic periods (American Psychiatric Association 2013).

Today, the VA offers treatment for mental health symptoms in a variety of settings, including short-term inpatient care, outpatient care in a psychosocial rehabilitation and recovery center, regular outpatient care (e.g., psychotherapy), residential rehabilitation treatment programs, primary care, supported work settings, and various other options (Hankin et al. 2014). In the literature, effective treatment of mood disorders combines two components: psychotherapy and medication. Treatment is effective within a few weeks to a couple of months, and research suggests that treatment also prevents future depressive episodes (Nemeroff and Owens 2002). Although research demonstrates conflicting views, psychotherapy can be an effective method for treating mood disorders, particularly for first episodes of depression (Nemeroff and Owens 2002; Scott et al. 2006). However, when psychotherapy alone is not effective or when functioning is greatly impaired, medication treatment may be necessary (Nemeroff and Owens 2002). Most of the time, the first line of medication treatment is typically an antidepressant, most commonly a selective serotonin reuptake inhibitors (SSRIs), because of their selective response to the neurotransmitter serotonin (Sachs et al. 2000).

In the VA, department policy requires an annual depression screening for veterans using VA health care (Hankin et al. 2014). Depression and bipolar are both treated with medication, psychological interventions, or both. The VA also utilizes two evidence-based treatments for depression: cognitive behavioral therapy (CBT) and acceptance and commitment therapy (ACT). Cognitive behavioral therapy is a form of psychotherapy based on decades of research, identifying the strong relationship between thoughts, emotions, and behaviors and how the culmination of thoughts, emotions, and behaviors leads to depression. Cognitive behavioral therapy helps patients learn new patterns of thinking and to develop new positive behaviors (Hughes 1988; Meichenbaum 1975; Rothbaum et al. 2000; Thase 1997). Acceptance and commitment therapy is also supported by clinical research and is based on the relationship between thoughts, feelings, and behaviors. It helps individuals overcome their struggle with emotional pain and worry and take active steps to move forward and achieve what matters most to them (Hayes et al. 1999).

Although the efficacies and modalities of mental health treatments vary by condition, most evidence for treatment in the VA supports the provision of psychotherapy as a secondary treatment, especially for mood disorders, anxiety, and PTSD (Lambert and Ogles 2004; Westen and Morrison 2001). Despite the importance of psychotherapy as a treatment modality and evidence indicating that patients often prefer psychotherapy (57%) to medication (43%; Gum et al. 2006), research on the quality of mental health care has largely focused on pharmacotherapy (Busch et al. 2004; Charbonneau et al. 2003, 2004). Furthermore, research shows that there are many barriers that stop veterans from engaging in psychotherapy that oftentimes lead them to request medications over psychotherapy. Research shows that veterans often believe they will get better on their own; have problems with getting care, finding a therapist, or transportation; believe that treatment costs too much; believe that treatments work but that services only work for other people and will not work for them; and most significantly, show concern for stigma associated with receiving mental health treatment as a veteran (Hoge et al. 2004; Ouimette et al. 2011). Furthermore, research shows that military members worry that talking about mental health symptoms with doctors, other soldiers, or commanding officers will hurt their career (Pietrzak et al. 2009).

Current Understandings of Etiology and Mechanisms

Accumulated findings over the past few decades converge on the view that depression results from a dysregulation of brain systems and associated brain chemistry as a maladaptive response to stress. This maladaptive response may be more or less likely to develop depending on each person's genetic disposition. The maladaptive response may be expressed as changes in cognitive and emotional behavior, for example, "cognitive biases," where a person will experience daily hassles as extremely negative and struggle to get a context about life events. The symptoms expressed as a result of this brain system dysregulation will vary in each person. Across individuals, the types of symptoms that have been linked to underlying brain system changes include rumination (an excessive focus on one's own thoughts and worries), negative biases (a tendency to dwell on or avoid negative information), anhedonia (a loss of a sense of pleasure and difficulty getting motivated), and problems concentrating and suppressing unwanted distractions to stay on task (for review: Williams, in revision; Williams and Gordon 2010).

Because there are a number of different lines of evidence that contribute to the current understanding of depression, the following sections are organized according to an overview of the theoretical context for a brain-stress model of depression, followed by a summary of the areas of evidence that contribute to this understanding.

Theoretical Context

The current understanding of depression is consistent with a biopsychosocial or diathesis-stress model. From this approach, it is relevant to integrate biological, psychological, and life experience factors that contribute to the development or maintenance of the disorder. This approach also accounts for individual differences in the risk for depression and in the way it might unfold. For example, one person may be resilient (excellent social support) and also have no genetic disposition for depression, and in this case it would take high levels of stress to activate symptoms, and these symptoms are likely to resolve once the stressor is dealt with. Another person may have a gene-brain disposition to depression and be more sensitive to daily stresses and thus have a lower threshold for developing active symptoms.

This diathesis-stress approach to understanding depression is consistent with the holistic care approach being developed within VA. Unique stressors and scenarios might serve to enhance risk for depression in veterans. Military personnel, both active and veteran status, are often forced to perform under uniquely stressful conditions (e.g., combat scenarios). Stress exists for service members not only in hostile situations but also in peacekeeping missions and through the demands of their daily jobs. There are various stressors that affect veterans on a daily basis. Some stressors include being away from home or family, uncertainty of return date, sanitation, lack of privacy, lack of time off, being injured, being ambushed or attacked, and close living quarters (Hoge et al. 2004). These environmental factors can reduce the threshold for vulnerability of developing a mood disorder. In addition, veterans are often faced with drastically changing environmental impacts as they acclimate to civilian life following a deployment.

There are various other stressors that affect active and veteran military personnel. One of the most important is residential mobility. Research shows that relocations in the military are frequent. For example, some researchers found that the average military family experiences six to seven moves in a 20-year military service period (Gill et al. 1994). This can be stressful due to the exhaustion of the move, creating a new life for oneself and one's family, and changes in social networks (e.g., friends, neighbors, etc.). The service member's absence from their family may occur not only during deployment but also when a nonmilitary spouse has a steady job and cannot follow their military partner. Yet another major stressor that occurs in the military is sleep deprivation. Lack of sleep is not uncommon, due to operational requirements or high-operations tempo training (Miller et al. 2008). Fatigue, along with constant stress, can undermine resilience and may factor into mood disorders, PTSD, and suicidal thoughts. Research also shows that stress levels among active military and veteran populations often leads to divorce in approximately 3.7% of the population (*Military Divorce Rate Hits Lowest Level in 10 Years*). Data from the Army STARRS study shows that enlisted soldiers are more at risk for attempting suicide as well (Schoenbaum et al. 2014). Therefore, it is important to understand these stressors and to find individualized treatments and precision medicines for those at risk.

It is also important to consider how stress interacts with biological factors and might lead to risk for mood disorder in the veteran population. For instance, a veteran may have adequate psychosocial support during deployment, but the occurrence of a traumatic brain injury, which changes the biological functioning of the brain, may increase the risk of developing depression. Similarly, a veteran with depression who acquires a traumatic brain injury may not heal as quickly as a veteran without symptoms of a mood disorder.

A diathesis-stress biopsychosocial model of depression does not provide a specific explanation of cause but does provide framework for guiding a deeper investigation of each contributing factor. We consider each factor in more detail in the following subsections.

Psychological Stressors Stressors occurring early in life and in current daily life can both contribute to risk for depression (Chu et al. 2013). Early life events that can be experienced as psychologically traumatic and that can enhance later risk for depression in adulthood include abuse, neglect, difficult family situations, severe illness, and bullying (Chu et al. 2013). In adulthood, the impact of particular stressors varies across individuals, and depression can develop when normal daily "hassles" feel especially stressful or when a traumatic event (such as death of a loved one) occurs. Death or losses, such as a job layoff, relationship difficulties (e.g., divorce), as well as normal milestones such as marriage or retirement, can be powerful enough to act as a catalyst for depressive symptoms in someone with other risk factors.

Depression often follows stressful experiences. The brain interprets events and decides whether they are threatening and then controls the behavioral and physiological responses to those events (Somers et al. 2006; Valenstein 2002; Parker and Hadzi-Pavlovic 1996). The brain's reaction to stress is useful in that it supplies extra energy to help a person act on or flee from dangerous situations (Somers et al. 2006;

Valenstein 2002). Sometimes, however, brain chemical levels that increase during stressful situations stay at high levels and cause problems such as depression (Williams and Gordon 2010).

Genetic Predisposition Meta-analyses suggest that the short allele of the serotonin transporter (*5-HTTLPR)* gene is a marker of risk for depression (Kiyohara and Yoshimasu 2010). Other genetic markers related to monoamine neurotransmission are polymorphisms of serotonin 2A and 1A receptors, and the Met allele of catechol-o-methyltransferase (COMT) Val108/158Met (Levinson 2006). The COMT Met allele is associated with risk for depression and with emotional brain markers (Williams et al. 2010). Another set of genetic markers reflects alterations in brain plasticity (the Met allele of BDNF Val66Met polymorphism) and overactivity of the hypothalamic-pituitary-adrenal axis (HPA) (tryptophan hydroxylase, or TPH). These studies suggest there is no one genetic cause of depression, and the viability of these candidate genetic risk factors requires replication in large independent studies.

There is increasing evidence that genetic disposition interacts with psychological stress to increase risk for depression. For example, in a seminal study Caspi et al. (2003) found that individuals possessing either one or two copies of the short variant of the 5-HTTLPR (serotonin transporter) gene, which is not transcriptionally as effective as the long form, experienced higher levels of depression and suicidality following a recent life stressor.

There is also evidence that depression is heritable, even though no single gene is involved in its cause. First-degree relatives of a patient with recurrent major depression have 1.5–3 times higher risk of depression themselves as compared to the general population (Fava and Kendler 2000). Of children with one parent with a mood disorder, 27% will develop a mood disorder themselves, and that rate increases to 50–75% if both parents are affected (Nadkarni and Fristad 2012). Of course, family history is not in itself sufficient to account for depression in everyone. Depression also occurs in people with no family history of mood disorders, consistent with the role of other multiple risk factors.

Brain Chemistry In terms of brain chemistry, the focus has been on monoamines, which include serotonin, norepinephrine, and dopamine (Krishnan and Nestler 2008). More recently, other neurotransmitters—such as acetylcholine, histamine, y-aminobutyric acid (GABA), and glutamate—have also been implicated in risk for depression (Augeraud et al. 2015). Most of the commonly used antidepressants are based on a monoamine understanding of depression. For example, the medications known as selective serotonin reuptake inhibitors (SSRIs) have an action that modulates serotonin uptake. Mood disorders are associated with a functional decrease in serotonin neurotransmission, which may be due to the excessive reuptake of the serotonin released by the presynaptic cell.

Over the past few years, the role of serotonin in the physiology of major depressive disorder has been intensively studied. There are various categories of depression medications (antidepressants) used to treat depression and conditions that have depression as a component (e.g., bipolar disorder). Currently available medications improve symptoms of depression by increasing the availability of neurotransmitters. The major antidepressants that exist are tricyclic antidepressants (TCAs), monoamine oxidase inhibitors (MAOIs), selective serotonin reuptake inhibitors (SSRIs), and serotonin norepinephrine reuptake inhibitors (SNRIs) (Kato and Serretti 2010).

Brain Structure There is increasing evidence that stress and depression may involve structural changes in the brain (Drevets et al. 2008). Changes, known as remodeling, can be prevented and potentially reversed with the right treatment, such as antidepressant and mood-stabilizing medications, as well as various forms of psychotherapy (Golden et al. 2005). Brain imaging studies show that brain areas involved in mood, memory, and decision-making may change in size and function in response to depressive episodes (Morey et al. 2008). Studies on animal models show that there may be many physical changes in the brain when it is unable to effectively respond or adapt to stress.

Three brain structures—the hippocampus, amygdala, and prefrontal cortex—help the brain determine what is stressful and how to respond. The hippocampus stores memories of events and responds to stress hormones in the blood. Many mental disorders, including depression, may cause the hippocampus to shrink or weaken. In the dentate gyrus, part of the hippocampal formation, new neurons (brain cells) are produced throughout adult life. Repeated stress slows the production of new neurons in the dentate gyrus and may also cause neurons in the hippocampus to shrink.

The prefrontal cortex, a key structure in emotional regulation, decision-making, and memory, may also shrink with depression. The amygdala, where emotional memories are stored, becomes more active in depressive illness and post-traumatic stress disorder. Repeated stress may enlarge the amygdala. A hyperactive amygdala, along with abnormal activity in other brain regions, leads to disrupted patterns of sleep and physical activity. It can also cause abnormal secretion of hormones and other chemicals that affect many systems of the body.

Animal studies have also shown that the stress hormone cortisol plays an important role in the remodeling of neurons in response to depression. A person's normally low evening levels of cortisol are increased in depression. Elevated cortisol is also a symptom of Cushing's disease, a disorder of the endocrine system. Studies of this illness have brought to light current knowledge about cortisol and depression, hippocampal shrinkage, and memory impairment. The good news is that after correction of the excess cortisol with treatment, the hippocampal shrinkage and subsequent memory impairment are partially, or in some cases completely, reversible, along with the depressive symptoms. This suggests that brain structural changes in major depression can be prevented or even reversed with the right treatments.

Brain Function Emerging research has identified brain function as a key contributor to depression and anxiety symptoms. Within this literature, intrinsic and task-specific neural circuits have been identified that support passive and active cognitive processes in humans (Seeley et al. 2007; Oosterwijk et al. 2012; Spreng et al. 2013; Cole and Schneider 2007; Haber and Knutson 2010; Williams et al. 2006). Specific circuits that appear to have specific dysfunctions in individuals with mood disorders, such as anxiety and depression, include the default mode, salience, negative affect, positive affect (reward), attention, and cognitive control. In general, findings tend to be inconsistent, revealing profiles of neural hypo-reactivity and hyper-reactivity, and both hypo-connectivity and hyper-connectivity, within the broad diagnostic categories of depression and anxiety. It is important to note that these inconsistencies are likely to emerge due to difference in defining samples for these studies, as well as the vast heterogeneity between individuals with depression and anxiety.

Several studies have reported evidence for hypo-connectivity of the default mode circuit in major depressive disorder. Functionally, hypo-connectivity of default mode regions has been correlated with clinical indicators of over-general autobiographical memory (Zhu et al. 2012) and some suggestion of treatment sensitivity (Dichter et al. 2015). Yet other studies have revealed a distinct profile of functional over-activation and hyper- (rather than hypo-) connectivity of the default mode circuit in depression (Veer et al. 2010; Sheline et al. 2010).

Regions responsible for the detection of salient changes in the environment (Korgaonkar et al. 2014) include the anterior cingulate cortex (ACC), anterior insula, and sublenticular extended amygdala (Seeley et al. 2007; Oosterwijk et al. 2012). Amygdala hypo-connectivity with has been specifically correlated with avoidance symptoms (Liao et al. 2010). Hypo-connectivity between the amygdala and anterior cingulate cortex has also been observed in social anxiety disorder (Arnold Anteraper et al. 2014), relevant to symptoms of avoidance. Hypo-connectivity between the insula and amygdala has been reported in major depressive disorder (Veer et al. 2010) and correlated with overall symptoms (Manoliu et al. 2014) and may reflect withdrawal from interoceptively salient stimulation.

Negative affect is a core feature of mood disorders, and the neural regions activated by stimuli such as facial expressions of fear, anger, and sadness (Lindquist et al. 2012) include the amygdala, brainstem regions, hippocampus, insula, rostral and subgenual anterior cingulate cortex, and medial prefrontal cortex (mPFC) (Williams et al. 2006; Kober et al. 2008). Amygdala over-reactivity elicited by nonconscious processing of threat-related stimuli has been reported in current depressive disorder (Jaworska et al. 2014), generalized anxiety disorder (Fonzo et al. 2015), generalized social phobia/anxiety disorder (Fonzo et al. 2015), specific phobia (Killgore et al. 2014), and panic disorder (Fonzo et al. 2015; Killgore et al. 2014). Heightened insula activity has been observed in major depressive disorder in response to expressions of sadness and disgust (Stuhrmann et al. 2011). Individuals with generalized social anxiety disorder also show exaggerated insula reactivity when attending to salient emotional faces (Klumpp et al. 2013). Mood-congruent hyper-responsivity of the amygdala has also been observed in response to sad faces (Victor et al. 2010; Arnone et al. 2012). A complementary profile of poor connectivity between the insula and anterior cingulate cortex has been observed in generalized anxiety states during the processing of negative expressions (Klumpp et al. 2013).

The ability to process positive affect, or rewarding stimuli, has also been implicated in mood disorders. Dysfunctions of the striatum, along with projections to the orbitofrontal cortex (OFC) and mPFC (Haber and Knutson 2010), have distinct profiles in individuals with depression and anxiety. Striatal hypo-activation in these depressed patients is apparent in response to socially rewarding stimuli (such as happy faces) and during reward-motivated decision-making (Treadway and Zald 2011). Anhedonia has also been associated with greater activation of the orbitofrontal cortex (ventral medial PFC) during the processing of happy faces (Keedwell et al. 2005) and reward outcomes (Dichter et al. 2012), which might reflect compensation for striatal hypo-activation. In remitted depression, over-activation of the anterior cingulate and mid-frontal region has been observed during the anticipation of primary rewards (Zhang et al. 2013). Consistent with emotional context insensitivity and the interplay of negative and positive affective circuits, other studies have observed amygdala hypo-reactivity to happy faces across disorders, including unmedicated major depressive disorder (Williams et al. 2015), generalized anxiety disorder (Blair 2008), panic disorder (Ottaviani et al. 2012), and obsessive compulsive disorder (Cannistraro et al. 2004).

Attentional abilities are crucial for alertness, sustained attention, and the support of recollection (Fornito et al. 2012), and the regions associated with the attentional circuit include the superior frontal cortex, anterior insula, anterior inferior parietal lobule, and precuneus (Fornito et al. 2012). Several studies have observed hypo-connectivity within the frontoparietal circuit in major depressive disorder (Veer et al. 2010) and social anxiety (Qiu et al. 2011), suggesting an "inattention" type. Frontoparietal circuit hypo-connectivity has been correlated with a specific behavioral profile of false alarm errors in anxiety (Sylvester et al. 2012). Other recent findings suggest that hyper- (rather than hypo-) connectivity of the frontoparietal circuit and its interactions with the striatal regions of the reward circuit contribute to experiences of hypervigilance and social anxiety (Arnold Anteraper et al. 2014).

The cognitive control circuits, comprised of the dorsolateral prefrontal cortex (DLPFC), anterior cingulate cortex (ACC), dorsal parietal cortex, and precentral gyrus, support functions of working memory and selective attention (Niendam et al. 2012). Hypo-activation of the DLPFC and dorsal anterior cingulate cortex (dACC) has been observed across diagnoses, including depression (Korgaonkar et al. 2013; Siegle et al. 2007; Elliott et al. 1997) and social anxiety (Koric et al. 2012) during tasks requiring cognitive control. Alternative dysfunction can be seen in hyper-activation of the DLPFC during working memory and executive function tasks in medicated major depressive disorder (Rose and Ebmeier 2006) and unmedicated major depressive disorder (Matsuo et al. 2007). Hyper-activation of the anterior cingulate cortex has also been observed in major depressive disorder when participants are performing similarly to controls (Rose and Ebmeier 2006).

It is important to consider changes in brain function following treatment as well. Various studies document changes in the brain after psychotherapy for depression, anxiety, and borderline personality disorder. In one of the first studies to document changes in the brain after psychotherapy for depression (Baxter et al. 1992), researchers compared behavior therapy with fluoxetine treatment. Medication management and psychotherapy produced similar changes in the brain, specifically in the caudate nucleus. Research suggests that cognitive behavioral therapy (CBT), dialectical behavior therapy (DBT), psychodynamic psychotherapy, and interpersonal psychotherapy alter brain function in patients suffering from mood disorders, obsessive-compulsive disorder, panic disorder, social anxiety disorder, specific phobias, PTSD, and borderline personality disorder.

The majority of these studies have reported similar brain changes after psychotherapy and medication. However, some recent studies have also shown clear differences among these treatment modalities. In the study by Goldapple et al. (2004), treatment response for cognitive behavioral therapy in patients with major depressive disorder was associated with increases in metabolism in the hippocampus and dorsal cingulate and decreases in the dorsal, ventral, and medial frontal cortex. This pattern was distinct from the pattern caused by paroxetine, which included increases in metabolism in the prefrontal areas and decreases in the hippocampus and subgenual cingulate. Furthermore, in a recent study by Karlsson et al. (2010), clear differences emerged between short-term psychodynamic psychotherapy and fluoxetine among patients with major depressive disorder.

Cognitive Factors

Negative Bias Beck's (2008) cognitive model of depression is seminal in detailing the thinking patterns associated with major depressive disorder and to proposing the idea that cognitive patterns are causal to the onset of major depressive disorder. According to this model, major depressive disorder is characterized by a pervasive negative bias in cognitions. This negative bias entails pessimistic thinking about expectations of the future and future consequences and about the interpretation of current events. There is selective screening of information for elements consistent with negatively held beliefs and expectations. Beck also identifies the tendency to make attributions toward the self and personal faults as characterizing depressive thinking.

Negative biases are thought to arise from negative schemas (or "thinking patterns") that are activated automatically. Examples of negative schemas are the thought that "I will always fail" or "If I lose someone close to me, I am helpless." These thinking patterns are heightened following stressful live events, hence the interaction of stress and thinking. In this regard, Beck's model is consistent with a diathesis-stress model.

The negativity bias self-report measure includes the criteria that surround endophenotypic risk markers of depression (Watters and Williams 2011). Negativity bias is accurate in identifying individuals suffering from major depression and furthermore accurately identifies major depression from various other mental health illnesses. The endogenous nature of negativity bias, and therefore its relative stability, is evidenced in its correlation with specific genetic variations (e.g., 5HTT-LPR short allele) and brain and physiological markers. Negativity bias begins as a genetic predisposition and eventually interacts with stress in one's life, which then leads to an individual automatically appraising a situation(s) negatively. Finally, this negativity manifests as behavioral symptoms of major depression (Watters and Williams 2011).

Repeated activation of negative thinking schemas leads over time to their predominance over more effective thinking patterns and a downward "spiral" of negativity to depression. Severe major depressive disorder is described by Beck (2008) as a state where negative schemas are constantly active. This concept is synonymous with symptoms of rumination. It is also complementary to the theory of "learned helplessness."

Psychologist Martin Seligman proposed the idea that depression results from learned helplessness or a tendency to give up passively in the face of unavoidable stressors. Seligman pointed out that people who have a pessimistic explanatory style are likely to experience depression. In early 1965, Seligman and his colleagues "accidentally" discovered an unexpected phenomenon related to human depression while studying the relationship between fear and learning in dogs. Through a series of experiments, Seligman demonstrated fear conditioning and learned helplessness in dogs. This research formed Seligman's subsequent theory of learned helplessness, which was then extended to human behavior as a model for explaining depression. According to Seligman, depressed people have learned to be helpless. In other words, depressed people feel that whatever they do will be futile and that they have no control over their environments.

Useful as it was for explaining why some people became depressed, the initial learned helplessness theory could not account for or explain why many people did not become depressed even after experiencing many unpleasant life events. With further study, Seligman modified the learned helplessness theory to incorporate a person's thinking style as a factor determining whether learned helplessness would occur. He suggested that depressed people tended to use a more pessimistic explanatory style when thinking about stressful events than did nondepressed people, who tended to be more optimistic in nature.

Individuals who tend to view the causes of negative events as internal, global, and stable (e.g., people who use explanations #1, #2) are said to have a pessimistic attributional style. Individuals who tend to view the causes of negative events as external, specific, and unstable (e.g., explanation #7) have an optimistic attributional style. Individuals who become depressed are more likely to have pessimistic attributional styles than optimistic attributional styles. According to the revised learned helplessness theory, a pessimistic attributional style increases the likelihood of developing learned helplessness. In addition, prolonged exposure to uncontrollable and inescapable events can lead people to develop a pessimistic attributional style, and to become apathetic, pessimistic, and unmotivated, even if they are not that way to begin with.

An adaptation of this theory argues that depression results not only from helplessness but also from hopelessness. The hopelessness theory attributes depression to a pattern of negative thinking in which people blame themselves for negative life events, view the causes of those events as permanent, and overgeneralize specific weaknesses to many areas of their life (e.g., "I am not good at creative things, so I am therefore not a good mother, therefore my relationship with my child is undoubtedly doomed").

Other cognitive behavioral theorists suggest that people with "depressive" personality traits appear to be more vulnerable than others to depression. Examples of depressive personality traits include neuroticism, gloominess, introversion, self-criticism, excessive skepticism and criticism of others, deep feelings of inadequacy, and excessive brooding and worrying. In addition, people who regularly behave in dependent, hostile, and impulsive ways appear at greater risk for depression.

Interventions and Clinical Care

Treatments Offered Protocols are in place for the treatment of military personnel who develop symptoms of a mood disorder during his or her service. The Department of Defense follows the privacy guidelines set down by HIPAA and the Privacy Act. These guidelines ensure the privacy of one's mental health records in most situations. However, if one's provider discovers that one's mental health condition may endanger oneself, others, or the mission, the provider is obligated to disclose this information to the chain of command. The precise definition of danger to self, others, or the mission is different for each branch of the armed forces (National Alliance on Mental Illness 2017).

If a medical officer or military care provider observes that one's health condition poses a danger, the officer will share the person's medical profile with commanding officers. The information they are allowed to share includes one's diagnosis and the medically recommended duty limitations. Unit commanders will decide what duties to assign until the condition improves.

If commanders or supervisors observe behaviors that appear to compromise safety or job performance, they can request a command-directed behavioral health evaluation. A command-directed evaluation does not guarantee as much confidentiality as a medical consultation one seeks oneself (National Alliance on Mental Illness 2017).

VA offers several options to veterans seeking treatment for mental health concerns, including mood disorders, both at VA facilities and outside the VA system. Often individuals are identified in primary care. The Veterans Health Administration requires annual screening for depressive symptoms in veterans, and this is completed via health reminders in the veteran's electronic medical record (Kirchner et al. 2004). Once identified by the physician or self-referred by the veteran, typically a veteran is referred to a mental health coordinator. From there, individuals complete a number of orientation and assessment sessions to determine the best course of care. Treatment options, which are typically a combination of medication and psychotherapy treatments, include:

- Short-term, inpatient care
- Outpatient care in a psychosocial rehabilitation and recovery centers (PRRC)
- Regular outpatient care, which may include telemedicine services
- Residential Rehabilitation Treatment Programs (RRTP)
- Primary care
- Residential care
- Supported work settings

Pharmacological Treatments Within these settings, veterans may receive medications under the management of a psychiatrist, psychotherapy, or a combination of both. Medication management follow-up sessions for outpatients are typically conducted once per month. Medications offered are antidepressant medications, antianxiety medications, and medications to improve sleep and other problems associated with depression and/or anxiety symptoms. For veterans presenting with PTSD, antidepressant medications, antianxiety medications, mood-stabilizing medications, and other medications to ease nightmares, irritability, sleeplessness, depression, and anxiety may be recommended. Veterans with bipolar disorder often receive antidepressant medications, mood-stabilizing medications, antipsychotic medications, and other medications to stabilize mood, organize thoughts, reduce hallucinations (if present), and ease related symptoms. Psychotherapy options at VA can be delivered by psychologists, psychiatrists, social workers, and case managers. Frequency and modality are determined by the provider following an assessment intake interview with the veteran.

Psychotherapy Interventions A veteran that presents with symptoms of depression or anxiety will often be offered psychotherapy, which can be conducted individually or in a group therapy setting. Common interventions include cognitive behavioral therapy, acceptance and commitment therapy, dialectical behavior therapy, and interpersonal therapy. Cognitive behavioral therapy (CBT) helps veterans understand the relationship between thoughts, emotions, and behaviors, learn new patterns of thinking, and practice new positive behaviors (relaxation techniques, using calming tapes to improve sleep, exercising, or socializing with friends). Acceptance and commitment therapy (ACT) helps veterans overcome their struggles with emotional pain and worries. It helps them recognize, commit to, and achieve what is important to them, in a nonjudgmental manner. Dialectical behavior therapy (DBT) helps veterans develop and practice skills related to mindfulness, emotion regulation, distress tolerance, and interpersonal effectiveness. Lastly, interpersonal therapy (IPT) helps veterans promote positive relationships and resolve relationship problems.

Veterans that present with symptoms of PTSD often have similar psychotherapy options. Evidence-based treatments for PTSD also include additional therapies that are specifically targeted to address the issues that arise with PTSD. These include cognitive processing therapy (CPT) and prolonged exposure (PE) therapy. Cognitive processing therapy is a form of cognitive behavioral therapy that involves correcting negative thought patterns so that memories of trauma do not interfere with daily life. It may also include writing about one's traumatic experience. Clinical guidelines strongly recommend cognitive processing therapy for PTSD treatment, as it is a non-exposure evidenced-based treatment. The other evidence-based treatment is prolonged exposure (PE) therapy, which helps veterans reduce fear and anxiety triggered by reminders of the trauma. In this form of therapy, veterans confront (or are exposed to) trauma reminders in a safe treatment environment until they are less troubling. In this way, individuals can stop avoiding and reacting to trauma reminders and live their lives more fully in the present with greater freedom from the past. Clinical guidelines strongly recommend prolonged exposure for PTSD treatment (Foa et al. 2008).

While the majority of mental health treatment is conducted in an outpatient setting, some circumstances warrant more intensive, residential programs of treatment. For example, individuals who do not respond to outpatient PTSD treatment may be referred to a residential rehabilitation treatment program for more intensive, specialized treatment within a structured, 24/7 care setting.

Lastly, veterans diagnosed with bipolar disorder receive psychotherapeutic care consistent with models that address serious mental illness. These include Psychosocial Rehabilitation and Recovery Services (PRRS) to optimize functioning, work therapies to promote and support recovery, social skills training, and Mental Health Intensive Case Management (MHICM). MHICM is a team of mental health physicians, nurses, psychologists, and social workers that treat veterans in their homes and community. MHICM helps veterans experiencing symptoms of severe mental illness cope with symptoms and live more successfully at home and in the community.

Electroconvulsive Therapy in the VA In rare instances of severe and treatment-resistant depression, a veteran may be referred for electroconvulsive therapy (ECT). Electroconvulsive therapy has been shown to be the most effect treatment for severe or treatment-resistant depression (Carney and Geddes 2003); however, the lack of widely accepted methods for determining when it is indicated may contribute to disparities and variation in use (Youssef and McCall 2015). Response rates with electroconvulsive therapy are 50–70% among patients who have not responded to prior antidepressant treatment (Rose et al. 2003). Within the Veterans Health Administration, there are approximately 1 in 613 patients that receive electroconvulsive therapy (Burnett-Zeigler et al. 2012). However, it is difficult to contextualize these findings with prior work in the VA and the general US population because the data relies heavily on survey methods and assessed populations other than those with major depression (Hermann et al. 1995; Srinivasaraghavan and Weiner 1997).

Although the efficacy and safety of electroconvulsive therapy has a well-established evidence base, there has been extensive variation in its availability and use. In the United States, the most recent nationwide data regarding electroconvulsive therapy use from a 1988 to 1989 survey filled out by psychiatrists estimated the rate of ECT use at 4.9 patients per 10,000 people (0.05%), with 36.3% of metropolitan areas reporting no ECT use (Hermann et al. 1995). The variability on electroconvulsive therapy use was not explained by the prevalence of depression; rather, the number of psychiatrists and primary care physicians and state regulations were the strongest predictors of ECT use.

The literature recommends electroconvulsive therapy after three or four failed psychotropic medication trials, and as many as one in three depressed patients may be candidates for ECT after receiving sequenced antidepressant treatment (Rush et al. 2006; Trivedi and Kleiber 2001). Due to the high rates of comorbidity among depressed VA patients, as well as hospitalization and suicide, it is unlikely that this population has less clinical need for electroconvulsive therapy than more broadly representative depressed populations (Valenstein 2002; Zivin et al. 2007). Current research findings suggest underutilization of electroconvulsive therapy in veteran populations.

New and Alternative Treatments for Mood Disorders

In efforts to provide quality care to the largest number of veterans in need of mental health care, the Veterans Health Administration has created more than 700 community-based outpatient clinics (CBOCs) across the country to reach veterans who are unable or find it difficult to travel to regional medical centers. However, those nearby clinics may not have the specialty services and providers that are found at the larger, regional medical centers. Therefore, VA incorporated into its mission the advancement of new and alternative treatments, including technologically delivered modes of therapy and telehealth programs across national VA medical centers (Godleski et al. 2012).

Technologically delivered modes of therapy include mobile applications that can be downloaded to the veteran's smart phone and utilized outside of the medical center facility. Some VA developed applications include:

ACT Coach ACT Coach was designed for veterans, service members, and others who are in acceptance and commitment therapy (ACT) with a mental health professional and want to use an ACT mobile application (app) in conjunction with their therapy. The app is designed to improve rates of patient participation in treatment and, as a result, treatment outcomes. Additionally, the app is designed to help providers adhere to published treatment protocol.

CBT-i Coach The CBT-i Coach app was designed for use by veterans and others who are having difficulty sleeping and are also engaged in cognitive behavioral therapy for insomnia (CBT-I) treatment guided by a health-care professional. With CBT-I, patients are taught to recognize how their thoughts and sleep-related behaviors affect their sleep patterns. Patients are provided with education about how sleep works. They are also guided on how to adjust both their sleep routines and their approach to sleep in order to enhance sleep quality and duration.

Mindfulness Coach Mindfulness Coach was designed to help veterans, service members, and others learn how to practice mindfulness. Mindfulness means paying attention, on purpose, to whatever is going on in the present moment without passing judgment on it.

Moving Forward With the Moving Forward app, one can access on-the-go tools and learn problem-solving skills to overcome obstacles and deal with stress. The app is designed for veterans and service members but is useful for anyone with stressful problems. It is especially helpful in managing challenges such as returning to civilian life, balancing school and family life, financial difficulties, relationship problems, difficult career decisions, and coping with physical injuries. It may be used alone or in combination with the free Moving Forward online course (www.Veterantraining.va.gov/movingforward/). The Moving Forward mobile app and online course were developed by the Department of Veterans Affairs, Department of Defense, and mental health subject matter experts across the country.

Transcranial Magnetic Stimulation Transcranial magnetic stimulation (TMS) is a noninvasive, nonconvulsive, neurostimulation treatment. The FDA granted approval for a repetitive transcranial magnetic stimulation (rTMS) device in October 2008. The approval was for 10 Hz stimulation of the left dorsolateral prefrontal cortex (DLPFC) as a treatment for major depression in patients who have not responded to only one antidepressant. rTMS has rather benign adverse effects—the most frequent are mild headache, nausea, and irritation at point of stimulation. The most serious adverse effect is the induction of a seizure—which is exceedingly rare, with an estimated incidence of less than 1 in 1,000 patients. Systematic review and meta-analysis of the studies to date, which are typically small, appear to show a positive effect in individuals with treatment resistant depression (Martin et al. 2003). Given the relative rarity of side effects and adverse effects compared with electroconvulsive therapy, transcranial magnetic stimulation has been shown to have the potential for significant advancement in the care of depression. However, few studies to date have examined the efficacy in veterans specifically, who often have high rates of comorbidities. Currently, a multisite investigation of the effectiveness of rTMS for the treatment of depression in VA patients is underway and demonstrates another important advancement in alternative treatments for depression in veterans. It is important to note that other stimulation therapies exist in the literature; however, most are newer and still experimental methods.

Another stimulation therapy discussed in the literature is vagus nerve stimulation (VNS), which was originally developed to treat epilepsy, but some research shows that it has favorable effects in mood disorders (Howland 2014). Magnetic seizure therapy (MST), another form of stimulation therapy, utilizes aspects from electroconvulsive therapy and rTMS to stimulate a precise target in the brain. Although magnetic seizure therapy is in the early stages of testing for mood and other mental health disorders, initial results are promising. For instance, a recent review article examined evidence form eight clinical studies of magnetic seizure therapy and found that it triggered remission from major depression or bipolar disorder in 30–40% of individuals (Lisanby et al. 2003).

Alternative Therapies for Mood Disorders Various other alternative options exist in the literature for treatment of mood disorders. For example, acupuncture is increasingly offered as an alternative therapy for depression along with other illnesses including anxiety and chronic pain (Leo and Ligot 2007). Another alternative and complementary treatment for mood disorders is exercise. In 2012, a clinical trial of heart failure patients found that regular exercise helped alleviate depressive symptoms. It is thought that exercise increases hormones (e.g., serotonin, dopamine), which subsequently helps people feel better (Strohle 2009). Additionally, a plethora of research exists documenting mindfulness as a treatment for mood disorders, specifically depression (Morgan 2003; Teasdale et al. 2000). Finally, eye movement desensitization reprocessing (EMDR) has been shown to directly affect the way the brain processes information, which exposes an individual to distressing material in a less stressful environment (Shapiro 2009; Bae et al. 2008). Although eye movement desensitization reprocessing studies focus on PTSD for the most part, recent literature has begun to assess this form of treatment for mood disorders.

Implications for the Future

Individuals who serve in the military may be prone to depression, at least partially as a result of exposure to combat, separation from family during deployment or training, and other traumatic factors (Hoge et al. 2006). People with depression may experience depressed mood or feel down, sad, or disinterested for extended periods of time. Depression may also interfere with daily life and normal functioning. People with bipolar disorder may experience unusual mood changes from feeling very "up" and energized to very "down" and depressed. Overall, mood disorders may cause significant distress or impairment in an important area of functioning (e.g., social, occupational). Veterans are twice as likely to die from suicide than non-veterans in the general population (Kaplan et al. 2007).

Though mood disorders have been documented for centuries, the label of specific criteria for diagnosis of these symptoms is relatively recent (American Psychiatric Association 2013). The Department of Veterans Affairs (VA) recognizes and serves both active military and veteran personnel suffering from mood disorders, although the overwhelming majority of literature on veterans and VA care is focused on PTSD specifically. The Department of Defense recently published a guidance memorandum that explains the armed forces' response to the deployment of individuals with psychiatric conditions. The stated goal is one of restoration, but if an individual's condition does not respond to treatment within 1 year or is not anticipated to respond, then the person would be referred to a medical evaluation board for a possible medical discharge. Since 2014 the VA has outlined a vision for the future of mental health care that is patient-centered and driven by a holistic approach that integrates physical and emotional well-being (US Department of Veterans Affairs 2014).

Advances in brain imaging and a greater understanding of the underpinnings of the brain shine light on the fact that brain circuits are an underlying complexity of cognitive, emotional, and self-reflective functions (Williams and Gordon 2010). Mental health disorders have been, and continue to be, treated with psychotherapeutic and psychopharmacological interventions, in the military, Veterans Health Administration settings, and with civilian providers. The direction of current research on mood disorders is heading toward clearly identifying biomarkers of depression, anxiety, and PTSD. Within that context, information gathered by advances in science, medicine, and technology have already provided new insights into the complex interplay between behavior, symptoms, genetics, and the brain.

Regardless of new treatments and medication regiments, clinicians and medical professionals still struggle with the complexity of predicting which therapeutic interventions will work best with individual patients, including the unique needs of veterans. Unfortunately, because it is so difficult to ascertain which treatment modality will work best, patients end up suffering most. Coupled with the symptoms they already experience from their mental health diagnosis, they are also subjected to trial-and-error treatment in order to establish the best course of treatment (Williams 2016; Williams and Gordon 2010). The goal of the new pattern of personalized medicine is to develop and use knowledge that will individualize treatments.

Over the past 10 years, the field of mental health has seen the emergence of a paradigm shift toward personalized medicine (Williams in press; Williams and Gordon 2010). This new paradigm provides treatment solutions for each individual's biological profile. By utilizing personalized medicine, the quality of health care depends on matching the right treatment to the right patient at the right time. It also requires a focus on proactive prevention and quality of life. Even though there are many benefits of standardized personalized medicine, this particular approach cannot address all needs within the field.

Additionally, future clinical practice has been focusing on identifying diagnostic and personalized treatment markers for brain disorders, which will require a taxonomy that extends the current *DSM* classifications based on signs and symptoms. The value of incorporating brain- and gene-based biological information into the diagnostic taxonomy has been recognized in the plans for additional editions of the *DSM*. Recently, the focus has been on identifying markers that support diagnostic decisions (Williams 2016; Williams and Gordon 2010).

As always, the field of mental health will continue to change and grow over the next few decades. The field has become very progressive over the past few years, and research indicates that it will continue to evolve and become more medically focused as time goes by. As discussed in this chapter, the major goal of new paradigms and the shift in current treatment approaches is to find a way to individualize treatment so that it is unique to every person suffering from mental health diagnoses and will evolve the current strategy of pharmacological and/or psychological interventions.

Key Concepts

1. Military service members and veterans have higher rates of mood disorders than the general population, likely due to circumstances associated with military service, including exposure to combat, being away from family and loved ones, and high pressures of service.
2. Different people experience mood disorders in different ways, and an individual's background should be considered when assessing for symptoms, including gender and age factors.
3. Evaluation and treatment of mood disorders for service members and veterans have evolved over time, and these individuals have

more options in terms of assessment and intervention for their mental health concerns.

4. Current knowledge of the etiology of mood disorders suggests a complex interaction of psychosocial factors, cognitive abilities, genetics, and brain chemistry, structure, and function.
5. Treatments for mood disorders include psychopharmacological intervention, psychotherapeutic treatments, and in severe cases, electroconvulsive therapy.
6. New and alternative therapies for mood disorders in veterans include mobile apps, noninvasive brain stimulation techniques, acupuncture, exercise, and mindfulness training.

References

Arnold Anteraper S, Triantafyllou C, Sawyer AT, Hofmann SG, Gabrieli JD, Whitfield-Gabrieli S (2014) Hyper-connectivity of subcortical resting-state networks in social anxiety disorder. Brain Connect 4(2):81–90

Arnone D, McKie S, Elliott R, Thomas EJ, Downey D, Juhasz G et al (2012) Increased amygdala responses to sad but not fearful faces in major depression: relation to mood state and pharmacological treatment. Am J Psychiatry 169(8):841–850

Augeraud E, Tassou P, Pollet C (2015) Treating depression in 2015

Blair RJR (2008) The amygdala and ventromedial prefrontal cortex: functional contributions and dysfunction in psychopathy. Philos Trans R Soc Lond B Biol Sci 363(1503):2557–2565

Carney S, Geddes J (2003) Electroconvulsive therapy: recent recommendations are likely to improve standards and uniformity of use. BMJ Br Med J 326(7403):1343

Deimling GT, Sterns S, Bowman KF, Kahana B (2005) The health of older-adult, long-term cancer survivors. Cancer Nurs 28(6):415–424

Dichter GS, Damiano CA, Allen JA (2012) Reward circuitry dysfunction in psychiatric and neurodevelopmental disorders and genetic syndromes: animal models and clinical findings. J Neurodev Disord 4(1):19

Dichter GS, Gibbs D, Smoski MJ (2015) A systematic review of relations between resting-state functional-MRI and treatment response in major depressive disorder. J Affect Disord 172:8–17

Fonzo GA, Ramsawh HJ, Flagan TM, Sullivan SG, Letamendi A, Simmons AN et al (2015) Common and disorder-specific neural responses to emotional faces in generalised anxiety, social anxiety and panic disorders. Br J Psychiatry 206(3):206–215. https://doi.org/10.1192/bjp.bp.114.149880

Fornito A, Harrison BJ, Zalesky A, Simons JS (2012) Competitive and cooperative dynamics of large-scale brain functional networks supporting recollection. Proc Natl Acad Sci 109(31):12788–12793

Jackson SW (1986) Melancholia and depression: From hippocrate times to modern times. Yale University Press, New Haven

Kirchner JE, Curran GM, Aikens J (2004) Datapoints: detecting depression in VA primary care clinics. Psychiatr Serv 55(4):350–350

Kober H, Barrett LF, Joseph J, Bliss-Moreau E, Lindquist K, Wager TD (2008) Functional grouping and cortical–subcortical interactions in emotion: a meta-analysis of neuroimaging studies. Neuroimage 42(2):998–1031

Korgaonkar MS, Grieve SM, Etkin A, Koslow SH, Williams LM (2013) Using standardized fMRI protocols to identify patterns of prefrontal circuit dysregulation that are common and specific to cognitive and emotional tasks in major depressive disorder: first wave results from the iSPOT-D study. Neuropsychopharmacology 38(5):863

Korgaonkar MS, Fornito A, Williams LM, Grieve SM (2014) Abnormal structural networks characterize major depressive disorder: a connectome analysis. Biol Psychiatry 76(7):567–574

Lambert MJ, Ogles BM (2004) The efficacy and effectiveness of psychotherapy. In: Lambert MJ (ed) Bergin and Garfield's handbook of psychotherpy and behavior change, 5th edn. Wiley, New York, pp 139–193

Manoliu A, Meng C, Brandl F, Doll A, Tahmasian M, Scherr M et al (2014) Insular dysfunction within the salience network is associated with severity of symptoms and aberrant inter-network connectivity in major depressive disorder. Front Hum Neurosci 7:930

Meichenbaum D (1975) Self-instructional methods. In: Kanfer FH, Goldstein AP (eds) Helping people change. Pergamon Press, New York, pp 357–391

Morey RA, Petty CM, Cooper DA, LaBar KS, McCarthy G (2008) Neural systems for executive and emotional processing are modulated by symptoms of posttraumatic stress disorder in Iraq War veterans. Psychiatry Res Neuroimaging 162(1):59–72

Murray CJ, Lopez AD, World Health Organization (1996) The global burden of disease: a comprehensive assessment of mortality and disability from diseases, injuries, and risk factors in 1990 and projected to 2020: summary

National Alliance on Mental Illness (2017) https://www.nami.org/Find-Support/Veterans-and-Active-Duty

Qiu C, Liao W, Ding J, Feng Y, Zhu C, Nie X et al (2011) Regional homogeneity changes in social anxiety disorder: a resting-state fMRI study. Psychiatry Res. Neuroimaging 194(1):47–53

Rose EJ, Ebmeier KP (2006) Pattern of impaired working memory during major depression. J Affect Disord 90(2):149–161

Seeley WW, Menon V, Schatzberg AF, Keller J, Glover GH, Kenna H et al (2007) Dissociable intrinsic connectivity networks for salience processing and executive control. J Neurosci 27(9):2349–2356

Sheline YI, Price JL, Yan Z, Mintun MA (2010) Resting-state functional MRI in depression unmasks increased connectivity between networks via the dorsal nexus. Proc Natl Acad Sci 107(24):11020–11025

Spreng RN, Sepulcre J, Turner GR, Stevens WD, Schacter DL (2013) Intrinsic architecture underlying the relations among the default, dorsal attention, and frontoparietal control networks of the human brain. J Cogn Neurosci 25(1):74–86

Thase ME (1997) Psychotherapy of refractory depressions. Depress Anxiety 5(4):190–201

Treadway MT, Zald DH (2011) Reconsidering anhedonia in depression: lessons from translational neuroscience. Neurosci Biobehav Rev 35(3):537–555

Williams LM (2016) Precision psychiatry: a neural circuit taxonomy for depression and anxiety. The Lancet Psychiatry 3(5):472–480

Williams LM, Kemp AH, Felmingham K, Barton M, Olivieri G, Peduto A et al (2006) Trauma modulates amygdala and medial prefrontal responses to consciously attended fear. Neuroimage 29(2):347–357

Williams LM, Gatt JM, Grieve SM, Dobson-Stone C, Paul RH, Gordon E, Schofield PR (2010) COMT Val 108/158 Met polymorphism effects on emotional brain function and negativity bias. Neuroimage 53(3):918–925

World Health Organisation (2010) Mental health and development: Targeting people with mental health conditions as a vulnerable group. WHO Press, Geneva. http://www.who.int/mental_health/policy/development/en/index.html and http://www.psychiatry.uct.ac.za/mhapp/

American Psychiatric Association (2000) Diagnostic criteria from dsM-iV-tr. American Psychiatric Pub. American Psychiatric Association, Washington, DC

American Psychiatric Association (2013) DSM 5. American Psychiatric Association, Arlington

Ariyo AA, Haan M, Tangen CM, Rutledge JC, Cushman M, Dobs A, Furberg CD (2000) Depressive symptoms and risks of coronary heart disease and mortality in elderly Americans. Circulation 102(15):1773–1779. https://doi.org/10.1161/01.CIR.102.15.1773

Bae H, Kim D, Park YC (2008) Eye movement desensitization and reprocessing for adolescent depression. Psychiatry Inv 5(1):60–65. https://doi.org/10.4306/pi.2008.5.1.60

Bagalman E (2013) Mental disorders among OEF/OIF Veterans using VA health care: facts and figures. Congressional Research Service Report For Congress: Congressional Research Service. https://fas.org/sgp/crs/misc/R41921.pdf

Baxter LR, Schwartz JM, Bergman KS, Szuba MP, Guze BH, Mazziotta JC, Phelps ME (1992) Caudate glucose metabolic rate changes with both drug and behavior therapy for obsessive-compulsive disorder. Arch Gen Psychiatry 49(9):681–689. https://doi.org/10.1001/archpsyc.1992.01820090009002

Beck AT (2008) The evolution of the cognitive model of depression and its neurobiological correlates. Am J Psychiatry 165(8):969–977. https://doi.org/10.1176/appi.ajp.2008.08050721

Beck AT, Alford BA (2009) Depression: causes and treatment. University of Pennsylvania Press. University of Pennsylvania Press, Philadelphia

Burnett-Zeigler I, Zivin K, Ilgen M, Szymanski B, Blow FC, Kales HC (2012) Depression treatment in older adult veterans. Am J Geriatr Psychiatry 20(3):228–238. https://doi.org/10.1097/JGP.0b013e3181ff6655

Busch SH, Leslie D, Rosenheck R (2004) Measuring quality of pharmacotherapy for depression in a national health care system. Med Care 42(6):532–542

Cannistraro PA, Wright CI, Wedig MM, Martis B, Shin LM, Wilhelm S, Rauch SL (2004) Amygdala responses to human faces in obsessive-compulsive disorder. Biol Psychiatry 56(12):916–920. https://doi.org/10.1016/j.biopsych.2004.09.029

Caspi A, Sugden K, Moffitt TE, Taylor A, Craig IW, Harrington H, Poulton R (2003) Influence of life stress on depression: moderation by a polymorphism in the 5-HTT gene. Science 301(5631):386–389. https://doi.org/10.1126/science.1083968

Charbonneau A, Rosen AK, Ash AS, Owen RR, Kader B, Spiro A III, Miller DR (2003) Measuring the quality of depression care in a large integrated health system. Med Care 41(5):669–680. Retrieved from: http://journals.lww.com/lww-medicalcare/Abstract/2003/05000/Measuring_the_Quality_of_Depression_Care_in_a.14.aspx

Charbonneau A, Rosen AK, Owen RR, Spiro III A, Ash AS, Miller DR, ..., Berlowitz DR (2004) Monitoring depression care: in search of an accurate quality indicator. Medical care 42(6):522–531. Retrieved from: http://journals.lww.com/lww-medicalcare/Abstract/2004/06000/Monitoring_Depression_Care__In_Search_of_an.4.aspx

Chu DA, Williams LM, Harris AW, Bryant RA, Gatt JM (2013) Early life trauma predicts self-reported levels of depressive and anxiety symptoms in nonclinical community adults: relative contributions of early life stressor types and adult trauma exposure. J Psychiatr Res 47(1):23–32

Cole MW, Schneider W (2007) The cognitive control network: integrated cortical regions with dissociable functions. NeuroImage 37(1):343–360. https://doi.org/10.1016/j.neuroimage.2007.03.071

Department of Defense (2006) Policy guidance for deployment-limiting psychiatric conditions and medications. http://www.ha.osd.mil/policies

Department of Defense (2013) Mental health evaluations for members of the military service. https://health.mil/Policies. Accessed on 10 Apr 2017

Depression Guideline Panel (1993) Clinical practice guideline, number 5: depression in primary care, 2: treatment of major depression. US Dept of Health and Human Services, Agency for Health Care Policy and Research, Rockville. AHCPR publication 93-0551

Drevets WC, Price JL, Furey ML (2008) Brain structural and functional abnormalities in mood disorders:

implications for neurocircuitry models of depression. Brain Struct Funct 213(1–2):93–118. https://doi.org/10.1007/s00429-008-0189-x
Elliott R, Sahakian BJ, Herrod JJ, Robbins TW, Paykel ES (1997) Abnormal response to negative feedback in unipolar depression: evidence for a diagnosis specific impairment. J Neurol Neurosurg Psychiatry 63(1):74–82. Retrieved from: http://jnnp.bmj.com/content/63/1/74.full
Fava M, Kendler KS (2000) Major depressive disorder. Neuron 28(2):335–341. https://doi.org/10.1016/S0896-6273(00)00112-4
Foa EB, Keane TM, Friedman MJ, Cohen JA (eds) (2008) Effective treatments for PTSD: practice guidelines from the International Society for Traumatic Stress Studies. Guilford Press, New York
Gadermann AM, Engel CC, Naifeh JA et al (2012) Prevalence of DSM-IV major depression among U.S. Military personnel: meta-analysis and simulation. Mil Med 177(8 Suppl):47–59
Gill HL, Haurin DR, Phillips J (1994) Mobility and fertility in the military. Soc Sci Q 75(2):340–353. Retrieved from: http://www.popline.org/node/290853
Glenn MB, O'Neil-Pirozzi T, Goldstein R, Burke D, Jacob L (2001) Depression amongst outpatients with traumatic brain injury. Brain Inj 15(9):811–818. https://doi.org/10.1080/02699050120330
Godleski L, Darkins A, Peters J (2012) Outcomes of 98,609 US Department of Veterans Affairs patients enrolled in telemental health services, 2006–2010. Psychiatr Serv 63:383–385. https://doi.org/10.1176/appi.ps.201100206
Goldapple K, Segal Z, Garson C, Lau M, Bieling P, Kennedy S, Mayberg H (2004) Modulation of cortical-limbic pathways in major depression: treatment-specific effects of cognitive behavior therapy. Arch Gen Psychiatry 61(1):34–41. https://doi.org/10.1001/archpsyc.61.1.34
Golden RN, Gaynes BN, Ekstrom RD, Hamer RM, Jacobsen FM, Suppes T, Nemeroff CB (2005) The efficacy of light therapy in the treatment of mood disorders: a review and meta-analysis of the evidence. Am J Psychiatr. https://doi.org/10.1176/appi.ajp.162.4.656
Goodwin FK, Jamison KR (2007) Manic-depressive illness: bipolar disorders and recurrent depression, vol 1. Oxford University Press, New York
Grob GN (1991) Origins of DSM-I: a study in appearance and reality. Am J Psychiatr 148(4):421–431. https://doi.org/10.1176/ajp.148.4.421
Gum AM, Areán PA, Hunkeler E, Tang L, Katon W, Hitchcock P, Unützer J (2006) Depression treatment preferences in older primary care patients. The Gerontologist 46(1):14–22. https://doi.org/10.1093/geront/46.1.14
Haber SN, Knutson B (2010) The reward circuit: linking primate anatomy and human imaging. Neuropsychopharmacology 35(1):4–26. https://doi.org/10.1038/npp.2009.129
Hankin CS, Spiro A III, Miller DR, Kazis L (2014) Mental disorders and mental health treatment among US Department of Veterans Affairs outpatients: the Veterans Health Study. Am J Psychiatr. https://doi.org/10.1176/ajp.156.12.1924
Haskell SG, Gordon KS, Mattocks K, Duggal M, Erdos J, Justice A, Brandt CA (2010) Gender differences in rates of depression, PTSD, pain, obesity, and military sexual trauma among Connecticut war Veterans of Iraq and Afghanistan. J Women's Health 19(2):267–271. https://doi.org/10.1089/jwh.2008.1262
Hayes SC, Strosahl KD, Wilson KG (1999) Acceptance and commitment therapy: an experiential approach to behavior change. Guilford Press, New York
Hermann RC, Dorwart RA, Hoover CW, Brody J (1995) Variation in ECT use in the United States. Am J Psychiatr 152(6):869–875. https://doi.org/10.1176/ajp.152.6.869
Hofmann SG, Litz BT, Weathers FW (2003) Social anxiety, depression, and PTSD in Vietnam Veterans. J Anxiety Disord 17(5):573–582. https://doi.org/10.1016/S0887-6185(02)00227-X
Hoge CW, Castro CA, Messer SC, McGurk D, Cotting DI, Koffman RL (2004) Combat duty in Iraq and Afghanistan, mental health problems, and barriers to care. N Engl J Med 351(1):13–22. https://doi.org/10.1056/NEJMoa040603
Hoge CW, Auchterlonie JL, Milliken CS (2006) Mental health problems, use of mental health services, and attrition from military service after returning from deployment to Iraq or Afghanistan. JAMA 295(9):1023–1032
Hopkins J (1986) Elvis: the final years. Berkley Publishing Group. Simon & Schuster, New York
Howland RH (2014) Vagus nerve stimulation. Curr Behav Neurosci Rep 1(2):64–73. https://doi.org/10.1007/s40473-014-0010-5
Hughes JN (1988) 3. Cognitive-behavioral school psychology: current issues and document resume. p 34
Jaworska N, MacMaster FP, Yang XR, Courtright A, Pradhan S, Gaxiola I, Ramasubbu R (2014) Influence of age of onset on limbic and paralimbic structures in depression. Psychiatry Clin Neurosci 68(12):812–820
Kaplan MS, Huguet N, McFarland BH, Newsom JT (2007) Suicide among male veterans: a prospective population-based study. J Epidemiol Community Health 61(7):619–624. https://doi.org/10.1136/jech.2006.054346
Karlsson H, Hirvonen J, Kajander J, Markkula J, Rasi-Hakala H, Salminen JK, Hietala J (2010) Research letter: psychotherapy increases brain serotonin 5-HT 1A receptors in patients with major depressive disorder. Psychol Med 40(03):523–528. https://doi.org/10.1017/S0033291709991607
Kato M, Serretti A (2010) Review and meta-analysis of antidepressant pharmacogenetic findings in major depressive disorder. Mol Psychiatry 15(5):473–500. https://doi.org/10.1038/mp.2008.116

Keedwell PA, Andrew C, Williams SC, Brammer MJ, Phillips ML (2005) A double dissociation of ventromedial prefrontal cortical responses to sad and happy stimuli in depressed and healthy individuals. Biol Psychiatry 58(6):495–503. https://doi.org/10.1016/j.biopsych.2005.04.035

Kessler RC, Berglund P, Demler O, Jin R, Koretz D, Merikangas KR, Wang PS (2003) The epidemiology of major depressive disorder: results from the National Comorbidity Survey Replication (NCS-R). JAMA 289(23):3095–3105. https://doi.org/10.1001/jama.289.23.3095

Kessler RC, Heeringa SG, Stein MB et al (2014) Thirty-day prevalence of DSM-IV mental disorders among nondeployed soldiers in the US Army: results from the Army study to assess risk and resilience in service members (Army STARRS). JAMA Psychiat 71(5):504–513

Killgore WD, Britton JC, Schwab ZJ, Price LM, Weiner MR, Gold AL, Rauch SL (2014) Cortico-limbic responses to masked affective faces across PTSD, panic disorder, and specific phobia. Depress Anxiety 31(2):150–159

Kiyohara C, Yoshimasu K (2010) Association between major depressive disorder and a functional polymorphism of the 5-hydroxytryptamine (serotonin) transporter gene: a meta-analysis. Psychiatr Genet 20(2):49–58. https://doi.org/10.1097/YPG.0b013e328335112b

Klumpp H, Post D, Angstadt M, Fitzgerald DA, Phan KL (2013) Anterior cingulate cortex and insula response during indirect and direct processing of emotional faces in generalized social anxiety disorder. Biol Mood Anxiety Disord 3(1):7. https://doi.org/10.1186/2045-5380-3-7

Koric L, Volle E, Seassau M, Bernard FA, Mancini J, Dubois B, Levy R (2012) How cognitive performance-induced stress can influence right VLPFC activation: an fMRI study in healthy subjects and in patients with social phobia. Hum Brain Mapp 33(8):1973–1986. https://doi.org/10.1002/hbm.21340

Krishnan V, Nestler EJ (2008) The molecular neurobiology of depression. Nature 455(7215):894–902. https://doi.org/10.1038/nature07455

Kruger PA (2005) Depression in the Hebrew bible: an update. J Near East Stud 64(3):187–192. https://doi.org/10.1086/491574

LeardMann CA, Powell TM, Smith TC et al (2013) Risk factors associated with suicide in current and former US military personnel. JAMA 310(5):496–506

Leo RJ, Ligot JSA (2007) A systematic review of randomized controlled trials of acupuncture in the treatment of depression. J Affect Disord 97(1):13–22. https://doi.org/10.1016/j.jad.2006.06.012

Levinson DF (2006) The genetics of depression: a review. Biol Psychiatry 60(2):84–92. https://doi.org/10.1016/j.biopsych.2005.08.024

Liao W, Qiu C, Gentili C, Walter M, Pan Z, Ding J, Chen H (2010) Altered effective connectivity network of the amygdala in social anxiety disorder: a resting-state FMRI study. PLoS One 5(12):e15238. https://doi.org/10.1371/journal.pone.0015238

Lindquist KA, Wager TD, Kober H, Bliss-Moreau E, Barrett LF (2012) The brain basis of emotion: a meta-analytic review. Behav Brain Sci 35(03):121–143. https://doi.org/10.1017/S0140525X11000446

Lisanby SH, Luber B, Schlaepfer TE, Sackeim HA (2003) Safety and feasibility of magnetic seizure therapy (MST) in major depression: randomized within-subject comparison with electroconvulsive therapy. Neuropsychopharmacology 28(10):1852–1865. https://doi.org/10.1038/sj.npp.1300229

Management of Major Depressive Disorder Working Group (2009) VA/DoD clinical practice guideline for management of major depressive disorder

Martin JLR, Barbanoj MJ, Schlaepfer TE, Thompson E, Pérez V, Kulisevsky J (2003) Repetitive transcranial magnetic stimulation for the treatment of depression. Br J Psychiatry 182(6):480–491. Retrieved from: http://bjp.rcpsych.org/content/bjprcpsych/182/6/480.full.pdf

Matsuo K, Glahn DC, Peluso MAM, Hatch JP, Monkul ES, Najt P, Fox PT (2007) Prefrontal hyperactivation during working memory task in untreated individuals with major depressive disorder. Mol Psychiatry 12(2):158–166. https://doi.org/10.1038/sj.mp.4001894

McEwen BS (2005) Glucocorticoids, depression, and mood disorders: structural remodeling in the brain. Metabolism 54(5):20–23. https://doi.org/10.1016/j.metabol.2005.01.008

Miller NL, Matsangas P, Shattuck LG (2008) Fatigue and its effect on performance in military environments. Perform Under Stress 2007:231–249. Burlington, VT: Ashgate Publishing Company

Morgan D (2003) Mindfulness-based cognitive therapy for depression: a new approach to preventing relapse. Psychother Res 13(1):123–125. https://doi.org/10.1080/713869628

Nadkarni RB, Fristad MA (2012) Stress and support for parents of youth with bipolar disorder. Isr J Psychiatry Relat Sci 49(2):104. Retrieved from: http://www.ncbi.nlm.nih.gov/pmc/articles/PMC4348006/

National Council for Behavioral Health (2012) Meeting the behavioral health needs of veterans. https://www.thenationalcouncil.org/wp-content/uploads/2013/02/Veterans-BH-Needs-Report.pdf

Nemeroff CB, Owens MJ (2002) Treatment of mood disorders. Nat Neurosci 5:1068–1070. https://doi.org/10.1038/nn943

Niendam TA, Laird AR, Ray KL, Dean YM, Glahn DC, Carter CS (2012) Meta-analytic evidence for a superordinate cognitive control network subserving diverse executive functions. Cogn Affect Behav Neurosci 12(2):241–268. https://doi.org/10.3758/s13415-011-0083-5

Oosterwijk S, Lindquist KA, Anderson E, Dautoff R, Moriguchi Y, Barrett LF (2012) States of mind: emo-

tions, body feelings, and thoughts share distributed neural networks. NeuroImage 62(3):2110–2128. https://doi.org/10.1016/j.neuroimage.2012.05.079
Ottaviani C, Cevolani D, Nucifora V, Borlimi R, Agati R, Leonardi M, Brighetti G (2012) Amygdala responses to masked and low spatial frequency fearful faces: a preliminary fMRI study in panic disorder. Psychiatry Res Neuroimaging 203(2):159–165. Retrieved from: https://www.researchgate.net/profile/Cristina_Ottaviani/publication/230790091_Amygdala_responses_to_masked_and_low_spatial_frequency_fearful_faces_A_preliminary_fMRI_study_in_panic_disorder/links/0912f50c8c0fab6859000000/Amygdala-responses-to-masked-and-low-spatial-frequency-fearful-faces-A-preliminary-fMRI-study-in-panic-disorder.pdf
Ouimette P, Vogt D, Wade M, Tirone V, Greenbaum MA, Kimerling R, Rosen CS (2011) Perceived barriers to care among veterans health administration patients with posttraumatic stress disorder. Psychol Serv 8(3):212. https://doi.org/10.1037/a0024360
Padesky CA, Hammen CL (1981) Sex differences in depressive symptom expression and helpseeking among college students. Sex Roles 7(3):309–320. https://doi.org/10.1007/BF00287545
Parker G, Hadzi-Pavlovic D (1996) Melancholia: a disorder of movement and mood: a phenomenological and neurobiological review. Cambridge University Press, Cambridge/New York. https://doi.org/10.1017/S0033291704004210
Piccinelli M, Wilkinson G (2000) Gender differences in depression. Br J Psychiatry 177(6):486–492
Pietrzak RH, Johnson DC, Goldstein MB, Malley JC, Southwick SM (2009) Perceived stigma and barriers to mental health care utilization among OEF-OIF veterans. Psychiatr Serv 60(8):1118–1122. https://doi.org/10.1176/ps.2009.60.8.1118
Reynolds CF III, Dew MA, Pollock BG, Mulsant BH, Frank E, Miller MD, Kupfer DJ (2006) Maintenance treatment of major depression in old age. N Engl J Med 354(11):1130–1138. https://doi.org/10.1056/NEJMoa052619
Ritschel LA, Gillespie CF, Arnarson EO (2013) Major depressive disorder. In: Craighead WE Psychopathology: history, diagnosis, and empirical foundations. John Wiley & Sons, p 285
Rose D, Fleischmann P, Wykes T, Leese M, Bindman J (2003) Patients' perspectives on electroconvulsive therapy: systematic review. BMJ 326(7403):1363. https://doi.org/10.1136/bmj.326.7403.1363
Rothbaum BO, Meadows EA, Resick P, Foy DW (2000) Cognitive-behavioral therapy
Rush AJ, Kraemer HC, Sackeim HA, Fava M, Trivedi MH, Frank E, Schatzberg AF (2006) Report by the ACNP Task Force on response and remission in major depressive disorder. Neuropsychopharmacology 31(9):1841–1853. https://doi.org/10.1038/sj.npp.1301131
Ryan RM, Deci EL (2001) On happiness and human potentials: a review of research on hedonic and eudaimonic well-being. Annu Rev Psychol 52(1):141–166. https://doi.org/10.1146/annurev.psych.52.1.141
Sachs GS, Printz DJ, Kahn DA, Carpenter D, Docherty JP (2000) The expert consensus guideline series: medication treatment of bipolar disorder. Postgrad Med 1:1–104
Sansone RA, Sansone LA (2009) Dysthymic disorder: forlorn and overlooked. Psychiatry (Edgmont) 6(5):46
Schoenbaum M, Kessler RC, Gilman SE, Colpe LJ, Heeringa SG, Stein MB, Cox KL (2014) Predictors of suicide and accident death in the Army Study to Assess Risk and Resilience in Service members (Army STARRS): results from the Army Study to Assess Risk and Resilience in Servicemembers (Army STARRS). JAMA Psychiat 71(5):493–503. https://doi.org/10.1001/jamapsychiatry.2013.4417
Scott JAN, Paykel E, Morriss R, Bentall R, Kinderman P, Johnson T, Hayhurst H (2006) Cognitive–behavioural therapy for severe and recurrent bipolar disorders. Br J Psychiatry 188(4):313–320. https://doi.org/10.1192/bjp.188.4.313
Shapiro R (2009) EMDR solutions II: for depression, eating disorders, performance, and more. WW Norton & Company, New York
Siegle GJ, Thompson W, Carter CS, Steinhauer SR, Thase ME (2007) Increased amygdala and decreased dorsolateral prefrontal BOLD responses in unipolar depression: related and independent features. Biol Psychiatry 61(2):198–209. Retrieved from: http://www.wpic.pitt.edu/research/biometrics/Publications/Biometrics%20Archives%20PDF/892-2007%20Siegle%20Increases%20amygdala%20and%20decreased%20dorsolateral%20Biol%20Psychiatry.pdf
Simbayi LC, Kalichman S, Strebel A, Cloete A, Henda N, Mqeketo A (2007) Internalized stigma, discrimination, and depression among men and women living with HIV/AIDS in Cape Town, South Africa. Soc Sci Med 64(9):1823–1831. https://doi.org/10.1016/j.socscimed.2007.01.006
Somers JM, Goldner EM, Waraich P, Hsu L (2006) Prevalence and incidence studies of anxiety disorders: a systematic review of the literature. Can J Psychiatr 51(2):100. Retrieved from: http://ww1.cpa-apc.org/Publications/Archives/CJP/2006/february/sommers-RP.asp
Srinivasaraghavan J, Weiner R (1997) 13. Utilization of ECT in veterans affairs medical centers. J ECT 13(1):58. Retrieved from: http://journals.lww.com/ectjournal/Citation/1997/03000/13__Utilization_of_ECT_in_Veterans_Affairs_Medical.35.aspx
Ströhle A (2009) Physical activity, exercise, depression and anxiety disorders. J Neural Transm 116(6):777–784. https://doi.org/10.1007/s00702-008-0092-x
Stuhrmann A, Suslow T, Dannlowski U (2011) Facial emotion processing in major depression: a systematic review of neuroimaging findings. Biol Mood Anxiety Disord 1(1):10. https://doi.org/10.1186/2045-5380-1-10
Sylvester CM, Corbetta M, Raichle ME, Rodebaugh TL, Schlaggar BL, Sheline YI, Lenze EJ (2012) Functional

network dysfunction in anxiety and anxiety disorders. Trends Neurosci 35(9):527–535. https://doi.org/10.1016/j.tins.2012.04.012

Takeuchi DT, Chung RCY, Lin KM, Shen H, Kurasaki K, Chun CA, Sue S (2014) Lifetime and twelve-month prevalence rates of major depressive episodes and dysthymia among Chinese Americans in Los Angeles. doi:https://doi.org/10.1176/ajp.155.10.1407

Teasdale JD, Segal ZV, Williams JMG, Ridgeway VA, Soulsby JM, Lau MA (2000) Prevention of relapse/recurrence in major depression by mindfulness-based cognitive therapy. J Consult Clin Psychol 68(4):615. https://doi.org/10.1037/0022-006X.68.4.615

Trivedi MH, Kleiber BA (2001) Algorithm for the treatment of chronic depression. J Clin Psychiatry. Retrieved from: http://psycnet.apa.org/psycinfo/2001-06383-004

U.S. Department of Veterans Affairs (2014) Capturing personalized, proactive, patient-driven care across VA

Valenstein E (2002) Blaming the brain: the truth about drugs and mental health. Simon and Schuster, New York

Veer IM, Beckmann C, Van Tol MJ, Ferrarini L, Milles J, Veltman D, Rombouts SA (2010) Whole brain resting-state analysis reveals decreased functional connectivity in major depression. Front Syst Neurosci 4:41. https://doi.org/10.3389/fnsys.2010.00041

Veterans Health Administration Mental Health Services (2015) Preliminary findings regarding prevalence and incidence of major depressive Disorder (MDD), non-MDD depression diagnoses, and any depression diagnosis in FY2015 among veterans. Veterans Health Administration Mental Health Services. Washington DC

Victor TA, Furey ML, Fromm SJ, Öhman A, Drevets WC (2010) Relationship between amygdala responses to masked faces and mood state and treatment in major depressive disorder. Arch Gen Psychiatry 67(11):1128–1138. https://doi.org/10.1001/archgenpsychiatry.2010.144

Watters AJ, Williams LM (2011) Negative biases and risk for depression; integrating self-report and emotion task markers. Depress Anxiety 28(8):703–718. https://doi.org/10.1002/da.20854

Westen D, Morrison K (2001) A multidimensional meta-analysis of treatments for depression, panic, and generalized anxiety disorder: an empirical examination of the status of empirically supported therapies. J Consult Clin Psychol 69:875–899. https://doi.org/10.1037/0022-006X.69.6.875

Williams LM, Gordon E (2010) Personalized medicine and integrative neuroscience: toward consensus markers for disorders of brain health. In: Koslow SH, Gordon E (eds) Integrative neuroscience and personalized medicine. Oxford University Press, England

Williams JW Jr, Barrett J, Oxman T, Frank E, Katon W, Sullivan M, Sengupta A (2000) Treatment of dysthymia and minor depression in primary care: a randomized controlled trial in older adults. JAMA 284(12):1519–1526. https://doi.org/10.1001/jama.284.12.1519

Williams LM, Barton MJ, Kemp AH, Liddell BJ, Peduto AP, Gordon E, Bryant RA (2005) Distinct amygdala-autonomic arousal profiles in response to fear signals in healthy males and females. NeuroImage 28(3):618–626. PMID:16081303. https://doi.org/10.1016/j.neuroimage.2005.06.035

Williams LM, Korgaonkar MS, Song YC, Paton R, Eagles S, Goldstein-Piekarski A, Etkin A (2015) Amygdala reactivity to emotional faces in the prediction of general and medication-specific responses to antidepressant treatment in the randomized iSPOT-D trial. Neuropsychopharmacology 40(10):2398–2408. https://doi.org/10.1038/npp.2015.89

Youssef NA, McCall WV (2015) Continuation antidepressant strategies after electroconvulsive therapy: ultrabrief pulse versus cognitive-behavioral therapy. Biol Psychiatry 77(3):e7. https://doi.org/10.1016/j.biopsych.2014.05.027

Zhang WN, Chang SH, Guo LY, Zhang KL, Wang J (2013) The neural correlates of reward-related processing in major depressive disorder: a meta-analysis of functional magnetic resonance imaging studies. J Affect Disord 151(2):531–539. https://doi.org/10.1016/j.jad.2013.06.039

Zhu X, Wang X, Xiao J, Liao J, Zhong M, Wang W, Yao S (2012) Evidence of a dissociation pattern in resting-state default mode network connectivity in first-episode, treatment-naive major depression patients. Biol Psychiatry 71(7):611–617. https://doi.org/10.1016/j.biopsych.2011.10.035

Zivin K, Kim HM, McCarthy JF, Austin KL, Hoggatt KJ, Walters H, Valenstein M (2007) Suicide mortality among individuals receiving treatment for depression in the veterans affairs health system: associations with patient and treatment setting characteristics. Am J Public Health 97(12):2193–2198. https://doi.org/10.2105/AJPH.2007.115477

Understanding and Treating Posttraumatic Stress Disorder (PTSD) in Veterans

15

Shannon McCaslin, Kile M. Ortigo, Erica Simon, and Josef I. Ruzek

Introduction

Public awareness of posttraumatic stress disorder (PTSD), particularly among veterans, has risen dramatically due to increased media attention. However, accurate knowledge about the diagnosis, functional impact, and treatment of PTSD is frequently lacking among the general population. The requirement of exposure to a traumatic event that precipitates the development of symptoms makes PTSD unique among psychiatric disorders. However, while the majority of people will experience at least one potentially traumatic event in their lifetime, only a minority will go on to develop PTSD. Four clusters of symptoms characterize the current PTSD diagnosis: reexperiencing, avoidance, hyperarousal, and negative changes in cognitions (see Table 15.1 for specific diagnostic criteria). PTSD is often associated with profound difficulties in social, occupational, and physical health functioning and quality of life (e.g., Koenen et al. 2008; Schnurr et al. 2006; Zatzick et al. 1997).

Serving in the military, particularly in combat, can increase the likelihood of trauma exposure. Combat service has been associated with higher rates of PTSD, depression, and alcohol misuse (Hoge et al. 2004; Kang et al. 2003; Kulka et al. 1990). Potentially traumatic military and combat-related experiences can include events occurring during rigorous training, life-threatening situations, being physically injured, bearing witness to death and dying, death and injury of comrades, interpersonal violence (e.g., sexual harassment and assault), and participation in actions that result in the injury or death of another. This chapter will provide an overview of PTSD, military and combat-related aspects, and clinical guidelines and treatments.

S. McCaslin (✉)
National Center for PTSD Dissemination & Training Division, VA Palo Alto Health Care System, 795 Willow Road, Menlo Park, CA 04025, USA
e-mail: Shannon.mccaslin@va.gov

K.M. Ortigo • E. Simon
Palo Alto Veterans Institute for Research (PAVIR), Palo Alto, CA, USA

National Center for PTSD Dissemination & Training Division, VA Palo Alto Health Care System, 795 Willow Road, Menlo Park, CA 04025, USA

J.I. Ruzek
National Center for PTSD Dissemination & Training Division, VA Palo Alto Health Care System, 795 Willow Road, Menlo Park, CA 04025, USA

Department of Psychiatry and Behavioral Sciences, Stanford University, Palo Alto, CA, USA

L.W. Roberts, C.H. Warner (eds.), *Military and Veteran Mental Health*,
https://doi.org/10.1007/978-1-4939-7438-2_15

Table 15.1 Core PTSD criteria clusters by version of DSM

Version of DSM			
DSM-III	DSM-III-TR	DSM-IV	DSM-5
A. Exposure to a stressor that would cause significant distress in majority of people	A. Exposure to a stressor unusual for most humans to experience and that would be significantly distressing to most people	A. Exposure to a traumatic stressor (witnessed, experienced, or learned about) and experienced intense emotional distress (fear, horror, helplessness)	A. Exposure to a traumatic stressor (witnessed, experienced, or learned about) that involved risk for or actual death, severe injuries, or sexual assault
B. Reexperiencing symptoms related to trauma (1+ of 3 criteria)	B. Reexperiencing symptoms related to trauma (1+ of 4 criteria)	B. Reexperiencing symptoms related to trauma (1+ of 5 criteria)	B. Intrusive symptoms related to trauma (1+ of 5 criteria)
C. Numbing symptoms and reduced interactions with external world after trauma (1+ of 3 criteria)	C. Avoidance of trauma-related stimuli and numbing symptoms (3+ of 4 criteria)	C. Avoidance of trauma-related stimuli and numbing symptoms (3+ of 7 criteria)	C. Avoidance of trauma-related stimuli symptoms (1+ of 2 criteria)
D. Hyperarousal and reactivity present after trauma (2+ of 6 criteria)	D. Hyperarousal and reactivity present after trauma (2+ of 6 criteria)	D. Hyperarousal and reactivity present after trauma (2+ of 5 criteria)	D. Negative changes in thoughts and mood starting or worsening after trauma (2+ of 7 criteria)
			E. Hyperarousal and reactivity starting or worsening after trauma (2+ of 6 criteria)

DSM-III criteria (p. 238), *DSM-III-R* (pp. 250–251), *DSM-IV-TR* criteria (pp. 467–468), and *DSM-5* criteria (pp. 271–280). *DSM-IV-TR* and *DSM-5* criteria exclude criteria specific to children and adolescents

Historical Overview of PTSD

Conceptual Precursors

Although the PTSD diagnosis did not enter the *DSM* until its third edition in 1980, the concept of maladaptive posttraumatic reactions can be traced back to at least the ancient Greeks. Drawing attention to the similarities between post-deployment reactions some veterans face and the experiences of select characters in the ancient Greek epic poems the *Iliad* and the *Odyssey*, psychiatrist Jonathan Shay (King et al. 1999; Shay 1994) makes a compelling case for viewing ancient Greek warriors from a modern-day lens. However, the recognition of such a postwar or posttraumatic syndrome has only recently been examined from a psychological standpoint. Over two millennia later, in the American Civil War, "soldier's heart" (or Da Costa's syndrome) was observed as a condition characterized by cardiac abnormalities such as palpitations, chest pain, and difficulty exerting energy (Renshaw 2011).

Eventually professionals began to view this condition as more psychological in nature. The attention to trauma in psychiatry first gained significance through Pierre Janet's (1889) book, *L'automatisme psychologique*, in which he explored how trauma can lead to severe dissociated states (van der Kolk et al. 1989). In World War I, the term "shell shock" referred to a collection of symptoms displayed by soldiers exposed to explosions from artillery rounds, combat weaponry, or other explosives (Renshaw 2011). Some of these soldiers expressed severe anxiety symptoms, others were dissociative or mute, and others had primarily psychosomatic complaints. Debate raged about whether there was an underlying physical origin of these symptoms, but many soldiers' claims for disability, in Britain at least, were approved.

By World War II, phrases such as "combat fatigue," "combat stress reaction," and "battle neurosis" began replacing older terms as common vernacular for similar syndromes. Still, the symptoms and theories behind these conditions remained diverse and little understood. One camp argued for physiological underpinnings, whereas others blamed mental processes. Edward Strecker, an American psychiatrist and consultant to the military, even blamed mothers for weakening their sons with letters from home that undermined their motivation for combat (Koenen et al. 2003). The US military leadership did not know what to think of these soldiers. Unfortunately, in 1943, Army General George Patton infamously struck in anger two Army soldiers suffering from "exhaustion" at a military medical facility (McCarthy and Petrakis 2010). Though his superior General Dwight Eisenhower, future president of the United States, made him apologize, the incident became emblematic of how some in the military view soldiers with less visible wounds. These attitudes and controversies continued into the Korean and Vietnam wars.

Treatments for these war-related conditions were as diverse as the theories of etiology. Generally afflicted soldiers were sent to a medical facility. Military psychiatrists were trained to treat combat fatigue or neurosis with a variety of methods ranging from rest to more invasive treatments like sodium amytal (a barbiturate derivative now known as amobarbital) and even electric shock in more severe cases (for a historical training video, see Pittman et al. 2012).

Case Study

Former US Army Staff Sergeant (Sgt.) Darren Smith (pseudonym) had just started his second semester at the local community college, after recently separated from military service. Although only 26 years old, Darren had already seen and dealt with situations that required him to take on a tremendous amount of responsibility. During his combat deployment in Afghanistan, he faced a number of situations where he or one of his comrades could have been injured or killed, including exposure to an improvised explosive device (IED) that hit his Humvee. He had needed to be aware, careful, and disciplined in his job to make sure that he was an asset to his team, not placing anyone else at risk. He had been in ambiguous situations where he was unsure of the best option but needed to make a decision. He made the best decision he could at the time but still sometimes pondered whether he could have done something different, if another decision would have been the better one.

Darren was unprepared for the anxiety and edginess he experienced soon after separation from the military, and he felt it even more acutely on the crowded busy campus. He wondered why he was unable to sleep until late hours at night, sometimes not falling asleep at all, and disturbed by the nightmares that would sometimes wake him once he did manage to fall asleep. Memories from his deployment often replayed in his mind, and he had trouble pushing them aside. He found himself easily angered by other students in his classes, who were texting or not pulling their weight during group assignments. He was determined to achieve his goal to transfer to a 4-year school and graduate in a healthcare-related area, as he wanted to pursue a career where he could make a difference in the lives of people. He was careful to turn in assignments on time, and he studied hard for his tests; however, he had trouble focusing during class and remembering information. There were even times he had to abruptly get up and leave the classroom, triggered by something someone said—usually about politics, war, or veterans. Finally, there were times that feelings of anxiety and depression became overwhelming, and he was unable to leave his apartment for the day or days at a time.

His grades during his first semester had been disappointing and he was at risk of academic probation. He wondered how much longer he would be able to continue to keep it together with little sleep and the frequent and vivid intrusive memories. Darren wasn't sure what was wrong with him. He felt alone and missed the camaraderie of the military. Darren had heard of posttraumatic stress and he thought perhaps this was what he had. He wondered whether he should talk to someone, such as a doctor, but was ambivalent, as he had been able to handle worse situations and felt like he should be able to handle this on his own as well.

Modern Conceptualizations and Diagnosis

In 1980, the American Psychiatric Association published the first criteria for the newly coined posttraumatic stress disorder in the *DSM-III*. Criterion A, the traumatic event, was defined as "a recognizable stressor that would evoke significant symptoms of distress in almost everyone" (p. 238) and was described as "generally outside the range of usual human experience" (p. 236). The symptom criteria set the stage for decades of the three cluster conceptualization of PTSD: (1) reexperiencing, (2) avoidance and numbing, and (3) hyperarousal and hypervigilance (though not initially labeled as such). *DSM-III* also introduced subtypes and specifiers—acute (onset of symptoms within 6 months of trauma and present for less than 6 months), chronic (symptoms lasting longer than 6 months), and delayed (onset at least 6 months after trauma). *DSM-III-R* (American Psychiatric Association 1987) added greater specification of Criterion A with examples. *DSM-IV* and its text revision (DSM-IV, American Psychiatric Association 1994, 2000) attempted to address continued Criterion A controversy by removing the language "outside the range of usual human experience" and adding requirements of emotional reactions during the trauma of intense fear, helplessness, or horror. Changes to this definition raised rates of meeting the trauma criterion by 22 % (Jakupcak et al. 2009).

In 2013, the current *DSM-5* made significant changes to the PTSD diagnosis (American Psychiatric Association 2013). First, it separated PTSD from the anxiety disorder section and created a new domain on trauma- and stress-related disorders. Criterion A was tweaked again by clarifying specific types of trauma that would or would not count (e.g., voluntarily watching violent YouTube videos does not count as traumatic, no matter how horrific) and removing the emotional reaction requirements. Importantly, the three clusters of symptoms were divided into four clusters: (1) intrusion, (2) avoidance, (3) negative alterations in cognition or mood, and (4) arousal and reactivity. The delayed onset specifier was maintained and joined by a "with dissociative symptoms" one. For a comparison of the various *DSM* criteria for PTSD, see Table 15.1.

Importantly, the PTSD diagnosis has had a fair share of criticisms over the years (Bodkin et al. 2007; Rosen and Lilienfeld 2008; Rosen et al. 2008, 2010) (cf., Yehuda and McFarlane 2009). Even Robert Spitzer, one of the architects of the *DSM-III* (APA 1980) that introduced PTSD, has recognized how controversial it has been in terms of its uniqueness (high comorbidity), specific criteria, overall validity, and use in practice (Spitzer et al. 2007).

Epidemiology of PTSD

Prevalence

Understanding the epidemiology of PTSD is an ongoing and vital task for researchers (Blanco 2011). In the first National Comorbidity Survey with a general US population sample, lifetime exposure to *DSM-III-R*-defined trauma was 55.7 % (60.7 % in men, 51.2 % in women), and the lifetime prevalence of PTSD was 7.8 % (5.0 % in men, 10.4 % in women) (Kessler et al. 1995). In a replication using *DSM-IV* criteria, lifetime PTSD prevalence was similar at 6.8 % (3.6 % in men; 9.7 % in women), and unlike the first study, the replication reported 12-month prevalence, which was at 3.6 % (1.8 % in men, 5.2 % in women) (Kessler et al. 2005; National Comorbidity Survey 2005).

In military and veteran populations, studies have shown a greater prevalence of PTSD and a reduced gender difference. Three large studies have looked at PTSD by era (see Table 15.2). The National Vietnam Veterans Readjustment Study (NVVRS) conducted in the 1980s (thus on *DSM-III* criteria) found a lifetime prevalence of 30.9 % in men and 26.9 % in women veterans (Kulka et al. 1988, 1990). At the time of the study, 15.2 % of male and 8.1 % of female veterans were diagnosed with PTSD. Marmar et al. (2015) conducted a follow-up study of veterans who had participated in the NVVRS, the National Vietnam Veterans Longitudinal Study (NVVLS). Over two decades following the original study, a significant number of male and female veterans continued to meet criteria for a full diagnosis or subthreshold PTSD symptoms (11.2 % and 8.7 %, respectively). Among deployed Gulf War veterans, Kang et al. (2003) found 12.1 % met the cutoff score based on self-reported symptoms. This was a threefold increase of risk compared to non-deployed Gulf War era veterans. For Operation Enduring Freedom/Operation Iraqi Freedom veterans, the most recent era of combat veterans, a similar current prevalence rate of PTSD (13.8 %) has been reported (Tanielian and Jaycox 2008). Predominately male (over 75 %), risk by gender for the Gulf War and Operation Enduring Freedom/Operation Iraqi Freedom veteran samples was not reported. More recently, a meta-analysis of 33 studies involving 4,945,897 veterans estimated PTSD prevalence to be 23 % among Operation Enduring Freedom, Operation Iraqi Freedom, and Operation New Dawn veterans (Fulton et al. 2015).

Risk and Resilience Factors

Research has identified multiple risk and resilience factors for the development of PTSD. These factors include characteristics of the trauma survivor, his or her reactions, and the event itself. For one, risk factors for higher trauma exposure, such as gender, age, socioeconomic status, and area of residence (violent neighborhoods, war-torn countries), tend to overlap with risk factors for developing PTSD (e.g., Gapen et al. 2011; Johnson and Thompson 2008; Norris et al. 2002). Of factors preceding the trauma, meta-analyses have shown female gender, family history of mental illness, previous trauma exposure, prior adjustment, adverse childhood events (particularly abuse), and lower socioeconomic status to be correlated with PTSD (Brewin et al. 2000; Ozer et al. 2003). The most powerful predictors were related to current factors—trauma severity, perceptions of life threat, and emotional intensity. The strongest predictor overall was whether the individual dissociated during or in the immediate aftermath of the trauma (Ozer et al. 2003).

Interestingly, military and veteran samples showed several differences in the Brewin et al. (2000) meta-analysis. The following characteristics were stronger risk factors for PTSD in military populations: younger age, lack of education, minority ethnicity, other adverse child-

Table 15.2 Major representative studies of deployed military veterans' rates of PTSD

Study	Era	PTSD diagnosis	Assessment method	Sample size
Kulka et al. (1990)	Vietnam	Lifetime: 30.9 % (men); 26.9 % (women) Current: 15.2 % (men); 8.5 % (women)	Multi-method composite diagnosis	2348–3016 (68.7 % male)
Kang et al. (2003)	Gulf War	Current: 12.1 %	Self-report (PCL)	11,441 (81.4 % male)
Tanielian and Jaycox (2008)	Iraq and Afghanistan	Current: 13.8 %	Self-report (PCL)	1965 (88.5 % male)

PCL PTSD Checklist

hood experiences, trauma severity, and lack of social support. Unlike in the civilian samples, gender was not associated with risk in military and veteran samples.

The above meta-analyses unfortunately omitted other important factors such as attachment, personality, and genetic variables that have also been shown to play important roles. First, attachment variables, especially considering their relation to childhood experiences, social support, and beliefs about oneself and others, may be potentially important factors to consider in the context of PTSD. While attachment insecurity may act as a risk factor (Benoit et al. 2010; Besser et al. 2009; Scott and Babcock 2010), it can also result from trauma exposure (Bogaerts et al. 2008; Cloitre et al. 2008; Sandberg et al. 2010; Twaite et al. 2004). One clear connection between attachment and PTSD lies in how they both involve social cognition and object relations—namely, views and representations of self and others (Westen 1991). One recent study found that object relation variables of self-esteem and qualitative representations of others partially mediated the relationship between adult attachment and PTSD symptoms (Ortigo et al. 2013). These theoretical and empirical connections among attachment, social cognition, and PTSD have led some theorists to incorporate attachment-based frameworks into treating trauma (Allen 2005; Stein and Allen 2007).

Second, of the personality characteristics identified, general negative emotionality, lack of constraint, and unstable self-esteem have been implicated in risk for PTSD and its comorbid disorders (e.g., Kashdan et al. 2006; Miller 2003; Miller et al. 2006). Finally, and likely intersecting with attachment and personality factors, genetic influences and gene-environment combinations have been identified as risk factors (e.g., Binder et al. 2008; Gillespie et al. 2009; Heim et al. 2009; Jovanovic and Ressler 2010; Norrholm and Ressler 2009). In sum, findings have generally supported the role of main effect and interactions among genetic, biological, environmental, and individual difference variables in how an individual responds to trauma and their subsequent risk for PTSD.

Veteran-specific research has also looked at risk factors. Using data from the National Vietnam Veterans Readjustment Study (NVVRS), Kulka et al. (1988, 1990) summarized that the most consistent prewar risk factors for PTSD development included the number of problem behaviors in childhood, antisocial personality disorder (before age 18), lower socioeconomic status in family of origin, and family history of mental illness. Controlling for these factors reduced the observed greater risk for PTSD in African-American and Latino American service members, but it did not completely eliminate this observed difference. In a reanalysis of the data, King et al. (1999) found an important gender difference. For men, war zone stressors (e.g., perceived threat, atrocities) were most predictive of PTSD, but for women, postwar factors (e.g., social support) were most important. In a longitudinal study of Vietnam veterans, Koenen et al. (2003) found predictors of a more chronic course of PTSD included high combat exposure, reports of negative community response returning from deployment, ethnic minority status, depression symptoms, and anger. Social support was again found as a protective factor.

In looking at more limited variables in a Gulf War sample, Kang et al. (2003) found greater risk for female, ethnic minority, and older veterans as well as those that had experienced multiple forms of combat stress. For Operation Enduring Freedom/Operation Iraqi Freedom veterans, one study found that combat experiences and perceived threat predicted PTSD and that low predeployment preparedness resulted in higher perceived life threat across levels of actual combat experience (Renshaw 2011). Increased risk for PTSD has also been associated with longer deployments and higher levels of combat exposure (Schell and Marshall 2008). Finally, Ramchand et al. (2015) conducted an extensive review of studies of risk factors among veterans who served in Afghanistan and Iraq, finding generally that individuals with lower levels of education and younger age, higher combat exposure and more deployments, and deployment-related injury were at increased risk for PTSD. Moreover, predeployment and deployment factors found to be of importance in this review included prior stressors and childhood adversity, preparedness for and leadership during deployment, concerns for family during deployment, and social support.

Type of Traumatic Stressor

The type of trauma experienced is also a crucial variable in predicting risk for PTSD. In addition to life-threatening stressors, several types of events particular to military and combat service have gained attention as important to consider. These include the death or injury of military comrades which can lead to profound grief, participation in or witnessing events that conflict with one's morals and values (i.e., moral injury), and military sexual trauma (MST) (see for review McCaslin et al. 2015).

Loss of Comrades Bonds formed during military training and combat are uniquely strong. These bonds, including a strong sense of responsibility for one's comrades, are cultivated during military and combat service (Papa et al. 2008). Thus, losses of comrades can profoundly impact service members, resulting in symptoms of posttraumatic stress and grief for years and even decades following the death. Significant numbers of combat veterans experience such losses. Between 63 and 80 % of US service members who served in Afghanistan and Iraq reported knowing someone who had been seriously injured or killed, and a smaller (20–25 %) but significant number reported having a buddy shot or hit close by (Thomas et al. 2010; Hoge et al. 2004; Toblin et al. 2012).

Notably high levels of grief symptoms, distinct from symptoms of PTSD and depression, have been reported in samples of Vietnam veterans who had lost comrades during their military service (Pivar and Field 2004). Indeed, levels of grief reported by these veterans were comparable to individuals who had recently experienced the death of a spouse. Grief symptoms can manifest in various ways and have been associated with poorer physical health, occupational functioning, sleep disturbance, fatigue, and pain—including musculoskeletal and back pain and headaches (Toblin et al. 2012). In addition to loss-related grief symptoms, veterans may also experience feelings of guilt for surviving when their comrade did not and/or self-blame stemming from a belief that the death was preventable (Currier and Holland 2012).

Moral Injury Exposure to or participation in events that conflict with one's core values and moral beliefs has been shown to increase the risk for PTSD over and above exposure to other combat stressors (Currier et al. 2013; Litz et al. 2009). Exposure to these kinds of stressors has been termed "moral injury," and research on this phenomenon has dramatically increased during the past decade. The types of events that can lead to moral injury are broad, including betrayal by others (e.g., leaders and peers), participation in events that lead to the injury or death of civilians or enemy combatants, helplessness in the face of suffering, and situations that present an ethical or moral dilemma for service members (see Litz et al. 2009; Maguen and Litz 2012 for reviews; Currier et al. 2013; Stein et al. 2012). In one study of veterans who had served in Afghanistan and Iraq, the most common types of experiences endorsed were betrayal from leaders and of personal values, overly harsh treatment of civilians, and survivor guilt (Currier et al. 2013). Other surveys of this era of service members found that approximately half reported directing fire at or shooting enemy combatants and witnessing ill or injured women or children whom they were unable to help (50 % and 48 % to 60 %, respectively), approximately a third reported responsibility for the death of an enemy combatant (23–32 %), and over 5–9.7 % reported responsibility for the death of a noncombatant (Thomas et al. 2010; Hoge et al. 2004).

Moral injury can lead to psychiatric symptoms including feelings of shame and guilt, and functional difficulties, as well as having profound existential and spiritual impact (e.g., loss of meaning). Killing or injuring others in the context of combat has been associated with increased PTSD symptoms among veterans who have served in Iraq and Afghanistan, over and above exposure to other combat stressors (Currier et al. 2013; Maguen et al. 2010, 2013;

Litz et al. 2009 for review). Stein et al. (2012) examined the relationship of the type of moral injury event with symptom type. The authors reported that reexperiencing symptoms were best predicted by moral injury acts committed by the individual, whereas state anger was most related to acts committed by others, such as enemy violence or betrayal. Litz et al. (2009) discussed the cognitive processes related to the development of moral injury, suggesting that the morally injurious events do not fit with preexisting moral schemas, resulting in emotional responses to the event.

Assessment instruments have been developed that can assist the clinician in better understanding the veteran's experience. These include the Moral Injury Events Scale (Nash et al. 2013) and the Moral Injury Questionnaire – Military Version (Currier et al. 2013). An eight-step treatment for moral injury was proposed by Litz et al. (2009). The treatment addresses various components including cognitive processing, therapeutic alliance, education, and other areas such as social connection and self-forgiveness.

Military Sexual Trauma (MST) Military sexual trauma (MST) is a term that refers to potentially traumatic events such as sexual harassment and assault. The Department of Veterans Affairs (VA) definition of MST is the following: "psychological trauma, which in the judgment of a VA mental health professional, resulted from a physical assault of a sexual nature, battery of a sexual nature, or sexual harassment which occurred while the Veteran was serving on active duty or [on] active duty for training" (US Code 1720D of Title 38) (see for review McCaslin et al. 2015). Sexual harassment events include a range of behaviors such as offensive sexual comments and display of pornographic materials. MST can occur at any point in military training and service, not only during combat service. Military sexual trauma has been associated with increased risk for physical health problems (Frayne et al. 1999; Kimerling et al. 2007; Kimerling et al. (2010) Turchik et al. 2012); psychological problems including PTSD, depression, anxiety, substance use disorders, and sexual dysfunction (e.g., Kang et al. 2005; Kimerling et al. 2007, 2010; Turchik et al. 2012; Yaeger et al. 2006); and other functional impairments (Skinner et al. 2000).

Annual prevalence rates of sexual assault within the military have been estimated at 6.8 % in females and 1.8 % for male service members. Rates of sexual harassment were reported to range between 9–31% for women and 3–7% for men, depending on the type of harassment (Lipari et al. 2008). Although a greater percentage of women report such events than men, the actual numbers impacted are equivalent because of the higher percentages of men serving in the military. Rates of MST are likely underreported because of barriers to reporting MST within the military. These barriers include the potential repercussions of reporting an incident perpetrated by a fellow service member who may be higher in rank or against fellow comrades from the same unit and the stigma associated with such events (e.g., perceptions that the individual should have been able to stop or may have contributed to the event; Turchik and Wilson 2010). Turchick and Wilson (2010) discussed the factors that can contribute to difficulties in recognizing and reporting sexual harassment and assault while serving in the military. In particular, the authors noted that the interaction between having a minority of women (approximately 20 %) service members and a strong masculine orientation can lead to an environment that condones such behaviors.

Resilience

Resilience, in addition to risk, is also essential to understand. Meta-analyses have identified perceived social support to be a strong predictor of decreased likelihood of PTSD development (Brewin et al. 2000; Ozer et al. 2003). Level of perceived social support has been found to prospectively predict the development of PTSD (Dinenberg et al. 2014). Cross-sectional and longitudinal studies have shown social support also predicts greater likelihood for recovery from PTSD (Charuvastra and Cloitre 2008). Similarly, just as insecure attachment is a risk factor, secure attachment can be protective (Ortigo et al. 2013). Additional factors found in previous studies to be related to resilience include optimism, cognitive flexibility, and active coping skills (for review, see Iacoviello and Charney 2014).

Resilience to trauma, though, may be conceptually broader than simply not developing PTSD. Some individuals experience personal growth as well, not just despite of but *because* of experiencing a trauma (Pals and McAdams 2004; Wilson 2006). Tedeschi et al. (1998) coined the term "posttraumatic growth" (PTG) to describe any positive psychological changes such as "an increased appreciation for life in general, more meaningful interpersonal relationships, an increased sense of personal strength, changed priorities, and a richer existential and spiritual life" (Tedeschi and Calhoun 2004, p. 1). Previous research has reported mixed findings regarding the relationship of posttraumatic growth to PTSD, with various studies reporting a linear relationship (For review see Shakespeare-Finch and Lurie-Beck 2014). Moreover, some research has suggested that this relationship may be curvilinear, with highest levels of posttraumatic growth developing when PTSD symptoms are moderate (e.g., Butler et al. 2005; McCaslin et al. 2009). Finding meaning from the trauma can be a fundamental component of posttraumatic growth. If posttraumatic growth exists (for a critical review, see Zoellner and Maercker 2006), then its predictors may have both overlapping and independent factors compared to PTSD.

Comorbidity of PTSD

Comorbidity of PTSD with other disorders is a complex issue that involves distinguishing between truly co-occurring disorders and seemingly comorbid conditions that are due to symptom overlap (Keane and Wolfe 1990). The overlap of PTSD symptoms with other disorders is particularly problematic for some critics (Bodkin et al. 2007; Rosen and Lilienfeld 2008). They argue that instead of a discrete disorder, current PTSD criteria just collect various reactions people may have after a trauma. PTSD's high comorbid rates with mood and anxiety disorders (e.g., major depressive disorder, phobias, generalized anxiety, and panic disorder), substance abuse, and personality pathology (Deering et al. 1996; Keane and Wolfe 1990; Southwick et al. 1993) point to this issue. Nevertheless, comorbidity is an issue for many psychiatric conditions.

In veteran populations, PTSD is also highly comorbid with other conditions. The National Vietnam Veterans Readjustment Study (NVVRS) (Kulka et al. 1988) showed higher rates of mood and anxiety disorders in male and female Vietnam veterans, but one of the highest comorbid conditions was lifetime alcohol use disorder—almost three-quarters of the male Vietnam veterans with PTSD had met criteria for alcohol dependence or abuse in their lifetime. For Operation Enduring Freedom/Operation Iraqi Freedom veterans, Tanielian and Jaycox (2008) narrowed in only on depression, traumatic brain injury (TBI), and PTSD and reported that the 13.8 % of Operation Enduring Freedom/Operation Iraqi Freedom veterans who had PTSD included 5.5 % who likely had all three conditions, 3.6 % with PTSD and depression, 1.1 % with PTSD and TBI, and 3.6 % with only PTSD. In another sample of Operation Enduring Freedom/Operation Iraqi Freedom veterans, Pittman et al. (2012) reported a high correlation ($r = 0.77$) between PTSD symptoms and depression symptoms. A similarly high correlation between PTSD symptoms and depression was found in recent studies of Operation Enduring Freedom/Operation Iraqi Freedom/Operation New Dawn Veterans (e.g., McCaslin et al. in press; Larson and Norman 2014). Unfortunately, screening positive for PTSD is associated with a fourfold increase in risk for suicidal ideation as well (Jakupcak et al. 2009).

Biology of PTSD

Since PTSD as a diagnosis emerged in the late 1970s, researchers have been working to better understand its pathophysiological and neurological underpinnings. Given the devastating impact that trauma symptoms can have on functioning and well-being, both for the person living with PTSD and others in their life such as significant others and family members, much attention has been given to identifying predictive and diagnostic PTSD biomarkers. This is especially true for military populations where trauma is often a necessary and unavoidable consequence of war. However, identifying relevant biomarkers is difficult because many studies cannot disentangle whether a biological abnormality is a risk factor for developing PTSD or a consequence of the disorder or of the trauma itself. Nevertheless, predicting who might be more susceptible to developing PTSD is particularly salient for military populations where a predictive biomarker would have significant value. In addition, psychophysiological and neurological indices of resilience to the development of PTSD could be beneficial and facilitate interventions aimed at preventing PTSD in vulnerable populations.

Neuroanatomy

Research generally points to three areas of the brain implicated in the development and maintenance of PTSD: the amygdala, hippocampus, and prefrontal cortex. The amygdala is relevant to PTSD due to its role in the formation and storage of emotion-laden memories, including fear-based memories. Probably not surprisingly, research consistently shows that amygdala abnormalities are present with PTSD (e.g., Huang et al. 2014), although at this time, research has not yet disentangled whether this is a cause or a consequence of PTSD. The hippocampus is another important brain region due to its role in the consolidation of memories, with a number of studies demonstrating that veterans with PTSD have smaller hippocampi and impaired hippocampal functioning, with some research suggesting that this is both a risk factor (e.g., Gilbertson et al. 2002) and a consequence of PTSD (Woon et al. 2010). Research also points to reductions in the size and impairment of functioning of the prefrontal cortex (e.g., Arnsten et al. 2015), which is the part of the brain that assists with making decisions and with planning behavior. It is important to note that cortisol, adrenaline, and noradrenaline, which will be discussed in subsequent sections, all play a critical role in these areas of the brain for the formulation of emotional memories, including trauma-related memories.

Autonomic Dysregulation

Dysregulation of both the sympathetic nervous system (SNS) and the parasympathetic nervous system (PNS) has been implicated in military-related PTSD. These two branches of the autonomic nervous system (ANS) exert influence over the organs of the body, maintaining important bodily functions and assisting in adaptive responding to changes in the environment, including stressful situations. The sympathetic nervous system is particularly important for quickly responding to threatening situations through catecholamine release (e.g., adrenaline and noradrenaline) in what is called the fight-or-flight response, which is an automatic response that maximizes the likelihood of successfully handling a physically dangerous situation. It thus makes sense that abnormalities in this defense mechanism could be either a cause or a consequence of PTSD. Indeed, some evidence suggests that a particularly heightened sympathetic nervous system response immediately following the trauma could be a risk factor for developing PTSD (e.g., Apfel et al. 2011), in addition to contributing to PTSD symptomatology, which has informed some pharmacologic interventions for PTSD (e.g., Boehnlein and Kinzie 2007). Consistent with these findings, elevations in cardiovascular indices have been observed in combat veterans with PTSD, which is particularly important given the higher risk of developing cardiovascular issues such as heart disease in this population (e.g., Coughlin 2011).

The literature on parasympathetic nervous system activity has been less extensive. The parasympathetic nervous system is under the control of the vagus nerve, which influences the heart and every bodily organ to maintain homeostasis. The parasympathetic nervous system controls the restorative features of the autonomic nervous system and has been called the rest-and-digest response (in direct contrast to the fight-or-flight response of the sympathetic nervous system). Although still in preliminary stages, some studies suggest that veterans with PTSD might have lower than normal basal levels of parasympathetic activity (e.g., Lakusic et al. 2007) and might not show typical autonomic nervous system responses to stressful situations (e.g., Sahar et al. 2001). It is important to note that not all findings have been consistent across the autonomic nervous system literature for PTSD, which might be attributable to individual differences in other factors that influence autonomic functioning.

Neuroendocrine Functioning

The hypothalamic-pituitary-adrenal (HPA) axis produces and excretes cortisol, which is often called "the stress hormone" because of its role in facilitating the body's adaptive response to a stressor. When faced with a threat of some kind, the body must maximize the use of energy and resources to most effectively cope with the stressor, and the HPA axis plays a central role in this process. It is important to note that although cortisol is central to the body's stress response, it is also important for a variety of other important processes, with levels naturally waxing and waning across the day in a predictable pattern (also called the "diurnal rhythm"). In general, findings for cortisol related to a diagnosis of PTSD have been extremely mixed, with studies showing higher or lower than normal levels of cortisol, as well as both an exaggerated and blunted diurnal pattern. However, somewhat consistently, veterans with PTSD generally show a blunted response (e.g., Wahbeh and Oken 2013) but not always. A recent meta-analysis is suggestive that depression might be exerting an influence on these findings (Morris et al. 2012), but in general, more research is needed to disentangle the literature on cortisol in PTSD and evaluate the effects of other potential contributors to aberrant cortisol activity. It is possible that cortisol plays an indirect role in the onset and maintenance of PTSD through increased inflammation in the body, which has been noted in a number of studies identifying inflammatory biomarkers in veterans with PTSD (see Zoladz and Diamond 2013, for a review).

PTSD Assessment and Treatment

Given the high rates of comorbidity and often profound psychosocial consequences of PTSD among veterans, conducting a comprehensive assessment is essential prior to commencing treatment. Such an assessment should include information about military background and experience, and it should elicit information about PTSD-related conditions and functioning. Moreover, co-occurring physical conditions should be assessed. The co-occurring presence of chronic pain and traumatic brain injury (TBI) is of particular importance to inquire about during the assessment process. During the recent conflicts in Afghanistan and Iraq, the use of improvised explosive devices (IEDs) by the enemy and increased survival rates for veterans with severe injuries due to better protective gear and medical care have led to an increase in co-occurring PTSD, pain, and TBI—indeed, these particular injuries have been coined the "signature wounds" of this era of veterans (Clapp et al. 2010; Gironda et al. 2006; Sharp and Harvey 2001). Providing referrals for these co-occurring cognitive and physical conditions is extremely important in ensuring that patients receive needed comprehensive care.

Best Practices for Clinical Care

The VA/DoD Clinical Practice Guidelines for The Management of Posttraumatic Stress were first developed in 2004 as a collaborative effort between the Department of Veterans Affairs (VA) and the Department of Defense (DoD) to guide healthcare professionals who treat veterans or military personnel with acute stress and PTSD. The guidelines were updated in 2010 and then again in 2017 to reflect the current state of the literature. The working group, which consisted of researchers and expert clinicians in the area of trauma as well as experts in relevant fields and specialties, used review of empirical evidence and expert consensus to formulate a set of clinical practice guidelines (CPGs) to guide clinical decision-making when treating military trauma populations.

The guideline discusses a range of best practices for the ongoing assessment and management of acute stress responses and PTSD. This encompasses appropriate screening, assessment, diagnosis, treatment, and follow-up for trauma-related symptoms and common comorbid conditions within a collaborative care model for medical and mental health treatment settings. Each practice is given a rating using the Grading of Recommendations Assessment, Development and Evaluation (GRADE) system (Andrews et al. 2013). Evidence is weighed based on factors such as the quality of the research (e.g., randomized controlled trial versus uncontrolled trial), number of available studies, relative benefit versus harm to the patient, and alignment with patient and provider preferences and values. Recommendations are then made based on the strength and direction of the evidence either for or against the practice and are provided on a continuum as follows: (1) "strong for," (2) "weak for," (3) "no recommendation for or against," (4) "weak against," and (5) "strong against.".

The guidelines also include algorithms for facilitating care, including for acute stress reaction/disorder, assessment and diagnosis of PTSD, and management of PTSD. Recommendations are provided for pharmacotherapy and psychological interventions, as well as complementary and integrative treatments and other types of adjunctive approaches. Practices are presented within the context of time since the trauma and include early preventative interventions and interventions for PTSD. The guidelines address common comorbidities and co-occurring concerns that influence the overall patient presentation and can interfere with treatment outcome, such as substance use issues, chronic pain, persistent sleep difficulties, and relationship distress. It is important to remember that the clinical practice guidelines are intended to guide clinical decision-making within the context of good clinical judgment regarding specific patient needs and preferences. Prior to treating veterans with PTSD, it is suggested that providers consult the clinical practice guidelines to become familiar with recommended treatments. Further, it is extremely important that clinicians become familiar with military culture and context. The military has a distinct culture, and within this larger umbrella, there are unique cultural aspects of each military branch. The Department of Veterans Affairs and Department of Defense have developed online resources that provide education about military culture (see Table 15.3). Understanding the unique aspects of military culture can help the clinician to better appreciate the veteran's experience, can improve therapeutic alliance, and can lead to a more accurate and comprehensive treatment formulation.

Exposure-Based Treatments for PTSD

The most recommended individual behavioral treatments highlighted in the clinical practice guidelines for PTSD are based on cognitive behavioral principles and employ some component of exposure (i.e., actively talking or writing about the traumatic event). These include prolonged exposure (PE) (Foa et al. 2007) and cognitive processing therapy (CPT) (Resick and Schnicke 1993), both treatments that have been formally disseminated ("rolled out") in VA Medical Centers across the nation. Fear conditioning models provide the basis for exposure-based therapies. Fear conditioning has been proposed as a main process by which PTSD symptoms develop (e.g., Orr et al. 2000). Generally, fear conditioning draws on behavioral principles wherein an individual learns to pair an aversive stimulus with neutral stimulus. For example, when a stressor occurs, this constitutes an unconditioned stimulus (UCS) which leads to an unconditioned response (UCR) of anxious arousal and fear. The stimuli and cues that were present in the environment at the time of the stressful or traumatic event then become associated with this event (conditioned stimulus, CS) and also elicit anxious arousal and fear (conditioned response, CR). If a veteran was in danger and witnessed his comrades killed in combat, the sensory contextual cues in the environment (e.g., what was seen, heard, felt) at the time of the event may become associated with a sense of fear and danger. After separating from the military, these contextual cues (e.g., what was seen, such as type of landscape, and heard, such as explosions or screaming) can themselves elicit anxious arousal or other emotions even in the absence of the original stressor. Even thoughts about the traumatic event may trigger intense emotional reactions. The experience of these intense emotional

Table 15.3 Websites, mobile applications (apps), and web-based trainings for patients and providers (Websites active at time of publication)

	Veterans	Providers
Websites: education and resources	National Center for PTSD: public http://www.ptsd.va.gov/public/index.asp	National Center for PTSD: providers http://www.ptsd.va.gov/professional/index.asp Community provider toolkit www.mentalhealth.va.gov/communityproviders Center for deployment psychology http://deploymentpsych.org/
Mobile applications	PTSD coach http://www.ptsd.va.gov/public/materials/apps/PTSDCoach.asp Mindfulness coach http://www.ptsd.va.gov/public/materials/apps/mobileapp_mindfulness_coach.asp	Cognitive processing therapy (CPT) coach http://www.ptsd.va.gov/public/materials/apps/cpt_mobileapp_public.asp Prolonged exposure (PE) coach http://www.ptsd.va.gov/public/materials/apps/pecoach_mobileapp-public.asp
Online trainings	PTSD coach online http://www.ptsd.va.gov/public/treatment/cope/index.asp	Military culture training http://deploymentpsych.org/military-culture Skills Training in Affective and Interpersonal Regulation (STAIR) http://www.ptsd.va.gov/apps/STAIR/STAIROrientation/wrap_menupage.htm Cognitive processing therapy (CPT) and prolonged exposure (PE) training http://deploymentpsych.org/online-courses

reactions can be extremely disruptive and can then lead the individual to avoid thoughts, places, people, and activities that have potential to elicit these reactions. Treatments such as cognitive processing therapy and prolonged exposure aim to create new learning through "exposing" the individual to the trauma in a safe environment and through providing space and tools for the individual to process through (e.g., cognitive restructuring) the event. These treatments can promote a better understanding of the event and disentangle the contextual cues and thoughts from the traumatic event itself, such that it no longer elicits such intense emotional reactions (i.e., fear extinction)—enabling individuals to engage more fully in life. Recent research has found greater fear conditioning in women (Inslicht et al. 2013). As noted earlier, women have been found to develop PTSD at higher rates than men, and the authors propose that differences in fear conditioning may be one mechanism through which women are at higher risk (Inslicht et al. 2013).

While cognitive processing therapy (CPT) and prolonged exposure (PE) have been shown to be effective in treating PTSD in veterans (Department of Veterans Affairs & Department of Defense 2010), not all veterans will necessarily be a match for the treatments or may not want to start with a treatment that requires a focus on the traumatic event. Cognitive processing therapy has also been shown to be effective even without the trauma exposure component (Resick et al. 2008), making this an attractive option for some veterans. Further, recent research has shown that for individuals with emotional regulation difficulties, providing a course of treatment focused on building emotional regulation skills may increase the acceptability and effectiveness of subsequent trauma-focused treatment (Cloitre 2015). One such treatment is Skills Training in Affective and Interpersonal Regulation Narrative Therapy (STAIR; Cloitre et al. 2006). This treatment targets the development of emotional regulation skills and increased social connectedness. Dialectical behavior therapy (DBT; Linehan 1993) is another stage-based skills building treatment shown to be helpful for individuals with a more complex presentation (Landes et al. 2013). As noted earlier, PTSD is often comorbid with other conditions such as depression. Acceptance and commitment therapy (ACT) is a widely used treatment for depression for civilians and has been shown to reduce symptoms of anxiety and depression in veterans (e.g., Walser et al. 2013).

Veterans with PTSD report more psychosocial functioning difficulties including poorer family relationships (Koenen et al. 2008) and higher rates of divorce and separation (Riggs et al. 1998; Cook et al. 2004). Given the important role of social connectedness and support in recovery from PTSD and in various domains of functional improvement, family and peer support interventions are important to consider, in addition to individual or group psychotherapies. Including a family or peer component to a veteran's treatment plan has been found to be acceptable to many veterans and may increase engagement in psychotherapy (e.g., Khaylis et al. 2011; Jain et al. 2013).

Conclusion

Posttraumatic stress disorder (PTSD) is regarded as a "signature wound" of combat service among the most recent cohort of veterans who served in Afghanistan and Iraq. While a minority will develop a full diagnosis of PTSD, even subthreshold levels of symptoms can be destructive to veterans' social, occupational, and health functioning. Moreover, without intervention, symptoms can endure throughout one's lifetime. Recent decades have seen a proliferation in PTSD research and treatment development. There are now evidence-based treatments that have promised to alleviate PTSD symptoms and to improve the quality of life of those who have survived often profoundly difficult events during military service. It is a privilege to serve the men and women who have served our country, and they are owed the very best treatment and support that can be provided.

Key Concepts

1. While more than half of the general population will experience a potentially traumatic event in their lifetime, only a minority will develop posttraumatic stress disorder (PTSD). Reported rates of PTSD are higher among veteran samples.
2. Risk factors for PTSD include trauma/event characteristics (e.g., level of trauma exposure), demographic and biological variables (e.g., gender, age, previous trauma exposure, history of mental illness), and psychosocial variables (e.g., social support).
3. Military sexual trauma (MST) and moral injury have been found to be predictive of PTSD in veteran samples and require additional attention during treatment.
4. Clinical practice guidelines (CPGs) are valuable in providing information about the recommended treatments for PTSD including evidence-based treatments such as prolonged exposure (PE) therapy, cognitive processing therapy (CPT), and eye movement desensitization and reprocessing (EMDR) therapy.

References

Allen JG (2005) Attachment in coping with trauma: hope through understanding. American Psychiatric Publication, Washington, DC

American Psychiatric Association (1980) Diagnostic and statistical manual of mental disorders, 3rd edn. American Psychiatric Association, Washington, DC

American Psychiatric Association (1987) Diagnostic and statistical manual of mental disorders, 3rd edn. American Psychiatric Association, Washington, DC

American Psychiatric Association (1994) Diagnostic and statistical manual of mental disorders, 4th edn. American Psychiatric Association, Washington, DC

American Psychiatric Association (2000) Diagnostic and statistical manual of mental disorders, 4th edn. American Psychiatric Association, Washington, DC

American Psychiatric Association (2013) Diagnostic and statistical manual of mental disorders, 5th edn. American Psychiatric Association, Washington, DC

Andrews J, Guyatt G, Oxman AD, et al. (2013) GRADE guidelines: 14. Going from evidence to recommendations: The significance and presentation of recommendations. J Clin Epidemiol 66(7):719–725

Arnsten AF, Raskind MA, Taylor FB, Conner DF (2015) The effects of stress exposure on prefrontal cortex: translating basic research into successful treatments for post-traumatic stress disorder. Neurobiol Stress 1:89–99

Apfel BA, Otte C, Inslicht SS, McCaslin SE, Henn-Haase C, Metzler TJ, Makotkine I et al (2011) Pretraumatic prolonged elevation of salivary MHPG predicts peritraumatic distress and symptoms of post-traumatic stress disorder. J Psychiatr Res 45:735–741

Benoit M, Bouthillier D, Moss E, Rousseau C, Brunet A (2010) Emotion regulation strategies as mediators of the association between level of attachment security and PTSD symptoms following trauma in adulthood. Anxiety, Stress Coping 23(1):101–118

Besser A, Neria Y, Haynes M (2009) Adult attachment, perceived stress, and PTSD among civilians exposed to ongoing terrorist attacks in Southern Israel. Personal Individ Differ 47(8):851–857

Binder EB, Bradley RG, Liu W, Epstein MP, Deveau TC, Mercer KB, …, Ressler KJ (2008) Association of FKBP5 polymorphisms and childhood abuse with risk of posttraumatic stress disorder symptoms in adults. J Am Med Assoc 299(11): 1291–1305

Blanco C (2011) Epidemiology of PTSD. In: Stein DJ, Friedman MJ, Blanco C (eds) Post-traumatic stress disorder (evidence and experience in psychiatry, volume 24). Wiley-Blackwell, Oxford, pp 49–74

Bodkin JA, Pope HG, Detke MJ, Hudson JI (2007) Is PTSD caused by traumatic stress? J Anxiety Disord 21(2):176–182. https://doi.org/10.1016/j.janxdis.2006.09.004

Boehnlein JK, Kinzie JD (2007) Pharmacologic reduction of CNS noradrenergic activity in PTSD: the case for clonidine and prazosin. J Psychiatr Pract 13:72–78

Coughlin SS (2011) Post-traumatic stress disorder and cardiovascular disease. Open Cardiovasc Med J 5:164–170

Bogaerts S, Daalder AL, Van Der Knaap LM, Kunst MJJM, Buschman J (2008) Critical incident, adult attachment style, and posttraumatic stress disorder: a comparison of three groups of security workers. Soc Behav Personal Int J 36(8):1063–1072

Brewin CR, Andrews B, Valentine JD (2000) Meta-analysis of risk factors for posttraumatic stress disorder in trauma-exposed adults. J Consult Clin Psychol 68:748–766. https://doi.org/10.1037//0022-006X.68.5.748

Butler LD, Blasey CM, Garlan RW, McCaslin SE, Azarow J, Chen XH, ..., Spiegel D (2005) Posttraumatic growth following the terrorist attacks of September 11, 2001: cognitive, coping, and trauma symptom predictors in an internet convenience sample. Traumatology 11(4): 247

Charuvastra A, Cloitre M (2008) Social bonds and posttraumatic stress disorder. Annu Rev Psychol 59:301–328. https://doi.org/10.1146/annurev.psych.58.110405.085650

Clapp JD, Masci J, Bennett SA, Beck JG (2010) Physical and psychosocial functioning following motor vehicle trauma: relationships with chronic pain, posttraumatic stress, and medication use. Eur J Pain 14:418–425

Cloitre M (2015) The role of emotion regulation in adult responses to traumatic stress. Symposium presented at the 31st annual meeting of the International Society for Traumatic Stress Studies (ISTSS), New Orleans, LA

Cloitre M, Cohen LR, Koenen KC (2006) Treating survivors of childhood abuse: psychotherapy for the interrupted life. The Guilford Press, New York

Cloitre M, Stovall-McClough C, Zorbas P, Charuvastra A (2008) Attachment organization, emotion regulation, and expectations of support in a clinical sample of women with childhood abuse histories. J Trauma Stress 21:282–289. https://doi.org/10.1002/jts.20339

Cook JM, Riggs DS, Thompson R, Coyne JC, Sheikh JI (2004) Posttraumatic Stress Disorder and current relationship functioning among World War II ex-prisoners of war. J Fam Psychol 18:36–45

Currier JM, Holland JM (2012) Examining the role of combat loss among Vietnam War veterans. J Trauma Stress 25:102–105

Currier JM, Holland JM, Drescher K, Foy D (2013) Initial psychometric evaluation of the moral injury questionnaire-military version. Clin Psychol Psychother. https://doi.org/10.1002/cpp.1866

Deering CG, Glover SG, Ready D, Eddleman HC, Alarcon RD (1996) Unique patterns of comorbidity in posttraumatic stress disorder from different sources of trauma. Compr Psychiatry 37(5):336–346

Department of Veterans Affairs & Department of Defense (2010) VA/DoD clinical practice guideline for management of post-traumatic stress. http://www.healthquality.va.gov/ptsd/cpg_PTSD-FULL-201011612.pdf

Dinenberg RE, McCaslin SE, Bates MN, Cohen BE. (2014) Social support may protect against development of posttraumatic stress disorder: Findings from the Heart and Soul Study. American Journal of Health Promotion. 28(5):294–7

Foa E, Hembree E, Rothbaum B (2007) Prolonged exposure therapy for PTSD: emotional processing of traumatic experiences. Oxford University Press, Oxford

Frayne SM, Skinner KM, Sullivan LM, Tripp TJ, Hankin CS, Kressin N, Miller D (1999) Medical profile of women veterans administration outpatients who report a history of sexual assault occurring while in the military. J Womens Health Gend Based Med 8(6):835–845

Fulton JJ, Calhoun PS, Wagner HR, Schry AR, Hair LP, Feeling N, Elbogen E, Beckham JC (2015) The prevalence of posttraumatic stress disorder in Operation Enduring Freedom/Operation Iraqi Freedom (OEF/OIF) veterans: a meta-analysis. J Anxiety Disord 31:98–107

Gapen M, Cross D, Ortigo KM, Graham A, Johnson E, Evces M, …, Bradley B (2011) Perceived neighborhood disorder, community cohesion, and PTSD symptoms among low-income African Americans in an urban health setting. Am J Orthopsychiatry, 81(1): 31–37

Gilbertson MW, Shenton ME, Ciszewski A, Kasai K, Lasko NB, Orr SP, Pittman RK (2002) Smaller hippocampal volume predicts pathologic vulnerability to psychological trauma. Nat Neurosci 5:1242–1247

Gillespie CF, Phifer J, Bradley B, Ressler KJ (2009) Risk and resilience: genetic and environmental influences on development of the stress response. Depress Anxiety 26(11):984–992

Gironda RJ, Clark ME, Massengale JP, Walker RL (2006) Pain among veterans of Operations Enduring Freedom and Iraqi Freedom. Pain Med 7:339–343

Heim C, Bradley B, Mletzko TC, Deveau TC, Musselman DL, Nemeroff CB, …, Binder EB (2009) Effect of childhood trauma on adult depression and neuroendocrine function: sex-specific moderation by CRH receptor 1 gene. Front Behav Neurosci 3:1–10

Hoge CW, Castro CA, Messer SC, McGurk D, Cotting DI, Koffman RL (2004) Combat duty in Iraq and Afghanistan, mental health problems, and barriers to care. N Engl J Med 351:13–22

Huang M, Yurgil KA, Robb A, Angeles A, Diwaker M, Risbrough VB, Nichols SL et al (2014) Voxel-wise resting-state MEG source magnitude imaging study reveals neurocircuitry abnormality in active-duty service members and veterans with PTSD. NeuroImage: Clin 5:408–419

Iacoviello BM, Charney DS (2014) Psychosocial facets of resilience: implications for preventing posttrauma psychopathology, treating trauma survivors, and enhancing community resilience. J Psychotraumatology 5:23970

Inslicht SS, Metzler TJ, Garcia NM, Pineles SL, Milad MR, Orr SP, Marmar CR, Neylan TC (2013) Sex differences in fear conditioning in posttraumatic stress disorder. J Psychiatr Res 47:64–71

Jakupcak M, Cook J, Imel Z, Fontana A, Rosenheck R, McFall M (2009) Posttraumatic stress disorder as a risk factor for suicidal ideation in Iraq and Afghanistan war veterans. J Trauma Stress 22(4):303–306. https://doi.org/10.1002/jts.20423

Jain S, McLean C, Adler EP, Lindley SE, Ruzek JI, Rosen CS (2013) Does the integration of peers into the treatment of adults with posttraumatic stress disorder improve access to mental health care? A literature review and conceptual model. J Trauma Stress Disord Treat 2:1–9

Janet P (1889) L'automatisme psychologique: Essai de psychologie experimentale sur les formes inferieures de l'activite humaine. Felix Alcan, Paris

Johnson H, Thompson A (2008) The development and maintenance of post-traumatic stress disorder (PTSD) in civilian adult survivors of war trauma and torture: a review. Clin Psychol Rev 28(1):36–47

Jovanovic T, Ressler KJ (2010) How the neurocircuitry and genetics of fear inhibition may inform our understanding of PTSD. Am J Psychiatr 167(6):648–662

Kang HK, Natelson BH, Mahan CM, Lee KY, Murphy FM (2003) Post-traumatic stress disorder and chronic fatigue syndrome-like illness among Gulf War veterans: a population-based survey of 30,000 veterans. Am J Epidemiol 157(2):141–148. https://doi.org/10.1093/aje/kwf187

Kang H, Dalager N, Mahan C, Ishii E (2005) The role of sexual assault on the risk of PTSD among Gulf War Veterans. Ann Epidemiol 15(3):191–195

Kashdan TB, Uswatte G, Steger MF, Julian T (2006) Fragile self-esteem and affective instability in posttraumatic stress disorder. Behav Res Ther 44(11):1609–1619

Keane TM, Wolfe J (1990) Comorbidity in post-traumatic stress disorder: an analysis of community and clinical studies. J Appl Soc Psychol 20:1776–1788

Kessler RC, Berglund P, Demler O, Jin R, Merikangas KR, Walters EE (2005) Lifetime prevalence and age-of-onset distributions of DSM-IV disorders in the National Comorbidity Survey Replication. Arch Gen Psychiatry 62(6):593–602. https://doi.org/10.1001/archpsyc.62.6.593

Kessler RC, Sonnega A, Bromet E, Hughes M, Nelson C (1995) Posttraumatic stress disorder in the National Comorbidity Survey. Arch Gen Psychiatry 52(12):1048–1060

Khaylis A, Polusny MA, Erbes CR, Gewirtz A, Rath M (2011) Posttraumatic stress, family adjustment, and treatment preferences among National Guard soldiers deployed to OEF/OIF. Mil Med 176:126–131

Kimerling R, Gima K, Smith MW, Street A, Frayne S (2007) The Veterans Health Administration and military sexual trauma. Am J Public Health 97:2160–2166

Kimerling R, Street A, Pavao J, Smith M, Cronkite R, Holmes T, Frayne S (2010) Military-related sexual trauma among Veterans Health Administration patients returning from Afghanistan and Iraq. Am J Public Health 100:1409–1412

King DW, King LA, Foy DW, Keane TM, Fairbank JA (1999) Posttraumatic stress disorder in a national sample of female and male Vietnam veterans: risk factors, war-zone stressors, and resilience-recovery variables. J Abnorm Psychol 108(1):164–170. https://doi.org/10.1037/0021-843X.108.1.164

Koenen KC, Stellman JM, Stellman SD, Sommer JF Jr (2003) Risk factors for course of posttraumatic stress disorder among Vietnam veterans: a 14-year follow-up of American legionnaires. J Consult Clin Psychol 71(6):980–986. https://doi.org/10.1037/0022-006X.71.6.980

Koenen KC, Stellman SD, Sommer JF, Stellman JM (2008) Persisting posttraumatic stress disorder symptoms and their relationship to functioning in Vietnam veterans: a 14-year follow-up. J Trauma Stress 21:49–57

Kulka RA, Schlenger WE, Fairbank JA, Hough RL, Jordan BK, Marmar CR, Weiss DS (1988) Contractual report of findings from the National Vietnam Veterans Readjustment Study. Research Triangle Institute, Research Triangle Park

Kulka RA, Schlenger WE, Fairbank JA, Hough RL, Jordan BK, Marmar CR, Weiss DS (1990) Trauma and the Vietnam war generation: report of findings from the National Vietnam Veterans Readjustment Study. Brunner/Mazel, New York

Lakusic N, Fuckar K, Mahovic D, Cerovec D, Majsec M, Stancin N (2007) Characteristics of heart rate variability in war veterans with post-traumatic stress disorder after myocardial infarction. Mil Med 172:1190–1193

Landes SJ, Garovoy ND, Burkman KM (2013) Treating complex trauma among veterans: three stage-based treatment models. J Clin Psychol In Session 69:523–533

Larson GE, Norman SB (2014) Prospective prediction of functional difficulties among recently separated veterans. JRRD 51:415–428

Linehan MM (1993) Cognitive-behavioral treatment of borderline personality disorder. The Guilford Press, New York

Lipari RN, Cook PJ, Rock LM, Matos K (2008) 2006 gender relations survey of active duty members. Department of Defense Manpower Data Center, Arlington

Litz BT, Stein N, Delaney E, Lebowitz L, Nash WP, Silva C, Maguen S (2009) Moral injury and moral repair in war veterans: a preliminary model and intervention strategy. Clin Psychol Rev 29:695–706

Maguen S, Lucenko BA, Reger MA, Gahm GA, Litz BT, Seal KH, Marmar CR (2010) The impact of reported direct and indirect killing on mental health symptoms in Iraq war veterans. J Trauma Stress 23:86–90

Maguen S, Litz B. Moral injury in veterans of war. PTSD Res Quart. 23(1):1–6. See more at: http://www. psychiatrictimes. com/articles/reactivation-ptsd-symptoms-resulting-sandy-hook-media-exposure/page/0/2# sthash. jNdeIlvy. dpuf. 2012.

Maguen S, Madden E, Bosch J, Galatzer-Levy I, Knight SJ, Litz BT, McCaslin SE (2013) Killing and latent classes of PTSD symptoms in Iraq and Afghanistan veterans. J Affect Disord 145:344–348

Marmar CR, Schlenger W, Henn-Haase C, Qian M, Purchia E, Li M, ..., Kulka RA (2015) Course of posttraumatic stress disorder 40 years after the Vietnam War: findings from the National Vietnam Veterans Longitudinal Study. JAMA Psychiatry 72(9): 875–881

McCarthy E, Petrakis I (2010) Epidemiology and management of alcohol dependence in individuals with posttraumatic stress disorder. CNS Drugs 24(12):997–1007. https://doi.org/10.2165/11539710-000000000-00000

McCaslin SE, de Zoysa P, Butler LD, Hart S, Marmar CR, Metzler TJ, Koopman C (2009) The relationship of posttraumatic growth to peritraumatic reactions and posttraumatic stress symptoms among Sri Lankan university students. J Trauma Stress 22(4):334–339

McCaslin SE, Maguen S, Metzler T, Bosch J, Neylan TC, Marmar CR (2016) Assessing posttraumatic stress related impairment and well-being: The Posttraumatic Stress Related Functioning Inventory (PRFI). J Psychiatr Res 31;72:104–11

McCaslin SE, Turchik JA, Hatzfeld JJ (2015) Considerations in the treatment of veterans with posttraumatic stress disorder. Evidence based treatments for trauma-related psychological disorders. Springer International Publishing, 413–430

Miller MW (2003) Personality and the etiology and expression of PTSD: a three-factor model perspective. Clin Psychol Sci Pract 10:373–393

Miller MW, Vogt DS, Mozley SL, Kaloupek DG, Keane TM (2006) PTSD and substance-related problems: the mediating roles of disconstraint and negative emotionality. J Abnorm Psychol 115(2):369–379

Morris MC, Compas BE, Garber J (2012) Relations among posttraumatic stress disorder, comorbid major depression, and HPA function: a systematic review and meta-analysis. Clin Psychol Rev 32:301–315

Nash WP, Marino Carper TL, Mills MA, Au T, Goldsmith A, Litz BT (2013) Psychometric evaluation of the moral injury events scale. Mil Med 178:646–652

National Comorbidity Survey (Producer) (2005) NCS-R appendix tables: table 1. Lifetime prevalence of DSM-IV/WMH-CIDI disorders by sex and cohort. Table 2. Twelve-month prevalence of DSM-IV/WMH-CIDI disorders by sex and cohort. Retrieved from http://www.hcp.med.harvard.edu/ncs/publications.php

Norrholm SD, Ressler KJ (2009) Genetics of anxiety and trauma-related disorders. Neuroscience 164(1):272–287

Norris FH, Friedman MJ, Watson PJ, Byrne CM, Diaz E, Kaniasty K (2002) 60,000 disaster victims speak: part I. An empirical review of the empirical literature, 1981–2001. Psychiatry: Interpersonal Biol Processes 65(3):207–239

Orr SP, Metzger LJ, Lasko NB, Macklin ML, Peri T, Pitman RK (2000) De novo conditioning in trauma-exposed individuals with and without posttraumatic stress disorder. J Abnorm Psychol 109(2):290

Ortigo KM, Westen D, DeFife JA, Bradley B (2013) Attachment, social cognition, and posttraumatic stress symptoms in a traumatized, urban population: evidence for the mediating role of object relations. J Trauma Stress 26:1–8. https://doi.org/10.1002/jts.21815

Ozer EJ, Best SR, Lipsey TL, Weiss DS (2003) Predictors of posttraumatic stress disorder and symptoms in adults: a meta-analysis. Psychol Bull 129:52–73. https://doi.org/10.1037/0033-2909.129.1.52

Pals JL, McAdams DP (2004) The transformed self: a narrative understanding of posttraumatic growth. Psychol Inq 15:65–69

Papa A, Neria Y, Litz B (2008) Traumatic bereavement in war veterans. Psychiatr Ann 38:686–691

Pittman JOE, Goldsmith AA, Lemmer JA, Kilmer MT, Baker DG (2012) Post-traumatic stress disorder, depression, and health-related quality of life in OEF/OIF veterans. Qual Life Res 21(1):99–103. https://doi.org/10.1007/s11136-011-9918-3

Pivar IL, Field NP (2004) Unresolved grief in combat veterans with PTSD. J Anxiety Disord 18:745–755

Ramchand R, Rudavsky R, Grant S, Tanielian T, Jaycox L (2015) Prevalence of, risk factors for, and consequences of posttraumatic stress disorder and other mental health problems in military populations deployed to Iraq and Afghanistan. Curr Psychiatry Rep 17:37

Renshaw KD (2011) An integrated model of risk and protective factors for post-deployment PTSD symptoms in OEF/OIF era combat veterans. J Affect Disord 128(3):321–326. https://doi.org/10.1016/j.jad.2010.07.022

Resick PA, Galovski TE, Uhlmansiek MOB, Scher CD, Clum GA, Young-Xu Y (2008) A randomized clinical

trial to dismantle components of cognitive processing therapy for posttraumatic stress disorder in female victims of interpersonal violence. J Consult Clin Psychol 76(2):243
Resick PA, Schnicke MK (1993) Cognitive processing therapy for rape victims: a treatment manual. Sage, Newbury Park
Riggs DS, Byrne CA, Weathers FW, Litz BT (1998) The quality of the intimate relationships of male Vietnam veterans: problems associated with posttraumatic stress disorder. J Trauma Stress 11:87–101
Rosen GM, Lilienfeld SO (2008) Posttraumatic stress disorder: an empirical evaluation of core assumptions. Clin Psychol Rev 28(5):837–868
Rosen GM, Lilienfeld SO, Frueh BC, McHugh PR, Spitzer RL (2010) Reflections on PTSD's future in DSM-V. Br J Psychiatry 197(5):343–344
Rosen GM, Spitzer RL, McHugh PR (2008) Problems with the post-traumatic stress disorder diagnosis and its future in DSM–V. Br J Psychiatry 192(1):3–4
Sahar T, Shalev AY, Porges SW (2001) Vagal modulation of responses to mental challenge in posttraumatic stress disorder. Biol Psychiatry 49:637–643
Sandberg DA, Suess EA, Heaton JL (2010) Attachment anxiety as a mediator of the relationship between interpersonal trauma and posttraumatic symptomatology among college women. J Interpers Violence 25(1):33–49
Scott S, Babcock JC (2010) Attachment as a moderator between intimate partner violence and PTSD symptoms. J Fam Violence 25:1–9. https://doi.org/10.1007/s10896-009-9264-1
Schell TL, Marshall GN (2008) Survey of individuals previously deployed for OEF/OIF. Invisible Wounds of War, 87
Schnurr PP, Hayes AF, Lunney CA, McFall M, Uddo M (2006) Longitudinal analysis of the relationship between symptoms and quality of life in veterans treated for posttraumatic stress disorder. J Consult Clin Psychol 74:707–713
Shakespeare-Finch J, Lurie-Beck J (2014) A meta-analytic clarification of the relationship between posttraumatic growth and symptoms of posttraumatic distress disorder. J Anxiety Disord 28(2):223–229
Sharp TJ, Harvey AG (2001) Chronic pain and posttraumatic stress disorder: mutual maintenance? Clin Psychol Rev 21:857–877
Shay J (1994) Achilles in Vietnam: Combat trauma and the undoing of character. New York, NY: Scribner
Skinner KM, Kressin N, Frayne S, Tripp TJ, Hankin CS, Miller DR, Sullivan LM (2000) The prevalence of military sexual assault among female Veterans' Administration outpatients. J Interpers Violence 15(3):291–310
Southwick SM, Yehuda R, Giller EL Jr (1993) Personality disorders in treatment-seeking combat veterans with posttraumatic stress disorder. Am J Psychiatr 150(7):1020–1023
Spitzer RL, First MB, Wakefield JC (2007) Saving PTSD from itself in DSM-V. J Anxiety Disord 21:233–241
Stecker T, Shiner B, Watts BV, Jones M, Conner KR (2013) Treatment-seeking barriers for veterans of the Iraq and Afghanistan conflicts who screen positive for PTSD. Psychiatr Serv 64:280–283
Stein H, Allen JG (2007) Mentalizing as a framework for integrating therapeutic exposure and relationship repair in the treatment of a patient with complex posttraumatic psychopathology. Bull Menn Clin 71(4):273–290
Stein NR, Mills MA, Arditte K, Mendoza C, Borah AM, Resick PA, Litz BT (2012) STRONGSTAR consortium. A scheme for categorizing traumatic military events. Behav Modif 36:787–807
Tanielian T, Jaycox L (eds) (2008) Invisible wounds of war: psychological and cognitive injuries, their consequences, and services to assist recovery. RAND Corporation, Santa Monica
Tedeschi RG, Calhoun LG (2004) Posttraumatic growth: conceptual foundations and empirical evidence. Psychol Inq 15(1):1–18
Tedeschi RG, Park CL, Calhoun LG (eds) (1998) Posttraumatic growth: positive changes in the aftermath of crisis. Lawrence Erlbaum, Mahwah
Thomas JL, Wilk JE, Riviere LA, McGurk D, Castro CA, Hoge CW (2010) Prevalence of mental health problems and functional impairment among active component and National Guard soldiers 3 and 12 months following combat in Iraq. Arch Gen Psychiatry 67:614–623
Toblin RL, Riviere LA, Thomas JL, Adler AB, Kok BC, Hoge CW (2012) Grief and physical health outcomes in US soldiers returning from combat. J Affect Disord 136:469–475
Turchik JA, Pavao J, Nazarian D, Iqbal S, McLean C, Kimerling R (2012) Sexually transmitted infections and sexual dysfunctions among newly returned veterans with and without military sexual trauma. Int J Sex Health 24:45–59
Turchik JA, Wilson SM (2010) Sexual assault in the US military: a review of the literature and recommendations for the future. Aggress Violent Behav 15:267–277
Twaite JA, Rodriguez-Srednicki O (2004) Childhood sexual and physical abuse and adult vulnerability to PTSD: the mediating effects of attachment and dissociation. J Child Sex Abuse 13:17–38. https://doi.org/10.1300/J070v13n01_02
van der Kolk BA, Brown P, van der Hart O (1989) Pierre Janet on post-traumatic stress. J Trauma Stress 2:365–378
Wahbeh H, Oken BS (2013) Salivary cortisol lower in posttraumatic stress disorder. J Trauma Stress 26:241–248
Walser RD, Karlin BE, Trockel M, Mazina B, Taylor C (2013) Training in and implementation of acceptance and commitment therapy for depression in the veterans health administration: therapist and patient outcomes. Behav Res Ther 51:555–563
Westen D (1991) Social cognition and object relations. Psychol Bull 109:429–455. https://doi.org/10.1037//0033-2909.109.3.429

Wilson JP (2006) Introduction and overview: a positive psychology of trauma and PTSD. In: Wilson JP (ed) The posttraumatic self: restoring meaning and wholeness to personality. Routledge, New York, pp 1–7

Woon FL, Sood S, Hedges DW (2010) Hippocampal volume deficits associated with exposure to psychological trauma and posttraumatic stress disorder in adults: a meta-analysis. Prog Neuro-Psychopharmacol Biol Psychiatry 34:1181–1188

Yaeger D, Himmelfarb N, Cammack A, Mintz J (2006) DSM-IV diagnosed posttraumatic stress disorder in women veterans with and without military sexual trauma. J Gen Intern Med 21(Suppl 3):S65–S69

Yehuda R, McFarlane AC (2009) PTSD is a valid diagnosis: who benefits from challenging its existence? Psychiatr Times 26(7):31

Zatzick DF Marmar CR, Weiss DS, Browner WS, Metzler TJ, Golding JM, …, Wells KB (1997) Posttraumatic stress disorder and functioning and quality of life outcomes in a nationally representative sample of male Vietnam veterans. Am J Psychiatr 154(12): 1690–1695

Zoellner T, Maercker A (2006) Posttraumatic growth in clinical psychology – a critical review and introduction of a two component model. Clin Psychol Rev 26(5):626–653

Zoladz PR, Diamond DM (2013) Current status on behavioral and biological markers of PTSD: a search for clarity in a conflicting literature. Neurosci Biobehav Rev 37:860–895

16 Combat and Operational Stress

Jill E. Breitbach, Yaron G. Rabinowitz, and Christopher H. Warner

History, Epidemiology, and Definitions of Combat and Operational Stress

Since the dawn of war, combat and operational stress has existed. It has been referred to by numerous names and captured in the earliest forms of written language. In the ancient epic poem the *Iliad* attributed to Homer, the warriors depicted in the midst of the Trojan War are described in situations in which the stress of battle and deployment negatively affects them. The first modern clinical descriptions of the psychological effects of combat were described during the US Civil War with the anxiety symptoms of "soldier's heart" (DaCosta syndrome) and then later in World War I with the advent of "shell shock." More recently, the immediate reaction to severe stress, trauma, or exhaustion associated with combat and military operations is called combat and operational stress (Hoge 2010). Combat and operational stress (COS) is considered normal for the context of a deployment and, as with any form of stress, can produce a positive or negative response. Service members can either experience growth or develop maladaptive responses, the latter of which are referred to as COS casualties.

COS casualties are not unique to US service members, as descriptions of COS have been recorded throughout history regardless of culture; Arab, Israeli, Chinese, British, French, and Russian forces have all noted COS as an outcome of various conflicts (Dailey and Ijames 2014). Starting in World War I, the treatment of COS casualties was outlined in the principles of forward psychiatry: proximity, immediacy, expectancy, and simplicity (PIES). At that time, "forward psychiatry" referred to a single psychiatrist located at the division level and "Training and Rehabilitation Centers" interspersed in the general area of operations (Bacon and Staudenmeier 2003). In the Vietnam War, combat and operational stress control (COSC) was further expanded, with both the number of behavioral health providers sent forward growing exponentially and the types of clinicians deployed broadening to include not only psychiatrists and neurospecialists but also psychologists, social workers, nurses, and enlisted personnel trained in behavioral health.

J.E. Breitbach (✉)
U.S. Public Health Service, US Northern Command, Colorado Springs, CO, USA
e-mail: jill.e.breitbach.mil@mail.mil; Jill.breitbach@hhs.gov

Y.G. Rabinowitz
Marine Special Operations School, Camp Lejeune, Jacksonville, NC, USA
e-mail: yaron.rabinowitz@socom.mil

C.H. Warner
US Army Medical Department Activity – Fort Stewart, Fort Stewart, GA, USA
e-mail: christopher.h.warner.mil@mail.mil

L.W. Roberts, C.H. Warner (eds.), *Military and Veteran Mental Health*, https://doi.org/10.1007/978-1-4939-7438-2_16

During the Vietnam War, the notion of "R&R" was also expanded, essentially providing an opportunity for all service members who were deployed at length—not only those with COS casualties—to "relax and regroup" in the theater of operations and then return to their units. R&R was promoted due to the known cost of prolonged combat engagements on the health of the individual and due to the recognized need for reprieve from the enduring stress of combat operations. However, R&R also brought to light that service members developed other maladaptive responses to the stress, including substance use/abuse and other high-risk behaviors, which were incongruent with traditional military conduct and potentially harmful to the overall mission.

COSC was further refined during the Persian Gulf War and the operations other than war of the 1990s, where COSC teams developed into two distinct entities with separate foci on prevention and rehabilitation. This culminated in COSC employment that closely mirrors that of today, with distinct prevention activities and restoration activities occurring in deployed theater of operations. As the understanding of COS has evolved, the responsibilities of the behavioral health providers assigned to military units have grown based on the requirements for management of COS during deployment.

Today, COSC describes a behavioral health capability that focuses on increasing the operational capabilities of forward deployed service members on the battlefield and preserving the fighting strength of the military. It is important to note that Army, Navy, Air Force, and Marine Corp components are all guided by the same Department of Defense policy regarding the prevention and management of COS (Reger and Moore 2006); however, how they employ these principles differs based on the needs of the organization. Current COSC doctrine calls for the forward deployment of all behavioral health personnel to engage in activities including prevention, education, treatment, and consultation services as close as possible to troops serving on combat, peacekeeping, and humanitarian assistance missions (*FM 4-02.51*). The current recommended provider to service member staffing ratio is between 1:700 and 1:800 to support delivery of care for highly dispersed units, with continued monitoring and adjustments of the staffing ratio relevant to the need of command (J-MHAT 2010). This ratio of behavioral health providers is the result of recommendations from numerous in-theater command-directed studies of COS casualties and behavioral health access to care in Iraq and Afghanistan.

Historically, estimates of COS casualties suggest rates ranging from 0% to 50% (Bacon and Staudenmeier 2003). Grossman (1996) notes that, at one point during World War II, psychiatric casualties were being discharged from the US Army faster than new recruits were being drafted. It is well established that the optimal outcome for psychiatric maladies is forward treatment, with evacuation being a known risk factor for further deterioration. Nonetheless, disease non-battle injuries continue to account for 80% of all aeromedical evacuations (Wilmoth et al. 2015), with high rates of psychiatric evacuations. Although the goal of COSC is to treat service members in theater and return them to duty, recent estimates of psychiatric evacuation rates show increasing trends, from 72.7 per 100,000 deployers in 2004 to 196.9 per 100,000 in 2010 (Wilmoth et al. 2015). This is not surprising, given the ample evidence that repeated exposure to military combat increases the risk of developing a range of mental health conditions, including posttraumatic stress disorder (PTSD), major depression, and substance abuse (Hoge et al. 2004; Wojcik et al. 2009). The sheer volume of operational requirements for the existing all-volunteer force strength necessitates repeated deployments and exponentially increases the risk for COS casualties.

Although most current literature focuses on the development of psychiatric conditions after deployment, there is a growing body of literature examining the epidemiology of COS responses during deployment, including the cumulative effects of deployments. Discussion of in-theater COSC efforts is feasible, as COS patient encounters are now documented by health-care providers in theater with increasing accuracy, thanks to the advancement of the theater medical integration platform, which allows electronic medical records to be maintained during deployment. Further, increasing command attention to the costs of COS has resulted in ongoing research efforts that have dramatically increased the understanding of deployment and associated COS reactions.

The US Army Surgeon General chartered the first Mental Health Advisory Team (MHAT) in July 2003, with a mission of assessing Operation Iraqi Freedom-related mental health issues and providing recommendations to medical and line commands after surveying soldiers during active combat (MHAT Executive Report 2005). This was the first time in history that the behavioral health of a force was assessed during active combat, and the undertaking was timely. Around the same time, Hoge and colleagues published a landmark study regarding the effects of deployment on mental health in 2004, noting deployment to Iraq was associated with an increased risk of a post-deployment anxiety or mood disorder, and those who screened positive were unlikely to seek mental health care. Following the publication of these two key items, the decision was made to continue the MHATs annually (they were discontinued in 2013) and to expand them from Iraq to Afghanistan as well as to multiple services, not just the Army. Also, each subsequent MHAT evolved beyond a narrow focus on only the epidemiology statistics to a broader focus on the impact of repeated deployments, the benefit of behavioral health care in theater, suicide (and suicide prevention), small unit leadership, mitigating risk factors, perceived stigma related to seeking behavioral health care, and concussion in the summary reports. This chapter focuses on the COS response during deployment and specific interventions the provider may choose to utilize if deployed.

Case Study, Part 1

Sergeant First Class (SFC) Harold Yamashita (pseudonym), a senior noncommissioned officer, approaches you outside the dining area on the forward operating base where you are deployed as a behavioral health provider in Afghanistan. You've seen him before; he was one of the leaders who came in a few nights ago after a vehicle-borne improvised explosive device blast killed two soldiers. That makes three deaths and two wounded in action who were evacuated from SFC Yamashita's battalion of 700 service members in the last 4 weeks. You were at the company's base of operations when they rolled back inside the base, exhausted, covered in dust and blood, chain smoking with sunken eyes. And then there's that smell—a mixture of dirt, diesel fuel, hot barbeque coals, sweat, blood, fear, and the heat of the summer. When you saw them, they still had another 2 h of debriefing to do with the intelligence officer (S2)—they had to complete an after action review of what happened and what went wrong. You were there when they had to review the details of the event, including how they tried to save their friends who burned to death inside their vehicle.

Combat and Operational Stress: Key Considerations

Risk Factors

Much of the current understanding of COS reactions is informed by the MHATs, and readers are strongly encouraged to read publicly available MHAT reports. The deployment experiences of each individual vary, and clinicians who work with service members during or after a deployment are encouraged to assess for various factors known to be associated with COS and subsequent behavioral health sequelae. There are many known factors that are associated with increased risk for COS and known protective factors that may ameliorate risk. In general, risk factors can be grouped into the following categories: (1) deployment experiences, (2) length and frequency of deployments, and (3) preexisting behavioral health conditions.

Deployment Experiences

Not all deployed service members have the same risk of behavioral health symptoms. While it is well established that environmental, leadership, and home-front factors impact whether service members develop healthy or maladaptive responses to COS, the level of combat exposure remains the single highest predictor of COS casualties. It is important that treating providers assess each individual's combat experiences by inquiring about the level of intensity and interpersonal violence experienced, the frequency of exposure to combat, and the perceived risk of harm to self during combat, which may correlate with frequency of combat casualties in an individual's unit. All of these factors are associated with higher levels of COS in theater and are risk factors for post-deployment behavioral health diagnosis (Phillips et al. 2010). Many providers will make an assumption that an individual's military occupational specialty will predict their level of combat exposure; this assumption is often misleading, as it is common for individuals who are in supporting roles to be tasked with different jobs during deployment. While combat arms occupational specialties, such as infantryman, gunner, pilots, or reconnaissance, are more frequently involved in the most intense and intimate fighting, it is often the case that vehicle drivers, military police/security forces, and medics are also exposed to stressful experiences. Further, the most commonly reported types of combat experiences will change with enemy tactics and time periods of deployment—even during the same theater campaign. For instance, in 2008, the MHAT reported that Brigade Combat Team Soldiers in Operation Enduring Freedom reported levels of combat exposure similar to or higher than levels reported by Brigade Combat Teams in Iraq. Also, the level of combat exposure reported in 2013 was significantly lower than in 2010 and 2012 but significantly higher than in 2009. The MHATs surveyed the same theaters of operation but with vast differences noted in combat experiences from 1 year to the next. Military activities in deployed theaters of operations will frequently change, along with the rules of engagement, making repeated deployers vulnerable to cognitive dissonance, frustration, and anger. What may have been allowed, or even encouraged, during a service member's previous deployment may result in Uniform Code of Military Justice action for a service member on the next deployment.

Length and Frequency of Deployments

The length of deployments and the frequency of deployments also contribute to the risk of an individual developing COS. Reports of work-related problems due to stress, mental health problems, and marital separations generally increase with each subsequent month of a deployment (MHAT-V 2008). For instance, in MHAT-IV, Marines had lower rates of noncombat problems when compared to Army soldiers who were deployed on average 3–4 months longer. Also, the longer an individual is deployed, the more risk they have of being exposed to a potentially significant combat event. Further, while many might presume that an individual could be inoculated from the effects of COS with previous deployment experience, this is not the case. MHATs have repeatedly found that the number of previous deployments remains a risk factor on many well-being indices. Soldiers on their third or fourth deployment have been shown to be at significantly higher risk than soldiers on their first or second deployment for mental health problems and work-related problems. While a majority of individuals evacuated for psychiatric reasons have been on their first deployment, Wilmoth et al. (2015) also found that the odds of psychiatric evacuation increase with a second and third deployment; interestingly, odds decreased for those deploying more than four times. When discussing the length of deployment, treating providers may also wish to inquire about the length of missions during deployment. For instance, many individuals may be deployed for only 3–6 months, but they may have been embedded with foreign nationals and "on mission," isolated from any source of support during the entire deployment. Further, in Air Force personnel, studies indicated that the interval between missions has a particularly important impact on risk for COS, with most flight surgeons agreeing that missions should not be flown more than three consecutive days (Rundell and Ursano 1990). For aviation personnel, there is a known risk of operational fatigue and subsequent human factors mishaps; thus, strict guidance limits the total flight hours an aviator can accumulate within a specified time period. It is unfortunate that this guidance is applied only to a few military occupational specialties. The cumulative effects of vigilance cannot be overstated; after 2–3 days of sleep disturbance and vigilance, a warfighter may be rendered essentially ineffective.

Preexisting Behavioral Health Conditions

The relationship of preexisting behavioral health diagnoses to post-deployment behavioral health problems is complex, but there is evidence to suggest that those with mental health diagnoses prior to deployment may be vulnerable to developing COS. Baseline rates of behavioral health conditions have been captured by research in training recruits (Monahan et al. 2013), entry level personnel (Warner et al. 2007), and in pre-deployment screenings (Monahan et al. 2013). It has been suggested that the Army has the highest overall incidence of mental disorders, with the Air Force having slightly higher rates for adjustment disorder and the Navy having higher rates of alcohol abuse-related disorders, posttraumatic stress disorder (PTSD), anxiety, other psychoses, and personality disorders (Monahan et al. 2013). The baseline level of anxiety symptoms is particularly salient, as Vasterling et al. (2010) have shown that combat severity is more strongly associated with symptom increases among active duty soldiers with higher baseline levels of PTSD symptoms. This finding was replicated in a study of Marines, where previous exposure to violence was considered a risk factor for developing PTSD after deployment (Phillips et al. 2010). Further, Larson et al. (2011) reported that 23% of Marines seen by an in-theater mental health provider had a prior ICD-9-CM mental health diagnosis; for service members with a prior diagnosis, the highest rates of re-diagnosis were for attention deficit disorder (57%) and PTSD (55%), suggesting that preexisting conditions are a risk factor for developing COS during deployment. Finally, it is important to note that recent data from the Army Study to Assess Risk and Resilience in service members (Army STARRS) consortium indicates that approximately one-third of post-enlistment suicide attempts are associated with pre-enlistment mental disorders, with post-enlistment attempts positively related to deployments (Nock et al. 2014). In general, a provider can surmise that deployment and combat experiences potentiate the risk for developing COS for an individual with preexisting behavioral health conditions.

Protective Factors

In addition to the current understanding of what can increase risk for COS, there is insight into protective factors, including (1) quality of leadership, (2) availability of behavioral health providers, and (3) pre-deployment training and screening.

Quality of Leadership

The importance of company-grade officer and noncommissioned officer (NCO) leadership cannot be understated. Leadership and leader development is a hallmark of all services. It impacts unit cohesion, morale, and esprit de corps and includes the development of subordinates in a unit and demonstration of core military values. Due to several high-profile events of ethical misconduct in Iraq in 2003–2005, concerns rose about the impact of COS and battlefield behaviors. A 2011 study showed that positive leadership can enhance soldiers' attitudes and behaviors regarding ethical conduct on the battlefield, which in turn decreases the level of COS (Warner et al. 2011b). To continue to enhance battlefield leadership, military training was adjusted to incorporate operational examples of positive and negative leadership, and leadership dilemmas were incorporated into training scenarios. Additionally, leaders were provided individual assessments and feedback regarding personal strengths and weaknesses, and all officers are now required to receive 360-degree feedback. Enhancing the development and progression of positive leaders is critical to the well-being of deployed service members.

Repeatedly, studies have found that small-unit leadership correlated with behavioral health, stigma, barriers to care, and unit effectiveness indices. Soldiers who perceived their NCOs and officers as ineffective were at highest risk for COS, whereas soldiers who rated their NCOs and officers as effective were at lowest risk. Effective leadership also appears to ameliorate intense combat experiences, which is the primary risk factor for development of COS. In both Operation Enduring Freedom and Operation Iraqi Freedom data, soldiers who report high levels of combat experience and poor leadership report very high levels of mental health problems. Leadership attitudes toward behavioral health, addressing stigma, breaking existing barriers to care, and overall unit cohesion have all been suggested to play a role in ameliorating COS. Further, leaders who place an emphasis on positive health behaviors, including emphasizing the importance of sleep and enforcing sleep standards, may buffer against COS.

Availability of Behavioral Health Providers

It is not surprising that the availability of behavioral health providers in a deployed theater of operations is considered a protective factor against COS. Since their inception, MHATs have examined both the dilemma of the ideal ratio of behavioral health providers to deployed service members and the methods for decreasing stigma in order to promote use of deployed behavioral health providers. In general, MHATs have found that when the numbers of behavioral health providers to service members increased (up to a ratio of 1:700 or 1:800), there was a corresponding reduction of reported stigma. Additionally, this increase in behavioral health providers was suggested to have had a positive impact on the well-being of deployed service members. These ratios also reduced the risk for burnout in deployed behavioral health providers, which was observed with ratios of 1:3000 or more. Ratios of providers to service members lower than 1:700 were not found to have been helpful and, in some cases, created confusion for commanders and low morale for the behavioral health providers who were deployed.

Despite concerted efforts to improve access to care, the relationship between perceived stigma and the utilization of resources remains complex. In 2008, soldiers reported difficulty accessing behavioral health services as numbers of behavioral health providers were beginning to increase but perceived less stigma when they did seek care. However, stigma remained a stable factor, even with more providers available. In other words, the availability of more providers, as a single variable, did not reduce the stigma of seeking behavioral health care, even though it reduced perceptions of barriers to care over time. These findings were replicated by Steenkamp and colleagues (2014) when they found that mental health treatment utilization in theater did not predict the course of stigma during a deployment. Interestingly, these findings persisted even as deployed behavioral health personnel reported significant increases in treatment encounters, as well as increased advising of commanders about soldier mental health issues. It is suggested that the presence of behavioral health providers, while improving access to care, may have also created a demand signal from commanders for the additional roles of consulting and advising. As behavioral health providers enter different professional roles during deployments (e.g., clinician, consultant, advisor), it may be challenging to simultaneously address the issues of stigma, as service members may lack clarity about how behavioral health providers negotiate these multiple roles professionally. Succinctly stated, service members may be more aware of behavioral health providers, but service members may be reluctant to seek behavioral health care if they perceive a provider to be "working for command."

Pre-deployment Training and Screening

Military branches have long focused pre-deployment training on unit tactics, marksmanship, leadership, and physical training. Now, increasing attention is focused on preparing for deployment from the human dimension perspective. This includes fostering positive health behaviors, emotional well-being, family resilience, and the prevention of sexual assault, as well as training in suicide prevention and stress management. Most recently, this program encompasses various total force fitness programs, such as the Comprehensive Soldier and Family Fitness Resilience (CSF2) training in the Army. While there is debate about the CSF2 program (Eidelson et al. 2011) and a paucity of data regarding its efficacy, questions related to aspects of the training (Performance Triad, Master Resilience Training, Sleep Hygiene) have been included in MHAT surveys of deployment epidemiology. More recent MHAT findings indicate not only that these force training programs are widely disseminated but also that there is a perception of improved training adequacy. Specifically, MHAT findings indicate that soldiers who report receiving resilience training before deployment demonstrate significantly lower rates of acute stress than soldiers who did not receive resilience training.

There are questions about whether larger Department of Defense (DoD) suicide prevention training programs have efficacy in preventing suicide, but few would question that robust training on managing suicidality has resulted from the larger initiatives. The DoD conducted force-wide analysis of suicide rates in 2012, and programs intended to prevent suicide have been measured against that report with some early indications that suicide rates are on a subtle decline, with the role of deployment as a questionable risk factor (DoD Suicide Event Report 2013). The efficacy of other military training initiatives, including those focused on prevention of sexual harassment and assault (DoD Report on Annual Sexual Assault in the Military 2014) and efforts to improve family well-being (CSF2), remains unknown for deployment and post-deployment well-being. Thus, while individual training programs that teach skills for building resiliency may prove helpful in preventing COS, many of the larger DoD training initiatives have unknown utility for prevention of COS.

Lastly, implementing a pre-deployment mental health screening and care coordination program has been shown to significantly reduce occupationally impairing mental health problems, medical evaluations, and suicide ideation (Warner et al. 2011c). This program was developed for two purposes: first, to identify those who did not meet minimum mental health criteria for deployment, either due to condition or medication requirements, and, second, to ensure continuity of care for those already engaged in treatment. This second purpose allowed those with preexisting conditions to continue to receive necessary treatment and monitoring in order to be successful even in an operationally stressful environment. The US Department of Defense now has a mandated pre-deployment screening program and system-wide mental health deployment requirements.

Etiology of Combat and Operational Stress Response

Given the known neuroendocrine consequences of prolonged stress, which can often be experienced during many deployments, it may be best to conceptualize COS reactions from a pathophysiological perspective prior to attending to psychological sequelae of COS. The basic understanding of the stress response dates back to the 1946 work of Hans Selye, whose general adaptation syndrome was viewed as a normal process all individuals endure in order to adjust to varying demands from themselves, other people, or their environment. Selye coined the "fight or flight" concept, and his work revealed that the body will respond to perceived changes or demands with a goal of maintaining homeostasis. Selye defined stress as any factor that creates a significant change in the body or the environment; however, the understanding of this process has been refined to include a person's perception of stress as impactful. Additionally, the concept has been expanded to include "fight, flight, or freeze" as potential stress reactions. As described by Gould (2006):

> General Adaptation Syndrome was thought to occur in three stages of stress response. In the alarm stage, physical defenses are mobilized through activation of the hypothalamus, sympathetic nervous system, and adrenal axis; we now commonly refer to this process as activation of the hypothalamic-pituitary-adrenal, or HPA, axis. This activation results in increased catecholamine release (e.g., norepinephrine), which facilitates recruitment of major muscle groups for a physical response. This activation further prioritizes for the individual what organ systems receive efferent attention from the central nervous system, and what organ systems (e.g., gastrointestinal) can be taken "off line." The consequence of this HPA activation is that the frontal lobes, or the "thinking" part of the brain, are also taken off-line; one does not need to be engaged in higher level cognitive processing when facing a life or death situation. In the resistance stage, hormone levels are elevated and essential body systems operate at peak performance. This can include the release of endorphins which often account for various descriptions of heroism, where an individual may have a physical injury but reports feeling no pain. This also includes release of aldosterone, which increases blood volume and blood pressure, which can help move oxygen and glucose to major organs involved in the stress response. This also includes release of cortisol which results in gluconeogenesis, or increasing the available glucose or energy for any required physical response, but also decreases inflammatory and immune responses. In the final stage of exhaustion, the body is unable to further respond to stressors and/or is damaged by increasing demands. This can be the result of prolonged stress hormone response, which can cause hypertension (prolonged vasoconstriction), headaches, insomnia, memory problems, fatigue, ulcers, and even diabetes mellitus and heart failure.

More recently, the work of Morgan and colleagues (2000, 2001, 2002) during Survival, Evasion, Resistance, and Escape (SERE) school has provided insights about changes in neuroendocrine functioning during observable periods of prolonged stress. SERE researchers have found heritable factors that serve to protect some military personnel in stressful situations, while making others more susceptible to stress reactions. For example, individuals with low levels of neuropeptide Y (NPY), a peptide related to the release of norepinephrine involved in the regulation of noradrenergic system functioning, fared worse on measures of performance at SERE (Morgan et al. 2004). Conversely, individuals with high levels of neuropeptide Y and dehydroepiandrosterone (DHEA), a hormone that can convert into estrogen and testosterone, performed better on military and cognitive tasks during SERE. Additional baseline indicators associated with poorer performance in SERE studies have included heart rate variability and baseline symptoms of dissociation (Morgan et al. 2000, 2001, 2002). In newer non-SERE research, anxiety and stress have been associated with lowered heart rate variability, thought to reflect autonomic nervous system function, causing a reduction in parasympathetic (vagal) activity and corresponding increase in sympathetic tone (Taylor et al. 2007). Additional studies of heart rate variability in Marines with and without a diagnosis of PTSD found that lower levels of high-frequency heart rate variability were associated with a diagnosis of PTSD (Minassian et al. 2014). In that study, an additional finding of note was that Marines with deployment experience had lower heart rate variability than did those with no experience. In summary, these evolving areas of research suggest there may be genetic predispositions that account for aspects of an individual's stress response, and the role of epigenetics (expression of these inherited vulnerabilities) is often not uncovered until environmental factors, such as a deployment, trigger a stress response.

Research to Practice

Given the physiological changes that occur with prolonged exposure to stressful environments, one must consider the associated behavioral consequences of the organism. How could these stress responses manifest on deployment? It is the experience of the authors that sleep difficulties are the most commonly reported COS symptom by deployed personnel, and many sleep problems represent a "safe" physical concern for which to seek assistance. Sleep difficulties can be related to initial onset insomnia, maintenance insomnia, or both. Individuals who receive fewer than 5 h of sleep per night are at risk for negative outcome, particularly during deployments when the ability to detect and determine threat levels and coordinate small unit tactics places a significant cognitive demand on the service member. The cumulative effects of partial sleep deprivation rapidly mimic the effects of total sleep deprivation, with 5–7 days of less than 5 h a night being virtually equivalent to 2 days of total sleep deprivation (US Department of the Army 2006). Further, the effects of sleep deprivation mirror the effects related to general adaptation syndrome previously discussed, namely, significant endocrine and metabolic changes, such as an increase in cortisol (Feng et al. 2015) and propensity for a subsequent depression (Finan et al. 2015).

Additional behavioral consequences include increased use of substances, such as nicotine, caffeine, prescribed medications, and alcohol, which represent attempts to calm the overactive hypothalamic-pituitary-adrenal axis. Unfortunately, these methods often exacerbate sleep disruption and physiological maladjustment. Nicotine use is associated with impaired night vision and delayed healing from injuries and wounds due to a reduced inflammatory response. Caffeine may be helpful in the short term, given the properties that facilitate alertness. However, caffeine products have been associated with unpleasant side effects and adverse events, including insomnia, mood swings, fatigue, dehydration, headaches, and cardiovascular complications. While some research suggests that caffeine may not be a significant contributor to insomnia (Waits et al. 2014), other data suggests that service members drinking three or more energy drinks per day were significantly more likely to report sleeping ≤4 h per night on average than those consuming two drinks or fewer (CDC 2012). Further, those who drank three or more drinks per day also were more likely to report sleep disruption related to stress and illness and were more likely to fall asleep during briefings or while on guard duty (CDC 2012). There are numerous cases in which temporary solutions to an array of these symptoms are treated but end up further complicating the clinical presentations in environments where risk for concussion or exposure to blast injury is extensive. Individuals who use prescription medications for sleep or alertness over prolonged periods of time may be at risk for abuse or even dependence on the medication. Finally, consumption of alcohol is generally prohibited by commanders in theater; however, service members may find creative solutions that facilitate alcohol consumption. Buying illicit drugs, including prescription medications, or alcohol in a foreign country where such substances are not subject to the same regulations as they are in the USA becomes incredibly risky for both the individual and the providers who may have to treat the side effects and withdrawal symptoms of an unknown substance. Assessing the use of substances, supplements, caffeine, nicotine, and prescription medications is essential in a deployed theater of operations.

Deployment will change the way one thinks and perceives one's environment, and this can contribute to other behavioral sequelae on deployment. While for many, the changes can be positive (e.g., positive self-reflection, thoughts of gratitude), for those with COS, cognitive changes may potentiate additional mood symptoms. For instance, COS is known to be associated with changes in attentional bias, including increased perception of threat. As anxiety, or "the pucker factor," increases, individuals may describe experiencing tunnel vision, or having a hyperfocus on one aspect of a situation, and thus ignoring what they perceive as extraneous variables. During deployments, this attentional bias can be functional. Individuals are often provided an inordinate amount of information in a brief period of time, with requirements for immediate decision-making devoid of traditional military decision-making processes. Often the consequences of decision-making can affect the life, or death, of individuals in the environment; delaying decision-making is not an option. Information overload, such as the sensory saturation that can occur during prolonged periods of combat, is what makes individuals vulnerable to maladaptive thinking patterns. Frequently, this equates to rigid thinking—that is, making quick decisions without consideration of all variables. While this can be helpful when engaged with the enemy when decisions require speed, engaging in this thinking pattern over prolonged periods of time can be habit forming and potentially harmful. Individuals become accustomed to going with their first thoughts or reactions and fail to consider the accuracy of their beliefs. It is not unusual for individuals who are many months into a deployment to begin to experience the consequences related to this way of thinking—namely, guilt, blame, shame, and interpersonal problems.

The etiology of cognitive changes relates to the previous discussion of general adaptation syndrome and specifically to the influx of catecholamines and stress hormones with noted downstream degradation of neurocognitive functioning. Namely, the hippocampus and its surrounding structures, richly populated with cortisol receptors, are particularly vulnerable to damage from glucocorticoids (i.e., cortisol) secreted by the HPA axis during chronic stress. The hippocampus is a critical area of the brain associated with memory and recall; thus, damage to this area by excess levels of glucocorticoids demonstrates a key neurobiological link between stress, memory (Taylor et al. 2007), and perception. Cortisol not only evokes suppressing effects on the hippocampus and degrades existing perceptual processes for encoding information (i.e., tunnel vision) but also impacts memory of salient information (Taylor et al. 2007). Clinically, this manifests as attention and concentration problems (encoding problems). Further, prolonged stress is associated with decreased hippocampal volume, which suggests that an additional complicating factor for those with COS may be memory difficulties. If individuals are unable to recall salient information from a stressful or traumatic event, they will often draw faulty conclusions that contribute to negative emotional states. Even executive dysfunction, as manifested by difficulties with abstract reasoning, problem solving, impulse control, and/or response inhibition, may be present in COS, as individuals struggle to attend to all information presented and develop solutions to life problems. These known cognitive correlates of prolonged stress are of additional concern for individuals with repeated deployments. Clinicians face an extraordinary challenge in differentiating the cognitive cluster of COS symptoms, which can be attributed to recent concussion and/or sleep deprivation; these comorbidities can be difficult to differentiate.

Psychological consequences of COS are as unique as the individual experiencing them and often include anxiety, grief, anger, and depression. The challenge for deployed providers is helping service members distinguish between a healthy emotional response to an atypical situation and a COS reaction warranting attention. For most individuals who are described as experiencing COS, it is the frequency, intensity, and duration of the emotional response that becomes problematic. Additionally, individuals with prolonged physiological stress responses will experience extreme mood lability and will report that their irritability, anger, or depression causes social and/or occupational problems. This could manifest as increased isolation from social supports, unit members, and withdrawal. COS is generally present when multiple attempts to self-soothe or engage in activities that previously helped with emotional regulation (i.e., exercise, talking with family) are no longer effective. As discussed by Grossman (1996), additional consequences may be present for individuals who have had intimate combat experiences involving using lethal means on others, having witnessed death, or having been confronted with situations where decisions had lethal consequences. It is known that 20% of soldiers reported difficulty coping with grief related to deployment experiences, and this difficulty was significantly associated with physical health outcomes and occupational impairment after deployment (Toblin et al. 2012).

It can be argued, then, that complicated grief reactions can also significantly impact individuals during deployment. Changes in thinking related to experiences of loss are common and can include an increasing focus on existential issues (i.e., Why me? Why not me?) and even morbid ideation (e.g., What's the point?) or suicide. It is well established that the rates of suicide in the military have seen an unprecedented increase. Many risk factors for suicidal behaviors are often experienced by deployed individuals, including being confronted with loss, chronic insomnia, isolation from social supports, thwarted belongingness, a stressful environment, engaging in risky behaviors, and consumption of substances (e.g., caffeine) that increase agitation (Bryan and Rudd 2006). Additionally, it is known that individuals exposed to prolonged stress will begin to shift their behaviors to match their mood state. Individuals who have intense anger will begin to behave aggressively, at times even committing misconduct. Individuals with a complicated grief reaction may develop survivor's guilt and entertain thoughts of suicide. It is not difficult to discern the relationship between prolonged physiological arousal, poor sleep, and emotional dysregulation; the challenge for the provider is how to differentiate the etiology of these responses so that an appropriate intervention can be cultivated for the individual.

Assessment of COS

Given the discussion of factors associated with COS, the known etiology of COS, and the ways that COS may manifest physically, behaviorally, and emotionally, it is recommended that deployed behavioral health providers engage in frequent assessment at the strategic, unit, and individual level. Thus, providers may wish to socialize the concept of battlefield circulation with their commanders. Providers may wish to share known indicators of risk for COS with command and discuss how to ensure appropriate assessment and treatment for deployed military personnel in the area of operations. For instance, providers may wish to engage particular focus on units that have seen high rates of combat, have been deployed for lengths greater than 6 months, who have high rates of repeat deployers, and/or units that have known leadership challenges. An additional consideration regarding the timing of battlefield circulation is the demonstrated incidence and prevalence of COS symptoms during a deployment. COS casualties are thought to follow a bimodal distribution, or a "U-shaped" curve (Campise et al. 2006), which is consistent with reports of provider experiences during deployments (Warner et al. 2007). It is recommended that behavioral health officers engage leadership prior to deployment to discuss how to meet the commander's intent during deployment, being mindful of critical periods and indicators that indicate a requirement for outreach to service members at more remote locations. As behavioral health officers infrequently have means to facilitate their own transportation, the importance of command support cannot be overstated.

Assessment methods can include large-scale unit needs assessments, formal leadership assessments, or more informal means such as "walkabouts." Unit needs assessments vary in scope, and behavioral health providers can use preexisting unit measures or develop their own based on the command environment. Generally, the unit NCO who is considered the Equal Opportunity point of contact has historical knowledge about Command Climate Surveys and can assist the behavioral health provider in construction of an appropriate unit and/or leadership assessment if it is indicated. For informal needs assessments, it is important to assess the following areas using whatever method the behavioral health provider deems appropriate: (1) environmental factors (Do troops have appropriate uniforms for the weather? Do they have heat if it's cold? Do they have protective gear for the area?) and housing conditions (Do they have an appropriate place to sleep? Is the area they are housed healthy and safe? Are they getting adequate nutrition and water? Is the housing area too crowded?); (2) equipment factors (Do they have sufficient protection from threat? Do they have communication that is adequate and consistent? Does their equipment function properly? Have they been trained on the equipment they are using?); (3) command climate (Do they feel supported by their leadership? Do they know how to communicate to their leadership? Do they believe their leadership is giving them clear guidance? Do they have a clear understanding of the rule of engagement and unit ethics? Are there signs of toxic leaders internal to the command); (4) access to health care and positive health behaviors (Do they know how to access medical care? Behavioral health care? Who can they contact for sexual harassment or assault reporting? Whom to report unethical/illegal behavior to? How much are they sleeping? Have they experienced any changes in health behaviors such as exercise, tobacco use, or sleep?); and, finally, (5) home-front concerns (Have any unforeseen home-front issue come up since you deployed? Does your family have adequate support? Do you believe your family could get ahold of you in a crisis? Have there been any concerning changes in the health of family?).

Additional sources of information and secondary assessments that may create a conduit for treatment of COS include the integrated health-care team (primary care providers, nurses, medics), unit chaplains, and unit intelligence officers (who conduct the post-event after action reviews). Unit chaplains and intelligence officers often have the first knowledge when a combat-related serious incident report occurs. It is incredibly important for behavioral health providers to be tied into these individuals for situational awareness, as frequently requests for behavioral health services follow these events. Further, many unit chaplains are licensed and credentialed master's level behavioral health professionals; while they may not be in that role on deployment, they can be a tremendous resource for behavioral health providers. Also, behavioral health providers will be coordinating care with primary care providers who are more likely to be engaged in the care of service members for the duration of the deployment. There will generally be more primary care providers and medics than behavioral health providers, and using these professionals as ancillary behavioral health points of care is imperative. Thus, it becomes important to have a discussion with the team of medical providers for the unit as to how COS signs and symptoms may present as physical maladies. Additionally, behavioral health providers would benefit from seeking constant feedback as to trends in disease and non-battle injuries observed at various treatment centers. Primary care providers must know how to communicate with the behavioral health providers in theater and coordinate for behavioral health care when it becomes necessary. Finally, it is of great importance to report disease and non-battle injuries statistics, including COS encounters, through theater consultants for reallocating behavioral health and/or medical resources in theater, or requesting additional backfill when needed.

Case Study, Part 2

SFC Yamashita follows up with you at the clinic on the base. It is 6 days after the event in which one of his squad members was killed. SFC Yamashita looks different now. Almost nervous, he's smoking again, and says "Doc, I need to talk to you." He describes how since you saw him he's been out on patrols. They had to immediately return after 6 h of sleep. They didn't have anyone else to rotate in, and if he didn't return to his unit as an example to his men, the alternative would have been worse. More soldiers would find ways to avoid returning to patrol; plus, there's a desire to hunt down those who planted the vehicle-borne improvised explosive device and killed their brothers in arms. But SFC Yamashita is not sleeping. "It doesn't matter what shift they put me on, I guess, I'm up all day anyways…," he smiles as he smokes and takes a swig from his energy drink. You hear him describe how he has only 5 months left—only five more until he can return to his family. Things aren't great on the home front, primarily because he hasn't been communicating back home: "It's just easier to call once a week and tell them what they want to hear." But the cost is he feels even more disconnected from his family. SFC Yamashita feels disconnected from everyone, except his men. So he continues to tell you, "I just need something to help me sleep, Doc, so I can take better care of my guys." You walk with him and ask him "tell me a little bit more so I know how I can best help you … with your sleep."

Treatment of COS

The early psychiatric treatment principles—proximity, immediacy, expectancy, and simplicity (PIES)—continue to guide the most effective treatment interventions for COS casualties and can be implemented in any situation—even during deployment. Treatment of COS involves basic reassurance, rest, and most importantly, restorative sleep, as soon as possible after COS is identified. "Three hots and a cot" is considered a true military intervention; simply taking a service member out of the fight long enough to get three hot meals and a good night's sleep is often restorative, allowing the sympathetic overdrive to shut off. However, it is not unusual for treatment of COS to involve differentiating between symptom clusters (e.g., does the patient have COS *and* an underlying psychiatric disorder?) and determining whether additional treatments are warranted. After providers have a sufficient understanding of the deployed environment and the service member's specific situation, it is important to consider which treatment approaches are (1) realistic and feasible given resources, (2) known to be effective (ideally during deployment), and (3) force enabling.

Given that poor sleep is the most often reported symptom of COS and also the body's natural way of restoring homeostasis, it makes logical sense for providers to focus initial efforts on improving sleep. In fact, most providers will hesitate to make a psychiatric diagnosis given that suboptimal sleep is virtually the norm among many deployed troops (Schmitz et al. 2012) and given that lack of sleep is known to cause psychological sequelae that can mirror anxiety and mood disorders. Sleep disturbances may actually necessitate an intervention with command/leadership, in which it is important to ensure that leaders are familiar with their service's specific guidance on sleep. It is important that leaders are held accountable for the sleep environment in their command, which ultimately determines the mission readiness and performance of their unit. Psychoeducation regarding the best ways to facilitate optimum sleep in an environment with continuous operations is strongly encouraged. For instance, this may include educating commanders on optimum times to shift schedules (a minimum of 30 days spent on a cycle before rotation), as well as the importance of shifting sleep *forward* on the clock when moving individuals from one shift to another. It could further include educational courses for all service members in the unit on basic sleep hygiene (i.e., addressing environmental concerns and misuse of caffeine), behavioral methods for improved sleep, and the importance of establishing a routine. First-line treatments of insomnia include behavioral interventions, such as stimulus control, sleep restriction, nightmare re-scripting, and cognitive-behavioral treatment for insomnia. Of note, there is some existing support for these behavioral interventions during deployment (Moore and Krakow 2007). Improving sleep is paramount for recovery of both physical and cognitive functioning. For individuals who are unable to successfully accommodate the requirements of deployment with their sleep schedule, short-term use of medications may be necessary and is a frequent focus of treatment (Schmitz et al. 2012). In general, medications that are not habit forming and are known to have short half-life (and thus lower risk for daytime sedation) are preferred.

Behavioral interventions targeting positive health behaviors are also common for treatment of COS and are considered realistic, effective, and force enabling. At a basic level, these interventions include examining the nutritional content of what deployed persons are consuming. For instance, it is known that deployed service members use *more* dietary supplements than those in garrison, with acknowledged changes to physical conditioning regimens (Austin et al. 2016) but with unknown consequences. Providers may wish to focus in particular on the use of caffeinated and sugary foods that can further cause disruption to an individual's homeostasis. Additional focus may also be warranted for the use of nicotine, given that tobacco use is known to increase during deployments, placing service members at risk for associated complications with healing and emotional dysregulation. The health benefits of exercise are extensive, including reduction in muscle tension, increase in circulation, improvement in the body's ability to burn more fats for energy and stabilize blood sugar levels, and improvement of blood supply to the brain to prevent mood swings. Even though deployments are often to austere environments, there are an increasing number of plyometric and/or cross-fitness exercises that are adaptable for the deployment environment. Engaging in mindfulness activities is known to increase distress tolerance and may include intentional distraction (e.g., reading a book), meditation, and yoga. Relaxation techniques, such as deep breathing, guided meditation, guided imagery, and progressive muscle relaxation, have also demonstrated utility in reducing stress and are feasible in a deployed environment. These skills can help alleviate the symptoms of COS and help soldiers return to baseline functioning.

When psychiatric diagnoses are warranted, anxiety disorders are the most commonly diagnosed psychiatric condition in theater (Schmitz et al. 2012). This is not surprising, as COS is thought to have a possible trajectory toward post-deployment anxiety disorders; however, what has been surprising is that while 63% of patients with a PTSD diagnosis were prescribed medications, only 40% had recommendations for psychotherapy or counseling (Schmitz et al. 2012), which are considered first-line treatment for anxiety disorders. This may be related to the view of medications as practical options for managing symptoms and psychiatric conditions in theater where behavioral health providers are scarce. Use of supportive psychotherapy and evidence-based treatments for PTSD are often applied during a deployment for individuals who have COS, as the symptoms are often quite similar in nature. The main difference is that PTSD is rarely diagnosed during a deployment, as the service member is not yet removed from the source of trauma (i.e., deployment), and COS that mimics acute stress and/or PTSD is considered normal while deployed. Veterans Affairs/Department of Defense clinical practice guidelines (2003) indicate that current evidence-based treatment for PTSD includes cognitive processing therapy, prolonged exposure, and eye movement desensitization and reprocessing therapy. These treatment modalities are generally completed in serial sessions, ranging in length from 8 to 16 sessions, which may not be realistic for most individuals who are deployed. Some providers, including the authors, have adapted aspects of these treatments down range with success (Cigrang et al. 2005; McLay et al. 2010). There is some growing evidence that supports a flexible model of these therapies (Galvoski et al. 2012), which permits providers to vary length of treatment, without disrupting the sequence of techniques utilized in treatment. Given that it can be incredibly challenging to consistently see a service member for treatment during deployment, providers may need to adopt a more solution-focused therapy model—that is, entering each treatment session with the expectation that it may be the only time the provider will be able to see the service member. Then, providers can utilize aspects of treatment known to be effective in a manner that accounts for environmental constraints. This may include using manualized treatments, or it may include using components of broader modalities, such as cognitive behavioral therapy, that are less sequential in nature.

Event-Driven Battlemind Psychological Debriefing is another potential intervention for individuals who have COS and who may be vulnerable to developing a more pronounced anxiety disorder. This intervention is a form of psychological debriefing that is designed for use in three contexts: in-theater event-driven situations where interventions follow potentially traumatizing events during deployment; in-theater time-driven debriefings that occur at specified times to address cumulative effects of stress; and immediate post-deployment briefings to facilitate transition from combat to home (Adler et al. 2008, 2009a, b). There is growing evidence that this form of debriefing that emphasizes posttraumatic growth and cognitive accommodation of traumatic events is helpful during deployment (Jones et al. 2013). This approach is a more flexible model than the Mitchell and Everly (2001) debriefing model (which is not recommended for use during deployment) and is thought to be more conducive to building unit cohesion, helping service members grieve losses, and facilitating normalization of combat experiences while still deployed (Jones et al. 2013).

Given the frequency at which debriefing is requested during deployment (Hung 2008; Jones et al. 2013), it is recommended that deploying providers be well versed in conducting Event-Driven Battlemind Psychological Debriefing.

After anxiety disorders, mood disorders—primarily depressive disorders—followed by occupational/relationship problems, accounted for the remaining majority of psychiatric diagnoses in theater (Schmitz et al. 2012). This is also consistent with research findings regarding post-deployment diagnoses (Hoge et al. 2004). When it comes to treating these conditions, the provider is often left to weigh the treatment options of evidence-based psychotherapy, with sometimes questionable continuity of care, use of psychotropic medications, or supportive psychotherapy. The use of psychotropic medications is not without risk; side effects of various medications, as well as withdrawal symptoms, requirements for medical monitoring, and availability and storage of medications, can be prohibitive. If medications are to be used in theater, the authors recommend the use of a longer half-life selective serotonin reuptake inhibitor or serotonin-norepinephrine reuptake inhibitor that is expected to be readily available in the theater of operations. For psychotherapy, cognitive behavioral therapy has the most robust evidence for treatment depression, although this therapy generally requires homework assignments that may be difficult for service members to complete on deployment. For soldiers who choose to bring their smart devices with them on deployment, use of data platforms or "apps" such as those developed by the Center for Deployment Psychology and Defense Centers of Excellence may prove helpful. It has been the author's experience that service members will complete homework assignments more readily with use of smart phone applications versus worksheets.

With regard to relationship counseling, deployed providers face even further challenges since, generally speaking, one of the persons in the relationship where treatment is indicated is deployed and the other is in the continental USA (i.e., CONUS). Though communication technology remains unreliable during deployment, use of telemedicine may prove helpful in this regard, for both marital and family counseling. Providers may choose to focus on how the service member can utilize strategies to create positive communication with loved ones. There is some research examining how poor communication during deployment can impact perceived depression and combat effectiveness (Cigrang et al. 2013). On the most basic level, relationship therapy addresses communication, cognitive distortions of individuals, and basic strategies to emotionally self-regulate when there is conflict. Service members can benefit from psychoeducation on these principles, and there are numerous books that are frequently housed in the unit chaplain's office that behavioral health providers can recommend for deployed service members struggling with relationship conflict. Additionally, there are several telehealth platforms available for family members who are facing challenges in relationships or child-rearing, in the form of apps, that are available from the Defense Centers for Health and Technology.

Finally, it is important to address suicidality during deployment, in terms of both preventative efforts and appropriate treatment interventions (Warner et al. 2011a). There is a growing body of literature that suggests brief cognitive behavioral therapy dramatically reduces suicide attempts (Rudd 2009) and is applicable in military treatment settings (Bryan et al. 2012). Brief cognitive behavioral therapy is a structured treatment model that focuses on suicide as a problem distinct from psychiatric diagnosis, with emphasis on a patient's mastery of specific skills for management of the "suicidal mode," or behaviors, cognitions, emotions, and physical symptoms that trigger suicidal thinking and subsequent acts (Bryan 2015). The treatment is divided into three phases, and the patient progresses through the phases based on demonstrated competency with skills. Phase I is focused on crisis management and distress tolerance; Phase II focuses on cognitive restructuring of the suicidal belief system, problem solving, and cognitive flexibility; and Phase III focuses on relapse prevention. Most behavioral health providers will facilitate evacuation from theater if service members present with acute suicidality, even if there is no resolved plan or preparation. However, for persons who present with chronic morbid ideation or difficulty with emotional regulation (e.g., borderline personality disorders) that must be managed in theater, this treatment provides an option that may be helpful when evacuation from theater is not possible.

It should be noted that there is no clear evidence about the relationship between COS casualties and treatment and the development of PTSD. The body of evidence of treatment for COS casualties has focused on service members' ability to return to combat rather than on the long-term development of PTSD. However, a recent RAND report noted that service members who had a COS reaction were more likely to later develop PTSD (Vaughn et al. 2015).

Case Study, Part 3

SFC Yamashita is willing to initially focus on his sleep. He is open to using some guided imagery and relaxation techniques and adjusts his caffeine use and intake times. He is unwilling to take any medications due to concern about being able to wake up and respond to an attack. SFC Yamashita's initial response is limited, and you talk with his platoon leader, recommending that he be given 2 days off to rest and recover. The platoon leader arranges for SFC Yamashita to take some items for the unit to the rear where he will have about 48–72 h before needing to return to the base. During this time, SFC Yamashita has the opportunity to take a hot shower, rest, eat several hot meals, and take some time to visit the Internet café to call his family. Upon return, his mood is improved and he is forward thinking. SFC Yamashita elects to continue coming to see you on a weekly basis and begins to establish a willingness to engage in therapy. Over the next 3 months, he completes a course of cognitive behavioral therapy, noting that he finds solace in some of the written exercises you ask him to complete regarding his grief and the loss of his peers. He begins to encourage others in his unit to seek assistance as well, and he works with the unit leadership to improve the unit work-rest cycle to maximize sleep effectiveness, including alternating patrol cycles and identifying better times for follow-up meetings. SFC Yamashita completes the deployment successfully.

Summary and Recommendations

Combat and operational stress is a condition that should be anticipated in all military actions. It will not be eliminated, but it can be mitigated by thorough pre-deployment screenings, behavioral health interventions during deployment, and thorough risk-reduction programs after deployment. Evolving research examining risk for and protective factors against the development of COS and subsequent post-deployment psychiatric conditions is in its infancy, but there are many valuable lessons that can inform the practice of future deploying behavioral health providers. The challenge is for providers to find balance as they negotiate their roles as consultants, advisors, and clinicians on multidisciplinary teams and across multiple echelons of the military unit to which they are assigned or that they are supporting.

Key Concepts

1. Sufficient knowledge about the combat and operational stress (COS) response is imperative. Providers must be able to explain to service members and commanders the etiology of COS and what kinds of preventions and treatments are possible.
2. Sufficient knowledge about the key nodes for assessment and the timing of assessments is critical. Providers must have an understanding of the command environment in which they operate, as well as knowledge of the critical signals/events that indicate assessment for possible intervention.

3. Interventions that are feasible within the operating environment, effective for the conditions treated, and force enabling are important to consider. Providers, like deployed service members, must adapt their way of thinking or risk falling into rigid thinking patterns that can compromise the integrity of a behavioral health unit. That is, providers must be flexible in their conceptualization of patients, in their role as providers, and in embracing the diversity that exists from one deployment experience to the next.
4. Effective COS treatment does not prevent posttraumatic stress disorder (PTSD). A recent review indicated that those who had a COS reaction were more apt to later be diagnosed with PTSD; therefore, it is recommended in future screenings to ask a veteran if they were treated for COS while deployed.

References

Adler AB, Litz BT, Castro CA, Suvak M, Thomas JL, Burrell L, McGurk D, Wright KM, Bliese PD (2008) A group randomized trial of critical incident stress debriefing provided to U.S. peacekeepers. J Trauma Stress 21(3):253–263

Adler AB, Castro CA, McGurk D (2009a) Time-driven battlemind psychological debriefing: a group-level early intervention in combat. Mil Med 174:21–28

Adler AB, Bliese PD, McGurk D, Hoge CW, Castro CA (2009b) Battlemind debriefing and battlemind training as early interventions with soldiers returning from Iraq: randomization by platoon. J Consult Clin Psychol 77:928–940

Austin KG, McLellan TM, Farina EK, McGraw SM, Lieberman HR (2016) Soldier use of dietary supplements, including protein and body building supplements, in a combat zone is different than use in garrison. Appl Physiol Nutr Metab 41:88–95

Bacon BL, Staudenmeier JJ (2003) A historical overview of combat stress control units of the U.S. Army. Mil Med 168:689–693

Bryan CJ, Rudd MD (2006) Advances in the assessment of suicide risk. J Clin Psychol Session 62:185–200

Bryan CJ, Gartner AM, Wertenberger E, Delano KA, Wilkinson E, Breitbach J, et al (2012) Defining treatment completion according to patient competency: a case example using brief cognitive behavioral therapy (BCBT) for suicidal patients. Prof Psychol: Res Pract 43:130–136

Bryan CJ (2015) Cognitive behavioral therapy for preventing suicide attempts: a guide to brief treatments across clinical settings. Routledge, New York

Campise RL, Geller SK, Campise ME (2006) Combat stress. In: Kennedy CH, Zillmer EA (eds) Military psychology: clinical and operational applications. Guilford Press, New York, pp 215–240

Centers for Disease Control and Prevention (CDC) (2012) Energy drink consumption and its association with sleep problems among U.S. service members on a combat deployment – Afghanistan, 2010. Morb Mortal Wkly Rep 61:895–903

Cigrang JA, Peterson AL, Schobitz RP (2005) Three American troops in Iraq: evaluation of a brief exposure therapy treatment for the secondary prevention of combat-related PTSD. Pragmat Case Stud Psychother 1(2):1

Cigrang JA, Talcott W, Tatum J, Baker M, Cassidy D, et al (2013) Intimate partner communication from the war zone: a prospective study of relationship functioning, communication frequency, and combat effectiveness. J Marital Fam Ther 40:332–343

Dailey JI, Ijames VL (2014) Evolution of the combat and operational stress control detachment. Army Med Dept J 2014:8–13

Department of Defense Suicide Event Report (DoDSER) (2013) Annual report. Defense centers of excellence for psychological health & traumatic brain injury (DCoR). Available at: http://t2health.dcoe.mil/sites/default/files/DoDSER-2013-Jan-13-2015-Final.pdf, 2014. Accessed Mar 2016

Department of Defense Annual Report on Sexual Assault in the Military (2014) Office of the under secretary of defense. Washington, DC. Available at: http://sapr.mil/public/docs/reports/FY14_Annual/FY14_DoD_SAPRO_Annual_Report_on_Sexual_Assault.pdf. Accessed Apr 2016

Eidelson R, Pilisuk M, Soldz S (2011) The dark side of the comprehensive soldier fitness. Am Psychol 66:643–644

Feng L, Wu HW, Song GQ, Lu C, Li YH, Qu LH, Chen SG, Liu XM, Chang Q (2015) Chronical sleep interruption-induced cognitive decline assessed by a metabolomics method. Behav Brain Res 30:60–68

Field Manual No. 6-22 Leader Development (2015) Headquarters department of the army. Washington, DC, 30 June. Available at: http://www.milsci.ucsb.edu/sites/secure.lsit.ucsb.edu.mili.d7/files/sitefiles/fm6_22.pdf. Accessed Mar 2016

Finan PH, Quartana PJ, Smith MT (2015) The effects of sleep continuity disruption on positive mood and sleep architecture in health adults. Sleep 38:1735–1742

Galvoski TE, Blain LM, Mott JM, Elwood L, Houle T (2012) Manualized therapy for PTSD: flexing the structure of cognitive processing therapy. J Consult Clin Psychol 80:968–981

Gould BE (2006) Pathophysiology for the health professions, 3rd edn. Elsevier Saunders, St. Louis

Grossman D (1996) On killing: the psychological cost of learning to kill in war and society. Hachette Book Group, New York

Hoge CW (2010) Once a warrior always a warrior: navigating the transition from combat to home, including combat stress, PTSD, and mTBI. Globe Pequot Press, Guilford

Hoge CW, Castro CA, Messer SC, McGurk D, Cotting DI, Koffman RL (2004) Combat duty in Iraq and Afghanistan, mental health problems, and barriers to care. N Engl J Med 351:13–22

Hung B (2008) Behavioral health activity and workload in the Iraq theater of operations. US Army Med Dept J 3:39–42

Joint Mental Health Advisory Team 7 (J-MHAT-7): Operation Enduring Freedom (2010) Afghanistan: report, p 81, Office of the Surgeon General United States Army medical command and Office of the Command Surgeon HQ, CENTCOM, and the Office of the Command Surgeon United States Forces Afghanistan (USFOR-A), February 22, 2011. Available at http://www.armymedicine.army.mil/reports/mhat/mhat_vii?j_MHAT_7.pdf. Accessed Feb 2016

Jones DE, Hammond P, Platoni K (2013) Traumatic event management in Afghanistan: a field report on combat applications in regional command south. Mil Med 178:4–10

Koffel E, Polusny MA, Arbisi PA, Erbes CR (2013) Pre-deployment daytime and nighttime sleep complaints as predictors of post-deployment PTSD and depression in National Guard troops. J Anxiety Disord 27:512–519

Larson GE, Hammer PS, Conway TL, Schmied EA, Galarneau MR, Konoske P, et al (2011) Predeployment and in-theater diagnoses of American military personnel serving in Iraq. Psychiatr Serv 61:15–21

McLay RN, McBrien C, Wiederhold MD, Wiederhold BK (2010) Exposure therapy with and without virtual reality to treat PTSD while in the combat theater: a parallel case series. Cyberpsychol Behav Soc Netw 13:37–42

Mental Health Advisory Team II: Executive Summary (2005) Washington, DC, U.S. Army Surgeon General, Jan 20

Mental Health Advisory Team (MHAT) V Report: Executive Summary (2008) Washington, DC, ffice of the Surgeon General United States Army Medical Command and Office of the Command Surgeon HQ. Available at http://www.armymedicine.army.mil/news/mhat/mhat_V/mhat-v.cfm. Accessed Feb 2016

Mental Health Advisory Team (MHAT) 6: Operation Enduring Freedom 2009 Afghanistan: Executive Summary (2009) Washington, DC, Office of the Surgeon General United States Army Medical Command and Office of the Command Surgeon HQ, CENTCOM, and the Office of the Command Surgeon United States Forces Afghanistan (USFOR-A), November 6. Available at http://www.armymedicine.army.mil/reports/mhat/mhat_vi/MHAT_VI-OEF_Redacted.pdf. Accessed Feb 2016

Minassian A, Geyer MA, Baker DG, Nievergelt CM, O'Connor DT, Risbrough VB (2014) Heart rate variability characteristics in a large group of active-duty marines and relationship to posttraumatic stress. Psychosom Med 76:292–301

Mitchell JT, Everly GS (2001) The basic critical incident stress management course: basic group crisis intervention, 3rd edn. International Critical Incident Stress Foundation, Ellicott City

Monahan P, Hu Z, Rohrbeck P (2013) Mental disorders and mental health problems among recruit trainees, U.S. armed forces, 2000–2012. Med Surveill Mon Rep 20:13–18

Moore BA, Krakow B (2007) Imagery rehearsal therapy for acute posttraumatic nightmares among combat soldiers in Iraq. Am J Psychiatr 164:683–687

Morgan CA III, Wang S, Rasmusson A, Hazlett G, Hauger RL, Charney DS (2000) Plasma neuropeptide-Y concentrations in humans exposed to military survival training. Biol Psychiatry 15:902–909

Morgan CA III, Hazlett G, Wang S, Richardson EG Jr, Schnurr P, Southwick SM (2001) Symptoms of dissociation in humans experiencing acute, uncontrollable stress: a prospective investigation. Am J Psychiatr 158:1239–1247

Morgan CA III, Rasmusson AM, Wang S, Hoyt G, Hauger RL, Hazlett G (2002) Neuropeptide-Y, cortisol, and subjective distress in humans exposed to acute stress: replication and extension of previous report. Biol Psychiatry 15:136–142

Morgan CA III, Southwick S, Hazlett G, Rasmusson A, Hoyt G, Zimolo Z, Charney D (2004) Relationships among plasma dehydroepiandrosterone sulfate and cortisol levels, symptoms of dissociation, and objective performance in humans exposed to acute stress. Arch Gen Psychiatry 61:819–815

Nock MK, Stein MB, Heeringa SG, Ursano RJ, Colpe LJ, et al (2014) Prevalence and correlates of suicidal behavior among soldiers: results from the Army study to assess risk and resilience in service members (Army STARRS). J Am Med Assoc 51:514–522

Phillips CJ, Leardmann CA, Gumbs GR, Smith B (2010) Risk factors for posttraumatic stress disorder among deployed US male marines. BMC Psychiatry 10:52. https://doi.org/10.1186/1471-244X-10.52

Reger GM, Moore BA (2006) Combat operational stress control in Iraq: lessons learned during operation Iraqi freedom. Mil Psychol 18:297–307

Rudd MD (2009) Psychological treatments for suicidal behavior: what are the common elements of treatments that work. In: Wasserman D (ed) Oxford textbook of Suicidology. Oxford University Press, Oxford, pp 427–438

Rundell JR, Ursano RJ (1990) Combat stress disorders and the U.S. air force. Mil Med 155:515–518

Schmitz KJ, Schmied EA, Webb-Murphy JA, Hammer PS, Larson GE, Conway TL, Galarneau MR, Boucher WC, Edwards NK, Johnson DC (2012) Psychiatric diagnoses and treatment of U.S. military personnel while deployed to Iraq. Mil Med 177:380–389

Steenkamp MM, Boasso AM, Nash WP, Litz BT (2014) Does mental health stigma change across the deployment cycle? Mil Med 179:1449–1452

Taylor MK, Sausen KP, Mujica-Parodi LR, Potterat EG, Yanagi MA, Kim H (2007) Neurophysiologic methods to measure stress during survival, evasion, resistance, and escape training. Aviat Space Environ Med 78:224–230

Toblin RL, Riviere LA, Thomas JL, Adler AB, Kok BC, Hoge CW (2012) Grief and physical health outcomes in U.S. soldiers returning from combat. J Affect Disord 136:469–475

U.S. Department of the Army: Field Manual 4-02.51 (2006) (FM8–51). Combat and Operational Stress Control. Washington, DC, Department of the Army, Available at http://www.fas.org/irp/doddir/army/fm4-02-51.pdf. Accessed Feb 2016

VA/DoD Clinical Practice Guidelines for the Management of Post Traumatic Stress (2003) http://www.oqp.med.va.gov/cpg/cpg.htm. Accessed Feb 2016

Vasterling JJ, Proctor SP, Friedman MJ, Hoge CW, Heeren T, King LA, King DW (2010) PTSD symptom increases in Iraq-deployed soldiers: comparison with nondeployed soldiers and associations with baseline symptoms, deployment experiences, and post deployment stress. J Trauma Stress 23:41–51. https://doi.org/10.1002/jts.20487

Vaughn CA, Farmer CM, Breslau J, Burnette C (2015) Evaluation of the operational stress control and readiness (OSCAR) program. RAND Health Q 30:14

WaitsWM, Ganz MB, Schillreff T, Dell PJ (2014) Sleep and the use of energy products in a combat environment. US Army Med Dept J :22–28

Warner CH, Appenzeller GN, Barry MJ, Morton A, Grieger T (2007) The evolving role of the division psychiatrist. Mil Med 172:918–924

Warner CH, Appenzeller GN, Parker JR, Warner C, Diebold CJ, Grieger T (2011a) Suicide prevention in a deployed military unit. Psychiatry 74:127–141

Warner CH, Appenzeller GN, Mobbs A, Parker JR, Warner CM, Grieger T, Hoge CW (2011b) Effectiveness of a battlefield ethics training during combat deployment: a programme assessment. Lancet 378:915–924

Warner CH, Appenzeller GN, Parker JR, Warner CM, Hoge CW (2011c) Effectiveness of mental health screening and coordination of in-theater care prior to deployment to Iraq: a cohort study. Am J Psychiatry 168:378–385

Wilmoth MC, Linton A, Gromadzki R, Larson MJ, Williams TV, Woodson J (2015) Factors associated with psychiatric evacuation among service members deployed to operation enduring freedom and operation Iraqi freedom, January 2004 to September 2010. Mil Med 180:53–60

Wojcik BE, Akhtar FZ, Hassell LH (2009) Mil Med 174:1010–1018

17 Military Sexual Assault

David E. Johnson and Jennifer Yeaw

Introduction

Public interest in sexual assault and sexual harassment within the military and Department of Veterans Affairs (VA) exploded with the 1991 Tailhook scandal involving US Navy aviators. Attention and advocacy have remained high through subsequent high-profile events and investigations, resulting in significant changes in the way that both organizations respond to allegations of sexual assault. Converse to lay opinion, most sexual assaults do not involve a stranger using actual or threatened force against a victim. Rather, most occur between individuals known to each other and often involve incapacitation with alcohol. Victims often demonstrate little to no resistance due to a combination of blunted consciousness or fear of reprisal. Military law has undergone frequent updates to address these factors, while military and VA medical systems have made marked adjustments to bring treatment to sexual assault survivors. Despite these interventions, survivors face a host of adverse medical and psychological sequelae and often prematurely end their prospective military careers. This chapter examines how the complex interplay of medical and societal factors creates systemic challenges and large-scale solutions.

D.E. Johnson (✉)
Center for Forensic Behavioral Sciences, Walter Reed National Military Medical Center, Bethesda, MD, USA
e-mail: dejforensic@gmail.com

J. Yeaw
Benesh & Yeaw Consulting LLC, Upper Marlboro, MD, USA
e-mail: beneshyeaw@gmail.com

Case Study

Specialist (SPC) Ashley Smith (pseudonym) is a 20-year-old female soldier in first squad, second platoon of a hypothetical infantry company. She interacts daily with her direct supervisor, Sergeant (SGT) Michael Jones (pseudonym). SPC Smith, like most of the squad, attends a Friday night party at SGT Jones's residence. Copious quantities of beer and hard liquor are freely available, and all but a few become extremely intoxicated. SPC Smith interacts with SGT Jones multiple times throughout the evening, often laughing and having a good time. Several partygoers see her consume multiple shots throughout the night. She eventually vomits outside and requires assistance to walk back into the house. Her female battle buddy takes her upstairs to lie on a bed. The battle buddy leaves SPC Smith, fully clothed, turns the lights off, and goes back to the party.

SPC Smith experiences alcohol-induced anterograde amnesia, aka "a blackout,"

L.W. Roberts, C.H. Warner (eds.), *Military and Veteran Mental Health*,
https://doi.org/10.1007/978-1-4939-7438-2_17

during this period. She later recalls feeling repetitive movement against her. She recalls seeing a snippet of a male figure above her on the bed and realizes he is performing sexual intercourse on her. Her limbs feel heavy and her thinking is clouded. She wants to resist but feels unable to move or scream. She next remembers seeing the male leaving the room. Light shines in as he opens the door, and she recognizes SGT Jones, her squad leader and a good friend. Still unable to compel her body into action, she remains on the bed and falls asleep.

The next day she feels hungover and confused. Wondering if her memory in fact occurred, she eventually text-messages SGT Jones and asks him how the night was. He vaguely replies that it was a fun night for everyone. On Monday, at work, she sees him at formation and experiences twinges of fear and mistrust. She begins avoiding him at work, to the point that she is not completing her own work. She eventually confides in a trusted female friend. Her friend encourages her to report the incident to military police. She also reports to Behavioral Health (BH) for anxiety symptoms.

Despite assurances of confidentiality, rumors of her allegation spread through her squad and the entire company. SGT Jones tells peers that consensual sex occurred between him and SPC Smith and that this is a case of "buyer's remorse." SPC Smith receives both support and harassment. Her close-knit squad divides into two camps over the issue. Although the commander moves SGT Jones to a different working location pending the investigation, SPC Smith nonetheless requests her own transfer due to strained relationships with peers who side with SGT Smith. Per regulation, command approves her transfer. Upon arrival at a new duty station, her new supervisor informs her that the company is aware of why she is transferring in and that he hopes there will not be any "new trouble" in the future.

In discussion with the local Army prosecutor, she learns that there is a less than 50% chance that SGT Jones would be found guilty of sexual assault. Factors working against her include that the only evidence is her own alcohol-fogged memory. Another is SGT Smith's reputation as an upstanding, hardworking noncommissioned officer with no history of criminal behavior. She also learns that she must eventually testify about her traumatic memories at a public trial and that SGT Jones will be there. The prosecutor informs her that the defense attorney will likely seek access to her behavioral health records to search for evidence against her and tells her about another case in which a rape survivor's request for a transfer was grounds to release her records. She wonders if her statements to her therapist about her childhood sexual abuse by her father might become open information to the court and to SGT Smith. She visits the behavioral health clinic as an urgent walk-in twice that week due to panic attacks, brought on while pondering these legal uncertainties.

The Increasing Public Awareness of Military Sexual Assault

Scenarios like the one described in the case study occur all too commonly, despite over two decades' worth of legislative intervention. Federal legal, medical, and administrative systems have increasingly recognized that, as with this chapter's case study, most military sexual assaults occur between acquaintances and do not follow a "forcible rape" schema (Rosenstein and Carroll 2015; McKimmie et al. 2014; Castro et al. 2015). In 1992, Congress responded to Tailhook with Public Law 102–585 which authorized VA services for female veterans who experienced sexual assault or harassment, referred to as military sexual trauma (MST), while on active duty. Treatment for MST was extended to veterans not normally eligible for VA treatment. In 1994, Congress expanded treatment eligibility to male veterans. Legislation in 2004 made the MST program permanent and extended it to include reservists and guardsmen who experienced MST while on active duty status.

The military response to sexual assault accelerated with the Care for Victims of Sexual Assault Task Force in 2004. This led to Department of Defense (DoD) Directive 6496.01, the Sexual Assault Prevention and Response Policy, in October 2005, and the creation of the Sexual Assault Prevention and Response Office (SAPRO) to coordinate all efforts. Starting in fiscal year (FY) 2007, SAPRO released annual Sexual Assault Prevention and Response (SAPR) reports to the President of the United States. Parallel to these efforts, modifications to the military criminal definition of rape began in 2007 (Sameit 2013).

Operational and Statutory Definitions of Sexual Assault

Rape is a topic of interest to social scientists of multiple disciplines, including epidemiology and public health, clinical psychology and medicine, social psychology, criminal justice, cognitive psychology, and nursing. Widely studied, a Web of Science search using the topic "rape" returned over 33,000 publications in the past 10 years (Web of Science 2016). The volume of research makes identification of trends and consensus findings possible, but the variability of methodology across fields can make comparison difficult, particularly with regard to estimates of incidence and prevalence. Clinical research tends to focus on the needs of those who report a sexual assault and those who present with sequelae of sexual assault, whether or not a crime was reported to law enforcement. Operational definitions of "rape" or "sexual assault" tend to be broad and generally do not include any value judgment as to credibility or criminality. Perhaps the broadest example is "military sexual trauma" or MST, the term favored by the VA, which includes "sexual harassment…which is threatening in character" (Department of Veterans Affairs 2015b). In contrast, social psychology and criminal justice studies tend to use narrower operational definitions tied to a specific statutory scheme or to a successful prosecution. Additionally, though most scientific literature, legal statutes, and legal professionals use the term "victim," this chapter uses the term "survivor" due to the chapter's focus on interventions promoting recovery. Varying statutory definitions result in variability in how police classify crimes, how crimes are investigated, whether they are prosecuted, and the likelihood of criminal convictions. The primary nationwide database on sexual assault crimes, the Federal Bureau of Investigation (FBI) Uniform Crime Report (UCR), compiles criminal data from most of the states, yet until 2013 its definition of "rape" excluded male survivors, any survivors of non-vaginal penetration, and incapacitated survivors (Federal Bureau of Investigation 2016). Military law followed this FBI definition until late 2007.

Crimes committed by service members are prosecuted under the Uniform Code of Military Justice (UCMJ). The UCMJ Article 120 contains the military statutory definition of rape and other sex crimes. Article 120 has been updated several times in recent years, reflecting an intent to enable better prosecution of the wide range of rape or sexual assault scenarios that did not easily fit within the older, narrower framework of "forcible rape." Within the military, the 2012 Uniform Code of Military Justice subsumes four categories under the collective label Article 120 – "Rape and Sexual Assault generally." Depending on factors such as use of force, penetration, and incapacity to express consent, Article 120 defines four major categories: rape, sexual assault, aggravated sexual contact, and abusive sexual contact. However, prior to June 28, 2012, different categorization and statutory language existed and again prior to October 1, 2007. These changes, as well as changes in state laws, mean that survivors may have had different experiences in the prosecution of their sexual assault depending on the year in which it occurred. For example, the 2012 version now includes language that contact or penetration with the mouth or anus constitutes a sexual act and provides clearer definitions of consent in scenarios where survivors are intoxicated, do not forcibly resist, or have no memory of the alleged sexual act. Veterans who experienced a sexual assault in 1970 may have faced greater hurdles in bringing a claim forward than an active duty member would in 2017, due to older statutory limitations as well as prevention and response systems described later in this chapter.

This chapter defines the term "sexual assault" as any non-consensual sexual contact involving any body parts, with or without penetration, and excludes purely verbal sexual harassment. This is in keeping with the clinical and public health focus of the text. VA data tends to study MST, not just sexual assault, so some inclusion of sexual harassment numbers is unavoidable in this chapter. Readers should remain alert to the fact that references to MST data from the VA include sexual harassment survivors, not just sexual assault survivors. No matter how a jurisdiction defines sexual assault, clinicians are free to label any patient's traumatic sexual event as a sexual assault and intervene appropriately.

Epidemiology: Relevant Characteristics of Sexual Assault

Civilian Population

There is broad consensus that most sexual assaults are never reported to law enforcement and that crime statistics alone do not present an accurate view of incidence or prevalence of sexual assault. Population survey research capturing reported and unreported sexual assaults supplements law enforcement data to get the full picture of prevalence. Civilian studies provide large datasets that are directly applicable to active duty military and veteran populations. Even among reported crimes, charges may never be filed due to lack of evidence or doubts about achieving a guilty verdict in court. Prevalence varies depending on various factors such as population density and socioeconomic status. Many studies include child sexual abuse with adult sexual assault, though the dynamics and survivor psychology may be much different. Further complicating things, several studies have estimated that the reporting rate of sexual assault—however defined—in the US population is between 5% and 20% (Lonsway and Archambault 2012), meaning research from police databases undercounts survivors. Finally, so-called unacknowledged victims may not classify their own past experiences as an assault, even on anonymous surveys (Cleere and Lynn 2013; Krebs et al. 2011). Thus, the wording of survey questions may capture or exclude survivors if the question assumes that survivors recognize themselves as sexual assault survivors. With these factors in mind, lifetime prevalence rates for female sexual assault survivors often fall within a range of nearly 20% (Tjaden and Thoennes 1998; Elliott et al. 2004; Breiding 2014), though some studies find higher rates (Finkelhor et al. 1990). The Centers for Disease Control and Prevention (CDC) found that of female sexual assault survivors, 38% experienced the assault within the age range of 18–24. One recent study estimated that 20–25% of US college women experience a completed or attempted rate (Fisher et al. 2000). This age cohort more closely mirrors the age distribution of active duty women and supports the generalizability of data collected on college students. Further, it shows that the military is receiving a large number of sexual assault survivors into its ranks from the recruitment pool. Sexual assault occurring within ongoing sexual relationships, termed intimate partner violence, has its own extensive literature, which is not covered in this chapter.

Military Population

Starting with fiscal year 2011, Congress required that the Department of Defense (DoD) produce an annual report on the issue of sexual assaults to the Committee on Armed Services. The annual report provides the most comprehensive overview of DoD's Sexual Assault Prevention and Response (SAPR) program. SAPR annual reports use an evolving array of data sources, such as the Workplace and Gender Relations Survey of Active Duty Members (WGRA) in 2012, the RAND Military Workplace Study (RMWS) in 2014, and the Survivor Experience Survey (SES) in 2014. As with any survey, respondents may underreport, while others may give false or inaccurate answers. However, there has been consistent effort on the part of Sexual Assault Prevention and Response and Department of Defense to improve research methodology (Morral et al. 2015a) and address the pervasive lack of consistent terminology (Logan et al. 2013) in the sexual assault literature, though the definition has been aligned with the legal definition under the Uniform Code of Military Justice.

According to the 2014 annual report, 5121 active duty service members reported experiencing a sexual assault (Department of Defense 2014). Using additional survey data and statistical extrapolation, RAND estimated that approximately 10,600 men and 9600 women out of 1,317,561 service members were sexually assaulted in fiscal year 2014 (Morral et al. 2015b). This represents 1 in 20 women and 1 in 100 men or 4.9% of all active duty women and 1.0% of all active duty men. It does not count an estimated 1.4% of active duty personnel who experienced "unwanted sexual contact" not amounting to the Uniform Code of Military Justice definition of sexual assault. Approximately 90% of all sexual assaults were allegedly perpetrated by other active duty personnel or within military settings.

Considering that these data reflect 1 year of risk for active duty personnel, an individual's lifetime risk of sexual assault rises with each year of service. One survey of female VA veterans found that 23% reported a sexual assault during their active duty years (Skinner et al. 2000). Granted, this population includes veterans from past conflicts such as the Gulf War and the Vietnam War, when a number of environmental and systemic variables differed from the current active duty climate. Other studies have arrived at female sexual assault rates of 1 in 4–1 in 3 while on active duty (Suris and Lind 2008). This is roughly similar to the estimate for college women cited above. Studies of US women, by comparison, have found lower rates for women such as 16% (Kilpatrick et al. 2007). Perhaps the best study comparing the prevalence of sexual assault between women on active duty versus the general population found similar lifetime rates, 40% and 36%, respectively, for the age range 18–59 (Black and Merrick 2013).

As the military is predominately male, there were more male survivors than female survivors in 2014, but only 8% of male survivors reported the crime versus 22% of female survivors (Morral et al. 2015c). MST data from the VA shows that women are more likely to experience MST, but 54% of all VA patients who screen positive for MST are male (Turner and Frayne 2004) since men vastly outnumber women in the VA system. The topic of male sexual assault, mostly overshadowed by female sexual assault over the past decade, will likely receive greater scrutiny, especially following a 2015 General Accounting Office (GAO) report on the topic to the Secretary of Defense (United States Government Accountability Office 2015).

The military data parallels civilian data that many, if not most, sexual assaults are committed by non-strangers. According to the 2014 RAND survey, 85% of male survivors and 93% of female survivors knew their assailant, with 46% of male survivors and 67% of female survivors describing the assailant as a "friend or acquaintance." 80% and 90% reported that the "friend or acquaintance" was an active duty military member, with over 50% being of a higher rank than the survivor.

Alcohol use also figures prominently in a large number of military sexual assaults. Twenty-five percent of men and 41% of women report they were drinking at the time of the assault, and 24% of men and 50% of women reported the assailant was drinking. Nine percent of male survivors and 3% of female survivors reported suspicion that they were slipped a date rape drug. As referenced elsewhere in this chapter, alcohol's deleterious effects on memory and ability or willingness to consent may cause greater psychological burden and hinder prosecution efforts.

Systemic Challenges

Prosecution

A therapist attempting to understand a survivor's decision to not report a sexual assault, or their struggle to decide whether to press charges, must understand the systemic factors working against the survivor. Multiple factors explain the low numbers of sexual assault allegations that result in guilty verdicts in a court of law. Some factors are unique to military jurisdictions, while others are universal. The evidence in these cases often does not reach the "beyond a reasonable doubt" standard required for a criminal conviction. There is often no evidence other than a survivor's verbal report. The presence of DNA does not provide guilt, especially when the perpetrator claims consensual sex occurred. Investigations may halt because prosecutors decide the evidence is insufficient to secure a guilty verdict at court-martial. The defense often presents "reasonable doubt" in terms of contradictory statements made by the survivor to different interviewers or witnesses. In many cases, the memory-impairing effect of alcohol or other substances clouds the survivor's ability to accurately report what happened (White 2003). Defenses seek to use survivors' personal history to imply that the allegation is false and serving an ulterior motive.

For military sexual assault allegations in fiscal year 2014, 15% of cases resulted in a sexual or nonsexual conviction, 10% resulted in a prison sentence, and 7% of defendants received mandatory registration as sex offenders. Less than 37% of cases proceeded to court-martial. Many cases were resolved through nonjudicial punishment, while over 500 were deemed "unfounded." By comparison, one study of the civilian legal system found a sexual assault felony conviction rate of 0.2–5.2% and an incarceration rate of 0.2–2.8%. Even then, only 0.2–2.9% of the convictions were for felony charges (Lonsway and Archambault 2012). Even without knowing these exact statistics, survivors often have intuitive understanding that pursuing full criminal prosecution may have a disappointing outcome.

Survivors cite many reasons for not reporting sexual assaults or refusing to participate in courts-martial after having initially reported the crime. The majority of men and women survivors state that they did not report due to their desire to "forget about it and move on." The second most common reason is they did not want anyone to know about the crime, while the third most common reason is that they thought the issue was not serious enough to report. Men were more fearful of being labeled homosexual, while women were more likely to feel partially to blame for the sexual assault. Significant numbers of both sexes feared outcomes such as retaliation, not being believed, having others blame them, career damage, and the system being unable to help them (Morral et al. 2015c).

Privacy Concerns

All forms of psychotherapy rely on a trusting, confidential relationship with a practitioner. For psychiatrists and psychologists, maintaining the confidentiality of a patient's communications is a primary ethical duty. Congress and the courts have recognized that the promise of privacy in psychotherapeutic relationships is of fundamental importance to advance the public interest of promoting the mental health of our citizens. Most patients recognize that there are some limits to confidentiality, and most practitioners can discuss how those limits apply in typical clinical settings. However, when the patient is a party to a criminal proceeding, the rules that govern psychotherapist-patient privilege, the legal enforcement of confidentiality, are unclear and unsettled (Fishman 2007). This is particularly true in military courts, for two reasons unique to the military (Zimmerman 2015). First, since psychotherapist-patient privilege was recognized in Military Rules of Evidence (MRE) 513, unique exceptions have been made allowing disclosure of information necessary to ensure a fit and effective fighting force (Department of Defense 2016). Second, military psychotherapist-patient privilege has been the subject of legislation and litigation over the past several years, and the clear impact of these changes for practitioners and their patients is likely several years off (Judicial Proceedings Panel 2015). This is troubling, because as the US Supreme Court noted, even the possibility of disclosure can impede development of a therapeutic relationship, and uncertain privilege is little better than no privilege at all (Redmond 1996).

In criminal law, privilege in general is based on recognition of a public interest so important that it overrides the general presumption that criminal defendants are entitled to present all relevant evidence. The landmark case in the Federal Courts is *Jaffee v. Redmond* (1996). In this case, the US Supreme Court recognized that psychotherapist-patient privilege serves the public interest by promoting mental health and that, as with attorneys and spouses, relationships between patients and psychotherapists have an "imperative need for confidence and trust." Psychotherapist-patient privilege has been a part of the Uniform Code of Military Justice since 1999 (Executive Order No. 13, 140, 64 1999).

Psychotherapist-patient privilege, MRE 513, is not an absolute privilege, because a military judge has the authority to review the records to determine whether or not the records contain an exception and can be released. It is helpful to compare MRE 513 with MRE 412, the military's version of the rape shield law. MRE 412 protects sexual assault survivors from invasive and degrading investigations into their sexual history. Both rules contain privacy protections for survivors of sexual assault, but MRE 412 is a rule of relevance, not of privilege. Generally, the sexual proclivities of an accusing witness are considered to be irrelevant to determine whether or not a particular accused committed sexual assault.

MRE 513 has exceptions that are similar to most civilian jurisdictions. However, there is a military-specific exception allowing disclosure: "when necessary to ensure the safety and security of military personnel, military dependents, military property, classified information, or the accomplishment of a military mission." The legal contours of military psychotherapist-patient privilege are actively changing. As of 2016, there were seven exceptions to MRE 513 psychotherapist-patient privilege (Department of Defense 2016).

There remains a risk that the mental health records of survivors of sexual assault will be reviewed as part of the assault prosecution. Clinicians should be aware of the potential legal relevance of the records being created as part of treatment. Attorneys may request mental health records for evidence to use to impeach the witness, usually to determine if the statements made to the psychotherapist are consistent with prior statements and statements expected at trial. Records are also requested as evidence of a mental disease or defect that would tend to make testimony less reliable or evidence of a motive to fabricate. Desire to preserve a relationship after infidelity has been seen as a motive to fabricate, and thus evidence of current or past relationship conflict could be relevant. Military survivors of sexual assault are afforded a number of protections to guard against retaliation and to ensure fitness for duty. For example, expedited transfers out of the unit may be requested, and a behavioral health provider can place temporary or permanent duty restrictions if occupational impairment is a concern. In some cases, this may amount to a motive to fabricate, as in suggestions that an allegation of sexual assault was falsely made to secure a change of duty location or requirement. In instances of alcohol-facilitated sexual assault, the records may contain information relevant to the plausibility of the survivor's reported level of impairment due to intoxication.

End of Military Career Due to Sexual Assault

Active duty survivors may face the end of their military career through a variety of mechanisms. Any psychiatric symptoms may compromise their ability to work, either stateside or in combat zones. This may result in a medical discharge from active duty, either with or without lifetime disability benefits depending on the severity. Harassment at work may contribute to the symptom severity or result in decreased work performance. Even without need for mental health treatment, the loss of trust for peers or the perception that the military did not stand by their side may lead the survivor to leave service at the end of their contract. In one study, one-third of female sexual assault survivors had left service soon after a sexual assault due to disability proceedings or a reason other than routine end-of-tour separation or retirement (Millegan et al. 2015).

The Feres doctrine prevents military members from suing other military members for civil damages (Kels 2012), partly on the basis that the military disability system provides money to survivors. A civil lawsuit requires a lower level of proof in a criminal trial, so survivors could potentially "win" more often. Ironically, many survivors leave service without disability despite having significant psychological trauma. Survivors may be hard-pressed to find civilian equivalent employment offering lifetime pension and health benefits. Male veterans with military sexual assault history have greater risk for being unemployed after their active duty service.

Systemic Improvements

Improvements in the Military

Prevention strategies include mandatory education and refresher training given to all active duty military members and increased emphasis on the role of the commander in promoting a safe climate. To improve reporting, the military allows survivors to make restricted reports, which prevents military law enforcement from learning about the report (Department of Defense 2015). A survivor may make restricted reports to a Sexual Assault Response Coordinator (SARC), a Sexual Assault Prevention and Response Victim Advocate (SAPR VA), or any medical provider who will pass on the information solely to the SARC or SAPR VA (Department of Defense 2015). The SARC or SAPR VA may refer patients to a sexual assault behavioral health provider, other medical providers, and a nurse case manager, all of whom are predesignated and trained for dealing with sexual assault survivors.

If the assault occurred during active duty service, then restricted reporting also provides access to Special Victims Counsel (SVCs), termed Victims' Legal Counsel (VLC) in the US Navy (Department of Defense 2013). The SVC/VLCs are experienced attorneys who provide survivors the legal perspective including pursuing charges, confidentiality of medical records, accused's rights, and the courtroom experience. SVCs are not part of the prosecution of the case, allowing them to remain focused on the survivor's needs and not the myriad of other components of a legal case. When survivors make an unrestricted report, their service's criminal investigative organization opens a case, and prosecution may ensue.

In 2011, military survivors gained the ability to request expedited transfer to a new duty station within 72 h of an unrestricted report, enabling survivors to escape uncomfortable work environments with the assailant or hostile coworkers (Department of Defense 2015). Other improvements since 2011 include the creation of confidential phone lines, apps, and chat rooms for survivors. The creation of a Victim Advocate-Victim privilege, termed Military Rule of Evidence 514, in the Uniform Code of Military Justice, ensured a degree of confidentiality from victim advocates being subpoenaed to testify about a survivor's statements to them, though it contains exceptions (Department of Defense 2016).

Congress has expressed its intent that military psychotherapist privilege be strengthened. The National Defense Appropriations Act of fiscal year 2015 (hereafter referred to as NDAA 2015) eliminated the "constitutionally required" exemption to privilege and codified procedural requirements that must be met before a witness' mental health records can be subjected to review by a judge (United States Senate 2015). There are a number of cases currently pending before the Court of Appeals of the Armed Forces, and the rulings will have implications for how military courts determine whether or not privilege must be pierced (Judicial Proceedings Panel 2015). Further analysis of the present state of privilege would be speculative and very likely outdated and inaccurate by the time this chapter is published.

Sexual assault medical forensic examiner (SAMFE) standards are promulgated by the US Department of Justice (DOJ) (United States Department of Justice Office of Violence Against Women 2013) and standardized for the military at the Department of Defense level (United States Senate 2015). The military services have established protocols by which their medical facilities have access to sexual assault medical forensic examiners (SAMFEs), also known as sexual assault nurse examiners (SANEs) to conduct sexual assault forensic examinations (SAFEs), either in-house or through memoranda of understanding with other local medical centers. For example, in overseas operational settings, the Army requires sexual assault medical forensic examiner capabilities at the combat support hospital (CSH) level, though it may exist when possible at smaller locations. Sexual assault survivors are transported to the combat support hospital emergently. Sexual Assault Response Coordinators (SARCs) and Sexual Assault Prevention and Response Victim Advocates (SAPR VAs) are stationed at the combat support hospital (Department of the Army 2014), and SAPR VAs may accompany survivors during travel, including back to the continental US (United States Army Medical Department 2015).

High-profile media reports and congressional inquiries have placed the spotlight on lack of military prosecution of sexual assault cases. Likely related to this, the number of alleged perpetrators for which commanders initiated the court-martial process rose from 30% in FY07 to 66% in FY14 (Department of Defense 2015). The military has seen annual increases in both reporting (Department of Defense 2015) and in survivors switching their reports from restricted to unrestricted (Department of Defense 2015). Promotion of sexual assault awareness and reporting options, as well as the number of confidential advisors now available to survivors, likely contributes to the increases in reporting. However, despite improvements, only 23% of active duty women and 43% of active duty men felt there were zero barriers to reporting sexual assault (Department of Defense Sexual Assault and Prevention Office 2012).

Military criminal investigative organizations (MCIOs) are also modifying their techniques. Survivors with spotty memory due to intoxicants or traumatic reactions may provide little useful information, may provide contradictory information on repeated interviews, and are vulnerable to generating false memories in response to leading questions. The traditional police approach of learning "just the facts" does not help improve this situation. All of the military criminal investigative organizations have adopted newer interview methods for sexual assault survivors. The Air Force utilizes the cognitive interviewing literature (Fisher and Geiselman 2010), while the Army and Navy use Forensic Experiential Trauma Interviewing (FETI) (Inspector General of the United States Department of Defense 2013).

Improvements in the Veterans Administration

As defined by Title 38 US Code 1720D, military sexual trauma (MST) is "psychological trauma resulting from a physical assault of a sexual nature, battery of a sexual nature, or sexual harassment which occurred while the Veteran was serving on active duty, active duty for training, or inactive duty training." Sexual harassment is defined as "repeated, unsolicited verbal or physical contact of a sexual nature which is threatening in character."

Since 2002, Veterans Affairs (VA) facilities offer free treatment for MST-related conditions for all VA-eligible veterans. Veterans who do not qualify for VA care may still sometimes receive care for MST-related conditions (Department of Veterans Affairs 2015a). Services include outpatient and inpatient care, and gender-specific treatment settings exist (Department of Veterans Affairs 2015b). The VA reports 1 in 4 women and 1 in 100 men respond affirmatively to screening questions for MST. Treatment for a MST-related condition remains optional. Screening for MST has led to higher treatment rates for both male and female veterans (Kimerling et al. 2008).

The VA further allows for relaxed evidentiary standards as far as verifying if a military trauma occurred while the service member was on active duty. This policy is consistent with the fact that most sexual assaults go unreported. Evidence of social or occupational dysfunction, sexual dysfunction, or collateral information from family and acquaintances may be used to support a VA claim for MST services. There need not be past documentation of a sexual assault or investigation. As with other medical conditions incurred while on active duty, a veteran may eventually qualify for formal disability status, with its attendant financial and medical benefits, due to the psychiatric sequelae of MST.

VA hospitals have protocols in place for the medical and forensic evaluation of emergency sexual assault survivors (Department of Veterans Affairs 2010a). As with the military, VA facilities may have internal capabilities or memoranda of understanding with other capable facilities. VA hospitals also have MST Coordinators as the point of contact for survivors for coordinating care and helping jump administrative hurdles (Department of Veterans Affairs 2010b). The VA relies on local civilian laws for reporting and investigation of sexual assault allegations. A universal system with survivor advocates and special victim counsels, as in the military, is not possible for the VA. However, MST Coordinators may have knowledge to make informed referrals of patients to local law enforcement.

Impact on Survivor

Both male and female survivors of military sexual assault have greater rates of psychological and physical sequelae than military non-survivors (Millegan et al. 2015, 2016). Some studies have found higher rates of PTSD due to military sexual assault than nonmilitary sexual assault (Yaeger et al. 2006). Approximately 50% of female sexual assault survivors develop PTSD (Creamer et al. 2001) and, in one study, 65% in male survivors (Millegan et al. 2016). The risk of PTSD following military sexual assault remains strong in both men and women, even when controlling for combat exposure (Kang et al. 2005).

Previous Sexual Assault Predicts Poorer Outcomes

Although discussion to this point has centered on sexual assaults occurring while on active duty status, 8.6% of sexual assault reports reported while on active duty involve incidents before the survivor entered the military (Department of Defense 2014). Further, one study found that 30.3% of active duty women reporting sexual assault also reported a previous sexual assault while still a civilian (Kimerling et al. 2007). A review of civilian studies concluded that two-thirds of sexual assault survivors may have previous sexual victimization history (Classen et al. 2005). Any sexual assault may lead to active duty service members seeking medical and psychiatric assistance. However, for veterans without VA eligibility, federal law currently only allows treatment for problems related to a sexual assault while on active duty status.

Some studies indicate that women in the military may have not only higher rates but also more severe experiences with childhood sexual assault than civilian control groups (Schultz et al. 2006). The combination of military sexual assault with previous childhood sexual assault is associated with more negative outcomes than nonmilitary sexual assault (Suris et al. 2007). In general, childhood sexual assault is a risk factor for later adult sexual victimization and assault (Lalor and McElvaney 2010; Desai et al. 2002).

Military-Specific Factors Predict Poorer Outcomes

The potential for combat exposure in today's military further complicates the medical sequelae of sexual assault. Co-occurring combat trauma may predict poorer outcomes, as might a sexual assault within a combat zone. Sexual harassment, independent of sexual assault, has much empirical support for worse psychological and physical sequelae. There is fair supporting evidence to hypothesize that military sexual harassment contributes to poor outcomes among military sexual assault survivors (Stander and Thomsen 2016; Settles et al. 2014). Veterans are at risk for developing PTSD due to multiple traumatic events, such as experiencing both sexual assault and seeing a colleague killed in action. Chronic pain may be secondary to psychological trauma but may very well have a physical source due to combat injury. Mild traumatic brain injury (mTBI) can occur in trauma survivors and brings its own host of medical comorbidities.

Tonic Immobility Predicts Poorer Outcomes

Another line of research ties tonic immobility during a sexual assault with poorer PTSD outcomes. Tonic immobility describes "freezing," such as inability to move or scream, during a sexual assault (TeBockhurst et al. 2015). Though tonic immobility is described as the human analog of the instinctual "freeze" reflex observed in some animals, others question whether it includes full or partial dissociation. Descriptions of survivor "freezing" are common in law enforcement reports. Intoxication by alcohol or date rape drugs may contribute to tonic immobility or simply create an alternative freezing mechanism. Survivors may experience greater degrees of self-blame due to their inability to resist. This may be particularly true of military members, who have increased confidence in their ability to resist a physical attack by virtue of their training, while the tendency to dissociate may indicate greater use of primitive defense mechanisms and thus greater resistance to therapy. Tonic immobility during child sexual assault experiences may affect as many as half of all child survivors (Heidt et al. 2005). Research into whether that childhood response might predict a similar immobility during military sexual assault has not been performed. Therapists should remain aware that untreated or latent PTSD from childhood sexual assault may cause a flashback experience during an adult-age sexual assault, hence a recurrent "freezing" as an adult.

Poorer Psychological and Physical Health After Sexual Assault

Sexual assault survivors are at risk for developing PTSD, major depression, anxiety disorders, somatoform disorders, and substance use disorders. Survivors may also experience secondary traumatization from involvement in investigative and judicial processes. The choice to not report at all may also impact psychological recovery, due to lack of punishment for the perpetrator or the realization that the perpetrator is free to assault others. Not all survivors seek psychiatric assistance, leading to worsening of symptoms or self-medication. Multiple sexual assaults, or overlap with combat trauma, may also lead to worse long-term outcomes.

Survivors report higher rates of physical symptoms compared to individuals with no sexual assault history. These symptoms are often not secondary with any physical harm sustained during the sexual assault, and studies have often found that physical health was normal until a sexual assault occurred (Koss et al. 1991). These symptoms also encompass a wider range, frequency and severity compared to non-traumatized individuals (McFarlane 2013; Frayne et al. 1999). The symptoms encompass virtually every body system, including muscular, cardiovascular, gastrointestinal, sexual, respiratory, and neurological systems.

Survivors with PTSD take on an additional burden of physical problems due to PTSD's association with several chronic physical complaints or conditions. Chronic pain is more common in trauma survivors and PTSD sufferers, though many studies lack information as to whether the pain preexisted before the traumatic event. In one study, 80% of women with a history of physical or sexual violence reported having chronic pain issues (Humphreys et al. 2010). Chronic pain may include headaches, lower back pain, arthritic pain, and fibromyalgia. Research indicates that PTSD is associated with hypertension, development of obesity and hyperlipidemia, and coronary heart disease. Naturally, some of these physiological changes could contribute to a variety of other physical ailments in non-cardiovascular systems including diabetes and arthritis. PTSD may increase the risk of future Alzheimer's dementia based on the common risk factors of stress and cortisol dysregulation (Yaffe et al. 2010; Tsolaki 2010).

The link between trauma, PTSD, and physical symptoms is multifactorial. Besides somatization, there may be direct effects from the assault such as injury, sexually transmitted disease, or pregnancy. Trauma survivors may engage in behaviors that may affect their health status, such as tobacco use, substance abuse, and high-risk sexual behavior (Turner and Frayne 2004). Multiple studies have found alterations in the hypothalamic-pituitary-adrenal (HPA) axis. Other endocrine systems, especially thyroid, may be affected directly or via HPA dysregulation.

Other Legal Stressors After Sexual Assault

Survivor participation in legal proceedings against the perpetrator does not necessarily result in alleviation of symptoms or psychological distress. Allegations often take 1–2 years or longer to reach court-martial, assuming the case even reaches that level. Survivors may find their sexual history or mental health records subject to questioning. Many alleged perpetrators may receive guilty findings only for nonsexual charges such as simply assault or conduct bringing discredit to the service. Without a guilty finding for sexual assault, perpetrators may receive punishment including confinement or hard labor yet still remain on active duty. Their command may choose to pursue separation at a later date or may not. A final verdict of not guilty on all charges could similarly result in stress to a survivor's psychological state.

Treatment of Survivors

Acute Treatment After Sexual Assault

Initial medical treatment may begin if a survivor seeks immediate care at an emergency department or other walk-in service for sexual assault-related issues. Depending on the recency of the assault, a sexual assault forensic examination (SAFE), conducted by a sexual assault medical forensic examiner (SAMFE), may be the next appropriate intervention. SAMFEs provide medical treatment for injuries and may contact sexual assault behavioral health specialists for immediate assistance. They also preserve legal evidence using secure protocols. A SAFE is potentially re-traumatizing due to the in-depth interview and invasive medical examination, especially if performed by inexperienced clinicians, so SAMFEs use appropriate bedside practices and have an understanding of the psychology of sexual assault. Even then, patients may report both "revictimization" and a sense of empowerment during SAFEs (DuMont et al. 2009). Patients report better outcomes when SAFMEs meet professional standards, and proper forensic examination may lead to improved prosecution rates (Campbell et al. 2012).

Screening and Referral for Sexual Assault

Both the military and the VA promote screening for sexual trauma among patients, though only the VA mandates it. Even so, the exact screening modality is left to the discretion of the facility or providers. Questions such as "Have you ever been the victim of sexual assault?" may elicit a negative response, but a question such as "Have you ever felt pressured into engaging in a sexual act?" may elicit a positive response. The survivor may believe their personal trauma does not meet the "definition" of rape or may be in a degree of denial. The VA has a publication with suggested screening tools, verbal screening techniques, and how to respond to a positive screen.

When positive screening occurs in a primary care setting, referral to a mental health provider is generally recommended unless that patient has received past counseling or psychiatric treatment. In recent years, the military services and VA have pushed forward a patient-centered medical home (PCMH) model. In PCMH, behavioral health providers are based within primary care settings to help alleviate patient anxiety about being referred to the "mental health clinic." This also improves communication between primary care and behavioral health, an important element considering the combined physical and psychological burden experienced by some sexual assault survivors. The military and VA both promote rapid appointment availability for sexual assault survivors. In addition, the sexual literature generally supports the idea that survivors' preference for the gender of their providers should be respected (Street et al. 2011).

Treatment of PTSD in Sexual Assault Survivors

A more complete description of PTSD treatment is found elsewhere in this textbook. SSRIs constitute the first-line psychopharmacological treatment for PTSD, anxiety disorders, and depressive disorders secondary to sexual assault. SSRIs may take 4–8 weeks to achieve an effect, so co-occurring treatment may assist in resolving associated physical complaints such as insomnia, nightmares, headache, anxiety, and sexual dysfunction. Benzodiazepines may provide immediate relief for sleep or anxiety but have no studies supporting a long-term benefit in resolving PTSD or major depression. Regarding benzodiazepine use, clinicians should remain vigilant that sexual abuse victims have greater risk for developing substance use problems.

Therapy options exist to target psychiatric conditions secondary to the sexual assault. Depression, anxiety, and PTSD all may respond to cognitive behavioral therapy (CBT). VA/Department of Defense Clinical Practice Guidelines promote prolonged exposure therapy (PET), cognitive processing therapy (CPT), eye movement desensitization and reprocessing (EMDR) therapy, and stress inoculation training (SIT) as having the best empirical support for providing significant benefit (The Management of Post-Traumatic Stress Working Group 2010). Other specialized therapies may be used for comorbid conditions such as substance abuse or personality disorders. Multiple civilian facilities now specialize in the treatment of active duty and veteran populations and may accept referrals from active duty medical centers and VA hospitals. Providers sometimes walk a fine line between wanting to start intensive therapy while risking re-traumatizing the survivor and having them drop out of treatment altogether. Thus, letting the survivor set the pace of treatment may be important.

Therapeutic Considerations Specific to Sexual Assault Survivors

Survivors with history of childhood sexual assault are at higher risk for repeat sexual victimization. These survivors, as well as some with such history, engage in behavioral patterns or use maladaptive coping strategies that increase their risk. Besides treating the sequelae of past assaults, therapists may need to address how to prevent future sexual assaults. Street, Bell, and Ready have written an excellent synopsis of these behavioral patterns (Street et al. 2011). Additionally, the military environment presents several unique risk factors that therapists should be aware of, as studied by Sadler (Sadler et al. 2003) and the aforementioned 2014 RAND survey.

Providers often grapple with questions as to whether their patient was truly sexually assaulted. The key dilemma is that to find out more about the sexual assault means opening the door to potential discovery by a court of law. Poorly written medical notes, or the discovery of contradictory information, may unintentionally provide reasonable doubt to a jury as to whether a sexual assault occurred. Patient confidentiality, once broken by subpoena, may also break a survivor's trust in the medical system. Fundamental therapies like prolonged exposure therapy (PET) depend on hearing the story of the trauma; yet documenting the patient's account may risk legal ramifications.

Clinicians are encouraged to remain cognizant of the uncertainty when treating survivors and witnesses of sexual assault. In making a determination about whether or not to release records, military judges must consider four competing interests: society's interest in promoting public health, the patient's interest in protecting privacy, the state's interest in seeing that crimes are prosecuted, and the accused's interest in confronting the witnesses against him or her. Less noted in legal writing are the professional interests of clinicians, who have an ethical mandate to maintain confidentiality and to inform patients in advance of any limits of confidentiality. Clinicians also have an interest in advancing best practices, which include fostering confidential relationships and providing prompt treatment of those in crisis.

The mental health records may be requested by the defense. The accused must show that the records will likely contain relevant and admissible evidence prior to any review of the records by the judge. The military judge will determine whether or not the records contain admissible evidence, and only those limited aspects will be released. Usually, the mere fact of treatment is not enough to establish that the records should be reviewed for relevance. The Special Victim's Counsel program has been instrumental in fighting to preserve the privacy of survivor's mental health records (Kastenberg 2013). Although the treating clinician can assert privilege on behalf of the patient, it is more common for the Special Victim's Counsel to advance the survivor's privacy interests in the court, before the appellate courts, and during appellate review.

The most recent statutes and case law have not provided guidance for review of mental health records by the military judge, and recent investigations have found inconsistent practices. Of concern to clinicians, military judges will determine whether or not psychotherapist-patient privilege should be pierced based on the judge's lay understanding and interpretation of the mental health records, and the decisions being made are questionable from a clinical perspective. Examples include a case in which adjustment disorder was found to be relevant to an argument that a witness was likely to have inaccurate recollection or perception of the event due to a mental disorder.

The Manual for Courts-Martial (MCM) emphasizes that MRE 513 is a *psychotherapist*-patient privilege, not a physician patient privilege, and covers only communications with psychiatrists, psychologists, clinical social workers, and their assistants. This is problematic, because in the military, as in most of American medicine, mental health evaluation, diagnosis, and treatment are regularly done by other medical providers. For example, primary care visits may include screening for depression, alcohol abuse, domestic violence, and sexual assault.

Compounding the provider's uncertainty, the survivor may harbor conflicting feelings about their degree of consent or the degree to which they wanted to have sex, even though they ultimately did not consent to engage in sex. Consent and wantedness may exist on a scale, rather than in a dichotomous present/not present fashion. Greater degrees of consent in survivors may be a risk factor for self-blame and maladaptive beliefs (Artime and Peterson 2015; Muehlenhard et al. 2016). Providers may find that therapy requires helping the patient distinguish and address these two concepts. Similar literature exists for sexual assault occurring within long-term relationships and marriages (Shotland and Goodstein 1992).

Providers may also question how to respond when the patient asks for advice on whether to report a sexual assault and seek legal remedy. The weighing of pros and cons to this question is different for each patient's scenario. The provider may not know sufficient facts or local legal factors to give an informed answer, and as previously mentioned, most investigations do not end in a sexual assault conviction or incarceration. The decision is probably best left to the patient. Active duty military clinicians may receive a restricted report and are under no obligation to disclose the allegation to command or law enforcement. Further, empowered decision-making following a sexual assault is associated with better health outcomes for the survivor (DuMont et al. 2009). Military providers are fortunate in that patients may receive extensive advice from their Sexual Assault Prevention and Response (SAPR) office and

Special Victims Counsel (SVC) or Victims' Legal Counsel (VLC) after making a restricted report. VA providers may consult with their Military Sexual Trauma Coordinator or hospital legal counsel to help patients make these difficult decisions.

Implications for the Future

Besides the military and VA, US colleges are also in the spotlight for their handling or mishandling of sexual assault cases. Colleges are responding with initiatives that parallel or complement military interventions of recent years (Institute on Domestic Violence and Sexual Assault 2016; The White House 2014). College populations are a similar age demographic as the military, though the ratio of men to women is less similar. Colleges also face similar cultural challenges, including social acceptability of the binge use of alcohol. Nationwide research and focus on colleges may fuel further improvements in military systems. Similarly, states may benefit from the investment in research and program development by the Department of Defense. As additional data on the impact of prevention efforts such as public health education and on the enhancements in support for survivors become available, civilian communities may be implementing innovative programs developed by the military. Examples with at least preliminary support include providing the option of restricted reporting and providing legal advocates such as Special Victims Counsel (SVCs) or Victims' Legal Counsel (VLCs).

Future improvements in the military will require greater understanding, by commanders and leaders, of the complexities facing male and female survivors. Non-survivors often lack understanding of the survivor experience, both across and within gender lines. Narrowing this gap will require policies and education that work toward changing the entire military culture. In this sense, the adjustments occurring at the college level and societal level may assist the military by modifying the recruitment pool. The military may benefit from implementing mandatory, universal sexual assault screening at its medical clinics, following the VA's lead. Addressing the needs of large numbers of male survivors will require robust funding for research into how to reduce reporting barriers and weaken military cultural stigmas.

Laws and system responses are converging on increased awareness of acquaintance rape, the effects of intoxication, bringing response networks to survivors instead of leaving it to them to find services, forensic examination and interviewing, and laws that go beyond the "forcible rape" stereotype. Enhanced prevention and creating a safe catch for survivors involve improving awareness of the variety of sexual assault scenarios, educating the community in order to reduce negative reactions to survivors, and creating user-friendly reporting mechanisms. Increasing focus on the large numbers of male military sexual assault survivors and very low reporting rates will lead to greater emphasis on awareness, prevention, and treatment. From a preventative standpoint, the short-term goal is communal vigilance against risk-increasing behaviors, while the ultimate goal is a universal shift in cultural definitions of consent and capacity to consent to sexual activity (Dinos et al. 2015).

Conclusions

In this chapter's case study, the female soldier experienced daunting personal and systemic events that are all too common among all sexual assault survivors. The legal system has a long-standing tradition of assuming innocence until proven guilty, such that a sexual assault trial will always require in-depth exploration of evidence to prove guilty beyond a reasonable doubt. Without a "guilty" verdict under their belt, survivors will face skepticism and ostracism from peers or leaders. They are more likely to be seen in medical settings than in courtroom settings, and their total population within military and VA settings is profound.

Medical providers both in psychological fields and in general medical fields need awareness of the prevalence of military sexual assault.

Sexual assault is a pervasive experience affecting both male and female veterans. Military service may increase the risk of exposure and the severity of outcomes. Many patients receiving medical care may have past sexual trauma they have not shared with their providers. Mandatory screening helps, but competent screening is also required. Overcoming patient resistance to opening up or receiving psychological treatment is another delicate skill set for providers.

Prevention of sexual assault, treatment of survivors, and the system response are all closely intertwined. Survivors must simultaneously cope with their own preconceptions of culpability, negative responses by family or peers, the uncomfortable realities of the legal system, and a host of medical disorders. Reporting of sexual assault crimes to authorities is an individual decision that may require advice from multiple types of professionals. Improved understanding of this web of factors will enable clinicians to understand their clients better and navigate a pathway to recovery.

Key Concepts

1. The US Congress and Department of Defense have prioritized awareness and availability of services to sexual assault survivors through a series of policy changes, criminal statute modifications, and an expanded network of sexual assault support and treatment professionals.
2. Sexual assault survivors are far more likely to seek support or treatment through nonlegal settings, and the experience at that first contact may positively or negatively affect the survivor's willingness to seek assistance.
3. Both the military and the Department of Veterans Affairs (VA) encourage or mandate screening for sexual assault due to survivors' reluctance to disclose and because the trauma may be contributing to other medical problems.
4. Sexual assault survivors are at risk for a host of psychological and physical problems, the combination of which can lead to profound impairment in multiple life domains.
5. Responders need to be aware of sexual assault and have the ability to refer survivors to professionals with specific training to address both medical and legal needs.

References

Artime TM, Peterson ZD (2015) Feelings of wantedness and consent during nonconsensual sex: implications for posttraumatic cognitions. Psychol Trauma: Theor Res Pract Policy 7(6):570–577

Black MC, Merrick MT (2013) Prevalence of intimate partner violence, stalking, and sexual violence among active duty women and wives of active duty men – comparisons with women in the US general population, 2010. Centers for Disease Control and Prevention. http://www.sapr.mil/public/docs/research/2010_National_Intimate_Partner_and_Sexual_Violence_Survey-Technical_Report.pdf. Accessed 13 Apr 2016

Breiding MJ (2014) Prevalence and characteristics of sexual violence, stalking, and intimate partner violence victimization—National Intimate Partner and Sexual Violence Survey, United States, 2011. http://www.cdc.gov/mmwr/preview/mmwrhtml/ss6308a1.htm?s_cid=ss6308a1_e. Accessed 10 Sep 2016

Campbell R, Patterson D, Bybee D (2012) Prosecution of adult sexual assault cases: a longitudinal analysis of the impact of a sexual assault nurse examiner program. Violence Against Women 18(2):223–244

Castro CA, Kintzle S, Schuyler AC et al (2015) Sexual assault in the military. Curr Psychiatry Rep 17(7):1–13

Classen CC, Palesh OG, Aggarwal R (2005) Sexual revictimization: a review of the empirical literature. Trauma Violence Abuse 6(2):103–129

Cleere C, Lynn SJ (2013) Acknowledged versus unacknowledged sexual assault among college women. J Interpers Violence 28:2593–2611

Creamer M, Burgess P, McFarlane AC (2001) Posttraumatic stress disorder: findings from the Australian National Survey of Mental Health and Well-being. Psychol Med 31(7):1237–1247

Department of Defense 2013) Special victim counsel handbook. http://responsesystemspanel.whs.mil/public/docs/meetings/sub_committee/20140226_vs/materials_related/03a_usa_specialvictimsconsel_handbook.pdf. Accessed 31 Aug 2016

Department of Defense (2014) Report to the President of the United States on sexual assault prevention and response, Appendix A. http://sapr.mil/public/docs/reports/ FY14_POTUS/FY14_DoD_Report_to_POTUS_Full_Report.pdf. Accessed on 1 Sep 2016

Department of Defense (2015) Department of Defense Instruction (DoDI) 6495.02: sexual assault prevention and response (SAPR) program procedures. Government Printing Office, Washington, DC

Department of Defense (2016) Manual for courts-martial. http://jsc.defense.gov/Portals/99/Documents/MCM2016.pdf?ver=2016-12-08-181411-957. Accessed 1 Nov 2016

Department of Defense Sexual Assault and Prevention Office (2012) Workplace and gender relations survey of active duty members. http://www.sapr.mil/public/docs/research/WGR_ActiveDuty_2012_Report.pdf. Accessed on 4 Sep 2016

Department of the Army (2014) Army regulation 600-20: Army command policy. Government Printing Office, Washington, DC

Department of Veterans Affairs (2010a) VHA directive 2010-014: assessment and management of veterans who have been victims of alleged acute sexual assault. Government Printing Office, Washington, DC

Department of Veterans Affairs (2010b) VHA directive 2010-033: military sexual trauma (MST) programming. Government Printing Office, Washington, DC

Department of Veterans Affairs (2015a) Military sexual trauma (MST). http://www.mentalhealth.va.gov/msthome.asp. Accessed 20 Aug 2016

Department of Veterans Affairs (2015b) Military sexual trauma (MST) general fact sheet. http://www.mentalhealth.va.gov/docs/mst_general_factsheet.pdf. Accessed 20 Aug 2016

Desai S, Arias I, Thompson MP et al (2002) Childhood victimization and subsequent revictimization assessed in a nationally representative sample of women and men. Violence Vict 17(6):639–653

Dinos S, Burrowes N, Hammond K et al (2015) A systematic review of juries' assessment of rape victims: do rape myths impact on juror decision-making? Int J Law Crime Justice 43(1):36–49

DuMont J, White D, McGregor M (2009) Investigating the medical forensic examination from the perspective of sexually assaulted women. Soc Sci Med 68:774–780

Elliott DM, Mok DS, Briere J (2004) Adult sexual assault: prevalence, symptomatology, and sex differences in the general population. J Trauma Stress 17(3):203–211

Executive Order No. 13, 140, 64 (1999) Fed Reg 55:115

Federal Bureau of Investigation (2016) Frequently asked questions about the change in the UCR definition of rape. In: CJIS, UCR, recent program updates. Federal Bureau of Investigation. https://www.fbi.gov/about-us/cjis/ucr/recent-program-updates/new-rape-definition-frequently-asked-questions. Accessed 21 Sep 2016

Finkelhor D, Hotaling G, Lewis I et al (1990) Sexual abuse in a national survey of adult men and women: prevalence, characteristics, and risk factors. Child Abuse Negl 14(1):19–28

Fisher RP, Geiselman RE (2010) The cognitive interview method of conducting police interviews: eliciting extensive information and promoting therapeutic jurisprudence. Int J Law Psychiatry 33:321–328

Fisher BS, Cullen FT, Turner MG (2000) The sexual victimization of college women. https://www.ncjrs.gov/pdffiles1/nij/182369.pdf. Accessed 3 Aug 2016

Fishman CS (2007) Defense access to a prosecution witness's psychotherapy or counseling records. Or L Rev 86:1

Frayne SM et al (1999) Medical profile of women Veterans Administration outpatients who report a history of sexual assault occurring while in the military. J Womens Health Gend Based Med 8(6):835–845

Heidt JM, Marx BP, Forsyth JP (2005) Tonic immobility and childhood sexual abuse: a preliminary report evaluating the sequela of rape-induced paralysis. Behav Res Ther 43:1157–1171

Humphreys J, Cooper BA, Miaskowski C (2010) Differences in depression, posttraumatic stress disorder, and lifetime trauma exposure in formerly abused women and mild versus moderate to severe chronic pain. J Interpers Violence 25(12):2316–2338

Inspector General of the United States Department of Defense (2013) Report No. DODIG-2013-043: evaluation of the military criminal investigative organizations' sexual assault investigation training. Government Printing Office, Washington, DC

Institute on Domestic Violence & Sexual Assault (2016) The blueprint for campus police: responding to sexual assault. http://sites.utexas.edu/idvsa/title-blueprint-for-campus-police-responding-to-sexual-assault. Accessed 14 Aug 2016

Judicial Proceedings Panel (2015) Report of the judicial proceedings since fiscal year 2012 Amendments Panel. http://jpp.whs.mil/public/docs/08-Panel_Reports/01_JPP_InitialReport_Final_20150204.pdf. Accessed 6 Sep 2016

Kang H, Dalager N, Mahan C et al (2005) The role of sexual assault on the risk of PTSD among Gulf War veterans. Ann Epidemiol 15(3):191–195

Kastenberg LRM V (2013) 72 M.J. 364

Kels CG (2012) Military medical malpractice and "the right to sue". Clin Dermatol 30(2):181–187

Kilpatrick DG, Resnick HS, Ruggiero KJ et al (2007) Drug-facilitated, incapacitated, and forcible rape: a national study. National Institute of Justice, Washington, DC

Kimerling R, Gima K, Smith MW et al (2007) The Veterans Health Administration and military sexual trauma. Am J Public Health 97(12):2160–2166

Kimerling R, Street AE, Gima K et al (2008) Evaluation of universal screening for military-related sexual trauma. Psychiatr Serv 59:635–640

Koss MP, Woodruff WJ, Koss PG (1991) Criminal victimization among primary care medical patients: prevalence, incidence, and physician usage. Behav Sci Law 9(1):85–96

Krebs CP, Lindquist CH, Warner TD et al (2011) Comparing sexual assault prevalence estimates obtained with direct and indirect questioning techniques. Violence Against Women 17:219–235

Lalor K, McElvaney R (2010) Child sexual abuse, links to later sexual exploitation/high-risk sexual behavior, and prevention/treatment programs. Trauma Violence Abuse 11(4):159–177

Logan TK, Walker R, Cole J (2013) Silenced suffering: the need for a better understanding of partner sexual violence. Trauma Violence Abuse 16(2):111–136

Lonsway KA, Archambault J (2012) The "justice gap" for sexual assault cases future directions for research and reform. Violence Against Women 18(2):145–168

McFarlane AC (2013) The long-term costs of traumatic stress: intertwined physical and psychological consequences. World Psychiatry 9:3–10

McKimmie BM, Masser BM, Bongiorno R (2014) What counts as rape? The effect of offense prototypes, victim stereotypes, and participant gender on how the complainant and defendant are perceived. J Interpers Violence 29(12):2273–2303

Millegan J, Milburn EK, LeardMann CA et al (2015) Recent sexual trauma and adverse health and occupational outcomes among US service women. J Trauma Stress 28(4):298–306

Millegan J, Wang L, LeardMann CA et al (2016) Recent sexual trauma and adverse health and occupational outcomes among men serving in the U.S. military. J Trauma Stress 29(2):132–140

Morral AR, Gore KL, Schell T et al (2015a) Sexual assault and sexual harassment in the U.S. military, annex to volume 2, tabular results from the 2014 RAND Military Workplace Study for Department of Defense service members. RAND Corporation. http://www.rand.org/pubs/research_reports/RR870z3.html. Accessed 30 Aug 2016

Morral AR, Gore KL, Schell T et al (2015b) Sexual assault and sexual harassment in the military, top-line estimates for active duty service members from the 2014 RAND Military Workplace Study. RAND Corporation. http://www.rand.org/pubs/research_reports/RR870.html. Accessed 30 Aug 2016

Morral AR, Gore KL, Schell T et al (2015c) Sexual assault and sexual harassment in the U.S. military, highlights from the 2014 RAND Military Workplace Study. RAND Corporation. http://www.rand.org/pubs/research_briefs/RB9841.html. Accessed 30 Aug 2016

Muehlenhard CL, Humphreys TP, Jozkowski KN et al (2016) The complexities of sexual consent among college students: a conceptual and empirical review. J Sex Res 53(4–5):457–487

Redmond JV (1996) 116 S.Ct. 1923

Rosenstein JE, Carroll MH (2015) Male rape myths, female rape myths, and intent to intervene as a bystander. Violence Gender 2(4):204–208

Sadler AG, Booth BM, Cook BL et al (2003) Factors associated with women's risk of rape in the military environment. Am J Ind Med 43:262–273

Sameit MD (2013) When a convicted rape is not really a rape: the past, present, and future ability of Article 120 convictions to withstand legal and factual sufficiency reviews. Mil L Rev 216:77

Schultz JR, Bell KM, Naugle AE et al (2006) Child sexual abuse and adulthood sexual abuse among military veteran and civilian women. Mil Med 171(8):723–728

Settles IH, Buchanan NT, Yap SCY et al (2014) Sex differences in outcomes and harasser characteristics associated with frightening sexual harassment appraisals. J Occup Health Psychol 19(2):133–142

Shotland RL, Goodstein L (1992) Sexual precedence reduces the perceived legitimacy of sexual refusal: an examination of attributions concerning date rape and consensual sex. Personal Soc Psychol Bull 18(6):756–764

Skinner KM, Kressin N, Frayne S et al (2000) The prevalence of military sexual assault among female Veterans' Administration outpatients. J Interpers Violence 15(3):291–310

Stander VA, Thomsen CJ (2016) Sexual harassment and assault in the U.S. military: a review of policy and research trends. Mil Med 181(1 Supplement):20–27

Street AE, Bell ME, Ready CB (2011) Sexual assault. In: Benedek DM, Wynn GH (eds) Clinical manual for management of PTSD. American Psychiatric Publishing, Washington, DC, pp 325–348

Suris A, Lind L (2008) Military sexual trauma a review of prevalence and associated health consequences in veterans. Trauma Violence Abuse 9(4):250–269

Suris A, Lind L, Kashner TM et al (2007) Mental health, quality of life, and health functioning in women veterans. J Interpers Violence 22(2):179–197

TeBockhurst SF, O'Halloran MS, Nyline BN (2015) Tonic immobility among survivors of sexual assault. Psychol Trauma: Theor Res Practice Policy 7(2):171–178

The Management of Post-Traumatic Stress Working Group (2010) VA/DoD clinical practice guideline: management of post-traumatic stress, version 2.0. http://www.healthquality.va.gov/guidelines/MH/ptsd/. Accessed 12 Aug 2016

The White House (2014) Not alone: the first report of the White House Task Force to protect students from sexual assault. https://www.justice.gov/ovw/page/file/905942/download. Accessed 9 Aug 2016

Tjaden P, Thoennes N (1998) Prevalence, incidence, and consequences of violence against women: findings from the national violence against women survey. Research in Brief. Available at https://www.ncjrs.gov/pdffiles/172837.pdf

Tsolaki M (2010) Posttraumatic stress disorder (PTSD) and Alzheimer's disease (AD). In: Sher L, Vilens A (eds) Neurobiology of post-traumatic stress disorder. Nova Science Publishers, New York, pp 201–216

Turner C, Frayne S (2004) Military sexual trauma. Department of Veterans Affairs. http://www.publichealth.va.gov/docs/vhi/military_sexual_trauma.pdf. Accessed on 5 Sep 2016

United States Army Medical Department (2015) Sexual assault medical forensic examiner adult and adolescent (SAMFE-A) curriculum. Available by email request to the authors

United States Department of Justice Office of Violence Against Women (2013) A national protocol for sexual assault medical forensic examinations – adults/adolescents, 2nd edn. Government Printing Office, Washington, DC

United States Government Accountability Office (2015) GAO-15-284: military personnel: actions needed to address sexual assaults of male service members.

http://www.gao.gov/assets/670/669096.pdf. Accessed 6 Sep 2016
United States Senate (2015) National Defense Authorizations Act. https://www.congress.gov/113/bills/hr4435/BILLS-113hr4435pcs.pdf. Accessed on 3 Aug 2016
Web of Science (2016) Thomson Reuters, New York. https://apps.webofknowledge.com. Accessed 1 Apr 2016
White AM (2003) What happened? Alcohol, memory blackouts, and the brain. Alcohol Res Health 27(2):186–196
Yaeger D, Himmelfarb N, Cammack A et al (2006) Posttraumatic stress disorder in female veterans with military and civilian sexual trauma. J Trauma Stress 19(6):837–846
Yaffe K, Vittinghoff E, Lindquist K et al (2010) Posttraumatic stress disorder and risk of dementia among US veterans. Arch Gen Psychiatry 67:608–613
Zimmerman M (2015) Rudderless: 15 years and still little direction on the boundaries of military rule of evidence 513. Mil L Rev 223:312

Ethical Challenges in Treating Detainees and Prisoners of War

18

Stephen N. Xenakis

All that is necessary for the triumph of evil is that good men do nothing.
—*Sir Edmund Burke*

Introduction

The fundamental conflict for military health professionals has been reduced to a question of dual loyalty: allegiance to the command and governmental authorities, in addition to duties and responsibilities to the individual and "to do no harm." Simply stated, the military practitioner feels tugged between prioritizing the demands of the military mission and prioritizing the needs of the patient, whether it is a warrior deploying to a combat zone or a detainee in Guantánamo. A competing perspective asserts that the military practitioner assumes dual responsibility to probe and discern facts, opinions, and assertions regarding clinical practice, command guidance, and Department of Defense (DoD) policy. This chapter explores the factors that constitute the elements of *dual responsibility* and reviews ethical dilemmas for military medical personnel as they relate to the treatment of detainees and prisoners of war.

Case Study

Mohammed Abu Wa'el (Jihad) Dhiab is a 45-year-old Syrian man detained at Guantánamo Bay Naval Base in 2002 and released in 2014. He was born in Lebanon to a Syrian father and Lebanese mother from Argentina. Dhiab spent his childhood in a small village east of Damascus and described his life as "normal," happy, and comfortable. Married for 21 years with four children, he has not seen his family since arriving in Guantánamo. His eldest son and six close family members have been killed in the war in Syria, several from chemical weapons.

His medical history is significant for he was in a serious motor vehicle accident while serving in the army, sustaining a painful back injury (possible undiagnosed vertebral fracture) when his car fell off the road and dropped 50 ft down into a ravine. He has no recollection of the details of the accident and the medical evaluation or if he lost consciousness. He has suffered continuous and chronic low back pain for 20 years.

American authorities apprehended Dhiab in Afghanistan and subsequently transported him to Guantánamo even

S.N. Xenakis (✉)
Uniformed Services University of Health Sciences, Arlington, VA, USA
e-mail: snxenakis@hotmail.com; snxenakis7@gmail.com

L.W. Roberts, C.H. Warner (eds.), *Military and Veteran Mental Health*,
https://doi.org/10.1007/978-1-4939-7438-2_18

though he insisted that he had never participated in any military or political activities against the United States. He is not aware of any basis for him to be considered an illegal belligerent, combatant, or enemy to the United States and its allies.

Dhiab found the conditions of confinement and treatment at Guantánamo to be harsh and abusive and aggravating to his medical conditions, state of mind, pain, and discomfort. Dhiab slept on a metal surface covered by one ISOMAT that was inadequate and uncomfortable. He had limited access to reading material or other media to occupy his attention and fill his time during waking hours.

Dhiab felt that the medical caregivers diminished the seriousness of his complaints and failed to provide him appropriate and adequate evaluation and treatment from the first days of his arrival. He refused food in 2006 or 2007 in objection to the harsh, inhumane, and abusive treatment and indignities by the Guantánamo authorities. Food refusal was the only peaceful means to express his grievances. He was subjected to forced cell extractions (FCEs) while being transported to enteral feedings that aggravated his back pain and assaulted his personal dignity. Dhiab repeatedly demonstrated his willingness to cease refusing food and agreed to stop his "hunger strike" after being informed of his potential transfer from Guantánamo.

An extensive evaluation and review of his medical conditions and treatment indicated that Dhiab suffers from chronic and debilitating back pain and diminished function and sensation in his right leg and arm. The physical and neurological examination indicated a physiologic and anatomic underlying cause for his symptoms and not a psychogenic basis as the medical record documented. There was no documentation that the US government had performed the appropriate diagnostic tests and evaluations.

Dhiab showed no signs of diagnosable neuropsychiatric disease. He exhibited attitudes and actions that are expectable under conditions of extreme stress, abusive treatment, and continuing confinement. There was no documentation and substantiating evidence to attribute his symptoms to a psychogenic cause. His actions, beliefs, and thoughts were culturally appropriate and understandable (Ritchie 2014; Petitioner's Notice of Filing, District Federal Court 2014).

The US government transferred Dhiab and five other detainees from Guantánamo to Uruguay in December 2014. The authorities had promised continuing medical care and reunification with his family. Over time, Dhiab became increasingly disillusioned as his family did not arrive in Uruguay, and he felt neglected by the medical care system. The media reported that he had slipped into Brazil during Ramadan and raised concerns about his activities. The Uruguayan foreign ministry confirmed in July 2016 that Dhiab abandoned the country in mid-June 2016; turned up at the Uruguayan consulate in Caracas, Venezuela; and requested he be sent to Turkey or another destination, but not Uruguay, to rejoin his family. There is no indication that he has engaged in terrorism. Since returning to Uruguay from Venezuela, Dhiab has staged public protests and is currently engaged in another hunger strike seeking transfer to Turkey and reunification with his family.

Ethical Principles for Military Health Professionals

The ethical standards that underlie medical practice in the military are anchored both in the fundamental practices and principles of clinical medicine and in military professionalism. For centuries, the medical profession has followed the cardinal ethical code of:

- "First, do no harm."
- Respect the autonomy of the patient.
- Provide treatment for the benefit and health of the patient.
- Act in the service of justice.

The American Medical Association (AMA) published its first update of the code of medical ethics in 50 years on June 13, 2016 (Brotherton et al. 2016):

1. A physician shall be dedicated to providing competent medical care, with compassion and respect for human dignity and rights.
2. A physician shall uphold the standards of professionalism, be honest in all professional interactions, and strive to report physicians deficient in character or competence, or engaging in fraud or deception, to appropriate entities.
3. A physician shall respect the law and also recognize a responsibility to seek changes in those requirements which are contrary to the best interests of the patient.
4. A physician shall respect the rights of patients, colleagues, and other health professionals and shall safeguard patient confidences and privacy within the constraints of the law.
5. A physician shall continue to study, apply, and advance scientific knowledge; maintain a commitment to medical education; make relevant information available to patients, colleagues, and the public; obtain consultation; and use the talents of other health professionals when indicated.
6. A physician shall, in the provision of appropriate patient care, except in emergencies, be free to choose whom to serve, with whom to associate, and the environment in which to provide medical care.
7. A physician shall recognize a responsibility to participate in activities contributing to the improvement of the community and the betterment of public health.
8. A physician shall, while caring for a patient, regard responsibility to the patient as paramount.
9. A physician shall support access to medical care for all people.

In light of the traditional principles undergirding clinical healthcare, military health professionals have framed ethical dilemmas of their medical practice in five principal areas:

1. Dual agency of the psychologist or psychiatrist (working for both the military and the service member)
2. Return to duty versus evacuation (whether to keep someone in the battlefield or return him or her home)
3. Retaining a service member in the military versus recommending the medical board (medical discharge)
4. Confidentiality versus what command needs to know
5. Disability and compensation issues for those diagnosed with PTSD (Ritchie 2014)

Military medical practitioners carry dual responsibilities and agency as clinicians and military officers. The physical and mental health of the entire force, including associated families, underlies the readiness of the military and its capability to execute the missions assigned to it. The military medical departments assume major responsibility to sustain the health of the force. In doing their assigned mission, military medical providers fulfill the oath taken by all officers of "protecting the nation against all enemies, foreign and domestic" (5 U.S.C. § 3331, Oath of Office 1966) and providing healthcare and sustaining the fitness of the force (Ethics Abandoned 2013). Many issues, problems, and missions encountered by military health professionals are ambiguous and complex. Ascertaining the proper course of action involves analysis and clarification of the core elements.

Primum Non Nocere: First, Do No Harm

The bedrock code of medical ethics has been "first, do no harm." The updated American Medical Association code elaborates and modifies this principle to providing competent care, upholding professional standards, and applying scientific knowledge (modernized AMA *Code of Medical Ethics* 1, 2, and 5). Examination of Dhiab's case identifies elements relevant to these principles and the ethical dilemmas confronting military practitioners when treating detainees:

1. The challenge of ascertaining the etiology of back pain, weakness, and impaired motor functioning that is not obviously organic and possibly an indication of psychological manipulation by an enemy combatant
2. Judging the impact of cultural background and conditions of confinement on severity and cause of symptoms
3. Managing the availability of standard diagnostic testing and other treatments constrained by environmental factors imposed by being in a prison facility outside of the continental United States
4. The acknowledgment that military professionals are expected to conduct medical practice independent of the authority of officials operating the prison facility

Military medical practitioners commonly assess patients, soldiers, and/or prisoners in detention facilities, with reports of back pain and neurological findings. With regard to Dhiab's case, repeated medical examinations recorded the symptoms and physical signs. The medical record had no documentation of appropriate radiological examinations or standard diagnostic testing. Like other remote installations, the medical clinic had limited radiological capabilities without the availability of an MRI, consistent CT scanning, and other sophisticated equipment. MRI scanning is standard diagnostic testing for conditions such as back pain and partial right-sided paralysis. The record documented that the medical staff regarded Dhiab as malingering and/or suffering from a psychogenic disorder. It annotated that he suffered from a "culturally bound syndrome" and that his symptoms were not secondary to injury or any organic process. The staff proposed that he willfully refused to comply with policies and could overcome his symptoms if he "really wanted to." They attributed his attitude and conduct to intentional opposition to military authorities because of his status as an "unlawful combatant."

The absence of standard radiological testing and other diagnostic capabilities compromised the thoroughness of evaluation and treatment planning and imposed an ethical dilemma on practitioners regarding confidence in diagnosis and therapy. To illustrate their challenge, it is reasonable to assume that practitioners would not have reliably excluded organic etiology had they evaluated a patient like Dhiab in almost any other clinical setting. The absence of appropriate diagnostic testing, evaluations by specialists, and provision of supportive care and treatment failed to meet standards of appropriate medical care and aggravated Dhiab's medical condition and state of mind.

Standard practice for complicated conditions, such as those that cross the boundaries of the physical and the psychological, dictates multidisciplinary approaches that rely on the expert opinions of specialists including physiatrists, neurologists, psychiatrists, and internists (Arehart-Treichel, 2013; Physicians for Human Rights and University of Cape Town Health Sciences Centre 2003; Unutzer, 2009). The medical staff practicing in a remote facility such as Guantánamo confronts ethical dilemmas and limitations imposed by "the realities of the war on terror" and detaining captives outside of the continental United States. Dhiab's case illustrates the challenges of upholding the medical code of "first, do no harm" and of providing competent care in compliance with the modernized AMA *Code of Medical Ethics*.

Physician Autonomy and Military Policy

The modernized American Medical Association *Code of Medical Ethics* amplifies the longstanding principle of autonomy by stipulating that physicians "shall respect the rights of patients, … and shall safeguard patient confidences and privacy within the constraints of the law, [and] … shall, while caring for a patient, regard responsibility to the patient as paramount." These principles inform the practice of military physicians at all times, including treatment of service members, families of active duty, and detainees and prisoners of war (POW). The status as an active combatant and the state of detention or incarceration impose ethical challenges upon military practitioners to comply with the inherent rights to exercise autonomy with respect to medical care.

Nonetheless, the Department of Defense (DoD) has asserted that the exigencies of combat and nature of asymmetrical warfare supersede the physician's traditional responsibility to the patient (Bloche and Marks 2005). In particular, DoD leadership has characterized opposition or challenges by detainees or illegal belligerents as military actions in support of asymmetrical warfare or as a form of terrorism. The Office of the Assistant Secretary of Defense of Health Affairs has advised that military physicians should subordinate their ethical principles of caring for patients to their duties as uniformed officers to act as warfighters in a combat role (Lazarus 2013).

The debate over the appropriate management of detainees who refuse food or who hunger-strike illustrates the ethical dilemma in military healthcare regarding exercising autonomy. The US government asserts that detainees are still agents of Al-Qaeda and continue to engage in asymmetrical warfare and that their tactics include participation in hunger strikes. Dhiab, like many other detainees, disclosed that refusing food was the only peaceful means to express his grievances over the harsh, inhumane, and abusive treatment and indignities carried out by the Guantánamo authorities. In other words, food refusal or hunger-striking was the best means for peaceful protest.

The principle of autonomy anchors the guidance for managing food refusal and hunger-striking, particularly force-feeding as an intervention. The American Medical Association's position on force-feeding is "Every competent patient has the right to refuse medical intervention, including life-sustaining interventions" (Crosby et al. 2007). Similarly, the Declaration of Tokyo (World Medical Association. Declaration of Tokyo 1975), dating from 1975, states:

> Where a prisoner refuses nourishment and is considered by the physician as capable of forming an unimpaired and rational judgment concerning the consequences of such a voluntary refusal of nourishment, he or she shall not be fed artificially. The decision as to the capacity of the prisoner to form such a judgment should be confirmed by at least one other independent physician. The consequences of the refusal of nourishment shall be explained by the physician to the prisoner.

The policies and procedures at Guantánamo Bay Naval Base contradict and fail to comply with accepted best practices for treatment of hunger strikers. These best practices (Crosby et al. 2007) include:

1. Establishing therapeutic relationship and rapport with the subject
2. Ascertaining the wishes of the subject with regard to supportive care, including end of life
3. Conducting an appropriate psychological and mental status evaluation
4. Ascertaining the presence of undue influence
5. Providing an independent second medical opinion

Guantánamo's policy of force-feeding contravenes accepted standards. Physicians are not independent and are instructed to follow a protocol for enteral feeding that overrides medical professionalism. They do not counsel detainees about options, much less help them prepare advance directives for the end-of-life stages of being on a hunger strike. According to published standard operating procedures (SOPs), healthcare providers participate in the coercive process, including being expected to order physical restraints for force-feeding (Medical Management of Detainees with Weight Loss 2013). Nurses are not allowed to act on a detainee's request to see a doctor or to change the content of the food used or the rate of flow—only to make a note in a chart.

Medical personnel are bound to respect the autonomy of their patients, irrespective of their status as detainees, prisoners of war, or active combatants. Traditionally, the standards of military medical care have acknowledged that active duty service members have the right to refuse recommendations for evaluation and treatment. Nonetheless, refusing to comply with recommendations for treatment may lead to administrative separation for the service member on the grounds that he/she cannot fulfill duty obligations. Service members exercising autonomy with regard to their healthcare do not escape the consequences of their decisions.

With regard to hunger-striking and food refusal, the AMA contends that the policies of the Department of Defense violate principles of medical ethics and have "weaponized" the provision of medical care. Particularly, the procedures for the management of hunger strikers undermine long-standing traditions and the unique role of military physicians. Medical personnel have the privilege of carrying specially recognized identification according to the Geneva Conventions and receive corresponding protection in combat (Chapter IV, Article 25 of the Geneva Convention 1966). Department of Defense policies violate the principles and intent of the Geneva Conventions by constricting the actions of military clinicians to the doctor-patient relationship. The Department of Defense has asserted that medics must act just like any other soldier at other times and are subject to orders of combatant commanders. These policies and procedures negate the acknowledged status of medical personnel as "healers" according to the Geneva Conventions and thrust them into action as warriors and combatants. Accordingly, US medical personnel lose traditional protections and diminish their unique status in times of combat. In adhering to the right for patients to exercise autonomy, including detainees and prisoners of war, military medical personnel underscore the increasingly important impact of individual and human rights on national security, peace, and stability.

The Benefit and Health of the Patient

All societies endow physicians and other clinicians with special trust and confidence in their role as healers, symbolically donning "the white coat." The role is anchored in the historic ethical principle that physicians provide treatment for the benefit and health of patients at all times. The modernized American Medical Association *Code of Medical Ethics* amplifies the traditional principles with the stipulations that physicians "regard responsibility to the patient as paramount"; "provide competent medical care, with compassion and respect for human dignity and rights"; and "recognize a responsibility to participate in activities contributing to the improvement of the community and the betterment of public health" (Brotherton et al. 2016). There are no qualifications or limitations to the overriding responsibility for the health and welfare of the patients entrusted to the clinician. The duty to provide care spans across the range of diagnosis, treatment, and discharge or aftercare. Military physicians learn early in a career that the soldiers and patients entrusted to them rely on their professionalism to provide the best care possible at all times, no matter the circumstances or constraints. The physician, like the chaplain and lawyer, is expected to provide aid unconditionally for the benefit and health of the warrior and patient. The expectations for and responsibilities of the clinician are not diminished by race, religion, ethnicity, or status, including designation as a detainee or prisoner of war.

Military practitioners confront ethical dilemmas imposed by nonmedical authorities and commanders enforcing restrictive and potentially harmful conditions. The involvement of health practitioners in interrogations is a poignant illustration of the challenges confronting military healthcare practitioners. The professional associations, including the American Medical Association, the American Psychiatric Association, the American Psychological Association, and the American Academy of Psychiatry and the Law, have published differing guidance and opinions. The American Medical Association and American Psychiatric Association admonish against the involvement of psychiatrists and physicians in interrogations and focus their policies and recommendations on the ethical responsibilities of the practitioner to the individual under questioning (Knoll 2010). The American Psychological Association has adopted broader, more controversial views condoning the involvement of psychologists in national security-related interrogations and other activities (Hoffman 2015).

Subjecting detainees to forced cell extractions (FCEs) for movement to enteral feedings falls in the domain of nonclinical activities that present ethical dilemmas for military clinical practitioners (forced cell extractions, or jail cell extractions, involve the use of controlled tactics by a team of law enforcement personnel for removing a non-compliant individual from a jail cell). The procedures and conduct of FCEs inflict undue harm and can aggravate conditions, such as chronic back and musculoskeletal pain. Detainees at Guantánamo concluded that FCEs and restrictions on bedding and reading material were conducted as a means to "break the hunger strikes" and induce compliance. They perceived the FCEs as means for overpowering detainees and graphically illustrating to them "who is in control." They perceived these actions, which they experienced as harsh and abusive treatment, as reactions to their refusal of food and decision to be on a hunger strike and not as actions by healthcare providers seeking to improve their quality of life or safeguard their lives. The dilemma that confronted medical professionals in this situation involved choosing between implementing the guidance and best practices for all the problems and conditions that Dhiab exhibited and complying with command authorities in actions justified as tactics in the conduct of asymmetrical warfare.

The professional associations agree that it is acceptable for medical practitioners to participate or assist in training, program design, and research on psychological issues as they apply to national security, if there is no real-time contact with subjects and if practitioners perform teaching, indirect consulting, or investigative roles not involving subjects. The disagreement and differences among the specialty associations apply to the direct involvement of practitioners in face-to-face engagement that are not regarded as clinical activities. Participation in interrogations and nonclinical activities is considered corrosive and undermining the professionalism of the discipline (Xenakis and Sherman 2015).

In the Service of Justice

The stipulation in the American Medical Association *Code of Medical Ethics* that the "physician shall respect the law and also recognize a responsibility to seek changes in those requirements which are contrary to the best interests of the patient" frames the dual responsibilities for military medical personnel. The Army stipulates guidelines for treating prisoners of war and other captives and holds military medicine accountable (Army Regulation 190-8 1997):

- All persons captured, detained, interned, or otherwise held in US Armed Forces custody during the course of conflict will be given humanitarian care and treatment from the moment they fall into the hands of US forces until final release or repatriation.
- All prisoners will receive humane treatment without regard to race, nationality, religion, political opinion, sex, or other criteria.
- First aid and medical treatment will be provided to the same extent that the United States provides to its own forces.

Military medical personnel cannot be expected to interpret or argue the letter of the law with commanders, attorneys, or other authorities. Nonetheless, they have the privilege and responsibility to interpret and implement the stipulations and intent of military regulations and policies as they apply to their professional domain. Military clinicians have the unique training and experience to operationalize guidelines for humane treatment and provide appropriate healthcare to patients that conforms to standard practice. Accordingly, military medical personnel carry the primary and unique responsibility of interpreting and executing the tasks and intent of the regulations and guidelines.

The tension between the traditional ethical codes of medicine, as amplified by the modernized AMA *Code of Medical Ethics*, pertinent Department of Defense regulations, and military procedures falls squarely on the shoulders of military medical personnel at all levels of command. The dual responsibilities of military medical personnel entail providing optimal healthcare, conforming to ethical standards, and fulfilling duties as military professionals. However, the duties and responsibilities of military personnel differ across the range of professional disciplines. Even though military professionals share a commitment to perform their duties to the utmost of their capability as well as some common skills, they are not interchangeable nor can they be expected to perform duties outside of their professional domain. Designating medical personnel as combatants and assigning principal duties outside the arena of healthcare violate principles of medical ethics and DoD guidelines. Military medical personnel are bound to uphold those principles and the intent of the laws as they apply in everyday practice.

Accordingly, the medical professionals at Guantánamo had the responsibility to advocate on behalf of detainees and to object to harsh and abusive treatments that harmed and aggravated their illnesses and conditions. The conditions of confinement and overriding control of the detention authorities interfered with the effective and appropriate delivery of medical care. Many detainees expressed no antipathy or hostility toward the United States or toward the authorities at Guantánamo Bay Naval Base; desired to establish a peaceful, normal, and productive life with their families; and did not present a terrorist threat before, during, or after their time in detention.

Summary: Providing Ethical Care During Twenty-First-Century Warfare

The case study of Mohammed Abu Wa'el (Jihad) Dhiab illustrates the ethical dilemma confronting military medical personnel. The Global War on Terror and warfare in the twenty-first century have thrust military medical personnel into unique roles and have caused them to face unique challenges. The backdrop of changing social dynamics, business operations, and means of warfare has stimulated fundamental shifts in military tactics, operations, and strategy (Department of the Army 2006). In today's world, the professional domain of military clinicians intersects with growing social and political trends, particularly the power of individualism. Insurgency and counterinsurgency tactics pivot on the actions and capabilities of individual warriors. Since 9/11, military clinicians have been deeply engaged on the front lines of this brave new world. It may be an unprecedented era of individual and human rights and individual empowerment. The dominance of formal nation states has seemed to recede with the rise of individuals, social groups, businesses, and crime organizations.

Accordingly, the ethical principles of clinical medicine that affirm individual and human rights empower larger roles and responsibilities for military medical personnel. The ethical challenges and duties anchor the dual responsibilities of the providers. The principles rest on the time-honored tradition of "do no harm" and on the premise that all physicians endeavor to benefit the patient (Xenakis 2014). That is, doctors acknowledge the challenges of treating detainees and prisoners of war in the broader context of national security strategy. The goals and purposes of improving health, quality of life, and functioning of detainees and prisoners of war help support the security of the nation in the fluid battlefields of the twenty-first century. Military medics have a common duty—from corpsmen to physicians to senior leaders—to provide care according to high standards of medical practice to all who need it.

All US military officers take an oath on commissioning and promotion to abide by the US Constitution and to support the safety and security of the nation. The burden of leadership is to ensure that high moral and ethical practices are maintained in even the most demanding situations. Patients trust doctors, nurses, and medics because they expect them to do what is right—to put the needs of others over their own. Facing ethical dilemmas is a common element of everyday medical practice, military medicine, and senior leadership. It is expected that military medical personnel will ask hard questions about the ethical parameters guiding their conduct and professionalism. They are obligated to exercise courage, stand up for their principles, and not compromise professional standards for any political purpose or personal agenda.

Key Concepts

1. The central ethical dilemmas that military health professionals face involve the following principal areas: dual agency (working for both the military and the service member patient), the decision-making processes regarding return-to-duty or evacuation and retaining a service member or recommending medical board review, maintaining patient confidentiality versus understanding what command needs to know, and the disability and compensation issues for those diagnosed with post-traumatic stress disorder (PTSD).
2. When treating detainees and enemy combatants, military practitioners confront ethical dilemmas that can challenge their compliance with the principles of medical ethics, including the bedrock principle "first, do no harm"; the American Medical Association's (AMA) updated principles of providing competent care, upholding professional standards, and applying scientific knowledge; and the right to exercise autonomy.
3. Medical personnel are bound to respect the autonomy of their patients, irrespective of their status as detainees, prisoners of war, or active combatants.
4. The best practices for treatment of hunger strikes include establishing a therapeutic relationship and rapport with the detained subject, ascertaining the wishes of the subject with regard to supportive care, conducting psychological and mental status evaluation, ascertaining the presence of undue influence, and providing an independent second medical opinion.
5. The professional associations have published differing guidance and opinions on medical practitioners' face-to-face engagement with interrogations that are not regarded as clinical activities. Participation in interrogations and nonclinical activities is corrosive and undermining the professionalism of the discipline.
6. Military clinicians have the unique training and experience to operationalize military and medical guidelines for humane treatment.
7. Facing ethical dilemmas is a common element of everyday medical practice, military medicine, and senior leadership. It is expected that military medical personnel will ask difficult questions about the ethical parameters guiding their conduct and professionalism, and the burden of leadership is to ensure that high moral and ethical practices are maintained in even the most demanding situations.

References

5 U.S.C. § 3331, (1966) *Oath of Office*

Arehart-Treichel J (2013) Psychosomatic medicine becomes deeper and wider. Published online.

Army Regulation 190-8 (1997) Enemy prisoners of war, retained personnel, civilian internees and other detainees

Bloche MG, Marks JH (2005) When doctors go to war. Perspective. New England Journal of Medicine, p 3–6

Brotherton S, Audiey Kao A, Crigger BJ (2016) Professing the ethics of medicine: the modernized AMA *Code of Medical Ethics*. JAMA. Published online 14 July

Chapter IV, (1966) Article 25 of the Geneva Convention

Crosby SS et al (2007) Hunger strikes, force-feeding, and physicians' responsibilities. JAMA 298:5
Department of the Army (2006) FM 3–24. Counterinsurgency
Ethics Abandoned (2013) Medical professionalism and detainee abuse in the "War on Terror." A task force report funded by IMAP/OSF. Education and training of military physicians on treatment of prisoners
Hoffman DH (2015) Report to the special committee of the board of directors of the American Psychological Association independent review relating to APA ethics guidelines, National Security Interrogations, and Torture
Knoll J (2010) Interrogations-medical ethics vs. Mr. Big. Psychiatric Times. Vol. no
Lazarus J (2013) Letter to the secretary of defense
Medical Management of Detainees with Weight Loss. Joint Medical Group. Joint Task Force Guantanamo Bay, Cuba (2013)
Petitioner's Notice of Filing, District Federal Court. Expert report of Stephen N. Xenakis, M.D., LLC (2014)
Physicians for human rights and University of Capetown health sciences centre, dual loyalty and human rights in health professional practice: proposed guidelines and institutional mechanisms (2003) http://physiciansforhumanrights.org/library/reports/dual-loyalty-and-human-rights-2003.html
Ritchie EC (2014) Forensic and ethical issues in military behavioral health. Office of the Surgeon General, Department of the Army, p 6
Unutzer J (2009) Integrated mental care: mental health is part of overall health. University of Washington School of Medicine
World Medical Association. Declaration of Tokyo (1975) Adopted by the World Medical Association, Tokyo, Japan. Oct. 1975
Xenakis SN (2014) The role and responsibilities of military psychiatrists in the 21st century. J Am Acad Psychiatry Law 42:504–508
Xenakis SN, Sherman N (2015) Not just about the psychologists. Huffington post

Substance Use in Military and Veteran Populations

19

John D. Hunsaker and Robert Joel Bush

Prevalence of Substance Use in the Military

The US military is comprised of a patient population at high risk for substance use. According to the Substance Abuse and Mental Health Services Administration (SAMHSA), youth transitioning into adulthood have some of the highest rates of alcohol and substance abuse (SAMHSA 2016), and 43% of the armed force's 1,326,273 personnel are under the age of 25 (DoD 2014). Despite being significantly comprised of a population at high risk, the military has rates of illicit substance use that are lower than comparable populations in the civilian sector.

Prevention programs are a significant contributor to the low rates of illicit substance use in the military. The Department of Defense (DoD) mandates that all service members be tested for drug use, requiring that, on average, every service member be tested at least once yearly for illicit drug and prescription medication abuse (DoDI 1010.01 2012). In 2014, the Department of Defense drug-testing laboratories analyzed 4.88 million specimens, performing over 43.4 million screening assays for 11 classes of illicit drugs and prescription medications (DoD 2015). The frequency and randomness of drug testing, as well as the consequences for positive results, has led to an ever-decreasing number of positive samples through all branches of the armed services.

While the rates of substance use may be relatively low in the military, substance abuse certainly does not spare the men and women serving their country, both during their active service and in the years that follow. There are unique characteristics of the patterns of substance use in military and veteran populations, and to assist in understanding these characteristics, this chapter will address the prevalence of illicit drug and prescription medication abuse, alcohol abuse, and tobacco use separately.

Illicit Drug Use

According to the Department of Defense drug-testing program (DoD 2015), in fiscal year 2014, only 0.88% of US service members (Active, Reserve and Guard) tested positive for illicit drug or prescription medication abuse. This is the lowest rate since the initiation of the drug-

J.D. Hunsaker (✉)
Fort Belvoir Community Hospital,
Ft. Belvoir, VA, USA

Uniformed Services University of the Health Sciences (USUHS), Bethesda, MD, USA
e-mail: John.d.hunsake4.mil@mail.mil

R.J. Bush
William Beaumont Army Medical Center,
Fort Bliss, TX, USA

L.W. Roberts, C.H. Warner (eds.), *Military and Veteran Mental Health*,
https://doi.org/10.1007/978-1-4939-7438-2_19

testing program in 1981, from which time the trend has been a general decline (Fig. 19.1). According to Quest Diagnostics, which runs millions of drug tests for the civilian workforce, the military rate is one-fifth the rate of the general US workforce, which has a 4.7% positive rate (Quest Diagnostics 2015).

Rates of substance abuse vary by military services. In 2014 the Army had the highest rate of positive drug tests among active duty personnel, with 1.04%. The lowest was the Navy at 0.37%, with the Marines at 0.60% and the Air Force at 0.39% (DoD 2015). Reserve and National Guard units often tested at higher rates than their active duty peers. For example, 1.86% of service members not on active duty status in the Army Guard tested positive, and 1.78% of those not on active duty status in the Reserve tested positive, as compared to the active army rate of 1.04% (DoD 2015). All service components had a similar higher rate of positive samples in their guard and reserve components that are in active duty.

Of positive samples in the military population, marijuana was the most common substance of abuse, detected in 66% of positive samples. This trend parallels civilian numbers, in which marijuana is also the most commonly found substance in positive samples (Quest Diagnostics 2015). Prescription opiates were detected in 13.8% of positive samples, the second most common drug of abuse in the military, and cocaine was the third most common, found in 11.2% of positive samples (DoD 2015).

While there is no drug-testing program for veterans, we know that today's military members are tomorrow's veterans, and thus the information for active duty personnel can be applied loosely to veterans as well. However, there are unique factors to consider when assessing and treating veterans for substance use disorders. The high rates of PTSD, depression, and anxiety in veterans predispose them to substance use disorders. While the rates and consequences of these disorders are discussed elsewhere, it is important to note the strong correlation between the experiences of veterans and substance use. In a recent study involving Iraq and Afghanistan veterans seeking VA care for the first time between 2001 and 2009, 5% received a diagnosis of drug use disorder (Seal et al. 2011). Alcohol use disorders, drug use disorders, or both were three to four times more likely to occur in veterans with PTSD and depression.

Alcohol Use

The Department of Defense drug-testing program does not test urine samples for alcohol and tobacco. Even if random sampling were to be obtained, testing for metabolites of alcohol or nicotine would not necessarily indicate problematic use. Measuring the use of these substances relies on self-report surveys conducted periodically.

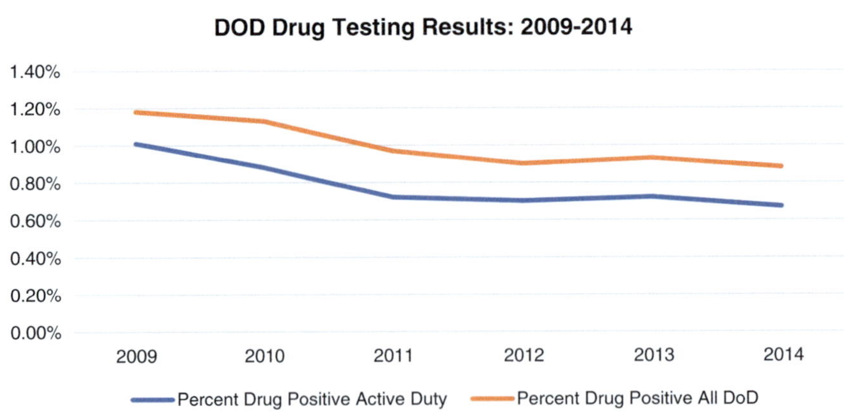

Fig. 19.1 DoD drug testing results, 2009–2014

According to a study conducted in 2014 by the National Institute on Alcohol Abuse and Alcoholism (NIAAA), 6.7% of people ages 18 and older engaged in heavy drinking within the past month (NIAAA 2016). Among all active duty service members in 2011, 8.4% were heavy drinkers (Barlas et al. 2013), where heavy drinking is defined as consuming five or more drinks on one or more occasions per week. When comparing these two studies, the rates of drinking appear to be higher in military populations, and the difference between military and civilian populations is also significant when it comes to alcohol use disorders. Among all US adults over the age of 18, 6.8% had an alcohol use disorder in 2014 (NIAAA 2016), while 10% of Iraq and Afghanistan veterans presenting to the VA for care for the first time between 2001 and 2009 were diagnosed with an alcohol use disorder (Seal et al. 2011).

The reasons for the higher rates of heavy drinking and alcohol use disorders among active duty personnel and veterans are multifactorial, but one strongly correlated finding is the association between combat stress and increased alcohol use. Recent studies have found that 12–15% of veterans returning from Operation Iraqi Freedom have endorsed problematic alcohol use in the 3–6 months following their return from combat (Milliken et al. 2007). These rates are double the national averages for heavy drinking in the civilian population.

The rate of drinking has been shown to differ among the branches of the military as well, as service culture influences the rate of substance use. For example, while the rate of heavy drinkers in the military is 8.4%, the Marine Corps has the highest rate of heavy drinkers at 15.5%, and the Air Force has the lowest rate of heavy drinkers at 3.8%. The Marine Corps also has the highest rate of binge drinking (5+ drinks for male service members and 4+ drinks for female service members in the last 30 days) at 48.2%, while the Air Force maintains the lowest rate of the services at 22.7% (Barlas et al. 2013).

Tobacco Use

Senator Richard Durbin, a member of the US Senate Committee on Appropriations, stated in a recent hearing to the Surgeons General of the Army, Air Force, and Navy, "The rate of tobacco use within our Military is higher than in civilian life, and we know what the costs are in terms of the health of the men and women who serve our nation. We need to be conscientious in reducing that number" (Durbin 2016). In 2011, 24% of all active duty military reported smoking cigarettes, compared with 19% of civilians. In addition, 12.8% of all military personnel reported using a smokeless tobacco product, compared to 3.2% of the general population. Over 52% of all service members endorsed using a nicotine product in the last 12 months (Barlas et al. 2013).

The use of tobacco products by service members is pervasive, and the stressors they encounter often lead to higher rates of use. Military personnel returning from Iraq and Afghanistan have 50% higher smoking rates than non-deployed personnel (IOM 2009). The effects of these increases do not resolve after military service: between 2007 and 2010, male veterans were more likely to be current smokers than nonveterans (CDC 2016).

As Senator Durbin emphatically pointed out, the rate of tobacco use in the military is higher than in civilian life, and there are not only health but also financial costs associated with this problem. The cost to the military health system from smoking is tremendous. In 2006 it was estimated that $564 million was spent treating tobacco-related illnesses. In 2008, the VA spent over $5 billion to treat chronic obstructive pulmonary disease (COPD), more than 80% of which is attributed to smoking (IOM 2009).

Much is known about the performance declines and health risks of tobacco use. Recent studies also point to significant behavioral health effects of tobacco use. Smoking cessation has been associated with significant decreases in anxiety and depression, with significant increases in quality of life (Taylor et al. 2014). In addition, tobacco use increases anxiety overall (McDermott et al. 2013), and when service members and veterans use this substance in higher amounts than the general population, the negative impact on the behavioral health of service members and veterans is significant.

The Impact of Military Life on Substance Use Issues

Substance use disorders within the military system require unique considerations and cannot be approached in the same way that a provider would approach any other substance use patient. Many of the unique aspects of substance use disorders within the military require knowledge of the history and culture of military populations, trends within specific populations, consequences of substance use in the service, and treatment programs available to service members.

Case Study, Part 1

Army Sergeant (SGT) Samuel Robison, a married, 24-year-old soldier, presents with a complaint of alcohol problems. He states that he has been drinking heavily and daily for about 2 years, more than five drinks at a time since returning from his first deployment. He states he has tried to slow down on his own, but has not been successful. He endorses mild withdrawal symptoms and some moderate cravings for alcohol use. His last drink was last night.

Military Culture

Understanding the culture of substance use and the military is critical to forming an approach to treatment. Military history has shaped the culture that permeates the different services and still plays a role in influencing the attitudes of members of the armed forces. Alcohol in particular has been widely used and even given in rations for soldiers as recently as World War II (Ross and Romanus 1992). Alcohol consumption has been encouraged within military cultures to promote unit cohesion and to boost morale. Although no rations of alcohol have been provided in the recent past, alcohol is currently available to service members at decreased cost at military installations (IOM 2013).

Social network facilitation, or when service members report that some or most of their friends use substances, has been reported as high as 89% for alcohol and 73% for nicotine. However, social network facilitation did not appear to be a factor for marijuana or prescription medication misuse, as only 6.5% and 4.5% endorsed peer use. In a recent study, 90% of service members felt that leaders somewhat or strongly discouraged the use of illegal substances, while only about 50% felt that leadership discouraged the use of alcohol or tobacco products (Barlas et al. 2013). In 2013, the Institute of Medicine reported, "Heavy drinking is an accepted custom that has become part of the military work culture and has been used for recreation, as well as to reward hard work, to ease interpersonal tensions, and to promote unit cohesion and camaraderie" (IOM 2013). This culture of alcohol use within the military has had an undesirable effect by increasing the rates of alcohol use within the armed forces.

Consequences of Substance Use in Military Service

It is not surprising that standards of performance are higher for those who are trained to fight, use weapons or explosives, and handle other sensitive items or information. What can result, for example, from an intoxicated soldier who must pack parachutes, handle missile systems, translate top-secret documents, or patrol with a loaded weapon? These implications create unique challenges for both diagnosing and treating substance use disorders. Although alcohol use among military members has long been tolerated, and even encouraged, by some cultures within the service, negative consequences of such use (i.e., driving while intoxicated, domestic violence, failure to meet work obligations) are not tolerated and can result in discipline and dismissal from the service.

Service members and veterans face strict regulations in regard to substance use. Zero tolerance policies that can result in dishonorable discharge or criminal prosecution are a deterrent, as well as a stressor and barrier to care for service members and veterans. For example, army regulations state that service members identified as illegal drug abusers or who have been involved in two serious incidents of alcohol-related misconduct will be processed for separation from the military (Army Regulation 600-85 2014). An additional barrier to care in the military system is the lack of confidentiality when seeking help for substance use disorders. The commanding officer of a service member seeking treatment is notified and updated regularly, and the commander also consults with the treating provider to decide on treatment plans. This type of oversight and exposure when seeking care can discourage service members from getting help. Fear of negative repercussions on their careers often results in service members not getting care until significant problems have developed.

Case Study, Part 2

SGT Robison presents as a routine case with minimal withdrawal and heavy alcohol use. He is offered medications for alcohol use to prevent consumption (such as disulfiram) or to reduce cravings for alcohol (such as naltrexone or acamprosate), but declines and reports that he thinks simple outpatient counseling would be sufficient to help him abstain. He is asked to return in 2 weeks. He returns again 34 days later and reports that he had not been completely open during his first visit and that since then he has increased his alcohol consumption and is now drinking on average one drink every 2 h and has not been able to stop. He has been going to his outpatient counseling sessions and reports learning a lot, but cravings are intense and withdrawal is difficult to deal with. SGT Robison reports that he is very anxious to start medications for alcohol use prevention and is started on outpatient detoxification protocol with abstinence-promoting medications and is asked to come back in 1 week to follow up.

Substance Use Disorder Treatment for Service Members

Addiction treatment within the Department of Defense and the Veterans Administration (VA) is similar to resources available in traditional healthcare systems. The American Society of Addiction Medicine (ASAM) lists the different levels of care and the placement criteria for each type of treatment (Table 19.1 and Fig. 19.2). These guidelines are utilized within the Military Health System (MHS) to direct care and resources.

Using ASAM Criteria Levels of Care as a guide, providers can speak the same language when communicating about the needs of treatment and plans for their patients. Across these levels of care, there are community, criminal justice, and traditional healthcare systems that provide an array of services. The military system of care follows the paradigm of the traditional healthcare system, but utilizes some of the same core concepts as the criminal justice system in its execution, as there are significant consequences for a soldier, airman, sailor, or marine who fails or refuses treatment.

The 2013 Institute of Medicine report found that the Military Health System "provides comprehensive health care to military service members" (IOM 2013). Service members and their families are covered for substance abuse care through an array of facilities located on military bases or through civilian facilities contracted to provide care if similar resources are unavailable on base.

Level I treatment is widely available in the Department of Defense, and resources for this level of treatment are located at virtually every single military installation, with few exceptions.

Table 19.1 American Society of Addiction Medicine (ASAM) criteria levels of care

ASAM PPC-2R description	Level	Notes
Detoxification levels for adults (Note: there are no separate detoxification services for adolescents)		
Ambulatory detoxification without extended onsite monitoring	I-D	Mild withdrawal with daily or less than daily outpatient supervision; likely to complete detoxification and to continue treatment or recovery
Ambulatory detoxification with extended onsite monitoring	II-D	Moderate withdrawal with all-day detoxification support and supervision; at night, has supportive family or living situation; likely to complete detoxification
Clinically managed residential detoxification	III.2-D	Minimal to moderate withdrawal, but needs 24-h support to complete detoxification and increase likelihood of continuing treatment or recovery
Medically monitored inpatient detoxification	III.7-D	Severe withdrawal and needs 24-h nursing care and physician visits as necessary; unlikely to complete detoxification without medical, nursing, monitoring
Medically managed inpatient detoxification	IV-D	Severe, unstable withdrawal and needs 24-h nursing care and daily physician visits to modify detoxification regimen and manage instability
Care levels (Note: same care levels of care for adolescents except level III.3)		
Early intervention (EI)	0.5	Assessment and education for at-risk individuals who do not meet diagnostic criteria for substance-related disorder
Outpatient services (OP)	I	Less than 9 h of service/week (adults); less than 6 h/week (adolescents) for recovery or motivational enhancement therapies/strategies
Intensive outpatient (IOP)	II.1	9 or more hours of service/week (adults); 6 or more h/week (adolescents) in a structured program to treat multidimensional instability
Partial hospitalization (PHP)	II.5	20 or more hours of service/week in a structured program for multidimensional instability not requiring 24-h care
Clinically managed low-intensity residential	III.1	24-h structure with available trained personnel with emphasis on reentry to the community; at least 5 h of clinical service/week
Clinically managed medium-intensity residential	III.3	24-h care with trained counselors to stabilize multidimensional imminent danger. Less intense milieu and group treatment for those with cognitive or other impairments unable to use full active milieu or therapeutic community
Clinically managed high-intensity residential	III.5	24-h care with trained counselors to stabilize multidimensional imminent danger and prepare for outpatient treatment. Able to tolerate and use full active milieu or therapeutic community
Medically monitored intensive inpatient	III.7	24-h nursing care with physician availability for significant problems in dimensions 1, 2, or 3. 16 h/day counselor availability
Medically managed intensive inpatient	IV	24-h nursing care and daily physician care for severe, unstable problems in dimensions 1, 2, or 3. Counseling available to engage patient in treatment
Opioid maintenance therapy	OMT	Daily or several times weekly opioid medication and counseling available to maintain multidimensional stability for those with opioid dependence

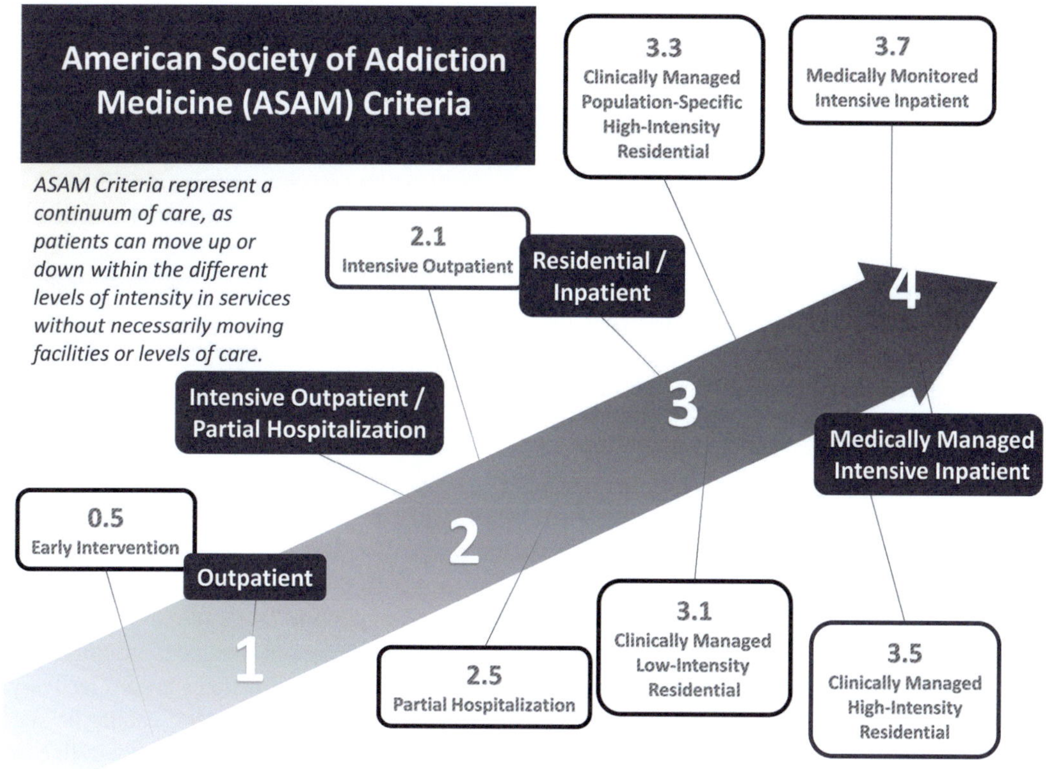

Fig. 19.2 ASAM criteria

Even aircraft carriers have programs that are integrated into their system of care. Many of the limitations on what is available are based on location and population. Very small locations tend to have fewer facilities and counselors, and larger installations tend to have robust programs with more intensive treatment. Based on need and population at installations, higher levels of care may be available, including intensive outpatient programs and partial hospitalization programs (IOP/PHP) and Level III residential programs. As needed, service members can travel to other bases for higher levels of care or utilize community resources for the same care as clinically indicated.

Each branch of the military has a similar portfolio of treatment capabilities. Larger bases, with more intensive resources, will lend support as needed to other facilities to ensure service members receive an optimal level of care. Communication and coordination between Department of Defense installations, even across services, is done when higher levels of treatment are needed but not available at an installation. Military leadership is working to expand treatment for this growing need, but creating new programs rapidly takes time and vast resources and programs are often outpaced by the demand.

Clinical care offered to service members does not differ from care available in the civilian model. Outpatient counseling is the general starting point, with abstinence-promoting medications available as needed. Referrals for comorbid behavioral health and medical disorders are readily available and often utilized, with coordinated care offered between providers. As discussed earlier, elevations in the levels of care are available as clinically indicated.

Differences between the Military Health System and civilian models rest primarily in the command and control aspect of military service. As noted earlier, commanders are notified when their service members seek care for substance use disorders. In addition, referrals for all levels of care must be acknowledged and agreed upon by the commander. This aspect of care limits confidentiality and clinical autonomy. Consequences for substance use also can deter service members from seeking care. However, oversight and supervision from a commander is not always a negative aspect of care. For example, the Department of Defense drug-testing program identifies substance abuse issues often before they come to clinical attention, allowing the commander to refer the service member to care early in the course of substance use and hopefully before serious consequences manifest. In addition, having the support and supervision of an employer (or commander) while receiving treatment for an alcohol use disorder can have a positive impact on recovery by offering additional resources, such as peer support and accountability, that may assist a service member in recovery. Experience working with commanders has shown that, first and foremost, they care about their service members and are motivated to help them pursue the necessary care. The dual role of commanders requires that they also satisfy the needs of the US military, but this loyalty does not mean that efforts to treat and care for those under their command are neglected.

Case Study, Part 3

SGT Robison does not follow up after the second visit, and his father contacts the provider 2 months later, reporting that the patient has been drinking again, expressing significant frustration about his relapse, and indicating thoughts of hopelessness. SGT Robison has not been taking his medication and has resumed daily heavy consumption. He is referred to Level IV residential treatment run by a nonmilitary facility in the local area. The patient returns to the provider after the 4-week inpatient treatment, reporting that he resumed alcohol consumption the very day he left and consequently has developed some thoughts of self-harm. He reports that he feels like a failure and knows he is letting everyone down. He has been drinking, heavily and daily, since he was released from his inpatient treatment. The patient's military unit commander decides to separate the soldier from active service based on failure to rehabilitate for alcohol use disorder. While the soldier awaits the process of separation, a referral for a partial hospital program (PHP) with co-occurring treatment capabilities is made. He engages in treatment at this level for 6 weeks.

Relapse is a defining characteristic of substance use disorders, and treatment must be flexible to accommodate individual circumstances. Engaging in multiple levels of care is common, and repeated courses of treatment are often necessary in order to assist patients toward recovery. However, service members who cannot be successfully treated and returned to their line of work within the armed forces may be separated from the service. The nature of service in the armed forces requires a sober mind and sound judgment, and when multiple attempts at treatment have failed, service members are often separated from the military. This heavy decision rests on the shoulders of the commander and is made with the service member's potential for rehabilitation in mind. When separation is the

Case Study, Part 4

SGT Robison returns 2 months later, after his release from Level II.5 treatment and reports that he has relapsed multiple times, both while in the program and again after release. His father travels to stay with him in the remaining weeks of his military service as he transitions to the VA system. SGT Robison continues to struggle with relapse over the subsequent weeks during his transition out of active military service.

course of action, the service member is often transitioned to treatment within the VA.

Institute of Medicine Report on Substance Abuse in the Armed Forces

In 2013 the Institute of Medicine published a report on substance abuse in the armed forces. Its thorough evaluation of the system resulted in recommendations for improvement in four main categories:

1. Increasing emphasis on prevention of substance use disorders (SUDs) in service members and their dependents
2. Developing and implementing evidence-based programs and best practices for SUD care
3. Increasing access to care
4. Strengthening the workforce of those treating SUDs in the armed services (IOM 2013)

While many specific findings and recommendations are provided in the Institute of Medicine report—too many to discuss individually here—these four categories encompass the major ideas and recommended changes. While some recommendations have solutions that are tangible and finite, others can be more difficult to approach and change across the Military Health System. A recommendation that is more easily addressed is access to care. Previous rules for TRICARE reimbursement limited access to residential programs to once yearly and a maximum of three treatments in a lifetime. After the publication of the Institute of Medicine report, TRICARE has changed this policy and no longer places limits on residential care, allowing clinical discretion and the needs of the patient to drive care recommendations.

Recommendations for the prevention of substance use disorders may require greater effort to effect change. For example, changing the culture in the military that often supports heavy alcohol use will take time and concerted effort. Even in the right circumstances, change within a culture—no matter how appropriate or necessary—will require patience and dedication. Efforts in this area are underway, with trainings and activities designed to educate new service members on the risks of substance use and the resources available to them. However, a complete shift in culture cannot be expected in days or months, as years will be required to see the effects of these new efforts. Recently, proposals have been put forward to enable service members to receive substance abuse care confidentially—an issue that was also addressed in the 2013 Institute of Medicine report. While this change has not yet been approved or taken effect, it is an example of further Military Health System efforts to bring the treatment of substance use disorders in the Department of Defense in line with the best standards of care.

Substance Use Disorder Treatment Within the Veterans Administration

The Army drug-testing program has been successful in deterring the abuse of substances. In the 1980 Department of Defense Survey of Health-Related Behavior Among Military Personnel, 30% of service members admitted to using illegal drugs in the past 30 days. More recently, in 2011, the same survey reported less than 1% admitting to illegal substance use in the last 30 days (Barlas et al. 2013). However, success in one area implies a cost in another. Filtered out of the military through dishonorable discharges, administrative separations, medical board reviews, and prohibition of reenlistment are veterans with substance abuse problems.

The transition from Department of Defense to VA treatment for substance use disorders is a process and can be difficult to navigate. There can be gaps in coverage when transitioning from the military to the VA, and facilities often have long wait times for initializing treatment. Generally, the VA has comprehensive treatments available throughout all levels of care.

Servicing the needs of veterans in every state, the VA offers a wide range of services and all levels of care for substance use disorders. Veterans transitioning to treatment for substance use disorders can receive care without limitations in time or resources. Members no longer able to serve in the military receive continued care in line with their needs.

Summary

Military and VA systems and facilities will continue to grapple with the need for substance use treatment for their patients. Barriers to care and limitations on resources result in unique challenges for patients, providers, and systems within both the Department of Defense and the VA. The 2013 Institute of Medicine report on Substance Use Disorders in the US Armed Forces made many recommendations for improvement in the care offered to service members. Many of these recommendations are being implemented, such as integrating care for substance use disorders with care for other mental health conditions, the recent expansion of TRICARE coverage for treatment of substance use disorders, the introduction of routine screening for unhealthy alcohol use in inpatient and outpatient settings, and the integration of technology into tracking and treating substance use disorders (IOM 2013).

Substance use disorder treatment for veterans and active duty service members requires knowledge of the history, culture, and trends of substance use behaviors within specific military populations. Familiarity with the consequences of continued substance use in the service and with available treatment programs for service members will assist providers as they seek appropriate treatment for service members (or veterans) of the armed forces.

Key Concepts

1. While illicit drug use is lower in the armed forces than in civilian populations, service members are at greater risk for alcohol and tobacco use disorders, which flourish in an environment and culture supporting their use.
2. Service members and veterans are subject to consequences and oversight when seeking care for substance use disorders, which can result in failure to seek care when needed.
3. All levels of care (from outpatient to full residential) are afforded to service members and veterans, both in the Department of Defense and the Veterans Administration, and are similar to community resources.
4. Recommendations have been made by the Institute of Medicine for improvements in care for service members and are being integrated into military and veterans systems of care to improve both access to and quality of care.

References

Army Regulation 600-85 (2014) The army substance abuse program, administrative revision

Barlas FM, Higgins WB, Pflieger JC, Diecker K (2013) 2011 Department of Defense Health Related Behaviors Survey of Active Duty Military Personnel. U.S. Department of Defense, TRICARE Management Activity, Defense Health Cost Assessment and Program Evaluation, and the United States Coast Guard

Centers for Disease Control and Prevention (2016) Current cigarette smoking among U.S. adults aged 18 years and older. http://www.cdc.gov/tobacco/campaign/tips/resources/data/cigarette-smoking-in-united-states.html. Accessed 13 May 2016

Department of Defense (DoD) (2014) 2014 Demographics: profile of the military community. Office of the Deputy Assistant Secretary of Defense (Military Community and Family Policy)

Department of Defense (DoD) (2015) Status of Drug Use in the Department of Defense (FOUO) Office of the Under Secretary of Defense for Personnel and Readiness. Data provided by Director, Drug Testing and Program Policy, Office of the Under Secretary of Defense for Personnel & Readiness

Department of Defense Instruction (DoDI) 1010.01 (2012) The Office of the Undersecretary of Defense for Personnel & Readiness

Durbin R (2016) Hearing to review FY17 budget request for the Defense Health Program. http://www.appropriations.senate.gov/hearings/hearing-to-review-fy17-budget-request-for-the-defense-health-program. Accessed 13 May 2016

Institute of Medicine (IOM) (2009) Combating tobacco use in military and veteran populations. The National Academies Press, Washington, DC

Institute of Medicine (IOM) (2013) Substance use disorders in the U.S. armed forces. The National Academies Press, Washington, DC

McDermott M, Marteau T, Hollands G, Hankins M, Aveyard P (2013) Change in anxiety following successful and unsuccessful attempts at smoking cessation: cohort study. Br J Psychiatry 202:62–67

Milliken CS, Auchterlonie JL, Hoge CW (2007) Longitudinal assessment of mental health problems among active and reserve component soldiers returning from the Iraq war. J Am Med Assoc 298(18):2141–2148

National Institute on Alcohol Abuse and Alcoholism (NIAAA) (2016) Alcohol facts and statistics. http://www.niaaa.nih.gov/alcohol-health/overview-alcohol-consumption/alcohol-facts-and-statistics. Accessed 21 May 2016

Quest Diagnostics (2015) Illicit drug positivity rate increases sharply in workplace testing. http://www.questdiagnostics.com/home/physicians/health-trends/drug-testing.html. Accessed 17 May 2016

Ross WF, Romanus CF (1992) The quartermaster corps: operations in the war against Germany. United States Army in World War II Reader's Guide. CMH Publication 11–9 Center of Military History. United States Army, Washington, DC

Seal K, Cohen G, Waldrop A, Cohen B, Maguen S, Ren L (2011) Substance use disorders in Iraq and Afghanistan veterans in VA healthcare, 2001–2010: implications for screening, diagnosis and treatment. Drug Alcohol Depend 116(1–3):93–101

Substance Abuse and Mental Health Services Administration (SAMHSA) (2016) Age- and gender-based populations. http://www.samhsa.gov/specific-populations/age-gender-based. Accessed 25 Apr 2016

Taylor G, McNeill Ann, Girling A, Farley A, Lindson-Hawley N, Aveyard P (2014) Change in mental health after smoking cessation: systematic review and meta-analysis. BMJ 2014; 348:g1151

Co-occurring Substance and Mental Health Disorders

20

Lantie Jorandby-Quinones, Ellen Edens, and Robert A. Rosenheck

Historical Context of Co-occurring Disorders

In 1981, Bert Pepper identified a new category of psychiatric patient (Pepper et al. 1981). A community psychiatrist, Dr. Pepper was working in Pomona, NY, in the late 1970s and early 1980s when he and his colleagues began to encounter a unique type of patient for that time. These were psychiatric patients from the ages of 18 to 35 with serious mental health diagnoses, frequently decompensating and presenting to local emergency rooms. They were simultaneously noncompliant with outpatient treatment and often used addictive substances (a growing fashion among young people of all types in those years) but consumed local mental health resources at a greater rate than the traditional psychiatric patient.

Dr. Pepper decided to study this group of patient. He theorized that this rise of the "young chronic," as he came to call them, originated from the deinstitutionalization movement in America, which depopulated the state mental health hospital systems by 76% from 1955 to 1977. Pepper coined the term "young chronic" to identify the first generation of seriously and persistently mentally ill patients to "grow up" in the community treatment era of mental health which now consisted of community mental health centers rather than state hospital systems. Pepper discovered that 85% of his study population were marginally housed with family or friends or living in single room occupancy hotels or homeless shelters, 24% had been incarcerated or had involvement with the legal system, and 42% could be considered a high suicide risk. An estimated 37% had a drug or alcohol problem (Pepper et al. 1982). Two main diagnostic threads were the demonstration of persistent and severe social and psychological impairments and the high consumption of costly mental and medical health services. These patients presented frequently in crisis to emergency rooms but did not follow up with outpatient care. In his seminal paper from 1981 and follow-up papers (Pepper et al. 1981), Dr. Pepper laid out a loosely formed strategy for treatment that involved a more integrated approach than the traditional one that was part of the mental health field at the time. This new strategy involved not only pharmacology but also housing support, family treatment, social skills training, vocational rehabilitation,

L. Jorandby-Quinones • E. Edens
Yale School of Medicine, New Haven, CT, USA

R. A. Rosenheck (✉)
Veterans Affairs New England Mental Illness Research, Education, and Clinical Center, West Haven, CT, USA

Yale University School of Medicine, New Haven, CT, USA
e-mail: Robert.rosenheck@va.gov

L.W. Roberts, C.H. Warner (eds.), *Military and Veteran Mental Health*,
https://doi.org/10.1007/978-1-4939-7438-2_20

outpatient community treatment, and substance abuse treatment.

Thirty-five years later, the newer, post-deinstitutionalization generation of psychiatrists are not familiar with this historical background or with the term "young chronic." The patient this term identifies, however, persists and is now called homeless or dually diagnosed and remains recognizable as a diagnostic and treatment challenge.

Case Study

Former First Lieutenant (1LT.) Santiago Jones (pseudonym) is a 57-year-old male with schizoaffective disorder, depressed type; HIV; cocaine, opioid, and nicotine use disorders; as well as a history of heavy drinking. Jones is currently on buprenorphine-naloxone maintenance for treatment of opioid addiction and is engaged in treatment, attending outpatient relapse-prevention groups in a VA clinic on a weekly basis. His last relapse to cocaine was 6 months ago. Jones hears voices commenting on his actions daily and has intermittent feelings that the television is sending him messages even during periods of prolonged abstinence from cocaine, opioids, and alcohol. He has been treated with an atypical antipsychotic which he will intermittently stop taking because he experiences sedation and is unconvinced that such medications help. Relapse to cocaine often occurs simultaneously with nonadherence to medications. His HIV is managed through the infectious disease clinic with three different antiretrovirals. He is treated in primary care for hypertension, hypercholesterolemia, and erectile dysfunction. He would like to stop smoking and has successfully cut down in the past but has had difficulty making steps to prepare for a quit date. He was an average student in school, dropping out before graduation to join the military. He earned his GED while on active duty. He served in the army for 3 years and was discharged honorably. He had no exposure to combat. Following discharge from the military, he had a difficult time finding jobs for which he was suited. He has been married several times. He has been incarcerated twice for drug-related charges. He has had several episodes of homelessness in the past, typically following release from prison or during a relapse to drug use. Currently, he resides with a family member.

Definition of Co-occurring Disorders and Reason for Concern

This chapter's case study and brief historical context highlight the complex nature of the health status of those with co-occurring mental health and substance use disorders and typically many other psychosocial challenges. Terminology has evolved since Dr. Pepper's study, and "dual diagnosis" is now considered one of several commonly used terms. Other terms include "co-occurring" disorders and "comorbidity"—and perhaps "homeless" should be included, because the numbers may be small but the impact is substantial. The term "dual diagnosis," however, is in some ways misleading. As can be seen in this chapter's case study, First Lieutenant Jones experiences multiple problems, not only mental health and medical but also legal, financial, and social—all of which converge to adversely impact his life. Although this chapter discusses the mental health treatment of the dually diagnosed veteran, Dr. Pepper's patients and Jones share many similarities. The multiple issues discussed in Dr. Pepper's work cross the boundary from civilian to veteran life and present similar challenges for providers with regard to treatment and management. These issues also represent a general clinical phenomenon that has emerged from changes in the culture and from acceleration of the policies of deinstitutionalization, the criminalization of substance abuse, and the reduced commitment to social welfare and income support programs in recent decades.

The terms "dual diagnosis" and "co-occurring" are used in their most limited sense to refer to patients with both psychiatric and substance use disorders, but recent research has broadened the concept to identify patients with the presence of any two or more medical conditions as well as numerous related psychosocial conditions that derive, to varying degrees, from the medical diagnoses. Traditionally, medical care for the dually diagnosed patient has focused treatment on the individual diseases and has involved a limited number of options for care (Drake et al. 1996). Historically, a *partial* treatment approach for dual diagnosis is an approach designed to treat only the most serious disease with which a patient presents. *Sequential* treatment has involved treating the primary disease first and then the secondary disease. *Parallel* treatment is defined as treatment with different specialists treating the varying disorders simultaneously but separately. All these approaches are often thought to fail to address the unintended consequences in patients with dual diagnoses, namely, the potential for high treatment burden (e.g., polypharmacy, frequent appointments, multiple procedures) or worsening of one disease by treatment of another. Within the mental health care system, this siloing (i.e., operating in isolation) of healthcare delivery has also been complicated by a systems procedure which insists that nonsubstance mental health diagnoses (e.g., depression, PTSD) be treated separately from addiction services, often with little coordination across treatment teams. This approach has led to fragmented and stymied mental health care delivery.

The co-occurrence of both substance abuse (SA) and other mental health conditions poses unique healthcare challenges. This chapter describes what these challenges are and why they are important to the treatment of the dually diagnosed veteran and how they have been addressed in both research and practice.

First, rates of dual diagnosis are substantial among the veteran population, and it is the consensus opinion that each condition is thought to worsen and increase the likelihood that the other will be present. For example, current data suggest that of veterans who served in Vietnam or later, 41.4% with a substance use disorder also have PTSD as well (Petrakis et al. 2011). Moreover, the veteran population is at high risk of having sustained a traumatic brain injury (TBI) with estimates of nearly 20% of Iraq and Afghanistan conflict veterans experiencing it (Hoge et al. 2008). PTSD, alcohol disorders, and mild TBI often co-occur, and veterans with these diagnoses have been dubbed the "triply diagnosed." Symptoms of each condition have commonalities, suggesting that they may cause each other or rather reflect different aspects of a single underlying problem.

Second, it has been shown that there are more medical, psychiatric, and social problems found in the dually diagnosed patient than in the patient with only one diagnosis. Administrative data on veterans receiving Veterans Health Administration services show that veterans with dual diagnoses of PTSD and substance use disorders demonstrate higher rates of bipolar diagnoses, liver problems, HIV infection, and homelessness. Additionally, they have increased rates of psychiatric hospitalizations and mental health outpatient visits compared with veterans with PTSD but without substance use disorders (SUDs) (Bowe and Rosenheck 2015). Studies within the field of infectious disease have shown that, among veterans with active hepatitis C infection waiting for treatment, an estimated 93% have at least one psychiatric disorder and 73% had two or more. An estimated 58% had a substance use disorder in addition to a mood disorder (Fireman et al. 2005). Additionally, mortality rates in veteran psychiatric patients have been estimated at 55% higher if the veteran has a co-occurring substance use and mood disorder (Rosen et al. 2008).

Recent studies evaluating veterans enrolled in methadone maintenance treatment (MMT) show that veterans receiving MMT have a high rate of severe mental illness (SMI), at 33.2%, including bipolar, schizophrenia, and major depressive disorder (MDD) diagnoses (McGovern et al. 2007). Veterans in this group also demonstrate higher rates of liver problems, HIV diagnoses, and higher homeless rates, compared to serious mental illness patients not enrolled in methadone maintenance treatment. Most importantly, there was a higher rate of fill for outpatient psychiatric medications among the methadone maintenance treatment/serious mental illness veterans. The authors theorized that this high rate could lead to both a risk of licit and illicit drug-drug interactions as well as a higher risk of sedation, falls, and respiratory depression. An additional study looking at psychotropic prescriptions filled by dually diagnosed veterans versus singly diagnosed veterans also found that dually diagnosed veterans with bipolar disorder filled more prescriptions than either dually diagnosed veterans with schizophrenia or the singly diagnosed veterans. The dually diagnosed veterans also demonstrated higher levels of medical comorbidities and higher consumption of mental health services (Marienfeld and Rosenheck 2013). Two VA studies have demonstrated substantially higher healthcare costs among dually diagnosed veterans as compared to those with a substance use disorder alone or a psychiatric disorder alone (Hoff and Rosenheck 1998, 1999).

Psychosocially, studies of supported housing programs within the VA have indicated that veterans with substance use disorders are more likely to have been recently homeless and have more episodes of homelessness and were more likely to have comorbid bipolar or other serious mental illnesses. Additionally, those with substance use disorders (SUDs) had improved housing but at a slower rate than those without SUDs (Tsai et al. 2014). Other studies, however, have shown that dually diagnosed veterans, once in a supported housing program, were just as likely to enter community housing as others (Edens et al. 2011). Other studies examining legal issues within the veteran population suggest that veterans with dual diagnoses are more likely to have been involved with the criminal justice system (Drebing et al. 2002; Tejani et al. 2014).

Third, along with the high frequency of dual diagnosis and its extensive comorbidity, a challenge to effective treatment is posed by the fact that the substance abuse, mental health, and medical fields typically encompass providers from different treatment traditions. The culture of substance abuse treatment has historically been inculcated with terminology such as "abstinence" and "willpower," focusing substance abuse treatment on volitional behavioral changes. Alternatively, psychiatric and medical treatment has increasingly focused attention on biological origins of disease and treatments that emphasize pharmacologic interventions. Subsequently, when more than one condition exists, treatment has been directed in a fragmented manner due to these differing philosophies, and some treatments may even impair the effectiveness of others.

Additionally, for many decades, substance abuse treatment has been considered the sole domain of the addiction psychiatrist or addiction provider, and treatment has been delayed or deferred by general mental health providers. This concept is complex and was highlighted in a large pharmaco-epidemiologic study of the use of naltrexone in alcohol-dependent veterans. The authors showed that naltrexone for alcohol relapse prevention was only used in <2% of veterans with the diagnosis of alcohol dependence (AD) treated nationally (Petrakis et al. 2003b). A more recent administrative study within the VA found that naltrexone for alcohol use disorders is still under-prescribed at a rate of 2.75% but that it is 69 times more likely to be prescribed if the veteran has an Axis I psychiatric disorder (Iheanacho et al. 2013). Additionally, evaluation of naltrexone prescribing in civilian populations has found that even among addiction providers, naltrexone is prescribed at a low rate of 13% for eligible patients with an alcohol use disorder (Harris et al. 2004). These findings underscore the multifaceted nature of dual diagnosis treatment in and outside the VA.

Finally, there is limited evidence-based research to guide the treatment of these most challenging cases. Most clinical trials are done in singly diagnosed individuals, and a co-occurring substance use disorder is often an exclusion criterion for various studies examining treatment modalities. For example, only very recently did the Department of Veterans Affairs, in coordination with the Department of Defense in 2010, revise their Clinical Practice Guidelines for treatment of PTSD and co-occurring substance use disorders. The revised guidelines specifically address the change of treatment approach within the VA from *exclusion* of veterans with substance use disorders from active treatment programs to the new standard of *inclusion* of these veterans in order to treat both disorders concurrently (Bernardy et al. 2011). However, the specifics of treatment for these co-occurring disorders remain loosely defined and at times unclear with some currently available treatments frequently used in the VA lacking a solid evidence base. As these guidelines evolve, more research and clinical caution is required given the limited evidence available to guide the practitioner.

In summary, the intricacies of dual diagnosis and co-occurring disorders clearly present providers and their patients with complicated and challenging problems. The complications extend beyond the medical comorbidities and involve psychosocial stressors and barriers as well. Furthermore, the current guidelines for treatment of this population continue to evolve. Within the veteran population, the intensity of these disorders is heightened due to the nature of military service and combat. When looking carefully at the young chronic patient defined 35 years ago, many similarities can be drawn to today's dual diagnosis patient. The spectrum of treatment starting from that original sketch of integrated care presented by Dr. Pepper to more comprehensive ones detailed today is leading the way for treatment models. Much of the new work in this area has focused on patient-centered care and a recovery model. One of many accepted definitions of *recovery* in mental health is *learning to live with and manage co-disorders to find a meaningful life*. This chapter will explore the current state of treatment interventions and the integrated care philosophy in more detail. Suffice to say, recovery should be the ultimate goal of treatment for the dually diagnosed patient.

Epidemiological Evidence

Determining the exact rate of co-occurring mental and substance use disorders among veterans is made difficult because recent major psychiatric epidemiologic studies, including replication of the National Comorbidity Study (NCS-R) and the National Epidemiologic Study of Alcohol and Related Conditions (NESARC), failed to document veteran status. The last large nationally representative study to include veteran status was the 1980 Epidemiologic Catchment Area (ECA) study. In a secondary analysis of this data, Norquist et al. found no differences in lifetime prevalences of psychiatric disorders among veterans of World War II, Korean, or Vietnam conflict eras and age-matched nonveteran men (Norquist et al. 1990). In contrast, however, veterans of the post-Vietnam era (the initial period of the All-Volunteer Force) showed a *greater* prevalence of lifetime mental disorder (54.6% of veterans vs. 40.9% of nonveterans [$p < 0.0001$]). Data on 6-month prevalence of mental disorder showed a similar pattern, although World War II era veterans had a significantly lower overall prevalence of mental disorder than nonveterans (11.8% vs. 17.7%, $p < 0.01$).

Examination of specific lifetime disorders revealed World War II era veterans had lower prevalences of any nonsubstance abuse disorder than nonveterans (12.2% vs. 18.5%, $p < 0.01$), Vietnam era veterans had lower prevalence of schizophrenic disorders (0.8% vs. 2.2%, $p < 0.05$) and affective disorders (4.4% vs. 8.3%, $p < 0.01$), and post-Vietnam veterans had *higher* lifetime prevalence of substance abuse disorders (47.4% vs. 30.6%, $p < 0.01$, including both alcohol and drug disorders) and antisocial personality disorder (14.9% vs. 5.8%) but lower prevalence of schizophrenic disorder than nonveterans (0.3% vs. 1.5%, $p < 0.01$).

Findings of greater rates of mental illness and especially substance abuse among veterans of the All-Volunteer Force (AVF) are consistent with several studies showing greater substance use among military personnel in the immediate post-Vietnam (Rosenheck and Fontana 1996), studies comparing heavy drinking rates between military and civilian populations (Ames and Cunradi 2004), and (Rosenheck and Director n.d.) studies that have demonstrated a three to four times greater risk of homelessness among post-Vietnam veterans as compared to nonveterans, as well as among female veterans (who have always served on a voluntary basis) (Gamache et al. 2000, 2001). The increased risk of homelessness is completely absent or not statistically significant among veterans of earlier eras in which the draft guaranteed a more representative military force. Thus, a major issue in the psychiatric epidemiology of US veterans appears to be the shift from the draft to the All-Volunteer Force. There have been far fewer veterans since the end of the Vietnam conflict, but they appear to have a greater risk of mental health and substance abuse problems, not because of the hazards of military service but because of self-selection processes among those who volunteer.

Rates of Dual Diagnosis Among Veterans

Outside the studies mentioned above, the majority of relevant data on rates of psychiatric and substance use disorders among military personnel comes primarily from veterans who utilize VA services, representing a minority of total veterans in the US. One of the earliest studies (Rosenheck and Director n.d.) on rates of co-occurring disorders among veterans being treated for a substance use disorder showed 24% had co-occurring psychiatric disorders and, over a 6-year period, incurred 37% higher mental health service costs than other substance abuse patients (Hoff and Rosenheck 1999). A more recent study showed 213,442 VA psychiatric patients (21% of the total) were dually diagnosed, including 22% of those with PTSD, 28% of those with schizophrenia, and 35% of those aged 35–54 (Petrakis et al. 2011). The highest rates of comorbidity occur among those with bipolar disorder and schizophrenia and in post-Vietnam era (1973–1991) veterans. The dually diagnosed are among those at greatest risk for homelessness, unemployment, and criminal justice involvement (Rosenheck et al. 2000). Among veterans dually diagnosed with PTSD and substance use disorders, there is evidence of greater medical comorbidity, mental health inpatient treatment, and homelessness than those with PTSD alone (Bowe and Rosenheck 2015).

Using fiscal year 2012 VA administrative data, the authors compared veterans using VA services with and without a dual diagnosis (see Table 20.1). Dually diagnosed veterans were six times more likely to experience homelessness during the year, four times as likely to use outpatient mental health services, and ten times as likely to use inpatient mental health services. Importantly, the authors found those with dual mental health and substance abuse diagnoses were twice as likely to be diagnosed with HIV and almost four times as likely to have hepatic disease, thus highlighting that veterans with dual diagnoses are not only psychosocially impaired but medically as well. Dual diagnosis is both highly prevalent among VA mental health patients and represents a high-cost, high-risk population.

Mechanisms of Disease

> "Wer sorgen Hat, hat auch Likor"
> (He who has cares, has brandy too)
>
> –Wilhelm Busch, German humorist and poet

Current theories regarding the mechanisms that lead to the frequent co-occurrence of psychiatric and substance use disorders remain speculative and largely descriptive but find their roots in the work of Sigmund Freud, a neurologist by training who also had an interest in substance use. Freud found cocaine, at least initially, both personally gratifying and professionally useful and wrote about alleviating the misery and psychic pain of everyday life with "intoxicating substances" (Freud 2005). In so doing, he was among the first to allude to the role of addictive substances in at least transiently relieving the pain of psychiatric disorders. Of note, he tempered such discussion by referring to the "punishments" that go hand in hand with substance

Table 20.1 Bivariate analysis of veterans receiving a psychiatric diagnosis[a] from the Veterans Health Administration in FY 2012 comparing veterans with and without co-occurring substance abuse or dependence (i.e., dual diagnosis)

	Psychiatric diagnosis only $N = 1{,}555{,}430$		Dual diagnosis $N = 381{,}507$		Ratio of dual diagnosis to non-dually diagnosed
	N/mean	%/SD	N/mean	%/SD	
Demographics					
Age	59.6	±16.2	52.8	±12.8	0.89
Male	1,412,521	90.8%	361,106	94.6%	1.04
Urban area residents	1,053,986	70.6%	284,875	76.7%	1.09
Operation Iraqi Freedom/Operation Enduring Freedom era veterans	198,841	12.8%	52,118	13.7%	1.07
VA pension	43,867	2.8%	25,801	6.8%	2.40
Service connected ≥50%	541,204	34.8%	102,291	26.8%	0.77
Service connected <50%	288,166	18.5%	65,019	17.0%	0.92
Homeless during the year	55,827	3.6%	87,094	22.8%	6.36
Medical diagnosis[b]					
Seizures	15,015	1.0%	5,295	1.4%	1.44
Insomnia	111,041	7.1%	31,420	8.2%	1.15
Narcolepsy	2,062	0.1%	269	0.1%	0.53
Pruritus	17,969	1.1%	5,187	1.4%	1.18
Myocardial infarction	23,201	1.5%	4,143	1.0%	0.73
Congestive heart failure	791,165	50.9%	192,021	50.3%	0.99
Peripheral vascular disease	82,577	5.3%	15,778	4.1%	0.78
Cerebrovascular accident	101,124	6.5%	16,583	4.3%	0.67
Dementia	42,675	2.7%	2,228	0.6%	0.21
Chronic obstructive pulmonary disease	241,888	15.6%	64,636	16.9%	1.09
Connective tissue disease	19,014	1.2%	2,804	0.7%	0.60
Peptic ulcer disease	14,078	0.9%	4,339	1.1%	1.26
Hepatic disease	39,472	2.5%	35,021	9.2%	3.62
Diabetes mellitus	400,265	25.7%	63,309	16.6%	0.64
Complications of diabetes	93,954	6.0%	12,898	3.4%	0.56
Paraplegia	14,039	0.9%	2,635	0.7%	0.77
Renal disease	88,660	5.7%	12,066	3.2%	0.55
HIV	7,526	0.5%	4,501	1.2%	2.44
Cancer	136,442	8.8%	23,621	6.2%	0.71
Pain diagnoses					
Headache	131,692	8.5%	31,940	8.4%	0.99
Diabetic pain	70,640	4.5%	10,429	2.7%	0.60
Musculoskeletal pain	418,030	26.9%	124,059	32.5%	1.21
Fibromyalgia	39,379	2.5%	9,050	2.4%	0.94
Skeletospasm pain	37,756	2.4%	9,714	2.5%	1.05
Herpetic pain	12,276	0.8%	3,326	0.9%	1.10
Any pain	825,490	53.1%	231,317	60.6%	1.14
Psychiatric diagnosis					
Organic brain syndrome	56,216	3.6%	2,278	0.6%	0.17
Schizophrenia	65,087	4.2%	24,095	6.3%	1.5
Bipolar disorder	74,794	4.8%	39,309	8.4%	2.14
Major depression	230,258	14.8%	79,116	20.7%	1.40
Other depression (e.g., dysthymia)	645,615	41.5%	187,191	49.1%	1.18

(continued)

Table 20.1 (continued)

	Psychiatric diagnosis only *N* = 1,555,430		Dual diagnosis *N* = 381,507		Ratio of dual diagnosis to non-dually diagnosed
	N/mean	%/SD	N/mean	%/SD	
Post-traumatic stress disorder	498,720	32.1%	139,731	36.6%	1.14
Anxiety disorder	366,582	23.6%	100,062	26.2%	1.11
Adjustment disorder	136,853	8.8%	40,266	10.6%	1.20
Personality disorder	26,406	1.7%	23,653	6.2%	3.65
Service use					
Any mental health inpatient Tx	18,429	1.2%	44,818	11.7%	9.92
Emergency room visits	0.53	±1.4	1.22	±2.8	2.29
Medical/surgical visits	9.3	±10.9	10.0	±11.3	1.08
Psych or substance abuse outpatient visits	4.6	±13.2	19.8	±38.7	4.34
All outpatient visits	13.8	±18.0	29.8	±31.8	2.16
Psychotropic medications					
Antidepressant	877,469	56.4%	248,025	65.0%	1.15
Antipsychotic	211,235	13.6%	94,152	24.7%	1.82
Anxiolytic/sedative/hypnotic	471,929	30.5%	120,681	31.6%	1.04
Stimulant prescriptions	23,488	1.5%	5,471	1.4%	0.95
Antiepileptic/mood stabilizer	297,489	19.1%	102,638	26.9%	1.41
Lithium	17,995	1.2%	9,259	2.4%	2.10
Received any psychotropic	1,081,912	73.7%	294,067	80.5%	1.09

[a]ICD-9290-312, excluding any substance abuse or dependence
[b]Medical and pain diagnoses as measured by the Charlson Medical Severity Index

use. Throughout the last century, psychodynamic theories of dual diagnosis have evolved. Wieder and Kaplan hypothesized that individuals with addiction choose specific drugs because of particular personality and ego impairments (Wieder and Kaplan 1968). Khantzian, in the 1980s, went further to argue that addicted patients seek out specific substances (e.g., opiates and cocaine) in "self-selection" efforts to medicate symptoms of rage, anger, depression, or attentional deficits (Khantzian 1987). Khantzian's theories remain provocative to this day though empirical evidence of such specificity is lacking. Identifying which came first—the drug abuse or the psychiatric disorder—is the holy grail of investigation regarding the etiology and mechanism of common co-occurring disorders. Is drug abuse a way to self-medicate specific effects or does drug abuse cause permanent neurobiological changes that can result in or predispose to a mood disorder? The answer continues to elude us with the best theoretical perspective involving a combination of factors including genetic vulnerabilities, environmental stressors, and pharmacological processes.

It is well known that all drugs of abuse modulate the dopamine systems of the brain, specifically in the limbic and nucleus accumbens (Koob and Bloom 1988). However, this does not explain why some drugs are more likely than others to contribute to comorbidity of psychiatric illness. For instance, nicotine has been shown in preclinical and clinical studies to modulate the dopamine system in the brain and also to inhibit monoamine oxidase, which has antidepressant effects. Though nicotine is legal in the US and widely available, it is not thought to be a major cause of severe psychiatric comorbidity. In light of the high prevalence of depression in nicotine-addicted individuals (Fowler et al. 2003), however, it is possible that nicotine contributes to the co-occurrence of addiction and depression more than other addictive substances (Picciotto et al. 2002). Similarly, excessive alcohol use is believed to result in or exacerbate depressive symptoms. More specifically, mechanisms that tie depression with use of alcohol, opiates, and stimulants may reflect modulation of dopamine, serotonin, and norepinephrine within the limbic systems of the brain (Markou et al. 1998; Koob 2008), but studies looking at genetic patterns related to depression in siblings and children of alcoholics have not supported the idea of a purely genetic link (Merikangas et al. 1994; Goodwin et al. 1977; Merikangas et al. 1988). Overall, available research supports that different drugs produce differing psychiatric symptoms with varying severity.

Clearly, the mechanisms that lead to psychiatric and substance use comorbidity are more complex than our current understanding of their genetics or neurobiology. The dually diagnosed patient, including the dually diagnosed veteran, presents with multiple complex problems—social, legal, and medical, among them. This chapter presents two proposed mechanisms of comorbidity to highlight the multifactorial processes involved: (1) the link between trauma and subsequent development of PTSD and substance use and (2) early cannabis use and the onset of psychotic disorders.

Trauma and Substance Use Disorders

A key theory in the development of PTSD and substance use disorders has been the "stress-induced" model. The stress-induced model has two proposed pathways. First, substance abuse precedes PTSD, and the act of procuring and using substances puts an individual into situations in which trauma is more likely to occur. Second, the trauma occurs first, leading to PTSD and then substance abuse as a form of self-medication (Jacobsen et al. 2001). Most published work supports the latter pathway, i.e., the trauma precedes substance abuse. Some evidence exists proposing that the type of substance abused derives from particular PTSD symptoms experienced—e.g., veterans with more arousal symptoms turning to alcohol to reduce or cope with discomfort. Other studies have suggested that withdrawal syndromes may mimic or exacerbate some PTSD symptoms leading to drug relapse. There is also evidence in both animal and human studies suggesting that the initiation and maintenance of stress lead to drug-seeking behaviors and continuation of drug use. In animal models (Koob 2008), introduction of physical and psychological stress has replicated both drug administration and drug relapse. Similarly in humans, stress has been shown to lead to cravings and drug use (Brady and Sinha 2007).

Preclinical studies have also demonstrated a link between corticotropin-releasing factor and induction of stress. During times of stress, the hypothalamus releases corticotropin-releasing hormone (CRH), which drives the neuroendocrine response to stress, by releasing cortisol from the adrenal glands. High levels of CRH have been found in the cerebrospinal fluid (CSF) of PTSD patients (Bremner et al. 1997). The end result of cortisol release leads to potentiated fear-related responses, such as the PTSD hyperarousal response, while pretreatment with anti-CRH molecules or antagonists have been shown to block or prevent the development of stress behaviors (Swerdlow et al. 1989). Withdrawal behaviors associated with cocaine or alcohol withdrawal can be blocked as well with the use of anti-CRH molecules or CRH antagonists (Sarnyai et al. 1995).

In concert with the CRH system, the neurotransmitter norepinephrine is released in regions of the brain with high turnover and increased metabolites during periods of stress (Tanaka et al. 1991; Southwick et al. 1999). The increased release of norepinephrine is driven by the increased action of CRH in the locus ceruleus (Chappell et al. 1986). This stress-induced release of norepinephrine is considered a dysregulation of the noradrenergic system and can be seen in substance abuse withdrawal as well. Supporting the role of norepinephrine in the stress pathway, norepinephrine appears to be an important catecholamine involved in laying down memories in the brain, specifically the amygdala and prefrontal cortex. Researchers have called for further investigations into treatment for PTSD and comorbid substance use disorders that can test this pathway more vigorously. This stress-induced model of comorbid PTSD and substance use along with the receptors and neurotransmitters involved is the leading area for current research into the neurobiological mechanisms underlying the emergence of the dually diagnosed patient.

Psychosis and Substance Use Disorders: The Cannabis Theory

Three main symptom clusters exist in schizophrenia including the positive, negative, and cognitive clusters. The positive cluster is characterized by paranoia, bizarre delusions, changes in time and space perceptions, and disorganized thinking. Negative symptoms include blunted affect, social and emotional withdrawal, and psychomotor slowing. Impairments with memory, attention, and executive function make up the cognitive cluster. Cannabis intoxication can replicate all three clusters, and there is growing evidence of a causal link between cannabis use and schizophrenia. Research has identified three main areas that appear to predispose a cannabis-using individual to psychotic disorders including (1) early heavy use, (2) genetic vulnerabilities, and (3) childhood trauma (Radhakrishnan et al. 2014).

Early and Heavy Use Several large longitudinal and cross-sectional studies have identified links between cannabis use and the development of schizophrenia. A Swedish study following a cohort of military conscripts found that if an individual had used cannabis at least once, their risk of developing schizophrenia was 2.4 times higher than if they had not. That risk rose sixfold if the individual had used heavy amounts of cannabis, i.e., at least 50 episodes of use (Andréasson et al. 1987). Additionally, a cohort study done in New Zealand demonstrated that earlier cannabis use, specifically starting as young as age 15, increased the risk of a schizophreniform illness by a factor of 4 (Arseneault et al. 2002). This was replicated in a study which found that cannabis use by age 14 increased the risk of development of an earlier onset psychotic illness (Schimmelmann et al. 2011). Animal studies appear to support this "window of vulnerability" with evidence of more harmful effects from cannabis seen in adolescence than in adult animal models. Researchers hypothesize that the adolescent brain is particularly vulnerable to cannabis given ongoing development and maturation (Radhakrishnan et al. 2014).

Genetic Vulnerabilities The two main genes that have been studied in the search for a causal link between cannabis and psychosis include catechol-O-methyltransferase (COMT) and AKT1. COMT is involved in the breakdown of dopamine in the prefrontal cortex. One study demonstrated that individuals with a specific allele expression of this gene, when exposed to cannabis, increased their risk of a psychotic disorder tenfold (Caspi et al. 2005). Further attempts have failed to replicate this finding, but a more recent investigation found an interaction among the allele, cannabis use, and a history of abuse in childhood conferring an increased risk of psychotic symptoms (Alemany et al. 2014). The gene AKT1 appears to have a stronger association with cannabis use and development of psychosis. Di Forti et al. (2012) found that a specific allelic expression of this gene in daily cannabis users increased their risk for psychosis by sevenfold. Family history is often used as a marker for genetic vulnerabilities, and studies that have examined patients hospitalized for acute psychosis who also tested positive for cannabis have found them to have a ten times greater likelihood of a positive family history of schizophrenia. Other studies have linked cannabis use to patients with family histories for schizophrenia. Thus, there is mounting evidence that genetic vulnerabilities modulate the link between cannabis use and psychosis.

Childhood Trauma Several studies have shown increased risk of developing psychosis among adolescents with a history of both childhood abuse and cannabis use (Houston et al. 2008; Harley et al. 2010; Konings et al. 2012), adding additional complexity to the genetic and environmental interplay that characterizes the link between cannabis and psychosis. In summary, though the mechanisms linking psychosis and cannabis are not clearly elucidated and apply only to a minority of cases of psychosis, the evidence is mounting to support an increased level of vulnerability to psychosis in some cannabis users.

Status of Interventions and Impact on Clinical Care

> Canst thou not minister to a mind diseased,
> Pluck from the memory a rooted sorrow,
> Raze out the written troubles of the brain,
> And with some sweet oblivious antidote
> Cleanse … that perilous stuff which weighs upon the heart?
>
> —William Shakespeare, *Macbeth* (Act 5, Scene 3)

Veterans with co-occurring mental health and substance use disorders have complex needs that require care extending beyond the traditional approach recommended for individual mental health and substance use disorders. This section will review the current state of treatments that are available for the dually diagnosed veteran, which range from pharmacologic, psychotherapeutic, and community treatments. It will further discuss how these current treatments are being used and specifically how they are being employed to target the dually diagnosed veteran.

Pharmacotherapy

There is a caveat regarding the status of pharmacologic interventions for dually diagnosed individuals and veterans: most available treatments were not developed specifically for the dually diagnosed individual. The information below highlights medications available for substance use disorders that have also been evaluated, even if only preliminary, in dually diagnosed populations.

Disulfiram Approved for treatment of alcohol use disorder since 1948, disulfiram was inadvertently discovered when patients receiving it for treatment of parasitic infections returned reporting severe symptoms after alcohol consumption. Disulfiram is considered an aversive medication and works by inhibiting the breakdown of acetaldehyde, a metabolite of ethanol, which leads to unpleasant side effects including flushing, nausea, and vomiting. In severe cases, it can lead to cardiovascular collapse and death and, therefore, is used only in select, highly motivated individuals. In addition to its effect on alcohol metabolism, however, disulfiram also inhibits dopamine dehydroxylase, leading to an increase in dopamine and, in some genetically vulnerable individuals, a worsening of psychosis. Much of the data for this worsening originated from older studies done prior to 1970 and with doses of 1–2 g, which exceed the current prescribed doses of 250–500 mg daily. Nonetheless, this concern has limited the use of disulfiram in the dually diagnosed.

In 2005, a 12-week study was conducted evaluating 254 veterans across three VA sites. The investigators looked at the impact of disulfiram, naltrexone, and the combination of both versus placebo in patients with dually diagnosed alcohol use disorder and Axis I disorders, including depression, bipolar, and schizophrenia diagnoses. They found no worsening of psychotic or depressive symptoms in the disulfiram or naltrexone groups, and those receiving either medication showed improved alcohol use outcomes versus the placebo group. Additionally, patients with a depression diagnosis showed improved depressive symptoms when treated with either medication, and specifically, the disulfiram/depression group demonstrated reduced cravings for alcohol. The authors concluded disulfiram and naltrexone safe and effective in dually diagnosed patients, more efficacious than placebo, and with some effect on depressive symptoms (Petrakis et al. 2005).

Naltrexone Naltrexone is an opioid antagonist acting on μ-opioid receptors in the brain to reduce cravings, the positive reinforcement of drinking, and the priming effect of a first drink, thereby reducing relapse to heavier drinking days (Volpicelli et al. 1992; O'Malley et al. 1992). Studies examining naltrexone use in dually diagnosed populations are limited but have shown no worsening of symptoms of schizophrenia (Sernyak et al. 1998) and no increase in adverse outcomes among a population of dually diagnosed patients versus patients with only substance use disorders (Croop et al. 1997). Additionally, a randomized placebo-controlled trial evaluating naltrexone augmentation in veterans with schizophrenia receiving neuroleptics demonstrated reduced drinking days, fewer heavy drinking days, and an increase in days abstinent versus a placebo group. There was no evidence of worsening psychotic symptoms with naltrexone use, though there was no improvement in symptoms either. Overall, the study authors argued that naltrexone was safe in the dually diagnosed population (Petrakis et al. 2004).

Additional randomized trials have looked at treatment of heroin users with naltrexone with and without fluoxetine to improve psychiatric symptoms, prevent HIV infection, and reduce relapse rates thought to be related to depressive symptoms. Results suggested that use of naltrexone, independent of fluoxetine, improved treatment retention, reduced relapse, and reduced HIV infection rates. The addition of fluoxetine to the naltrexone or to the naltrexone placebo group overall did not improve outcomes. Overall, naltrexone has proven effective in a population where maintenance therapy is not available, and there are mixed results when naltrexone is combined with antidepressants.

Naltrexone has probably best been studied in those with co-occurring alcohol use disorder and PTSD. Foa et al. (2013) conducted a randomized controlled trial evaluating the use of naltrexone plus exposure therapy in a 2×2 study of dually diagnosed veterans. Four treatment arms were evaluated: naltrexone with exposure therapy, naltrexone with supportive therapy, placebo with exposure therapy, and placebo with supportive therapy. Findings revealed that in all four arms, veterans showed reduction of percentage of drinking days, but those in the naltrexone treatment arms showed a greater reduction of drinking days even after a 6-month period. Additionally, prolonged exposure, which had initially been considered to cause a worsening of alcohol use disorders, did not show this effect. Surprisingly, the investigators also found that prolonged exposure therapy did not statistically reduce PTSD symptoms among the four groups as it had in non-dually diagnosed people with PTSD. Six months after treatment, all groups demonstrated increases in drinking days, but the naltrexone-treated groups showed the lowest percentage of increase. This study was one of the first of its kind examining treatment of co-occurring disorders by evidence-based medication and psychotherapy (Foa et al. 2013).

A multi-VA site study looked at the combination of naltrexone and disulfiram in co-occurring PTSD and alcohol use disorder and found that patients had both improved alcohol and PTSD outcomes when treated with medications for alcohol use disorders. There was no advantage found with the combination of naltrexone and disulfiram nor an advantage of one medication over the other, causing investigators to conclude that patient preference can be taken into account when treating dually diagnosed individuals (Petrakis et al. 2006c).

Embedded in this multisite VA study was a naltrexone-disulfiram treatment trial evaluating the subgroup of individuals with depression and alcohol use disorder. The veterans were divided into four groups: disulfiram treatment, naltrexone treatment, both medications, or placebo. The investigators found that individuals with depression treated with disulfiram reported lower alcohol cravings versus those on naltrexone, with primary outcomes looking at alcohol use and secondary outcomes examining depressive symptoms on the Hamilton Depression Rating Scale. More importantly, the study investigators found no significant side effect difference between the medication groups, and in fact, veterans in both medication treatment groups showed improved depressive symptoms over the course of the 12-week trial.

Looking specifically at alcohol use disorders in individuals with psychotic disorders, a randomized controlled 12-week trial examined naltrexone and disulfiram alone and in combination for treating individuals with psychotic spectrum disorders and alcohol use disorders. The investigators found that individuals with psychotic spectrum had overall worse alcohol outcomes than those without a psychotic spectrum disorder. However, they also found that those taking an active medication versus placebo had better overall alcohol use outcomes, though there was no clear advantage of naltrexone versus disulfiram, or the two in combination (Petrakis et al. 2006b). These authors and others investigating the dually diagnosed population continue to call for additional randomized controlled studies to be completed in order to confirm the results of these and other studies that can support consensus recommendations.

Acamprosate Acamprosate is hypothesized to act as a partial NMDA/glutamate agonist and partial antagonist at metabotropic glutamate receptors in the brain. Given this action, there have been some concerns that this medication could potentially cause worsening memory, learning, and cognitive impairments (Schneider et al. 1999). For dually diagnosed patients who already have cognitive impairments related to their psychiatric disorders and/or alcohol use, acamprosate was originally considered a confounding variable in treatment. Contrary to this, however, a study of a mixed civilian/veteran population with schizophrenia and alcohol use disorders showed clinically significant reductions in alcohol use without worsening or improvement of cognitive symptoms with use of acamprosate (Ralevski et al. 2011). The authors of the study theorized that the absence of cognitive impairments was possibly related to the relatively short term of the trial (12 weeks) and that longer treatment periods could result in impaired cognition in this population.

Selective Serotonin Reuptake Inhibitors (SSRIs) and Serotonin and Norepinephrine Reuptake Inhibitors (SNRIs) SSRIs and SNRIs are commonly used to treat depressive disorders, and major depression is the most common comorbid condition with substance use disorders (SUDs), conferring a poorer prognosis (Regier et al. 1990). It stands to reason, then, that SUDs and depressive disorders have been main areas of investigation when looking at dually diagnosed individuals, with a natural focus on SSRIs. Although SSRIs and SNRIs are standard classes of medication for major depressive disorder, no medication has been approved for treatment of both depression and substance use disorders. A 2003 review of VA administrative data (Petrakis et al. 2003a) evaluated the use of antidepressants in alcoholic and nonalcoholic veterans in mental health and nonmental health care settings. While dually diagnosed individuals were not specifically identified, the investigators found that veterans with alcohol dependence were less likely to be prescribed antidepressants in VA mental health clinics as compared to nonalcohol-dependent veterans and that a diagnosis of alcohol dependence is associated overall with a decreased likelihood of receiving antidepressant treatment. The authors of the study hypothesized that this finding might reflect a treatment culture of suspicion among VA mental health providers regarding treatment of potentially dually diagnosed veterans but might also reflect concerns about mixing antidepressants and alcohol on a clinical assumption that depressive symptoms would remit if the patient stopped or reduced alcohol consumption.

A study evaluating dually diagnosed individuals on sertraline at doses of 150 mg daily in a placebo-controlled trial found no significant difference between placebo and sertraline in reducing alcohol use or PTSD symptoms. However, the individuals with less severe alcohol use and earlier onset PTSD showed a greater reduction in alcohol use when treated with sertraline (Brady et al. 2005).

A randomized controlled trial comparing SSRIs and SNRIs with the addition of naltrexone found that the SSRI (paroxetine) was as effective as the SNRI (desipramine) in treatment for PTSD symptoms but that the SNRI (desipramine) was superior in reducing heavy drinking days and drinks per week as measured by gamma-glutamyl transferase (GGT) levels. Additionally, the investigators found that the combination of naltrexone and desipramine did not produce a robust effect for both disorders (Petrakis et al. 2012). This study is interesting for two reasons: first, the equivalent efficacy of a noradrenergic agent with the more standard serotonergic agent is a promising finding, and second, it can direct future research on the attenuation of noradrenergic hyperactivity as a target for PTSD treatment. Desipramine has also been investigated for treatment of cocaine-dependent individuals with schizophrenia, and one small open-label study demonstrated that individuals receiving desipramine had fewer cocaine-positive urines over the 12-week trial period (Ziedonis et al. 1992).

Buspirone Buspirone is a non-benzodiazepine anxiolytic that is considered clinically useful for populations diagnosed with alcohol use disorders and anxiety disorders. Many individuals with alcohol use disorders frequently report poorly controlled anxiety and often seek out benzodiazepines as treatment options, having received these medications in past detoxifications. Given the addictive potential of benzodiazepines, however, having a safer alternative to treating comorbid anxiety is greatly needed. Investigators have reviewed the use of buspirone in individuals with anxiety disorders and alcohol use and have found in three of four studies an improvement in treatment retention, a reduction of anxiety levels, and, in individuals with the highest levels of anxiety, a reduction in frequency of alcohol intake (Modesto-Lowe and Kranzler 1999).

Prazosin Prazosin is an α-1 adrenergic receptor antagonist that works to reduce noradrenergic output and, although not FDA-approved for PTSD, has been shown to reduce nightmares in both veteran and nonveteran populations (Raskind et al. 2007; Taylor et al. 2008). Additionally, there have been animal studies showing the benefit of prazosin in reducing alcohol self-administration (Rasmussen et al. 2009). Given this finding, and following on the heels of the theory that targeting noradrenergic systems may be useful in treating PTSD symptoms, there is a small body of research looking into prazosin as a potential treatment for individuals with both PTSD and alcohol use disorders. A recent pilot study examined the effect of prazosin on individuals with alcohol use disorders and co-occurring PTSD. The results showed the prazosin group had fewer drinking days versus the placebo group, but no difference was found in PTSD symptoms (Simpson et al. 2009). Currently there are ongoing trials at the New England Mental Illness Research Education Clinical Center (MIRECC) investigating the effects of prazosin on dually diagnosed veterans with PTSD and alcohol use disorders in order to fully explore and confirm benefits of prazosin for both disorders.

Antipsychotics The mainstay of treatment for patients with a psychotic or bipolar disorder, antipsychotics are also used to augment depression management. Most available literature and epidemiologic studies suggest that close to half of individuals with schizophrenia have a co-occurring substance use disorder, with a third having a co-occurring alcohol use disorder. This fact remains a significant obstacle for effective treatment in this population. Currently, there are no approved medications for both conditions, though there is a small and growing body of research examining the utility of antipsychotics in dually diagnosed patients.

One theory for the common co-occurrence of substance use with psychotic disorders is the idea that conventional antipsychotics cause "neuroleptic dysphoria," defined as sustained depression and negative symptoms stemming from dopamine blockade (Voruganti and Awad 2004). This theory holds that the neuroleptic-induced dysphoria drives a need for relief through dopamine release obtained from drug use. Due to this theory, along with the side effect profile of conventional antipsychotics, a general consensus has been built that conventional antipsychotics are not as effective for the dually diagnosed population. Some investigators have even suggested that conventional antipsychotics can worsen substance use in individuals with psychotic disorders (Voruganti and Awad 2004; McEvoy et al. 1995). Hence, more investigation has occurred with the newer atypical antipsychotics that work at a variety of neurotransmitter systems rather than primarily blocking dopamine receptors. Conflicting with this, however, investigators have discovered atypical neuroleptics were associated with no better outcomes than conventional neuroleptics for SUD in patients with schizophrenia (Petrakis et al. 2006a).

Other researchers have examined the use of specific neuroleptics and their efficacy in populations with alcohol, drug use, and schizophrenia. Initial case studies of clozapine demonstrated reduced use of substances among patients with schizophrenia on clozapine (Albanese et al. 1994; Marcus and Snyder 1995). An observational study of 118 patients with schizophrenia or schizoaffective disorder treated with clozapine showed reduced substance use (alcohol, cocaine, and marijuana). The authors also highlighted the finding that the history of substance use or active use did not negatively affect clozapine treatment in these individuals (Buckley et al. 1994). A later retrospective survey of 58 individuals with schizophrenia and substance use treated with clozapine found similar results (Zimmet et al. 2000). A prospective study on patients with schizophrenia 6 months into remission from any substance found the clozapine-treated patients had a significantly lower rate of relapse versus those on other atypical antipsychotic medications (8% vs. 40%) (Brunette et al. 2006). Open-label studies of other atypicals such as olanzapine and quetiapine have also found favorable results with remission rates from substance use disorders in dually diagnosed individuals (Littrell et al. 2001; Martinotti et al. 2008). These authors highlight the limitations of the observational studies and call for randomized controlled studies to confirm results.

Finally, future directions have focused on glycine and abnormalities of the glutamatergic neurotransmitter system as potential treatment for individuals with both schizophrenia and alcohol use disorders. In a proof of concept study, glycine, a glutamatergic amino acid, was used as treatment for both alcohol misuse and symptoms of schizophrenia and revealed preliminary results supporting previous research that glycine is effective for the negative symptoms of schizophrenia, but not alcohol consumption (Ralevski et al. 2012). It should be noted that the final data analysis is not yet complete.

Topiramate Topiramate is currently being studied for alcohol use disorders and, according to recent research, holds much promise. It is known to act at several sites in the nervous system, including calcium channels, gamma-aminobutyric acid (GABA), and glutamine receptors (Johnson and Ait-Daoud 2010). In one randomized controlled trial, topiramate reduced alcohol intake and cravings and improved quality of life and health (Johnson 2004), and a subsequent multisite trial of topiramate demonstrated reduced obsessional thoughts and compulsions about alcohol, reduced number of heavy drinking days, and reduced risk of relapse (Johnson et al. 2008).

Open-label studies of topiramate have suggested efficacy for PTSD symptoms such as nightmares and insomnia with adjunct topiramate treatment (Berlant 2000; Berlant and van Kammen 2002). More recent randomized controlled trials have demonstrated efficacy as an add-on treatment in treating PTSD symptoms as well as reducing high-risk alcohol intake in combat veterans (Alderman et al. 2009). A recent randomized controlled trial evaluated topiramate for use with veterans with co-occurring alcohol use and PTSD (Batki et al. 2014). Investigators found topiramate reduced alcohol use, cravings, and drinking days as well as amounts of alcohol consumed and also had a beneficial effect on PTSD symptoms—specifically hyperarousal. The authors noted the negative cognitive effects with topiramate (a common side effect) but also found these effects were transient and eventually tolerated. Overall, the limiting factors for topiramate appear to be the side effect profile, which can involve cognitive impairment (though this may be lower in patients with alcohol use disorder than in other treated populations) as well as risks of metabolic acidosis, acute glaucoma, and others.

Zonisamide Zonisamide can be considered a future direction worthy of evaluation. An antiepileptic in the category with topiramate but with a better side effect profile, zonisamide, is being studied in alcohol use disorders as well. One set of investigators conducted a double-blind randomized controlled trial evaluating zonisamide in 40 individuals with alcohol use disorders and found a significant effect in the zonisamide treatment group with reduced heavy drinking days, reduced drinks per week, and improved alcohol urge scores. Additionally, the medication was well tolerated (Arias et al. 2010). Future research should focus on topiramate and zonisamide for use in dually diagnosed individuals.

Ketamine A potent N-methyl-D-aspartate (NMDA) receptor antagonist, ketamine is gaining increasing interest among researchers as a potential treatment for individuals with co-occurring depression and alcohol use disorders. There is a growing body of evidence on ketamine's effect on depressive symptoms in mono-diagnosed individuals (Berman et al. 2000) but no definitive evidence of its effectiveness with comorbid populations. It has been studied in Operation Iraqi Freedom/Operation Enduring Freedom burn victims undergoing surgery showing a lower prevalence of PTSD in veterans treated with perioperative ketamine. This finding suggests that ketamine may have some possible role in mitigating development of PTSD via improved pain control and/or antagonism of the NMDA receptor (McGhee et al. 2008).

Efforts to study ketamine treatment in heroin users suggest promising results as well. A double-blind study examined the use of psychedelic doses of ketamine versus non-psychedelic doses both paired with psychotherapy. The outcome measures included improved abstinence rates, reduced relapse rates, and reduced depressive symptoms, labeled "syndrome of anhedonia" by the investigators. Results showed statistically significant improvement in rates of abstinence in the higher-dose ketamine group. Complicating the results is the exclusion of dually diagnosed individuals, though the results are provocative given that other measured findings included reduced anxiety, depression, and mood (Krupitsky et al. 2002). An attempt to replicate these results by the same group of researchers found mixed results, with improved abstinence after 1 year for heroin users who received multiple ketamine sessions versus one ketamine session, but no difference between groups regarding mood, depression, or anxiety (Krupitsky et al. 2007). Specifically targeting the dually diagnosed population, an ongoing double-blind, randomized controlled proof of concept study is currently recruiting in the VA New England Mental Illness Research Education Clinical Center to evaluate the effect of a single dose of ketamine administered IV on both mood and alcohol intake. Further studies are necessary to evaluate ketamine utility in the dually diagnosed.

Vivitrol (Alkermes) Vivitrol is a depot form of intramuscular naltrexone FDA-approved for both alcohol and opioid use disorders. At this time, there are no available randomized controlled studies looking at Vivitrol use in the dually diagnosed population, only sparse case reports. Further studies are needed.

Clonidine and Guanfacine Clonidine and guanfacine are both centrally acting α-2 agonists. Clonidine modulates the brain's noradrenergic system and is commonly used to treat opioid and alcohol withdrawal syndromes. There is little data evaluating the effectiveness of clonidine in the dually diagnosed population though a small body of research limited by open-label designs has examined clonidine's effectiveness in treating PTSD in children (Pfefferbaum 1997; Harmon and Riggs 1996) and co-occurring PTSD and alcohol use disorders in adults (Kolb 1991; Kinzie and Leung 1989; Boehnlein and Kinzie 2007; Boehnlein et al. 2004). Similarly, guanfacine has showed some promise in blocking stress-induced cocaine cues (Fox et al. 2012). However, in a small randomized study of guanfacine for PTSD treatment in a veteran population, no significant positive effect was found on any outcome measures such as PTSD symptoms, depression, or sleep quality (Neylan et al. 2006). Future trials evaluating the use of α-2 agonists in dually diagnosed populations and specifically in veteran populations are needed.

Buprenorphine A partial kappa agonist for μ-opioid receptors, buprenorphine is used in the treatment of opioid use disorders as maintenance therapy. It has been well studied as effective for opioid use disorders as maintenance therapy, but little study has been done to investigate the value of buprenorphine in dually diagnosed civilian or veteran populations.

Methadone A full μ-opioid receptor agonist, methadone is used as replacement therapy for heroin and other opioid dependence. Though there is ample evidence documenting the effectiveness of methadone as a replacement therapy for opioid-dependent individuals, there is only scant data looking at treatment in dually diagnosed populations. Marienfeld and Rosenheck identified the high rate of serious mental illness (33.2%) among those in methadone maintenance treatment (McGovern et al. 2007). Such findings highlight the need for appropriate screening for co-occurring disorders that will guide comprehensive treatment planning and optimal outcomes (Hien et al. 2000). Methadone has also been evaluated for antianxiety and antimanic properties in emergently hospitalized individuals showing effectiveness in acute psychiatric situations (Pacini and Maremmani 2005). Additionally, the same research group found that individuals with co-occurring disorders, such as depression or anxiety, may have better long-term outcomes with their substance treatment (Maremmani et al. 2007) but require higher doses of methadone to stabilize (Maremmani et al. 2000).

Results in treating individuals with depression and opioid use disorder with antidepressants remain mixed. A meta-analysis demonstrated ineffectiveness with antidepressants as a general category (Torrens et al. 2005). Two exceptions, however, are imipramine and doxepin. Nunes et al. (1998) found improvement in cocaine-related outcomes in methadone-maintained patients when treated with imipramine, suggesting that antidepressants can affect substance use indirectly by improving depression. Doxepin was also shown to improve depression in patients with opioid addiction (Titievsky et al. 1982) and was superior to placebo for reducing depressive symptoms and opioid use (Woody et al. 1975). Further studies are needed evaluating methadone in dually diagnosed populations.

Clearly the array of pharmacotherapy treatment available for the dually diagnosed veteran remains limited to a small but substantial group of medications as discussed above. The challenge lies in the fact that there are no medications currently approved for co-occurring conditions, given limited research in the area. Though there are promising areas of investigation, particularly with medications targeting the glutamatergic, noradrenergic, and serotonergic systems, as well as the μ-opioid receptors, there remains a great need for rigorous systematic studies to determine safe and effective pharmacologic treatment for those patients with co-occurring disorders.

Psychotherapies

The psychotherapies discussed below are office-based treatments and specifically include treatments developed for substance use disorders that have also been evaluated in patients. The research in this area remains limited, and further investigations are needed for this special population.

Motivational Interviewing/Motivational Enhancement Therapy Both of these therapies are patient-centered therapies developed to utilize the patient's own motivations, goals, and ambivalence to generate commitment to change. Motivational interviewing (MI) remains a key method for engaging individuals in initial treatment, providing a safe nonjudgmental therapeutic environment for the patient to seek treatment (Miller and Rollnick 1991). Motivational interviewing use in a dually diagnosed population is a key part of integrated treatment and will be discussed within this context below.

Cognitive Behavioral Therapy (CBT) Cognitive behavioral therapy (CBT) is a type of therapy that evaluates drug dependence as a learned behavior and investigates how an individual's thoughts affect their emotions and actions and subsequently their drug use. Cognitive behavioral therapy uses this information to facilitate change and improvement of behavior and coping skills. It incorporates a number of different types of therapies as noted below, which are modifications of the basic premise of reshaping cognitive habits.

Prolonged Exposure Dr. Edna Foa developed exposure therapy in 1998 as a specific cognitive behavioral therapy treatment for PTSD. It involves in vivo and imaginal exposure and re-experiencing of traumatic events with a goal of attenuating pathological reactions. It has been studied in both civilian and veteran populations and shows significant reduction of PTSD symptoms and related problems such as depression in both populations (Hembree and Foa 2000; Foa et al. 1999). The consensus statement by the International Consensus Group on Depression and Anxiety selected exposure therapy as the most appropriate form of psychotherapy for PTSD (Ballenger et al. 2000). Initially, Dr. Foa believed that use of this treatment in substance use disordered populations could be too destabilizing and distressing, causing a worsening of both substance use and PTSD symptoms. However, a preliminary study on a population with cocaine dependence and PTSD (Brady et al. 2001) demonstrated improvement in both substance use and PTSD symptoms without a risk of relapse, which was maintained over a 6-month period. The authors cautioned that results could not be interpreted as conclusive due to lack of a control group and a high drop-out rate. Since this study, exposure therapy has expanded to include other substance use disorders and has been noted above; the most recent study (Foa et al. 2013) examining alcohol use disorders and naltrexone as combination treatment groups showed mixed results, suggesting limited benefits for dually diagnosed patients with PTSD and alcohol disorder.

Cognitive Processing Therapy (CPT) Cognitive processing therapy is a cognitive behavioral therapy with some similarity to exposure therapy also initially developed for PTSD. A pilot study investigating the effects of cognitive processing therapy on PTSD symptoms and modified for heavy alcohol use found improvements in both (McCarthy et al. 2009).

Concurrent Treatment of PTSD and Cocaine Dependence (CTPCD) Concurrent treatment of PTSD and cocaine dependence is a form of cognitive behavioral therapy designed to treat PTSD and cocaine dependence but has since been modified for any substance. It is based on cognitive behavioral therapy and prolonged exposure techniques. Initial studies investigating the effect of this treatment have demonstrated improved outcomes in both cocaine use and PTSD symptom clusters which were maintained over a 6-month period (Brady et al. 2001).

Seeking Safety This therapy is the most studied intervention for alcohol use disorders and comorbid PTSD and was specifically developed for dually diagnosed patients. It is a form of cognitive behavioral therapy integrated with elements of other behavioral interventions. It bases its design in controlling and coping with present problems rather than past traumata, with the goal of preventing retraumatization while reducing PTSD symptoms and maintaining abstinence. It has been studied with good results in uncontrolled studies but has failed to demonstrate evidence of effectiveness when compared to control groups (Hien et al. 2009). Although seeking safety was originally designed to assist a civilian female population, it has been adapted to treat veterans and more specifically has been adapted to incorporate prolonged exposure as well. In fact, in a small pilot trial of five individuals in which seeking safety was combined with prolonged exposure for substance use disorders, multiple areas of functioning, drug use, trauma symptoms, meaningfulness, anxiety, and hostility improved (Najavits et al. 2005). It continues to be a main form of treatment within the VA system for veterans suffering from substance use disorders and PTSD. Pilot trials with Operation Iraqi Freedom/Operation Enduring Freedom veterans have shown some modest improvements in both substance use and PTSD symptoms, but high dropout rates have limited study validity (Norman et al. 2010). Evaluation of seeking safety in a homeless female veteran population has also shown modest improvements in clinical outcomes but not with substance use outcomes. Again, this study was limited by dropout and poor follow-up rates (Desai et al. 2008). A multisite study evaluating seeking safety compared with a health education group showed no difference between groups with regard to outcomes (Hien et al. 2009). Further and rigorous study with control groups is necessary to ascertain its utility and effectiveness for the dually diagnosed veteran population.

Future directions for research into psychotherapeutic treatment area should encourage inclusion rather than exclusion of dually diagnosed veterans, as well as combination trials investigating the effects of both psychotherapy therapy and medications together.

Psychosocial and Community-Based Treatments

Beyond the generally accepted medications and psychotherapies for dually diagnosed veterans, there is an additional category of well-defined treatments that includes psychosocial and community interventions. We will evaluate what is currently available. Ironically, recalling Dr. Pepper's work in the 1980s with the young chronics, this population remains understudied yet produces some of the greatest amount of work and monetary burden within communities as well as medical and mental health systems. It behooves our field to continue to investigate treatments that could improve care for this group in an integrated manner.

Residential and Supported Housing Programs Psychosocial treatment of dually diagnosed individuals is considered particularly difficult, due not only to the complex nature of the disorders but also to the frequent consequences that stem from uncontrolled substance use and undertreated mental illness. Frequently, individuals have legal entanglements and financial challenges that often lead to tenuous housing or even homelessness. The challenges of substance use and mental health disorders as well as social stressors add a significant layer of complexity to treatment.

Due to the fact that a high percentage of veterans with co-occurring disorders are also homeless, the VA has put effort and funding into studying and developing programs that can successfully house such veterans. In 1992, the Department of Housing and Urban Development created a memorandum of agreement with Veterans Affairs to create Housing and Urban Development-Veterans Affairs Supportive Housing (HUD-VASH) in order to grant permanent housing vouchers and case management services to homeless veterans with substance or psychiatric problems. Outcomes in supported housing for the chronically homeless with active substance use have demonstrated that these individuals can be successfully housed and that a "low-demand" housing program (one which does not require drug or alcohol sobriety for admission) is not required in order for successful housing (Edens et al. 2011). This low-demand type of program, also known as "housing first," models after a harm-reduction approach to substance treatment, where abstinence is encouraged but not required for entry into or continuation of treatment. More recently, investigators showed that veterans with substance and alcohol disorders can be housed successfully, though substance use and mental health disorders continue with little improvement (Tsai et al. 2014). Both of these studies argue for further integrated treatment into such housing models of care for the dually diagnosed homeless veteran.

Further studies have demonstrated improved outcomes with homelessness, specifically improvement in days housed along with fewer days homeless when individuals are not only enrolled in housing voucher programs but also exposed to intensive case management services as part of the voucher program (Rosenheck et al. 2003; Cheng et al. 2007).

Residential treatment—which is treatment given in a structured living setting—is one of the most costly programs set up for progress toward sober living. Residential treatment is often paired with housing when looking at outcomes. Studies evaluating multistage housing programs, where individuals are transitioned into housing programs through residential treatment, show little difference when compared with direct housing models, but both have produced improvement in outcomes for substance, housing, and mental health for homeless dually diagnosed individuals and veterans (Mares et al. 2004;

O'Connell et al. 2009). Initial studies examining residential and intensive outpatient treatment for homeless individuals with substance disorders have shown little benefit (Burnam et al. 1996), while others have shown better outcomes with utilization of more structured therapeutic communities (Nuttbrock et al. 1998). There has been little evaluation of self-help groups such as AA and NA in this population, but another study demonstrated that these groups are underutilized by dually diagnosed populations (Noordsy et al. 1996).

Other residential programs continue to provide beneficial outcomes for dually diagnosed veterans, specifically when paired with an integrated treatment approach. An examination of a dual diagnosis VA program in Cincinnati found that veterans who engage in the initial admission visits for the dual diagnosis treatment demonstrated a reduction in ER visits and shorter inpatient stays versus veterans who do not engage in the initial admission visits and were lost to drop-out (Sekerka et al. 1999). A direct head-to-head comparison of residential treatments for veterans that integrate care in a dual diagnosis model versus ones that focused only on substance treatment found that the integrated care/dual diagnosis residential programs led to more veterans entering directly into community housing versus more institutional settings. Social and vocational problems were seen improved among participants in the integrated residential program as well (Kasprow et al. 1999). Gonzalez and Rosenheck evaluated the effect of a 5-year, 18-site program on homeless individuals with substance use disorders and mental illness (the ACCESS program: Access to Community Care and Effective Services and Supports). Their findings support improved outcomes when homeless individuals with dually diagnosed disorders received extensive substance abuse services along with self-help groups (Gonzalez and Rosenheck 2002).

Contingency Management, Compensated Work Therapy, and Money Management Contingency management (CM) is a type of treatment that uses incentive or disincentive programming to modify behaviors, specifically in substance abuse treatment (Petry 2000). The majority of evidence for the effectiveness of this treatment has been positive. Various studies have demonstrated that the use of contingency management through monetary incentives or monetary reinforcement led to improved substance use outcomes, though mental health outcomes were either not measured or not improved across these studies (Sigmon et al. 2000; Bellack et al. 2006; Ries et al. 2004).

In addition to contingency management, there have been studies looking at vocational rehabilitation and combined contingency management as a treatment modality for dually diagnosed individuals. One study examined a small sample of dually diagnosed veterans entering into the Veterans Administration vocational rehabilitation program, Compensated Work Therapy (CWT) (Drebing et al. 2005). Compensated Work Therapy, the VA's version of vocational rehabilitation, was established as a program in 1957 and was designed to assist veterans identified as having vocational problems and clinical problems. Estimates have found 96% of participants in the VA program as having a psychiatric disorder and 76% as having a substance use disorder (Resnick and Rosenheck 2008). The investigators randomly assigned veterans to either Compensated Work Therapy alone or CWT paired with contingency management. Results showed improved vocational outcomes for the Compensated Work Therapy/contingency management group versus the Compensated Work Therapy alone group. Substance abuse outcomes were also improved within the Compensated Work Therapy/contingency management group, but mental health outcomes in this study were not measured. The findings were replicated in a larger veteran sample, again demonstrating improved vocational and substance abuse outcomes, though the authors cautioned that nuances regarding relapse once an individual is engaged with Compensated Work Therapy will need to be more thoroughly addressed in future studies (Drebing et al. 2007).

Innovative research has been done to examine money management within a substance abuse population. Though space precludes a thorough, in-depth discussion of this new area, a group of investigators have studied veterans voluntarily enrolled in money management that involved financial advisors holding checkbooks and check cards as well as education on money management skills. The investigators have been able to demonstrate reductions in Addiction Severity Index for subjects who engaged in the money management course (Rosen et al. 2009). A more recent study demonstrated that the same money management substance intervention led to a reduction in subjects' cocaine use (Black and Rosen 2011). This promising new area of treatment is currently being more thoroughly explored and holds the promise of a new type of treatment that could be extrapolated to the dually diagnosed individual.

An integrated model of treatment has been increasingly considered a gold standard approach for the dually diagnosed population due to demonstrated improved outcomes in substance use, mental health, and housing that have been consistently proven effective. Originally, in the early 1980s, when Dr. Pepper identified his population of "young chronics," available treatment for this population remained separate, parallel, fragmented, and ineffective. Early studies examining an integrated approach to treatment demonstrated limited results mainly due to the lack of recognition of the complexity of the population (Drake et al. 1998). A more comprehensive integrated approach for treatment has been refined and developed since the 1990s and has evolved into a well-studied and proven effective treatment. Robert Drake and colleagues have been intimately involved with developing this integrated treatment. There are now seven identified key components of the integrated approach for treating a dually diagnosed population built from previous studies of integrated treatment that had partial effectiveness. These components include staged interventions, motivational interviewing, assertive outreach, counseling, social support, comprehensiveness, and cultural sensitivity.

The first three components—staged interventions, motivational interviewing, and assertive community outreach—are considered the initial key elements of engaging a dually diagnosed individual in treatment. Initial engagement has been repeatedly identified as a treatment barrier for this population given their frequently difficult social settings, such as homelessness, their ambivalence toward substance treatment, and the significant impact that mental illness can have on their levels of trust toward a provider or treatment team. Counseling and social support incorporate multiple and individualized therapies, such as cognitive behavioral therapy and involvement with self-help groups and communities as well as family therapy. The final pieces of integrated care are sensitive treatment for an individual that incorporates their cultural identities and comprehensively addresses other aspects of their lives that can hinder their progress, such as finances or legal difficulties. Barriers for implementing this type of integrated care are many (Drake et al. 2001). The key barriers appear to be policy and programmatic ones. The scope and breadth of the VA's funding and resources has allowed for studying and developing programs for implementing integrated treatment at a continually larger audience of the dually diagnosed veteran.

Summary and New Directions

> The doctor of the future... will interest his patients in the care of the human frame...and in the cause and prevention of disease.
>
> –Thomas Edison

In this chapter's case study, First Lieutenant Jones is not only a patient of the past and present but also will continue to be the patient of the future. Multimorbidity, coined by geriatrician Mary E. Tinetti (Tinetti et al. 2012), is defined as the presence of two or more medical conditions in one person and is the more accurate term to define First Lieutenant Jones. Given his complexities, beyond diseases and extending into psychosocial issues, this term is more comprehensive than "dually diagnosed." As this chapter has reviewed, traditional medical care has historically focused on individual diseases, with multiple specialists treating each diagnosis separately. However, this approach can result in undertreatment or overtreatment, either of which can lead to harm rather than help for patients. This review of the status of interventions for dually diagnosed individuals and veterans has specified that treatment of "multimorbidities" should involve a coordinated effort in engaging ambivalent patients, identifying the biological and psychological diseases as well as the social complexities, and integrating a comprehensive strategy for individualized treatment.

The research evaluating this population has primarily been by single investigators. Their findings are relevant but will need to continue into wider replication studies. However, research is not the only area that demands expansion. Improved treatments that incorporate the integrated approach for the dually diagnosed are also imperative. Improved treatments require policy and program changes, as well as investment in changing the culture of mental health treatment for those with dual disorders. Rather than simply a call for more research, this chapter heralds a call for the development of innovative treatments that effectively integrate care for those with multimorbidities.

Key Concepts

1. Individuals with dual diagnoses have more severe illness trajectories.
2. Historically, treatment of dually diagnosed individuals has been fractured and sequential, leading to poor outcomes.
3. There are limited available trials evaluating medications for the dually diagnosed veteran.
4. Psychosocial and behavioral treatments are available and have demonstrated some measure of success in the dually diagnosed veteran population.
5. Treatment for the dually diagnosed veteran must include an integrated approach addressing medical, psychiatric, and psychosocial issues.

References

Albanese MJ, Khantzian EJ, Murphy SL, Green AI (1994) Decreased substance use in chronically psychotic patients treated with clozapine. Am J Psychiatry 151(5):780–781

Alderman CP, McCarthy LC, Condon JT, Marwood AC, Fuller JR (2009) Topiramate in combat-related posttraumatic stress disorder. Ann Pharmacother 43(4):635–641

Alemany S, Arias B, Fatjó-Vilas M, Villa H, Moya J, Ibanez M, Ortet G, Gasto C, Fananas L (2014) Psychosis-inducing effects of cannabis are related to both childhood abuse and COMT genotypes. Acta Psychiatr Scand 129(1):54–62

Ames G, Cunradi C (2004) Alcohol use and preventing alcohol-related problems among young adults in the military. Alcohol Res Health 28(4):252–258

Andréasson S, Engström A, Allebeck P, Rydberg U (1987) Cannabis and schizophrenia A longitudinal study of swedish conscripts. Lancet 330(8574):1483–1486

Arias A, Feinn R, Oncken C, Covault J, Kranzler HR (2010) Placebo-controlled trial of zonisamide for the treatment of alcohol dependence. J Clin Psychopharmacol 30(3):318

Arseneault L, Cannon M, Poulton R, Murray R, Caspi A, Moffitt TE (2002) Cannabis use in adolescence and risk for adult psychosis: longitudinal prospective study. BMJ 325(7374):1212–1213

Ballenger JC, Davidson JR, Lecrubier Y, Nutt DJ, Foa EB, Kessler RC, McFarlane AC (2000) Consensus statement on posttraumatic stress disorder from the International Consensus Group on Depression and Anxiety. J Clin Psychiatry 61(Suppl 5):60–66

Batki SL, Pennington DL, Lasher B, Neylan TC, Metzler T, Waldrop A, Delucchi K, Herbst E (2014) Topiramate treatment of alcohol use disorder in veterans with posttraumatic stress disorder: a randomized controlled pilot trial. Alcohol Clin Exp Res 38(8):2169–2177

Bellack AS, Bennett ME, Gearon JS, Brown CH, Yang Y (2006) A randomized clinical trial of a new behavioral treatment for drug abuse in people with severe and persistent mental illness. Arch Gen Psychiatry 63(4):426–432

Berlant JL (2000) Topiramate in posttraumatic stress disorder: preliminary clinical observations. J Clin Psychiatry 62:60–63

Berlant J, van Kammen DP (2002) Open-label topiramate as primary or adjunctive therapy in chronic civilian posttraumatic stress disorder: a preliminary report. J Clin Psychiatry 63(1):15–20

Berman RM, Cappiello A, Anand A, Oren DA, Heninger GR, Charney DS, Krystal JH (2000) Antidepressant effects of ketamine in depressed patients. Biol Psychiatry 47(4):351–354

Bernardy NC, Hamblen JL, Friedman MJ, Kivlahan DR (2011) Co-occurring posttraumatic stress disorder and substance use disorder: recommendations for man-

agement and implementation in the Department of Veterans Affairs. J Dual Diagn 7(4):242–261
Black AC, Rosen MI (2011) A money management-based substance use treatment increases valuation of future rewards. Addict Behav 36(1):125–128
Boehnlein JK, Kinzie JD (2007) Pharmacologic reduction of CNS noradrenergic activity in PTSD: the case for clonidine and prazosin. J Psychiatr Pract 13(2):72–78
Boehnlein JK, Kinzie JD, Sekiya U, Riley C, Pou K, Rosborough B (2004) A ten-year treatment outcome study of traumatized Cambodian refugees. J Nerv Ment Dis 192(10):658–663
Bowe A, Rosenheck R (2015) PTSD and substance use disorder among veterans: characteristics, service utilization and pharmacotherapy. J Dual Diagn 11(1):22–32
Brady KT, Sinha R (2007) Co-occurring mental and substance use disorders: the neurobiological effects of chronic stress. Focus 5(2):229–239
Brady KT, Dansky BS, Back SE, Foa EB, Carroll KM (2001) Exposure therapy in the treatment of PTSD among cocaine-dependent individuals: preliminary findings. J Subst Abus Treat 21(1):47–54
Brady KT, Sonne S, Anton RF, Randall CL, Back SE, Simpson K (2005) Sertraline in the treatment of co-occurring alcohol dependence and posttraumatic stress disorder. Alcohol Clin Exp Res 29(3):395–401
Bremner JD, Licinio J, Darnell A, Krystal JH, Owens MJ, Southwick SM, Nemeroff CB, Charney DS (1997) Elevated CSF corticotropin-releasing factor concentrations in posttraumatic stress disorder. Am J Psychiatr 154:624–629
Brunette MF, Drake RE, Xie H, McHugo GJ, Green AI (2006) Clozapine use and relapses of substance use disorder among patients with co-occurring schizophrenia and substance use disorders. Schizophr Bull 32(4):637–643
Buckley P, Psych M, Thompson P, Way L, Meltzer HY (1994) Substance abuse among patients with treatment-resistant schizophrenia: characteristics and implications for clozapine therapy. Am J Psychiatry 151(3):385–389
Burnam MA, Morton SC, McGlynn EA, Petersen LP, Stecher BM, Hayes C, Vaccaro JV (1996) An experimental evaluation of residential and nonresidential treatment for dually diagnosed homeless adults. J Addict Dis 14(4):111–134
Caspi A, Moffitt TE, Cannon M, McClay J, Murray R, Harrington H, Taylor A, Arseneault L, Williams B, Braithwaite A (2005) Moderation of the effect of adolescent-onset cannabis use on adult psychosis by a functional polymorphism in the catechol-O-methyltransferase gene: longitudinal evidence of a gene X environment interaction. Biol Psychiatry 57(10):1117–1127
Chappell P, Smith M, Kilts C, Bissette G, Ritchie J, Anderson C, Nemeroff C (1986) Alterations in corticotropin-releasing factor-like immunoreactivity in discrete rat brain regions after acute and chronic stress. J Neurosci 6(10):2908–2914
Cheng A-L, Lin H, Kasprow W, Rosenheck RA (2007) Impact of supported housing on clinical outcomes analysis of a randomized trial using multiple imputation technique. J Nerv Ment Dis 195(1):83
Croop RS, Faulkner EB, Labriola DF (1997) The safety profile of naltrexone in the treatment of alcoholism: results from a multicenter usage study. Arch Gen Psychiatry 54(12):1130–1135
Desai RA, Harpaz-Rotem I, Najavits LM, Rosenheck RA (2008) Impact of the seeking safety program on clinical outcomes among homeless female veterans with psychiatric disorders. Psychiatr Serv 59(9):996–1003
Di Forti M, Iyegbe C, Sallis H, Kolliakou A, Falcone MA, Paparelli A, Sirianni M, La Cascia C, Stilo SA, Marques TR (2012) Confirmation that the AKT1 (rs2494732) genotype influences the risk of psychosis in cannabis users. Biol Psychiatry 72(10):811–816
Drake RE, Mueser KT, Clark RE, Wallach MA (1996) The course, treatment, and outcome of substance disorder in persons with severe mental illness. Am J Orthop 66(1):42
Drake RE, Mercer-McFadden C, Mueser KT, McHugo GJ, Bond GR (1998) Review of integrated mental health and substance abuse treatment for patients with dual disorders. Schizophr Bull 24(4):589–608
Drake RE, Essock SM, Shaner A, Carey KB, Minkoff K, Kola L, Lynde D, Osher FC, Clark RE, Rickards L (2001) Implementing dual diagnosis services for clients with severe mental illness. Psychiatr Serv 52(4):469–476
Drebing CE, Fleitas R, Moore A, Krebs C, Van Ormer A, Penk W, Seibyl C, Rosenheck R (2002) Patterns in work functioning and vocational rehabilitation associated with coexisting psychiatric and substance use disorders. Rehabil Couns Bull 46(1):5–13
Drebing CE, Ormer E, Krebs C, Rosenheck R, Rounsaville B, Herz L, Penk W (2005) The impact of enhanced incentives on vocational rehabilitation outcomes for dually diagnosed veterans. J Appl Behav Anal 38(3):359–372
Drebing CE, Van Ormer EA, Mueller L, Hebert M, Penk WE, Petry NM, Rosenheck R, Rounsaville B (2007) Adding contingency management intervention to vocational rehabilitation: outcomes for dually diagnosed veterans. J Rehabil Res Dev 44(6):851–865
Edens EL, Mares AS, Tsai J, Rosenheck RA (2011) Does active substance use at housing entry impair outcomes in supported housing for chronically homeless persons? Psychiatr Serv 62(2):171–178
Fireman M, Indest DW, Blackwell A, Whitehead AJ, Hauser P (2005) Addressing tri-morbidity (hepatitis C, psychiatric disorders, and substance use): the importance of routine mental health screening as a component of a comanagement model of care. Clin Infect Dis 40(Supplement 5):S286–S291

Foa EB, Dancu CV, Hembree EA, Jaycox LH, Meadows EA, Street GP (1999) A comparison of exposure therapy, stress inoculation training, and their combination for reducing posttraumatic stress disorder in female assault victims. J Consult Clin Psychol 67(2):194

Foa EB, Yusko DA, McLean CP, Suvak MK, Bux DA, Oslin D, O'Brien CP, Imms P, Riggs DS, Volpicelli J (2013) Concurrent naltrexone and prolonged exposure therapy for patients with comorbid alcohol dependence and PTSD: a randomized clinical trial. JAMA 310(5):488–495

Fowler JS, Logan J, Wang G-J, Volkow ND (2003) Monoamine oxidase and cigarette smoking. Neurotoxicology 24(1):75–82

Fox HC, Seo D, Tuit K, Hansen J, Kimmerling A, Morgan PT, Sinha R (2012) Guanfacine effects on stress, drug craving and prefrontal activation in cocaine dependent individuals: preliminary findings. J Psychopharmacol 26(7):958–972

Freud S (2005) Civilization and its discontents. WW Norton & Company

Gamache G, Rosenheck R, Tessler R (2000) Choice of provider among homeless people with mental illness: veterans and the VA. Psychiatr Serv 51(8):1024–1017

Gamache G, Rosenheck R, Tessler R (2001) The proportion of veterans among homeless men: a decade later. Soc Psychiatry Psychiatr Epidemiol 36(10):481–485

Gonzalez G, Rosenheck RA (2002) Outcomes and service use among homeless persons with serious mental illness and substance abuse. Psychiatr Serv 53(4):437–446

Goodwin DW, Schulsinger F, Knop J, Mednick S, Guze SB (1977) Psychopathology in adopted and non-adopted daughters of alcoholics. Arch Gen Psychiatry 34(9):1005–1009

Harley M, Kelleher I, Clarke M, Lynch F, Arseneault L, Connor D, Fitzpatrick C, Cannon M (2010) Cannabis use and childhood trauma interact additively to increase the risk of psychotic symptoms in adolescence. Psychol Med 40(10):1627–1634

Harmon RJ, Riggs PD (1996) Clonidine for posttraumatic stress disorder in preschool children. J Am Acad Child Adolesc Psychiatry 35(9):1247–1249

Harris KM, DeVries A, Dimidjian K (2004) Trends in naltrexone use among members of a large private health plan. Psychiatr Serv 55(3):221

Hembree EA, Foa EB (2000) Posttraumatic stress disorder: psychological factors and psychosocial interventions. J Clin Psychiatry 61(Suppl 7):33–39

Hien DA, Nunes E, Levin FR, Fraser D (2000) Posttraumatic stress disorder and short-term outcome in early methadone treatment. J Subst Abus Treat 19(1):31–37

Hien DA, Wells EA, Jiang H, Suarez-Morales L, Campbell AN, Cohen LR, Miele GM, Killeen T, Brigham GS, Zhang Y (2009) Multisite randomized trial of behavioral interventions for women with co-occurring PTSD and substance use disorders. J Consult Clin Psychol 77(4):607

Hoff RA, Rosenheck RA (1998) Long-term patterns of service use and cost among patients with both psychiatric and substance abuse disorders. Med Care 36(6):835–843

Hoff RA, Rosenheck RA (1999) The cost of treating substance abuse patients with and without comorbid psychiatric disorders. Psychiatr Serv 50(10):1309–1315

Hoge CW, McGurk D, Thomas JL, Cox AL, Engel CC, Castro CA (2008) Mild traumatic brain injury in US soldiers returning from Iraq. N Engl J Med 358(5):453–463

Houston JE, Murphy J, Adamson G, Stringer M, Shevlin M (2008) Childhood sexual abuse, early cannabis use, and psychosis: testing an interaction model based on the National Comorbidity Survey. Schizophr Bull 34(3):580–585

Iheanacho T, Issa M, Marienfeld C, Rosenheck R (2013) Use of naltrexone for alcohol use disorders in the Veterans' Health Administration: a national study. Drug Alcohol Depend 132(1):122–126

Jacobsen LK, Southwick SM, Kosten TR (2001) Substance use disorders in patients with posttraumatic stress disorder: a review of the literature. Am J Psychiatr 158(8):1184–1190

Johnson BA (2004) Progress in the development of topiramate for treating alcohol dependence: from a hypothesis to a proof-of-concept study. Alcohol Clin Exp Res 28(8):1137–1144

Johnson BA, Ait-Daoud N (2010) Topiramate in the new generation of drugs: efficacy in the treatment of alcoholic patients. Curr Pharm Des 16(19):2103

Johnson BA, Rosenthal N, Capece JA, Wiegand F, Mao L, Beyers K, McKay A, Ait-Daoud N, Addolorato G, Anton RF (2008) Improvement of physical health and quality of life of alcohol-dependent individuals with topiramate treatment: US multisite randomized controlled trial. Arch Intern Med 168(11):1188–1199

Kasprow WJ, Rosenheck R, Frisman L, DiLella D (1999) Residential treatment for dually diagnosed homeless veterans: a comparison of program types. Am J Addict 8(1):34–43

Khantzian EJ (1987) The self-medication hypothesis of addictive disorders: focus on heroin and cocaine dependence. The Cocaine Crisis: Springer, p 65–74

Kinzie JD, Leung P (1989) Clonidine in Cambodian patients with posttraumatic stress disorder. J Nerv Ment Dis 177(9):546–550

Kolb LC (1991) PTSD: psychopathology and the startle response. Psychiatry Q 62(3):233–250

Konings M, Stefanis N, Kuepper R, De Graaf R, Have M t, Van Os J, Bakoula C, Henquet C (2012) Replication in two independent population-based samples that childhood maltreatment and cannabis use synergistically impact on psychosis risk. Psychol Med 42(01):149–159

Koob GF (2008) A role for brain stress systems in addiction. Neuron 59(1):11–34

Koob GF, Bloom FE (1988) Cellular and molecular mechanisms of drug dependence. Science 242(4879):715–723

Krupitsky E, Burakov A, Romanova T, Dunaevsky I, Strassman R, Grinenko A (2002) Ketamine psychotherapy for heroin addiction: immediate effects and two-year follow-up. J Subst Abus Treat 23(4):273–283
Krupitsky EM, Burakov AM, Dunaevsky IV, Romanova TN, Slavina TY, Grinenko AY (2007) Single versus repeated sessions of ketamine-assisted psychotherapy for people with heroin dependence. J Psychoactive Drugs 39(1):13–19
Littrell KH, Petty RG, Hilligoss NM, Peabody CD, Johnson CG (2001) Olanzapine treatment for patients with schizophrenia and substance abuse. J Subst Abus Treat 21(4):217–221
Marcus P, Snyder R (1995) Reduction of comorbid substance abuse with clozapine. Am J Psychiatry 152(6):959
Maremmani I, Zolesi O, Aglietti M, Marini G, Tagliamonte A, Shinderman M, Maxwell S (2000) Methadone dose and retention during treatment of heroin addicts with Axis I psychiatric comorbidity. J Addict Dis 19(2):29–41
Maremmani I, Pacini M, Lubrano S, Perugi G, Tagliamonte A, Pani PP, Gerra G, Shinderman M (2007) Long-term outcomes of treatment-resistant heroin addicts with and without DSM-IV axis I psychiatric comorbidity (dual diagnosis). Eur Addict Res 14(3):134–142
Mares AS, Kasprow WJ, Rosenheck RA (2004) Outcomes of supported housing for homeless veterans with psychiatric and substance abuse problems. Ment Health Serv Res 6(4):199–211
Marienfeld C, Rosenheck RA (2013) National psychotropic prescription dispensation among dually diagnosed patients. Advances Dual Diagn 6(1):34–44
Markou A, Kosten TR, Koob GF (1998) Neurobiological similarities in depression and drug dependence: a self-medication hypothesis. Neuropsychopharmacology 18(3):135–174
Martinotti G, Andreoli S, Di Nicola M, Di Giannantonio M, Sarchiapone M, Janiri L (2008) Quetiapine decreases alcohol consumption, craving, and psychiatric symptoms in dually diagnosed alcoholics. Hum Psychopharmacol Clin Exp 23(5):417–424
McCarthy E, Richardson G, Jane S, O'Brien E, Keegan K, Bassett G, Petrakis I (2009) Modified CPT-C for the treatment of veterans diagnosed with PTSD and alcohol dependence. Veteran's Administration Mental Health Conference
McEvoy JP, Freudenreich O, Levin ED, Rose JE (1995) Haloperidol increases smoking in patients with schizophrenia. Psychopharmacology 119(1):124–126
McGhee LL, Maani CV, Garza TH, Gaylord KM, Black IH (2008) The correlation between ketamine and post-traumatic stress disorder in burned service members. J Trauma Acute Care Surg 64(2):S195–S199
McGovern MP, Matzkin AL, Giard J (2007) Assessing the dual diagnosis capability of addiction treatment services: the Dual Diagnosis Capability in Addiction Treatment (DDCAT) index. J Dual Diagn 3(2):111–123
Merikangas KR, Prusoff BA, Weissman MM (1988) Parental concordance for affective disorders: psychopathology in offspring. J Affect Disord 15(3):279–290
Merikangas KR, Risch N, Weissman MM (1994) Comorbidity and co-transmission of alcoholism, anxiety and depression. Psychol Med 24(01):69–80
Miller W, Rollnick S (1991) Motivational interviewing: preparing people to change addictive behavior. Guilford, New York
Modesto-Lowe V, Kranzler HR (1999) Diagnosis and treatment of alcohol-dependent patients with comorbid psychiatric disorders. Alcohol Res Health 23(2):144–150
Najavits LM, Schmitz M, Gotthardt S, Weiss RD (2005) Seeking safety plus exposure therapy: an outcome study on dual diagnosis men. J Psychoactive Drugs 37(4):425–435
Neylan TC, Lenoci M, Samuelson KW, Metzler TJ, Henn-Haase C, Hierholzer RW, Lindley SE, Otte C, Schoenfeld FB, Yesavage JA, Marmar CR (2006) No improvement of posttraumatic stress disorder symptoms with guanfacine treatment. Am J Psychiatr 163(12):2186–2188
Noordsy DL, Schwab B, Fox L, Drake RE (1996) The role of self-help programs in the rehabilitation of persons with severe mental illness and substance use disorders. Community Ment Health J 32(1):71–81
Norman SB, Wilkins KC, Tapert SF, Lang AJ, Najavits LM (2010) A pilot study of seeking safety therapy with OEF/OIF veterans. J Psychoactive Drugs 42(1):83–87
Norquist GS, Hough RL, Golding JM, Escobar JI (1990) Psychiatric disorder in male veterans and nonveterans. J Nerv Ment Dis 178(5):328–335
Nunes EV, Quitkin FM, Donovan SJ, Deliyannides D, Ocepek-Welikson K, Koenig T, Brady R, McGrath PJ, Woody G (1998) Imipramine treatment of opiate-dependent patients with depressive disorders: a placebo-controlled trial. Arch Gen Psychiatry 55(2):153–160
Nuttbrock LA, Rahav M, Rivera JJ, Ng-Mak DS, Link BG (1998) Outcomes of homeless mentally ill chemical abusers in community residences and a therapeutic community. Psychiatr Serv 49(1):68–76
O'Connell MJ, Kasprow W, Rosenheck R (2009) Direct placement versus multistage models of supported housing in a population of veterans who are homeless. Psychol Serv 6(3):190
O'Malley SS, Jaffe AJ, Chang G, Schottenfeld RS, Meyer RE, Rounsaville B (1992) Naltrexone and coping skills therapy for alcohol dependence: a controlled study. Arch Gen Psychiatry 49(11):881–887
Pacini M, Maremmani I (2005) Methadone reduces the need for antipsychotic and antimanic agents in heroin addicts hospitalized for manic and/or acute psychotic episodes. Heroin Addict Relat Clin Probl 7(4):43–48
Pepper B, Kirshner MC, Ryglewicz H (1981) The young adult chronic patient: overview of a population. Hosp Community Psychiatry 32(7):463–469

Pepper B, Ryglewicz H, Kirshner MC (1982) The uninstitutionalized generation: a new breed of psychiatric patient. New Dir Ment Health Serv 1982(14):3–14
Petrakis IL, Leslie D, Rosenheck R (2003a) The use of antidepressants in alcohol-dependent veterans. J Clin Psychiatry 64(8):865–870
Petrakis IL, Leslie D, Rosenheck R (2003b) Use of naltrexone in the treatment of alcoholism nationally in the Department of Veterans Affairs. Alcohol Clin Exp Res 27(11):1780–1784
Petrakis IL, O'Malley S, Rounsaville B, Poling J, McHugh-Strong C, Krystal JH (2004) Naltrexone augmentation of neuroleptic treatment in alcohol abusing patients with schizophrenia. Psychopharmacology 172(3):291–297
Petrakis IL, Poling J, Levinson C, Nich C, Carroll K, Rounsaville B (2005) Naltrexone and disulfiram in patients with alcohol dependence and comorbid psychiatric disorders. Biol Psychiatry 57(10):1128–1137
Petrakis IL, Leslie D, Finney JW, Rosenheck R (2006a) Atypical antipsychotic medication and substance use-related outcomes in the treatment of schizophrenia. Am J Addict 15(1):44–49
Petrakis IL, Nich C, Ralevski E (2006b) Psychotic spectrum disorders and alcohol abuse: a review of pharmacotherapeutic strategies and a report on the effectiveness of naltrexone and disulfiram. Schizophr Bull 32(4):644–654
Petrakis IL, Poling J, Levinson C, Nich C, Carroll K, Ralevski E, Rounsaville B (2006c) Naltrexone and disulfiram in patients with alcohol dependence and comorbid post-traumatic stress disorder. Biol Psychiatry 60(7):777–783
Petrakis IL, Rosenheck R, Desai R (2011) Substance use comorbidity among veterans with posttraumatic stress disorder and other psychiatric illness. Am J Addict 20(3):185–189
Petrakis IL, Ralevski E, Desai N, Trevisan L, Gueorguieva R, Rounsaville B, Krystal JH (2012) Noradrenergic vs serotonergic antidepressant with or without naltrexone for veterans with PTSD and comorbid alcohol dependence. Neuropsychopharmacology 37(4):996–1004
Petry NM (2000) A comprehensive guide to the application of contingency management procedures in clinical settings. Drug Alcohol Depend 58(1):9–25
Pfefferbaum B (1997) Posttraumatic stress disorder in children: a review of the past 10 years. J Am Acad Child Adolesc Psychiatry 36(11):1503–1511
Picciotto MR, Brunzell DH, Caldarone BJ (2002) Effect of nicotine and nicotinic receptors on anxiety and depression. Neuroreport 13(9):1097–1106
Radhakrishnan R, Wilkinson ST, D'Souza DC (2014) Gone to pot–a review of the association between cannabis and psychosis. Front Psychol 5:54
Ralevski E, O'Brien E, Jane JS, Dean E, Dwan R, Petrakis I (2011) Effects of acamprosate on cognition in a treatment study of patients with schizophrenia spectrum disorders and comorbid alcohol dependence. J Nerv Ment Dis 199(7):499–505
Ralevski E, Gianoli MO, Russo M, Dwan R, Radhakrishnan R (2012) Cognitive deficits in schizophrenia and alcoholism: a review of the evidence and findings on the effects of treatment on cognitive functioning in patients with dual diagnoses. J Dual Diagn 8(3):205–217
Raskind MA, Peskind ER, Hoff DJ, Hart KL, Holmes HA, Warren D, Shofer J, O'Connell J, Taylor F, Gross C (2007) A parallel group placebo controlled study of prazosin for trauma nightmares and sleep disturbance in combat veterans with post-traumatic stress disorder. Biol Psychiatry 61(8):928–934
Rasmussen DD, Alexander LL, Raskind MA, Froehlich JC (2009) The α1-adrenergic receptor antagonist, prazosin, reduces alcohol drinking in alcohol-preferring (P) rats. Alcohol Clin Exp Res 33(2):264–272
Regier DA, Farmer ME, Rae DS, Locke BZ, Keith SJ, Judd LL, Goodwin FK (1990) Comorbidity of mental disorders with alcohol and other drug abuse: results from the Epidemiologic Catchment Area (ECA) study. JAMA 264(19):2511–2518
Resnick SG, Rosenheck RA (2008) Posttraumatic stress disorder and employment in veterans participating in Veterans Health Administration compensated work therapy. J Rehabil Res Dev 45(3):427–435
Ries RK, Dyck DG, Short R, Srebnik D, Fisher A, Comtois KA (2004) Outcomes of managing disability benefits among patients with substance dependence and severe mental illness. Psychiatr Serv 55(4):445–447
Rosen CS, Kuhn E, Greenbaum MA, Drescher KD (2008) Substance abuse–related mortality among middle-aged male VA psychiatric patients. Psychiatr Serv 59(3):290–296
Rosen MI, Carroll KM, Stefanovics E, Rosenheck RA (2009) A randomized controlled trial of a money management–based substance use intervention. Psychiatr Serv (Washington, DC) 60(4):498
Rosenheck R, Director V (n.d.) Appendix C, mental and substance-use health services for veterans: experience with performance evaluation in the Department of Veterans Affairs. Improving the quality of health care for mental and substance-use conditions: quality chasm series, p 423–482
Rosenheck R, Fontana A (1996) Race and outcome of treatment for veterans suffering from PTSD. J Trauma Stress 9(2):343–351
Rosenheck RA, Banks S, Pandiani J, Hoff R (2000) Bed closures and incarceration rates among users of Veterans Affairs mental health services. Psychiatr Serv 51(10):1282–1287
Rosenheck R, Kasprow W, Frisman L, Liu-Mares W (2003) Cost-effectiveness of supported housing for homeless persons with mental illness. Arch Gen Psychiatry 60(9):940–951
Sarnyai Z, Bíró É, Gardi J, Vecsernyés M, Julesz J, Telegdy G (1995) Brain corticotropin-releasing factor mediates 'anxiety-like' behavior induced by cocaine withdrawal in rats. Brain Res 675(1):89–97
Schimmelmann BG, Conus P, Cotton SM, Kupferschmid S, Karow A, Schultze-Lutter F, McGorry PD, Lambert M (2011) Cannabis use disorder and age at onset of psychosis—a study in first-episode patients. Schizophr Res 129(1):52–56

Schneider U, Wohlfarth K, Schulze-Bonhage A, Haacker T, Müller-Vahl K, Zedler M, Becker H, Dengler R, Emrich H (1999) Effects of acamprosate on memory in healthy young subjects. J Stud Alcohol Drugs 60(2):172

Sekerka R, Goldsmith RJ, Brandewie L, Somoza E (1999) Treatment outcome of an outpatient treatment program for dually-diagnosed veterans: the Cincinnati Veterans Affairs Medical Center. J Psychoactive Drugs 31(1):85–94

Sernyak MJ, Glazer WM, Heninger GR, Charney DS, Woods SW, Petrakis IL, Krystal JH, Price LH (1998) Naltrexone augmentation of neuroleptics in schizophrenia. J Clin Psychopharmacol 18(3):248–251

Sigmon SC, Steingard S, Badger GJ, Anthony SL, Higgins ST (2000) Contingent reinforcement of marijuana abstinence among individuals with serious mental illness: a feasibility study. Exp Clin Psychopharmacol 8(4):509

Simpson TL, Saxon AJ, Meredith CW, Malte CA, McBride B, Ferguson LC, Gross CA, Hart KL, Raskind M (2009) A pilot trial of the alpha-1 adrenergic antagonist, prazosin, for alcohol dependence. Alcohol Clin Exp Res 33(2):255–263

Southwick SM, Bremner JD, Rasmusson A, Morgan CA, Arnsten A, Charney DS (1999) Role of norepinephrine in the pathophysiology and treatment of posttraumatic stress disorder. Biol Psychiatry 46(9):1192–1204

Swerdlow NR, Britton KT, Koob GF (1989) Potentiation of acoustic startle by corticotropin-releasing factor (CRF) and by fear are both reversed by alpha-helical CRF (9-41). Neuropsychopharmacology 2(4):285–292

Tanaka T, Yokoo H, Mizoguchi K, Yoshida M, Tsuda A, Tanaka M (1991) Noradrenaline release in the rat amygdala is increased by stress: studies with intracerebral microdialysis. Brain Res 544(1):174–176

Taylor FB, Martin P, Thompson C, Williams J, Mellman TA, Gross C, Peskind ER, Raskind MA (2008) Prazosin effects on objective sleep measures and clinical symptoms in civilian trauma posttraumatic stress disorder: a placebo-controlled study. Biol Psychiatry 63(6):629–632

Tejani N, Rosenheck R, Tsai J, Kasprow W, McGuire J (2014) Incarceration histories of homeless veterans and progression through a national supported housing program. Community Ment Health J 50(5):514–519

Tinetti ME, Fried TR, Boyd CM (2012) Designing health care for the most common chronic condition—multimorbidity. JAMA 307(23):2493–2494

Titievsky J, Seco G, Barranco M, Kyle EM (1982) Doxepin as adjunctive therapy for depressed methadone maintenance patients: a double-blind study. J Clin Psychiatry 43(11):454–456

Torrens M, Fonseca F, Mateu G, Farré M (2005) Efficacy of antidepressants in substance use disorders with and without comorbid depression: a systematic review and meta-analysis. Drug Alcohol Depend 78(1):1–22

Tsai J, Kasprow WJ, Rosenheck RA (2014) Alcohol and drug use disorders among homeless veterans: prevalence and association with supported housing outcomes. Addict Behav 39(2):455–460

Volpicelli JR, Alterman AI, Hayashida M, O'Brien CP (1992) Naltrexone in the treatment of alcohol dependence. Arch Gen Psychiatry 49(11):876–880

Voruganti L, Awad A (2004) Neuroleptic dysphoria: towards a new synthesis. Psychopharmacology 171(2):121–132

Wieder H, Kaplan EH (1968) Drug use in adolescents. Psychodynamic meaning and pharmacogenic effect. Psychoanal Study Child 24:399–431

Woody GE, O'Brien CP, Rickels K (1975) Depression and anxiety in heroin addicts: a placebo-controlled study of doxepin in combination with methadone. Am J Psychiatry 132(4):447–450

Ziedonis D, Richardson T, Lee E, Petrakis I, Kosten T (1992) Adjunctive desipramine in the treatment of cocaine abusing schizophrenics. Psychopharmacol Bull 28(3):309–314

Zimmet SV, Strous RD, Burgess ES, Kohnstamm S, Green AI (2000) Effects of clozapine on substance use in patients with schizophrenia and schizoaffective disorder: a retrospective survey. J Clin Psychopharmacol 20(1):94–98

Psychosis: Schizophrenia and Related Disorders

21

Ronald J. Gurrera and Nicole L. Perry

Introduction

A comprehensive study of hospitalizations among all active-duty military service members from 1990 to 1999 found that psychiatric disorders were the leading cause of military discharge for men and the second leading cause (after pregnancy) for women (Hoge et al. 2002). Mental disorders accounted for 13% of all hospitalizations and 23% of all inpatient bed days. Among service members hospitalized for the first time for a psychiatric illness, 47% left military service within 6 months, compared to 12% for nonpsychiatric disorders (Hoge et al. 2002). Due to the common practice of documenting clinical encounters in military settings with diagnostic codes that emphasize situational factors rather than intrinsic psychopathology, which may reflect a reluctance to label active-duty service members in potentially stigmatizing and career-damaging ways (Hoge et al. 2004; Wilson et al. 2009), the true prevalence of mental disorders may be underestimated. According to Hoge et al. (2002), "mental disorders appear to represent the most important source of medical and occupational morbidity among active-duty U.S. military personnel." This fact is amplified by the observation that mental health encounters in the Department of Veterans Affairs (VA) have increased 71% from 10.5 million in 2005 to 18.0 million in 2013 (DoD/VA Report to the Congress 2014).

Psychosis is one of the severest mental disorders and can be conceptualized broadly as a state in which perceptions, experiences, and/or beliefs do not conform to consensus-based notions of reality. Perceptual disturbances usually take the form of hallucinations. Most often these are auditory and consist of one or more human voices conversing with one another, providing a running narrative of the individual's behaviors, making derogatory or threatening statements to or about the individual, or instructing the individual to carry out specific actions. Delusions are false beliefs about self or others and can include grandiose, persecutory, religious, somatic, or false identity elements. Individuals with certain forms of psychosis may feel that their thoughts are being removed from their heads or that others' thoughts are being inserted into their own thought process. Alternatively they may experience parts of their body as not belonging to them or under the control of another individual or an outside force. Symptoms and the individual's interpretation of them are often mutually reinforcing, making it more difficult for the patient to appreciate their unreality. For example, someone who

R.J. Gurrera (✉)
VA Boston Healthcare System, Harvard Medical School, Boston, MA, USA
e-mail: Ronald.gurrera@va.gov

N.L. Perry
VA Boston Healthcare System, Boston, MA, USA

L.W. Roberts, C.H. Warner (eds.), *Military and Veteran Mental Health*,
https://doi.org/10.1007/978-1-4939-7438-2_21

believes there is a conspiracy to harm him may also hear auditory hallucinations warning him of an impending attack or telling him he deserves to be punished for some past transgression. In other cases it may be difficult for an observer to discern a common theme linking reported symptoms, which may seem to consist of unrelated abnormal mental elements.

Most theories of psychosis assign an etiologic role to stress, and individuals who manifest psychosis may be relatively more prone to experience stress more intensely. General population studies have found that a variety of traumatic or stressful life events can lead to psychotic experiences (DeVylder et al. 2016). The diathesis-stress model hypothesizes that psychosis is triggered by an interaction between stressful life events and heightened individual vulnerability to psychosis and has been prominent in scientific thinking for decades. There is considerable evidence that the relationship between stress and psychosis is mediated by the hypothalamic-pituitary-adrenal (HPA) axis, specifically cortisol (Walker et al. 2008). Psychotic disorders have been linked to abnormalities in many different brain networks and physiological systems, some of them genetically based, and traumatic stress is obviously an important consideration with respect to the mental health of active service members and veterans (Hoge et al. 2004).

Case Study

Mark Chen, a 21-year-old male Operation Iraqi Freedom/Operation Enduring Freedom soldier, is brought in for psychiatric evaluation by the military police, who were called when the soldier began screaming at individuals on the military base. He had just returned from a combat mission. He was screaming that he needed to go back out in order to save everyone from the "end of the world." Following acute medical and psychiatric stabilization, which included emergent administration of intramuscular antipsychotic medication, a urine toxicology screen and basic blood tests were ordered.

During the interview with the treatment team, Chen describes hearing the voice of God telling him about his special mission and that he is a savior for the earth. He speaks rapidly, is difficult to interrupt, and makes illogical or incomprehensible statements; he appears internally preoccupied at times and paces around while talking. He is oriented to person and place but not to time. He denies any suicidal or homicidal ideation or plans. He denies use of illicit drugs and says he uses alcohol in moderation. He has no known history of psychiatric illness. He describes not having slept for the past week during his recent combat mission. His commanding officer says he did not think that the soldier had behaved abnormally on the mission and noted that, although they did not come under fire, they were constantly on the move, did not get much sleep—they did not sleep for three nights—and just returned yesterday.

Historical Background and Evolution of the Construct of Psychosis

The nosology of psychotic disorders is limited by a lack of biological markers or even widely accepted models of their disease processes. Conventional classification has divided psychoses pragmatically into syndromes associated with established medical disorders and those for which no clear anatomical or physiological basis is known. Those in the latter group have traditionally been designated psychiatric disorders, a classification that reflects the limits of a purely historical-descriptive methodology. The field of neuroscience is advancing at an accelerating pace, however, and it seems possible there will be sufficient evidence at some point to elevate each disorder from syndrome status to a disease whose pathophysiology and neuroanatomy are known in detail, rendering this traditional dichotomy obsolete. In fact, the need to reevaluate current psychiatric classification strategies so that clinical entities (and their treatments) are more readily aligned with likely underlying biological mechanisms is a focus of current scientific discourse (e.g., Carpenter 2016; Pearlson et al. 2016; Yee et al. 2015).

Formal systems for assigning clinical diagnoses to psychotic disorders will be described briefly below. This chapter focuses on psychotic syndromes representing primary and persistent psychiatric disorders, in contrast to psychotic symptoms stemming from a known neurological disorder or those arising in conjunction with extreme mood disturbances, which resolve when the mood disturbance is adequately treated (e.g., bipolar disorder); and distinct from cognitive or perceptual disorders secondary to an intoxicated state.

Schizophrenia-Related Disorders

Schizophrenia is the most commonly treated psychotic disorder. Clinical features vary considerably across individuals and include hallucinations, delusions, and disorganized thought processes or behaviors—the so-called "positive" symptoms; and diminished emotional expression, motivation, or spontaneous behaviors—collectively termed "negative" symptoms. Schizoaffective disorder was once viewed as distinct from schizophrenia and bipolar disorder, but more recently it is seen more as an intermediate or hybrid form of those disorders (Malhi et al. 2008). The current edition of the standard psychiatric diagnostic reference (*Diagnostic and Statistical Manual of Mental Disorders*, 5th edition) classifies schizoaffective disorder as a variant of schizophrenia, one in which either periodic or persistent mood disturbances also occur. It is differentiated clinically from major mood disorders with psychosis by the temporal dissociation between mood and cognitive symptoms. In addition, the valence of the psychotic symptoms is often incongruent. The ideational content in psychotic mood disorders tends to mirror the mood state, so a manic mood state may be accompanied by grandiose ideation, whereas the same individual may experience nihilistic or other morbid delusions when in a depressed state. In contrast, psychotic symptoms in schizoaffective disorder are typically present even when mood is within a normal range and often are not reflective of mood when it is outside the normal range (i.e., they are mood incongruent). Schizophrenia and schizoaffective disorder are severe illnesses that are often associated with substantial disability in social, educational, and vocational domains. Emergence of either disorder during active military service invariably leads to medical discharge, and this is often the point at which a veteran will enter the VA health-care system.

Other Psychotic Disorders

A few relatively uncommon psychotic disorders are characterized by persistent delusional beliefs in the absence of other signs of psychosis. The delusional ideation is typically organized around a dominant theme (e.g., grandiosity, persecution, etc.) and is relatively unchanging over time. These disorders are notoriously refractory to treatment, but they are generally less debilitating than schizophrenia and schizoaffective disorder and in many cases would not be apparent to a casual observer. An even rarer syndrome termed "brief psychotic disorder" may occur in otherwise psychiatrically healthy individuals who experience an extreme psychological stressor; symptoms are indistinguishable from those of schizophrenia at a descriptive level, but the syndrome has a very abrupt onset and is short-lived, the symptoms do not recur, and affected individuals have no known genetic or biological predisposition. These disorders are less likely to precipitate a discharge from military service because they resolve quickly or because the symptoms are not fully evident to observers.

Schizotypal Personality Disorder

The construct of schizotypal personality disorder was introduced by the American Psychiatric

Association's *Diagnostic and Statistical Manual of Mental Disorders*, third edition (*DSM-III*), in an attempt to integrate accumulated clinical observations of patients with severe personality psychopathology who did not display overt psychosis and family studies—including the well-known Danish adoption study (Tsuang and Tohen 2002)—which found that some nonpsychotic family members of patients with schizophrenia demonstrated subtle abnormalities of thought, communication, and social functioning (Rosell et al. 2014). A recent review of research in this area supports the view that schizotypal personality disorder is an intermediate schizophrenia-spectrum phenotype that shares many neurobiological abnormalities with schizophrenia (Rosell et al. 2014).

Diagnosis

Psychotic disorders share many features and may be genetically related (Jablensky 2006). Schizophrenia likely represents multiple etiologically distinct but interactive processes rather than a unitary process; a multifactorial disease model (e.g., cancer) is more consistent with the evidence, but research strategies to date generally have not incorporated this perspective (Jablensky 2006). There are no established biological markers for schizophrenia, so it is currently defined in terms of observable clinical attributes (Jablensky 2006).

The *Diagnostic and Statistical Manual of Mental Disorders* (*DSM*) is familiar to mental health clinicians everywhere, especially those who work with mental health clinician trainees in academic settings. The *DSM*, first published by the American Psychiatric Association in 1952, was based on the sixth edition of the *International Statistical Classification of Diseases and Related Health Problems* (*ICD-6*) (World Health Organization 2016), which included an inaugural section on mental disorders. The first edition of *DSM* also drew heavily upon War Department Technical Bulletin, Medical 203 (Office of the Surgeon General, Army Service Forces) and on a nomenclature created by VA (*DSM-I*, p vii). The fifth iteration of the *DSM* (*DSM-5*; APA 2013) is the first major revision since 1994. There were a number of changes in diagnostic criteria from the previous edition, including those for schizophrenia and schizoaffective disorder. While *DSM* is preferred by practicing clinicians, the tenth revision of the *ICD* (*ICD-10*) was recently adopted by VA as the coding standard for third-party billing.

Epidemiology

Data regarding the incidence of psychosis in active-duty service members are somewhat limited. A study of all first hospitalizations for psychosis of active-duty enlisted US Navy personnel during the period 1980–1988 found an incidence rate of 57 per 100,000 for schizophrenia (Gunderson and Hourani 1998). During that time period, the rate of first hospitalizations for schizophrenia[1] dropped from 92.1 to 29.2 per 100,000, but the incidence rate for affective psychoses nearly doubled. The practice at that time was to immediately discharge navy service members diagnosed with schizophrenia and transfer their care to VA (Gunderson and Hourani 1998). Cowan et al. (2011) examined initial hospitalization rates for all US military service members from 2000 to 2009 and reported a relatively unchanging incidence of 14/100,000 person-years for schizophrenia and schizoaffective disorder (combined) over that period. Notably, 38% of service members had more than one hospitalization for these disorders, indicating that in many cases the initial hospitalization did not result in an immediate medical discharge.[2] A

[1] It is interesting to note that the apparent drop in schizophrenia incidence among navy personnel followed the publication of *DSM-III* in 1980; this edition was the first in the series to provide objectively verifiable standardized diagnostic criteria for schizophrenia, which effectively narrowed its clinical definition (Tsuang and Tohen 2002).

[2] The customary practice is to hospitalize an actively psychotic service member promptly, and when clinically stable enough to be treated as an outpatient, transfer him/her to a medical holding company, where the service member will await the outcome of disability and physical evaluation board reviews. This process, which may take up to 1 year, determines whether the service member will be medically retired from military service.

similarly designed study of the period 1992–1996 found a comparable incidence rate for these disorders (16/100,000 person-years) (Herrell et al. 2006).

Given the rapid attrition of service members with a diagnosed psychotic disorder from the active-duty population, prevalence estimates are less meaningful. According to the VA National Psychosis Registry, during a 1-year period beginning October 1, 1998, there were 71,363 veterans diagnosed with schizophrenia and 14,717 diagnosed with schizoaffective disorder (Blow et al. 2004). Data from the National Center for Veterans Analysis and Statistics (http://www.va.gov/vetdata/Utilization.asp, downloaded 9/4/16) indicates a nearly linear annual increase in veteran enrollees from FY2000 through FY2014; extrapolating backward yields an estimated 2,942,906 enrolled veterans in FY1998, implying crude prevalence estimates of 2425 per 100,000 for schizophrenia and 500 per 100,000 for schizoaffective disorder. Mean ages and mean annual incomes for these groups were 53.9 and 50.2 years and $12,282 and $8915, respectively, illustrating the serious disability that often accompanies these disorders. Dually diagnosed substance abuse was slightly more prevalent in the schizoaffective cohort (25.6% vs. 32.6%) (Blow et al. 2004).

Data from the 1999 Large Health Survey of Veteran Enrollees ($n = 559{,}985$) indicate a prevalence for schizophrenia and schizoaffective disorder (combined, ICD-9 295.xx) of 3010 per 100,000 (Chwastiak et al. 2010); women comprised 5.1% of that patient group (Teh et al. 2008). Bauer et al. (2015) used administrative files from the VA Corporate Data Warehouse to examine prevalence of major mental health diagnoses during fiscal years 2003–2010. Using all but the most restrictive administrative case exclusion criteria, the prevalence of schizophrenia spectrum disorders (*ICD-9* codes 290.0-295.9) was between 1350 and 1660 per 100,000 in 2010, and this rate was relatively stable over the 7-year study period.

Successive versions of the *DSM* have defined schizophrenia in progressively more narrow terms (Tsuang and Tohen 2002). Prior to the third edition of the *DSM* (*DSM-III*, 1980), schizophrenia prevalence estimates in the general population ranged from 1000 to 7000 per 100,000, with more recent estimates centering on approximately 3000 per 100,000 (Tsuang and Tohen 2002, p. 368). Two large US epidemiological surveys using *DSM-III* diagnostic criteria found schizophrenia prevalence rates of 6400–6900 per 100,000 (the higher rate included all forms of psychosis except those related to mood disorders). A very recent study based on *ICD-9* clinical diagnoses obtained from the Mental Health Research Network (a nationwide consortium of US public domain research centers based in large not-for-profit health-care systems) found a schizophrenia prevalence of 2000 per 100,000 in a sample of more than 7.5 million enrollees (Coleman et al. 2016). The prevalence of other psychoses was 3100 per 100,000, but that group appears to have included psychotic mood disorders.

In systematic reviews of all studies published from 1965 to 2002, McGrath et al. (2004, 2008) found a median worldwide incidence of schizophrenia of 15.2 per 100,000 (10–90% quantile range 7.7–43.0 per 100,000). The incidence of schizophrenia was higher in men compared to women (median male/female ratio 1.4, 10–90% quantile range 0.9–2.4), higher in urban sites compared to mixed urban/rural sites, and higher in migrants compared to native-born individuals. This median incidence sex ratio is very similar to that obtained by a previous meta-analysis (Aleman et al. 2003). McGrath and colleagues also reported that corresponding median prevalence estimates (per 100,000 persons) for point, period, lifetime, and lifetime morbid risk (10–90% quantiles) for the distributions were 4600 (1900–10,000), 3300 (1300–8200), 4000 (1600–12,100), and 7200 (3100–27,100), respectively.[3]

[3]Prevalence measures the proportion of individuals who manifest a disorder at a specified time point, or during a specified time span. Point prevalence is the fraction of individuals at risk for a disorder who actually manifest that disorder at a narrow point in time (e.g., one or more days), whereas period prevalence references a longer time frame (e.g., 1 year). Lifetime prevalence is the fraction of individuals at risk for a disorder who manifest that disorder ever, who are alive on a given day. Lifetime morbid risk estimates the probability that a person will develop the disorder during a specified period in their life, or up to a particular age (Saha et al. 2005).

It is notable that in contrast to the preponderance of males in incident schizophrenia, males and females do not differ with respect to prevalence (Saha et al. 2005). The authors did not speculate on the reason for this discrepancy, but certainly one possibility is a higher mortality rate in males with schizophrenia.

The prevalence of schizotypal personality disorder in a US nonclinical community sample was estimated to be 3300 per 100,000 (Lenzenweger et al. 2007), and a recent estimate of the lifetime prevalence (per 100,000) of this disorder in the USA is 4200 for men and 3700 for women (Rosell et al. 2014). In contrast, in a large ($n = 693$) cohort of twin pairs from the Vietnam Era Twin Registry, the prevalence of schizotypal personality disorder in veterans was only 300 per 100,000 (Tsuang and Tohen 2002).

These data indicate that in veterans the prevalence of schizophrenia and schizoaffective disorder is lower than in the general population. One reason may be that the enlistment process preferentially selects for individuals who are at relatively reduced risk of developing one of these disorders. The difference in schizotypal personality disorder prevalence between veteran and nonveteran populations is even greater. A key feature of personality disorders, including schizotypal personality disorder, is that they are evident prior to adulthood. This feature could account for a relatively greater adverse selection effect on individuals with this disorder compared to those who are subsequently diagnosed with schizophrenia or schizoaffective disorder because the latter illnesses often do not manifest premorbid behavioral abnormalities.

Treatment

Antipsychotic medications are essential for treating psychotic symptoms, but psychosocial interventions are also very important (Chien and Yip 2013). The evidence base for the treatment of schizophrenia is the most developed, so our discussion will focus on that, beginning with medications. The treatment course can be divided into acute episode, maintenance or relapse prevention, and recovery stages. The acute episode can be further divided into acute and stabilization phases, and recently the prepsychotic or prodromal stage is receiving attention as a possible window of opportunity for early interventions that may alter the illness course (refer to Fig. 21.1 for an overview of schizophrenia treatment stages).

Prodromal Schizophrenia

The prodromal stage rarely begins before puberty and is characterized by mild positive symptoms and subjectively experienced disturbances in cognitive, somatic, and perceptual domains. This stage typically continues for 1–5 years before frank psychosis emerges, during which functioning rapidly declines (Mokhtari and Rajarethinam 2014). There are three levels of intervention for mitigating the disability that attends the prodromal stage: universal, selective, and indicated (Mrazek and Haggerty 1994, cited in Mokhtari and Rajarethinam 2014). Universal prevention addresses the general population (e.g., education of primary care providers and the public, access to mental health services, etc.); selective prevention focuses on individuals who evidence specific factors known to be associated with increased risk of developing schizophrenia; and indicated prevention targets individuals whose mild subsyndromal symptoms are progressing and have worsened to the point of causing them distress (Mokhtari and Rajarethinam 2014).

Early intervention (i.e., during the prodromal stage, prior to the first episode of frank psychosis) can improve outcome, but identifying individuals with prodromal schizophrenia is challenging because the symptoms at that point are nonspecific (McGorry et al. 2009). In order to direct preventive interventions more effectively, clinical criteria have been developed to identify individuals who are at "ultrahigh" risk for manifesting schizophrenia (Yung et al. 2003). There are several components to these criteria: attenuated or transient psychotic symptoms and trait and state risk factors. Attenuated psychotic symptoms include ideas of reference, odd beliefs, magical thinking, perceptual distortions, and odd speech,

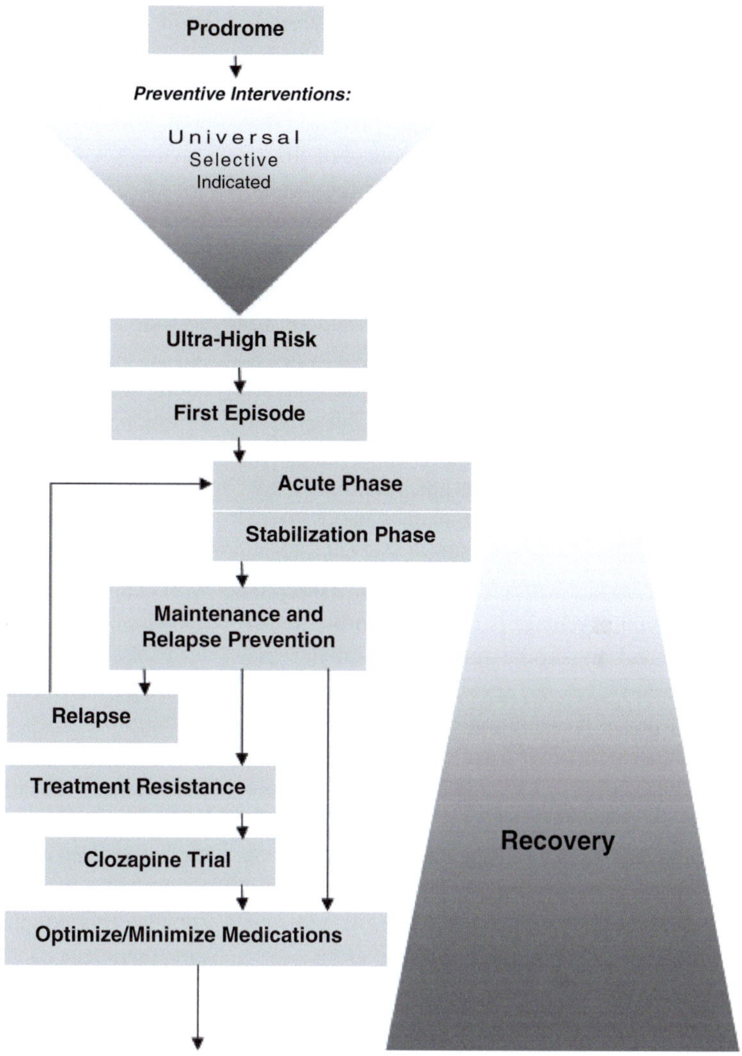

Fig. 21.1 Schizophrenia illness stages

behavior, or appearance (features that overlap with schizotypal disorder). Transient psychotic symptoms are brief, limited, and intermittent; they last less than 1 week or are very infrequent and resolve spontaneously. The trait and state risk factors consist of nonspecific symptoms such as anxious or depressed mood plus trait risk factors (e.g., schizotypal personality disorder or a family history of psychosis in a first-degree relative) (Yung et al. 2003). More than one-third of individuals who meet ultrahigh risk criteria and are not receiving antipsychotic medication will progress to first episode psychosis within 1 year (Mokhtari and Rajarethinam 2014).

During a 1-year period from 1999 to 2000, 10.2% of all active duty service members admitted to the Walter Reed Army Medical Center for a psychiatric disorder were subsequently readmitted at least once during the study period (Bobo et al. 2004). Logistic regression analysis revealed that a history of a previous psychiatric hospitalization and childhood onset of psychiatric problems were the strongest predictors of rehospitalization. Additional predictors were having less than a high school education, legal problems, and a history of substance abuse (Bobo et al. 2004). It is worth noting that many of these predictor variables are historical and thus potentially very accessible to a screening process. Service members are typically hospitalized within several weeks after symptom onset.[4]

Clinical staging is based on the principle that treatments offered earlier in the course of illness should be correspondingly safer, and their effectiveness should be evaluated in terms of remission and recovery rates (McGorry et al. 2009). The risks associated with antipsychotic medications, coupled with their uncertain benefit for prodromal illness (Marshall and Rathbone 2011), make the clinical staging model appropriate for the prodromal period. For example, some prodromal individuals may benefit from cognitive behavioral therapy without antipsychotic medication (McGorry et al. 2009; Galletly et al. 2016). Unequivocal psychotic symptoms, however, should be treated without delay because duration of untreated psychosis is linked to poorer symptomatic and functional recovery from the first episode and increased severity of negative symptoms at initial presentation (Perkins et al. 2005). The Department of Defense's culture of promptly hospitalizing service members with active psychosis minimizes treatment delay and places the service member in a setting where effective treatment is accessible. It is not known whether delayed treatment of the first episode is associated with increased risk of recurrence (Perkins et al. 2005).

The Acute Episode – Acute Phase

The goals of treatment during an acute psychotic episode include preventing harm, containing disturbed and dangerous behaviors, reducing psychotic and associated behavioral symptoms (e.g., agitation and aggression), addressing factors that contributed to the occurrence of the acute episode, expediting a return to the highest attainable level of functioning, developing an alliance with the patient and family, and connecting the patient with appropriate community aftercare (APA 2004).

Management of Behavioral Emergencies

Agitation is often present during the initial portion of the acute phase and must be addressed immediately because it is distressing for the patient and presents substantial risk of injury to the patient and others. Consensus guidelines generally agree that calming the patient is a priority because this attenuates immediate risk and permits therapeutic interactions to take place (Gould 2012a). Physical restraint is sometimes required in the most extreme behavioral emergencies, but it carries its own risks to patients and staff and should be reserved for behaviors that pose imminent threat of significant injury and are unresponsive to less restrictive alternatives (Allen et al. 2003). Consensus guidelines stress the importance of initial de-escalation techniques in minimizing the risk of injury (Allen et al. 2003). In 2006 VA rolled out the Prevention and Management of Disruptive Behavior (PMDB) training program nationally, which is mandated for all employees who occupy positions designated as high risk for potentially assaultive behaviors.

The VA Prevention and Management of Disruptive Behavior training program has four levels. Level I is an introductory course that is accessible online and addresses general work-

[4]Service members can access several mental health treatment options before entering psychiatric treatment. These are (a) the chaplain, who is also a trained counselor attuned to military lifestyle issues and able to offer confidential, professional assistance, and referral services; (b) combat stress control teams, which are a field resource capable of supporting the mental and emotional well-being of service members during deployments; and (c) nonmedical programs (Military One Source and Military and Family Life Counseling) whose counselors possess a masters or doctorate degree in a mental health field, are licensed or certified to practice independently and provide confidential, short-term counseling to active-duty, National Guard, and reserve service members (regardless of their activation status), and their families. These sessions are available in three formats: face to face, by telephone, or online in a secure real-time "chat" format. In addition, the Family Advocacy Program is a supportive resource for service members and their families that assesses, refers, and provides counseling for families experiencing domestic violence or child abuse. If FAP identifies someone as suicidal, they refer the individual to an MTF (a military treatment facility), TRICARE, or local community resource for immediate professional, medical, mental health treatment (http://www.militaryonesource.mil/casualty?content_id=268934).

place violence prevention and situational awareness; it is required for all VA employees. Levels II–IV are mandated for those who work in areas deemed high risk for violent behaviors (e.g., psychiatric inpatient units, emergency departments, etc.). Levels II and III are in-person training sessions that teach specific skills for identifying and verbally de-escalating disruptive behavior and for evading or escaping from grabs, chokes, hair pulls, bites, punches, and kicks. Level IV teaches participants evidence-based, specific therapeutic containment techniques utilizing a three-person team-based approach that physically contains violent behaviors.

Most states have laws that authorize involuntary medical assessment and hospitalization when individuals are too impaired to make a competent decision regarding their own need for treatment. VA medical centers generally defer to local state statutes governing involuntary mental health assessment and hospitalization. Forced administration of psychotropic medication to involuntarily hospitalized veterans must follow state law and meet constitutional due process requirements (VHA Handbook 1004.01, "Informed Consent for Clinical Treatments and Procedures," August 14, 2009). In the Department of Defense (DoD), the unit commander has the authority[5] to refer a service member for a mental health evaluation, and the clinician conducting that evaluation may in turn order involuntary hospitalization. Protections for the service member include "the right to contact a relative, friend, chaplain, attorney, any office of Inspector General, and anyone else the member chooses, as soon as the service member's condition permits, after admission to the hospital"; the expectation that the admission conforms to relevant clinical practice guidelines; and independent medical review of the need for hospitalization within 72 h of admission and again within five business days. Unlike state statutes, there is no specific limit on the length of involuntary hospitalization or any requirement for judicial review.

Medication is usually necessary to achieve adequate behavioral control when a patient is severely agitated. Oral treatment with olanzapine or risperidone, or an oral benzodiazepine added to oral haloperidol or risperidone, is preferred. If oral medication cannot be used, intramuscular haloperidol plus intramuscular benzodiazepine, or intramuscular olanzapine, can be administered (Gould 2012a). Alternatively, intramuscular ziprasidone with or without a benzodiazepine can be considered. Intramuscular lorazepam is usually preferred over other injectable benzodiazepines because of its consistent rapid absorption (Gould 2012a). Intramuscular preparations of aripiprazole, haloperidol, lorazepam, olanzapine, and ziprasidone are all superior to placebo, but it is not known if any of them is superior to another (Gould 2012b).

Psychopharmacologic Treatment of the Acute Episode

Although VA has not developed specific treatment guidelines for schizophrenia or schizoaffective disorder,[6] it has established a general imperative to utilize evidence-based treatments. The VA/Department of Defense Evidence-Based Practice Working Group (EBPWG) has been chartered by the VA/Department of Defense Health Executive Committee since 1998 to develop evidence-based practice guidelines for use within VA and Department of Defense (VA, http://www.healthquality.va.gov/policy/index.asp). The Evidence-Based Practice Working Group is co-chaired by the Assistant Deputy

[5]This authority is conferred by DoD Instruction 6490.04, "Mental Health Evaluations of Members of the Military Services" (March 4, 2013) (http://www.dtic.mil/whs/directives/corres/pdf/649004p.pdf), which incorporates and cancels the prior DoD Directive 6940.1, "Mental Health Evaluations of Members of the Armed Forces" (October 1, 1997) (http://biotech.law.lsu.edu/blaw/dodd/corres/pdf2/d64901p.pdf).

[6]As of September 18, 2016, there are no current VHA treatment guidelines for schizophrenia or schizoaffective disorder (http://www.healthquality.va.gov/). According to the VA/DoD *Clinical Practice Guideline for Management of Bipolar Disorder in Adults* (version 2.0, May 2010), the original VHA *Clinical Practice Guideline for the Management of Persons with Psychosis*, published in 2001, "was aimed to assist medical care providers in all aspects of mental health care for a cluster of medical conditions characterized as mood disorders" (p i).

Under Secretary for Health for Quality, Safety, and Value, and its scope includes the following: identify and assess further opportunities for improving the adoption of evidence-based clinical practices through the coordination and sharing of health-related services and resources between the departments; develop tools to assist with implementation of evidence-based clinical advances into practice; champion the integration of evidence-based clinical practice into current developing information systems; foster integration of evidence-based practice into VA/Department of Defense initiatives related to health promotion, disease prevention, and wellness initiatives; adopt or adapt, develop, and update evidence-based clinical practice guidelines; and identify opportunities and make recommendations for research related to evidence-based practice within VA/Department of Defense.

Published evidence-based clinical guidelines for the treatment of schizophrenia are widely available. Among the most recent are Galletly et al. (2016), National Institute for Health and Clinical Excellence (NICE) (2014), Barnes and the Schizophrenia Consensus Group of the British Association for Psychopharmacology (2011), Buchanan et al. (2010), and American Psychiatric Association (2004, updated 2009). All treatment guidelines recommend the use of antipsychotic medication, but choosing between a so-called first- and second-generation antipsychotic medication remains controversial. Second-generation antipsychotic agents (SGAs) were modeled on clozapine because of its unique efficacy, which was recognized more than 25 years ago; like clozapine, second-generation antipsychotic agents are "atypical" because they have lower dopamine D2 receptor affinity and higher affinity for other receptors, especially 5-HT2A (Lewis and Lieberman 2008). First-generation (FGA), or "typical," antipsychotic medications have greater affinity for D-2 and lower affinity for 5-HT2 receptors than second-generation antipsychotic agents (Meltzer et al. 1989).

D2 and 5-HT2 receptor affinities are significantly correlated in SGAs, such that a 5-HT2/D2 binding affinity ratio $\geq$1.12 differentiates second-generation antipsychotic agents from first-generation ones (Meltzer et al. 1989). Consequently, the principal adverse effects of FGAs are movement disorders, whereas for SGAs they are metabolic (Freudenreich et al. 2016). Another important clinical correlate of this pharmacokinetic profile is the avoidance of sustained hyperprolactinemia (Kapur and Seeman 2001). In addition to having distinct pharmacokinetic profiles, first-generation and second-generation antipsychotic medications were introduced to clinical practice during discrete historical periods. Haloperidol, the last FGA to be released for clinical use in the USA, was approved by the US Food and Drug Administration (FDA) in 1967; clozapine, approved by the FDA in 1989, was the first SGA released for clinical use (Freudenreich et al. 2016).

SGAs are now used widely and considered first-line treatments by many clinicians, but the evidence basis for their ascendancy has been challenged. One of the most influential studies comparing the effectiveness of antipsychotic medications was the NIHM-sponsored Clinical Antipsychotic Trials of Intervention Effectiveness (CATIE) study (Lieberman et al. 2005). In that study almost 1500 patients were recruited from 57 US cities and randomly assigned to treatment with olanzapine, perphenazine, quetiapine, risperidone, or ziprasidone. The most notable findings were the overall high rate of medication discontinuation (74%) and the equivalent efficacies of perphenazine (an FGA) and SGAs. Olanzapine was associated with a lower rate of discontinuation (64%) but greater increases in weight, glycosylated hemoglobin, cholesterol, and triglycerides. In a subsequent editorial (Lieberman and Stroup 2011), the lead authors summarize the import of the Clinical Antipsychotic Trials of Intervention Effectiveness study as follows: "The numerous antipsychotic drugs, however they might be classified, are more similar to than different from each other. To the extent that antipsychotics differ, it is more in their side effects than therapeutic effects. Nevertheless, there is variation in the effectiveness of antipsychotic medications, which for individual patients can be substantial, and what works for one person may not work for another. Consequently, treatments for schizophrenia must be individualized" (p. 772).

Another highly influential study known as CUtLASS 1 (Cost Utility of the Latest Antipsychotic Drugs in Schizophrenia Study) (Jones et al. 2006a) enrolled 227 patients from 14 community mental health clinics in the English National Health Service to test the hypothesis that SGAs other than clozapine were associated with improved quality of life compared to FGAs during a 1-year study period. Patients were randomly assigned to FGA or SGA treatment groups; within treatment groups, specific agents were selected pragmatically by the treating psychiatrist. FGAs were chlorpromazine, flupenthixol, haloperidol, loxapine, methotrimeprazine, sulpiride, trifluoperazine, zuclopenthixol, fluphenazine decanoate, flupentixol decanoate, haloperidol decanoate, pipothiazine palmitate, and zuclopenthixol decanoate. SGAs were risperidone, olanzapine, amisulpride, zotepine, and quetiapine. The responsible consultant psychiatrists (specialist physicians in secondary care) chose the individual medication in each class before randomization. The main result of this study was that treatment with SGAs was not associated with superior quality of life. In a commentary (Lewis and Lieberman 2008) on these two major studies, their senior authors provided the following response to the rhetorical question, "Where does this leave prescribers?": "Our conclusion must be that first-generation drugs, if carefully prescribed, are as good as most second-generation drugs in many if not most patients with established schizophrenia.... Careful prescribing of first-generation antipsychotics means using lower doses than was often done in the past and avoiding high-potency drugs.... Choosing which drug to switch to may depend on the reasons for switching in the first place: lack of efficacy might suggest a switch to olanzapine or clozapine, whereas lack of tolerability might suggest another choice" (p. 163).

In their update to the American Psychiatric Association guideline for the treatment of schizophrenia, Dixon et al. (2009) reviewed the outcomes of these and several other important studies that examined the comparative effectiveness and tolerability of antipsychotic medications. According to those authors, "The guideline ... states that for some patients, a first-generation agent may be an appropriate first-line option. This latter recommendation has been strengthened by the results of several recently published effectiveness studies that suggest that the first-generation antipsychotics perphenazine and molindone may be equally effective as second-generation agents. In fact, the distinction between first- and second-generation antipsychotics appears to have limited clinical utility" (p. 2).

The schizophrenia treatment guidelines referenced above agree on general principles for managing the acute phase of the illness but reflect a lack of consensus regarding initial treatment for the first episode. For example, the Royal Australian and New Zealand College of Psychiatrists (Galletly et al. 2016) recommends initiating treatment with an SGA other than olanzapine. If the response is insufficient, they suggest trying a different SGA, including olanzapine. Notably, FGAs are not recommended as either first- or second-line treatment (Galletly et al. 2016). In contrast, the National Institute for Health and Care Excellence (United Kingdom) guidelines contain no specific recommendations for first- or second-line medication choices but state the choice "should be made by the service user and health care professional together, taking into account the views of the carer if the service user agrees" (p. 9) (NICE 2014). Similarly, the British Association for Psychopharmacology guidelines indicate that the initial antipsychotic medication choice should be based on the relative liability for side effects and on the patient's preference and risk factors for side effects, including medical history (Barnes and the Schizophrenia Consensus Group of the British Association for Psychopharmacology 2011). The Schizophrenia Patient Outcomes Research Team (PORT) Psychopharmacology Evidence Review Group (University of Maryland) recommends "antipsychotic medications other than clozapine and olanzapine" as first-line treatment for first episode schizophrenia (Buchanan et al. 2010). According to the American Psychiatric Association guideline (APA 2004, updated 2009), "second-generation antipsychotics should be considered as first-line medications for patients in the acute phase of schizophrenia, mainly because of the decreased risk of extrapyramidal side effects and tardive dyskinesia" (p. 28).

Most treatment guidelines caution that first-episode patients are generally more responsive to antipsychotic medication and more sensitive to adverse effects and recommend that lower doses (as much as 50% lower than standard dosing for patients with recurrent episodes) be used. While guidelines differ with respect to suggested roles for FGAs and SGAs in the treatment of first-episode schizophrenia, they all concede there is insufficient evidence to establish superiority of one class of medication over the other. SGAs are no more effective than FGAs in the acute treatment of positive symptoms, and it is not clear that they are more effective in preventing relapse (cf. Galletly et al. 2016; Barnes and the Schizophrenia Consensus Group of the British Association for Psychopharmacology 2011).

While it is likely that marketing strategies by pharmaceutical companies have impacted prescribing practices, several meta-analyses have failed to find evidence that industry sponsorship has biased results of clinical trials (Barnes and the Schizophrenia Consensus Group of the British Association for Psychopharmacology 2011). The World Federation of Societies of Biological Psychiatry recommends first-line use of SGAs (except clozapine) or FGAs dosed at the lower end of the standard dose range, for treatment of first-episode schizophrenia (Falkai et al. 2005), and based on a World Health Organization study of the cost-effectiveness of psychiatric interventions for psychosis in developing countries, FGAs have been proposed as the first-line treatment of choice for low- and middle-income countries (Gadelha et al. 2012). Treatment guideline recommendations for management of recurrent acute episodes of psychosis are essentially the same as those for first episodes, except that the patient's past experience of treatment must also be considered.

The Acute Episode – Stabilization Phase

During the stabilization phase of the acute episode, treatment goals include stress reduction and support to prevent relapse, reintegration into the community, and further symptom improvement (APA 2004). Most first-episode patients experience full remission of psychotic symptoms within 3–4 months after treatment initiation and more than 80% within 1 year. Premature reduction or discontinuation of antipsychotic medication can precipitate symptom recurrence or clinical relapse, so a successful medication regimen should be maintained for at least 6 months in conjunction with ongoing supportive psychosocial interventions and illness education (APA 2004). It might be expected that SGAs are better than FGAs at preventing relapse because a lower rate of extrapyramidal side effects could improve treatment adherence. However, SGAs have not been shown consistently to improve long-term adherence (Barnes and the Schizophrenia Consensus Group of the British Association for Psychopharmacology 2011).

After a service member has been treated for the acute phase in the hospital and is sufficiently stable clinically to be managed as an outpatient, he/she is transferred to a medical holding company to continue treatment while awaiting the outcome of evaluations regarding fitness to return to duty. While assigned to the medical holding company, the service member is housed in barracks and receives outpatient services. In larger, regional mental health referral centers (e.g., the Walter Reed National Military Medical Center), a spectrum of services is available, including intensive outpatient treatment programs. Smaller local holding companies may only be able to offer group and individual treatment in addition to psychopharmacology. Generally, service members with serious mental illness (SMI) such as schizophrenia or schizoaffective disorder will be transferred to a regional medical center at this point in order to permit access to more intensive treatment. If a service member requires acute hospitalization and the local military hospital is unable to adequately manage the episode, the individual may be transferred temporarily to a geographically convenient VA medical center (under a formal Department of Defense-VA agreement regarding medical evacuations) for acute management; once stabilized, the service member will be returned to the custody of his/her command and from there may be transferred to a regional military facility for ongoing treatment until the case is adjudicated.

All branches of the military have explicit fitness for duty standards, and all consider a diagnosis of schizophrenia or schizoaffective disorder to be a disqualifying condition. Once a diagnosis has been assigned, the service member is referred for a disability evaluation, which considers the clinical information in terms of the fitness for duty requirements. If the board finds the service member to be medically disqualified, the individual is medically retired with or without an associated disability rating. Diagnoses of schizophrenia or schizoaffective disorder are generally awarded a 100% disability rating. When the service member is retired, his/her medical care is transferred permanently to VA, which conducts its own disability evaluation to determine eligibility for veteran benefits. Recently the VA and Department of Defense have been working to synchronize the disability examination process to eliminate unnecessary redundancies.

Maintenance and Relapse Prevention

Treatment guidelines for long-term maintenance or relapse prevention somewhat consistently advise against discontinuation of antipsychotic medication except for first episodes, but dose reduction recommendations following the acute phase vary (Takeuchi et al. 2012). Discontinuation within 5 years is generally inadvisable, but following a first episode, it might be considered after 1–2 years of continuous treatment. Intermittent or targeted treatment during the maintenance phase, a strategy of antipsychotic medication discontinuation coupled with prompt reinitiation when relapse appears imminent, is not advisable because it is associated with a significantly higher relapse rate. However, there is preliminary evidence that an extended dosing strategy, in which antipsychotic medication is administered continuously but less frequently (e.g., every other day) during the maintenance phase, may reduce adverse effects without increasing the likelihood of relapse (Takeuchi et al. 2012).

In contrast to discontinuation, dose reduction is generally a successful strategy, but the target dose is important. A meta-analysis examined standard, low, and very low dosing strategies during the maintenance phase and found no difference in outcomes for standard and low dosing, but very low dosing was associated with higher risk of treatment failure (Uchida et al. 2011). Standard dosing was defined as ≥1 "defined daily dose" (i.e., the average dose per day for a medication used for its main indication in adults), low dosing was ≥0.5 and <1 defined daily dose, and very low dosing was <0.5 defined daily dose. This study had insufficient clinical trial data, especially regarding SGAs, but it has been interpreted to suggest that maintenance phase antipsychotic medications should be reduced gradually to the lowest effective dose, with the target dose being not be less than one-half the dose needed during the acute phase (Takeuchi et al. 2012).

Depot Formulations

Since continuous treatment with antipsychotic medication is crucial to successful relapse prevention, it is imperative to promote and monitor patient adherence to the medication plan. Factors that make nonadherence more likely—such as active substance abuse, homelessness, impeded access to health care, etc.—must be addressed whenever possible. In many cases schizophrenia itself makes treatment adherence more difficult because of its effects on insight, judgment, and motivation. These are only some of the reasons that clinicians often turn to long-acting injectable (LAI) antipsychotic medications when persistent or recurrent treatment nonadherence complicates illness management.

In addition to infrequent administration (infrequent need for adherence) and the transparency with which adherence can be monitored (which allows for prompt intervention when needed), long-acting injectables also avoid first-pass hepatic metabolism. This means more consistent bioavailability, so effective dosing can be lower, and blood levels are more predicable (Brissos et al. 2014). However, psychiatrists' experience and attitudes regarding long-acting injectables can be barriers to their use. Psychiatrists tend to prefer long-acting injectables for chronic but not first-episode schizophrenia, to overestimate treatment adherence, to incompletely inform patients of the potential benefits of long-acting injectables, and to assume patients prefer oral medication (Brissos et al. 2014).

Evidence that long-acting injectables improve treatment adherence is inconsistent, but methodological issues may account for this (Olivares et al. 2013). For example, two meta-analyses of randomized controlled trials involving depot and oral preparations (Leucht et al. 2011, 2012) found that long-acting injectables were more effective in preventing relapse, but a subsequent meta-analysis by some of the same authors found no superiority of pooled long-acting injectables compared with oral antipsychotics in 21 studies of 4950 patients (Kishimoto et al. 2014). Publication bias in older studies, changing definitions of relapse over time, and increasing use of oral SGAs as comparators may have contributed to the inconsistent findings, but it is also possible that randomized controlled trials overrepresent patients with relatively greater treatment adherence and less severe illness (Olivares et al. 2013). A meta-analysis of mirror-image open studies, in which a period of oral treatment is compared with a subsequent period of long-acting injectable treatment for the same patients, seems consistent with that interpretation (Kishimoto et al. 2013). That analysis included 25 mirror-image studies involving almost 6000 patients from 28 countries and found strong superiority of long-acting injectable antipsychotics in preventing a next hospitalization and in reducing the number of hospitalizations. Kishimoto et al. (2013) concluded that for long-acting injectables, analyses of naturalistic studies may provide more accurate information because they are less likely to be affected by inadvertent subject enrollment biases stemming from disease features (e.g., low motivation, inattention, etc.). Indirect factors, such as frequency of contact between care providers and patients, may contribute to better adherence with long-acting injectables (Buckley et al. 2016).

Treatment Resistance

Unfortunately, many patients with schizophrenia do not respond well to medication. Depending on how response is defined and when the study was done, between 30% and 50% of patients with schizophrenia respond inadequately to treatment, with a trend suggesting that this rate may be gradually declining (Elkis and Buckley 2016). Inconsistency across studies in the definition of "treatment resistance" may explain some of the variance in estimates of its frequency. Suzuki et al. (2012) proposed operationalized criteria for treatment resistance which require treatment failure with trials of at least two different antipsychotic medications, each utilizing a chlorpromazine-equivalent dose of 600 mg per day and lasting at least 6 weeks. They also specify the response measures, which address psychopathological symptoms and global functioning. Another definition of treatment resistance also requires that persistent symptoms interfere significantly with functioning continuously for at least 5 years (Elkis and Buckley 2016). A 6-week trial may not always be necessary to establish treatment resistance because patients who do not show at least minimal improvement within 2 weeks are unlikely to respond later (Samara et al. 2015).

Recent treatment guidelines (Galletly et al. 2016; NICE 2014; Barnes and the Schizophrenia Consensus Group of the British Association for Psychopharmacology 2011; Buchanan et al. 2010; APA 2004/2009; see also Warnez and Alessi-Severini 2014) agree that a clozapine trial should be offered following treatment failures with at least two different non-clozapine antipsychotic medications; they differ only with respect to specifying a FGA or a SGA for one or both of the failed trials. Numerous studies, including the second phases of the Clinical Antipsychotic Trials of Intervention Effectiveness (CATIE) study and the Cost Utility of the Latest Antipsychotic

Drugs in Schizophrenia Study (CUtLASS) (Lewis et al. 2006b; McEvoy et al. 2006), have shown that clozapine is more effective than FGAs and other SGAs for the treatment of severe, refractory schizophrenia. A systematic review and meta-analysis that included 21 studies and 2364 patients with treatment-refractory schizophrenia found that clozapine was superior to other antipsychotics for reducing positive psychotic symptoms in both the short and long term, and superior for negative symptoms in the short term (Siskind et al. 2016). Between 30% and 60% of patients with schizophrenia who do not respond to other antipsychotics may respond to clozapine (Barnes and the Schizophrenia Consensus Group of the British Association for Psychopharmacology 2011; Remington et al. 2013); it may especially benefit patients with persistent aggression or hostility, and it reduces suicide risk (Barnes and the Schizophrenia Consensus Group of the British Association for Psychopharmacology 2011).

Clozapine

Clozapine was approved by the FDA in 1989 for treatment-resistant schizophrenia, and it is the only medication currently approved by the FDA for this indication (Christian et al. 2012, Appendix A). Its unusually arduous path to mainstream psychiatry has been recounted in detail elsewhere (Crilly 2007) and will be described only briefly here. It was discovered by the Swiss pharmaceutical company Sandoz in 1958, several years after chlorpromazine had been discovered in France, but their development tracks diverged almost immediately. Following successful clinical trials in North America, chlorpromazine was readily received into psychiatric practice, but clozapine was viewed skeptically because its lack of extrapyramidal side effects violated the paradigm that antipsychotic potency and extrapyramidal toxicity are inextricably yoked (Crilly 2007). Also, in contrast to the North American chlorpromazine clinical trials, which were tightly controlled by the FDA, clozapine clinical trials took place in Europe and Asia, where comparatively relaxed clinical trial standards created the opportunity for more dramatic adverse effects to accumulate before they could be addressed. This difference became important in 1975, within a year after the first US-based clinical studies had begun. Four months after clozapine marketing began in Finland, a series of patients had developed serious blood disorders, including agranulocytosis, with nine fatalities. These reports alarmed the medical community, and Sandoz's research and development program for clozapine was halted in 1976. This also caused a large trial underway in the USA to be suspended, which meant that the progress of a FDA new medication application for clozapine was blocked (Crilly 2007).

Over the next decade, clozapine was restricted to compassionate use for patients who had not responded to other antipsychotic medications, and in 1984 the FDA communicated its willingness to consider a new medication application on condition that Sandoz could prove clozapine worked in patients with treatment refractory schizophrenia and also that it worked better than standard antipsychotic medications. The landmark study that ensued, led by Dr. John Kane and published in 1988, satisfied those requirements.

Although reports of fatal agranulocytosis in Finland had caused its introduction to the USA to be aborted abruptly, contemporaneously available data suggested that the rate of agranulocytosis was not substantially greater with clozapine than it was for chlorpromazine (Crilly 2007). In fact, other clozapine adverse effects including aspiration pneumonia, ileus, and weight gain have subsequently caused more deaths than agranulocytosis (Nielsen et al. 2013). Nonetheless, this experience motivated the mandatory safety surveillance program that was established when clozapine was first approved by the FDA in 1989. This program, known as the Clozaril Patient Management System (CPMS), was operated by the manufacturer (Sandoz Limited) and tracked white blood cell counts based on federally mandated minimally acceptable parameters for the frequency and values of these determinations (Crilly 2007). As other manufacturers entered the market, they were also required to monitor clozapine prescribing according to these federally established standards.

The federally imposed monitoring requirements were costly to insurers and patients and ultimately led to an antitrust action against Sandoz by stakeholders. In this context VA argued it could perform all of the monitoring provided by the Clozaril Patient Management System at lower cost, and in 2008 the VA National Clozapine Coordinating Center (NCCC) was established. The National Clozapine Coordinating Center asserted control over clozapine prescribing throughout VA by creating a national registry for veterans receiving, and physicians prescribing, clozapine and implementing the Clozapine Patient Management Protocol (CPMP) (VHA Handbook 1160.62). The Clozapine Patient Management Protocol set forth the requirements for clozapine administration within VA, including the designation of a clozapine treatment manager (CTM) at each facility dispensing clozapine. The Clozapine Patient Management Protocol required the clozapine treatment manager to be a psychiatrist, and this individual was charged with "ensuring that clozapine is offered as an option to any VA patient diagnosed with schizophrenia or schizo-affective disorder, who has experienced two antipsychotic medication failures." The VA's electronic medical record, which gives any clinician at any VA facility access to a veteran's entire medical record, facilitates coordination between the National Clozapine Coordinating Center and individual clinicians. When an administrative override of the standard safety parameters is clinically indicated, communication between the clinician and the National Clozapine Coordinating Center can take place very efficiently using an internal, secure, and encrypted e-mail platform.

In late 2015 the US Food and Drug Administration (FDA) announced changes in its requirements for monitoring and prescribing clozapine, including a new system for monitoring clozapine utilization and outcomes known as Risk Evaluation and Mitigation Strategy (REMS) (USFDA 2015). The Risk Evaluation and Mitigation Strategy program replaced six existing clozapine registries maintained by individual clozapine manufacturers with a single centralized program and issued new guidelines for monitoring white blood cell counts. Clozapine is now prescribed in VA according to the Risk Evaluation and Mitigation Strategy guidelines, with compliance monitored and enforced centrally. In light of clozapine's history, it is significant that the Risk Evaluation and Mitigation Strategy guidelines have relaxed the thresholds for interrupting and stopping clozapine and have introduced separate (lower) thresholds for individuals with benign ethnic neutropenia.

Clozapine is more expensive to administer than other generic antipsychotic medications because the intensive clinical monitoring entails more frequent outpatient visits and more frequent and extensive laboratory monitoring (no less than every 28 days). However, the cost is offset by reduced hospitalization (Pollack et al. 1998) and lower lifetime treatment cost (Davies and Drummond 1993). Cost savings related to clozapine use in veterans are concentrated in those with very high rates of hospital utilization (Rosenheck et al. 1999). Clozapine presents a greater burden for patients, who must make more time in their schedules for appointments, endure frequent blood draws, and experience a number of significant adverse effects that may be only partly ameliorated by dosage adjustments and adjunctive medications. However, despite this additional burden, patients are less likely to discontinue this medication (McEvoy et al. 2006).

Clozapine is cost-effective, and its proven benefits for a substantial portion of patients with treatment-resistant schizophrenia are corroborated by better adherence. However, clinicians often prescribe a combination of two or more antipsychotic medications (other than clozapine) to treat refractory schizophrenia because they feel insufficiently knowledgeable about clozapine (Barnes and the Schizophrenia Consensus Group of the British Association for Psychopharmacology 2011). Psychiatrists' inexperience with clozapine is also responsible for many medically unnecessary treatment terminations (Nielsen et al. 2013). Consequently, clozapine is underutilized generally (Warnez and Alessi-Severini 2014) and in VA (Weissman 2002; Leslie and Rosenheck 2003). The magnitude of the underutilization deserves emphasis: If all patients with treatment-resistant schizophrenia should be offered clozapine, as current guidelines suggest, and up to 50% of individuals with schizophrenia are treatment-resistant, then *as many as half of all people with schizophrenia should receive a full trial of clozapine.* Other factors that may contribute to clozapine underutilization in VA are veterans' relatively greater social isolation, functional impairment (Leslie and Rosenheck 2003), and transportation obstacles related to accessing clozapine treatment at geographically distant VA clinics.

Buchanan et al. (2010) define an adequate clozapine trial as consisting of 300–800 mg/day for at least 8 weeks, whereas Barnes and the Schizophrenia Consensus Group of the British Association for Psychopharmacology (2011) recommend a trial of 3–6 months. Siskind et al. (2016) endorse ending the trial after 6 months in the absence of meaningful improvement, in consideration of the risks associated with clozapine. For patients who are only partial responders to clozapine, addition of a second antipsychotic medication can be modestly beneficial, and this is usually apparent within 6 weeks (Taylor et al. 2012). In particular, there is some evidence that augmentation with a more potent D2 antagonist, such as risperidone, may provide incremental benefit, but data are somewhat contradictory (Mouaffak et al. 2006). Data in support of antipsychotic medication augmentation of clozapine are weak overall and even weaker for other pharmacologic agents (e.g., mood stabilizers, antidepressants, tetrabenazine, and glutamatergic medications) (Tranulis et al. 2006; Miyamoto et al. 2014). Neurostimulation techniques (electroconvulsive therapy, repetitive transcranial magnetic stimulation, and transcranial direct current stimulation) have shown some promise in preliminary small trials but need further investigation (Tranulis et al. 2006; Miyamoto et al. 2014).

Management of Clozapine Adverse Effects and Risk

Clozapine side effects range from merely inconvenient and/or uncomfortable to life threatening. Many of these are also associated with other antipsychotic medications, but extrapyramidal side effects, including tardive dyskinesia, are rarely seen with clozapine (Lieberman 1998). Common and relatively benign side effects shared with other antipsychotic medications include sedation, hypersalivation, and urinary incontinence. Other shared side effects such as weight gain, metabolic syndrome, orthostatic hypotension, tachycardia, and constipation may seriously impact patient safety and health depending on their severity. Neutropenia may range from a transient medically inconsequential laboratory finding to a life-threatening medical emergency; agranulocytosis occurs in approximately 1% of clozapine-treated patients (Gardner et al. 2005). Other medically serious complications are seizures, with an incidence of approximately 5% at doses of 600 mg per day or greater, early myocarditis (≤0.19%), or late cardiomyopathy (≤0.1%) (Gardner et al. 2005). Clozapine has also been associated with other very rare and potentially medically serious conditions (De Fazio et al. 2015), including neuroleptic malignant syndrome (Karagianis et al. 1999).

Nielsen et al. (2013) systematically reviewed the literature for medically serious clozapine adverse drug reactions (ADRs). According to those authors, "the overwhelming majority of decisions to discontinue clozapine treatment are made on the basis of side effects … which, under normal circumstances, can be managed and should not lead to such a decision" (p. 604). The most common reasons given for medical decisions to discontinue clozapine are seizures (45.5%), severe constipation (36.4%), somnolence (27.3%), and neutropenia (18.2%). However, these and most other clozapine-induced side effects can be managed successfully with existing strategies (Nielsen et al. 2011). QTc interval prolongation is rarely seen with clozapine, and its actual frequency may be even lower because tachycardia is common with clozapine; the formula usually used to correct QTc interval for heart rate is valid only for rates below 80 beats/minute and yields overestimates of QTc prolongation at higher rates (Nielsen et al. 2013). Seizures occur in 4.4% of patients receiving doses greater than 600 mg per day, but discontinuation is rarely indicated because this risk can be managed by dose reduction or by adding an anticonvulsant such as valproate sodium (Nielsen et al. 2013). Clozapine-induced myoclonus may signal increased seizure risk (Nielsen et al. 2011). A systematic literature review found "clear evidence indicating a dose-related increased risk of seizures, at least to 500–600 mg/day" (p. 505), but insufficient data to demonstrate a relationship between plasma levels and clinical response, side effects or serious adverse effects (Remington et al. 2013).

Whereas most clozapine-induced adverse effects can be managed by dose reduction or supplemental medication strategies, vigilance for medically serious complications must be maintained. Myocarditis occurs within the first several months of treatment and is accompanied by flu-like symptoms, fever, fatigue, and dyspnea; ST-segment elevation and tachycardia, or elevated troponin levels, are diagnostic (Nielsen et al. 2013). Of special concern is that in most cases of fatal myocarditis, patients did not complain of symptoms before death, so frequent (e.g., weekly) monitoring of troponin levels may be warranted when myocarditis is suspected; troponin levels twice the upper limit of normal should prompt discontinuation, and rechallenge is not recommended. Later in the treatment course, a dilated cardiomyopathy may emerge with symptoms of fatigue, dyspnea, and tachycardia; it should be suspected if tachycardia arises after a month or more of unchanging treatment. EKG findings are nonspecific but often include T- and P-wave abnormalities and signs of left ventricular hypertrophy; if echocardiography confirms the diagnosis, clozapine should be discontinued (Nielsen et al. 2013).

Eosinophilia is usually transient but can herald serious conditions including myocarditis, agranulocytosis, and hepatitis. Agranulocytosis usually occurs within the first 6 months of treatment, whereas neutropenia can occur throughout the treatment course; rechallenge is not recommended after agranulocytosis. Elevated liver enzymes, in particular alanine transaminase (ALT, formerly serum glutamic pyruvic transaminase, SGPT), are common during the initial months of treatment but can portend fulminant hepatitis. If transaminase levels exceed three times the upper limit of the normal range, dose reduction or discontinuation is recommended; rechallenge may be considered once levels return to normal (Nielsen et al. 2013).

Constipation is a common antimuscarinic side effect of clozapine treatment that can progress rapidly to a life-threatening problem (Palmer et al. 2008; Hibbard et al. 2009). Constipation may represent a broader clozapine-induced gastrointestinal hypomotility syndrome that can affect any portion of the gastrointestinal tract and is correlated with plasma clozapine levels (Every-Palmer et al. 2016). It can be so severe that patients aspirate fecal material, and clozapine-associated dysphagia has also been implicated in a life-threatening case of aspiration pneumonia (Gurrera et al. 2016). Clozapine-induced diabetes mellitus may also be mediated by muscarinic M3 receptor blockade, which reduces insulin secretion (Nielsen et al. 2013). Clozapine plasma levels predict serum antimuscarinic activity better than dose (de Leon et al. 2003), so monitoring plasma therapeutic drug levels could help manage this risk more effectively.

The role of therapeutic drug blood levels more generally in clozapine treatment is unclear. Clozapine dose, blood level, and clinical response are all poorly correlated owing to its complex metabolism and a variety of physiologic factors such as smoking habits (Nielsen et al. 2011). Clozapine is oxidatively converted into the principal metabolites norclozapine (N-desmethylclozapine) and clozapine-N-oxide, in addition to at least six other minor metabolites. Like its parent compound, norclozapine has D2 and 5HT-2 receptor activity and has been associated with toxicity. The principal enzymes involved are CYP1A2 (norclozapine) and CYP3A4 (clozapine-N-oxide) (Khan and Preskorn 2005). Smoking increases metabolism through induction of CYP1A2, significantly lowering blood levels, and smoking reduction can raise levels, but smoking patterns contribute only modest variance to large intraindividual fluctuations in blood levels (Lee et al. 2016). Clozapine plasma concentration (whether it is measured as clozapine alone or combined with norclozapine) demonstrates a weak relationship with the number, but not the severity, of non-neurological side effects (Yusufi et al. 2007).

In addition to intraindividual factors that can cloud relationships between blood level, dose, and response threshold, studies have not consistently examined clozapine and norclozapine levels separately. For example, one review of this literature concludes that an adequate clozapine trial requires plasma levels above 350–420 ng/ml for at least 12 weeks (Nielsen et al. 2011), but a key study cited as a basis for that conclusion (Perry et al. 1991) found that clozapine plasma concentrations ≥350 ng/ml or concentrations of clozapine plus norclozapine *combined* ≥450 ng/ml were associated with treatment response. In their systematic review of the literature, Remington et al. (2013) found a lack of evidence linking plasma clozapine levels to serious side effects but suggested clinical benefits are unlikely above plasma levels of 600–838 ng/ml. Based on evidence for a therapeutic window and a strong relationship between seizure risk and dose, therapeutic drug monitoring is recommended (Khan and Preskorn 2005; Hiemke et al. 2011).

Many VA facilities manage clozapine outpatients in a designated clinic. Some clinics are managed primarily by a clinical pharmacy specialist, while others are staffed by an interdisciplinary team that may include psychiatrists, pharmacists, nurses, and health or peer support technicians (Williams and Purvis 2012). A clozapine clinic may manage only the patient's clozapine therapy, or it may provide comprehensive psychiatric care (Williams and Purvis 2012). A group therapy approach is sometimes employed in these clinics, which allows veterans to support one another while sharing experiences of, and offering suggestions for mitigating, adverse effects (Cone et al. 2008). We have found the multidisciplinary team approach to be very useful in our clozapine clinic because it is efficient (each member has specific responsibilities) and provides continuity for patients when one or more team members is absent. This model also facilitates cross-coverage for clozapine prescribing, which can seem challenging to psychiatrists who are unfamiliar with it. In particular, because clozapine has many adverse effects, some of which need to be treated with additional medications, and because many of our patients have complex comorbid medical disorders, it has been especially helpful to have a clinical pharmacy specialist on the team. The clinical pharmacist is typically well versed in the management of these adverse effects, utilizing both pharmacological and non-pharmacological strategies to improve the patient's experience (Dishman et al. 1994).

The metabolic risks of clozapine and other SGAs are well known. Metabolic syndrome has a prevalence of 30–60% in patients with serious mental illness (SMI), and in middle-aged veterans (mean age 50 years) with schizophrenia or schizoaffective disorder, it is 51–55% (Meyer et al. 2006). In a very large study of veterans, the hazard risk (i.e., the instantaneous risk at a specific point in time) of new-onset type 2 diabetes mellitus with risperidone, quetiapine, or olanzapine is 1.6–1.7 times that for haloperidol (Lambert et al. 2006). Metabolic syndrome is diagnosed if at least three of the following five criteria are met: obesity (waistline >40 in. for males, >35 in. for females), fasting serum triglycerides >150 mg/dL, serum HDL cholesterol <40 mg/dL (males) or <50 mg/dL (females), hypertension (>130/85 mmHg), and hyperglycemia (fasting serum glucose >110 mg/dL) (Sernyak 2007).

Expert consensus guidelines for monitoring the metabolic effects of antipsychotic medications were developed jointly by the American Diabetes Association, American Psychiatric Association, American Association of Clinical Endocrinologists, and the North American Association for the Study of Obesity (Clark 2004); they are currently a standard against which health-care quality is measured (Sernyak 2007). The American Diabetes Association/American Psychiatric Association guidelines recommend baseline monitoring of weight and body mass index (BMI), waist circumference, blood pressure, fasting blood glucose, and fasting lipid panel. Personal and family histories of diabetes, hypertension, dyslipidemia, and cardiovascular disease should also be obtained. The monitoring protocol includes monthly weights for the first 3 months, then quarterly for the first year, and annually thereafter. Other parameters are monitored at 12 weeks and then annually, except for the fasting lipid profile, which is monitored every 5 years (Clark 2004). Adherence to this monitoring protocol is especially important for patients being started on clozapine or olanzapine because of their ability to cause significant weight gain (McEvoy et al. 2005).

Veterans who demonstrate significant metabolic changes due to antipsychotic medications are often referred to a specialty clinic. For weight gain, veterans can be referred to MOVE!, a 16-week comprehensive weight management program. Veterans may also be referred to a registered dietician or to a telehealth monitoring program in which they can have their weight, blood sugar, blood pressure, and other vital signs monitored remotely from home. Clinical pharmacy specialists are embedded in primary care, and in some mental health programs, to manage patients with hyperglycemia, dyslipidemia, and hypertension. The VA has developed a decision support system of automated clinical reminders within the electronic medical record that prompt providers when metabolic screening is due, and there is also a reminder to administer the Abnormal Involuntary Movement Scale (AIMS) regularly.

Other Somatic Therapy Agents

Antipsychotic medications currently in use were developed in accord with the hypothesis that schizophrenia is caused by dysregulated central dopaminergic pathways, consisting of excess activity in mesolimbic circuits and reduced neurotransmission in mesocortical circuits; many SGAs were designed to also block serotonin 5-HT2A receptors based on their suspected role in causing extrapyramidal side effects (Miyamoto et al. 2012). However, enormously diverse neuropharmacological strategies are currently under investigation for schizophrenia treatment, including dopamine D1 agonists; D3 and D4 antagonists; 5-HT1A, 5-HT2C, and 5-HT4 agonists; 5-HT3, 5-HT6 and 5-HT7 antagonists; 5-HT-2A inverse agonists; a variety of glutamatergic, adrenergic, and cholinergic agents; hormones such as estrogen, oxytocin, and erythropoietin; fatty acids; and phosphodiesterase inhibitors (Miyamoto et al. 2012; Gopalakirshna et al. 2016). Despite showing initial promise in many cases, however, none have consistently demonstrated efficacy.

Schizoaffective Disorder

The discussion so far has focused on the treatment of schizophrenia because it is the most common and well researched of the psychotic disorders. There is no general consensus on the management of schizoaffective disorder because there are relatively few adequately designed studies (Lindenmayer and Kaur 2016). In practice, the management of schizoaffective disorder generally reflects evidence-based strategies for treating schizophrenia (cognitive symptoms) and major mood disorders (mood syndromes of depression or bipolar disorder).

Delusional Disorder

A recent literature review of delusional disorder pharmacotherapy (Mews and Quante 2013) found only scattered individual case reports and moderately large case series, with no controlled studies. Based on their own small series of cases and previously published reports, those authors concluded there is insufficient evidence to recommend a particular medication or treatment approach, but most clinicians manage it pragmatically as though it were a form of schizophrenia.

Other Medication Treatment Issues

Antipsychotic Polypharmacy

Antipsychotic monotherapy is the standard treatment for schizophrenia, but veterans with schizophrenia are more likely to be treated with polypharmacy (prescribing more than one antipsychotic medication) than are veterans with other diagnoses (Weissman 2002). Polypharmacy is highly prevalent, with rates as high as 20% in VA during fiscal year 2000, and up to 35–40% in patients being treated in non-VA public mental health systems (Sun et al. 2014). Even higher rates have been reported, and polypharmacy appears to be increasing worldwide (Fleischhacker and Uchida 2014). One recent critical review of the polypharmacy literature concluded that polypharmacy may benefit specific patients, in particular those who respond only partially to clozapine, but this should be the exception to the rule, and any conclusions regarding the usefulness of polypharmacy are constrained by a paucity of well-designed studies (Fleischhacker and Uchida 2014). In a recent longitudinal study of polypharmacy across VA and non-VA systems (2002- or 2005–2009), polypharmacy rates in VA were relatively higher and more stable, but the authors attributed this to better access to care and more complex clinical presentations (Sun et al. 2014). Veterans may have had more access to more medications more consistently over time, were less likely to drop out of treatment, and were more likely to have medical comorbidities necessitating more complex medication regimens due to their relatively greater age (Sun et al. 2014).

Polypharmacy may be justified during active cross-titration, when each agent is prescribed for a different comorbid disorder or when specific pharmacokinetic properties are exploited to enhance a regimen. However, it is inappropriate to stop cross-titration after the addition of the second agent or when a provider's preference takes priority over evidence-based literature. When adding a second antipsychotic before attempting a clozapine trial, the risks associated with clozapine need to be weighed against the potential risks of antipsychotic polypharmacy, which include excessive dosing, unanticipated and/or toxic drug interactions, and unnecessary cost (Correll and Gallego 2012; Fleischhacker and Uchida 2014). VA utilizes education targeted to prescribers with the aim of reducing inappropriate antipsychotic polypharmacy. The so-called academic detailing, which includes routine pharmacy reviews at both local and Veterans Integrated Service Network (VISN) levels, is an expanding program in VA and has been effective in reducing antipsychotic polypharmacy.

The Role of the Clinical Pharmacy Specialist

Incorporating a clinical pharmacy specialist (CPS) into a mental health service improves patient outcomes and satisfaction, improves prescribing practices, and reduces costs—benefits first recognized three decades ago in VA mental health ambulatory care clinics (Lobeck et al. 1989). Entry-level pharmacists now graduate with a doctor of pharmacy degree (Pharm.D.), and many pharmacy school graduates complete pharmacy practice residencies or fellowships for additional training. After that they may choose to specialize in a field by completing a second-year residency program and becoming board certified. In 1994 psychiatric pharmacy became a specialty recognized by the Board of Pharmaceutical Specialties (Finley et al. 2003). Board certified psychiatric pharmacists currently number more than 625 (CPNP 2016). Within VA a clinical pharmacy specialist can prescribe under an approved scope of practice with a designated supervising physician. A clinical pharmacy specialist can also hold a specialty scope of practice in psychiatry, oncology, infectious disease, etc. Clinical pharmacy specialists with a psychiatry scope of practice are able to prescribe medications for treating a number of psychiatric disorders and are considered mid-level practitioners. They can perform Abnormal Involuntary Movement Scale (AIMS) exams and other routine monitoring, including the ordering of laboratory tests, which reduces some of the time-consuming requirements associated with prescribing antipsychotic medications and other agents used in psychiatric practice (Cone et al. 2008; Williams and Purvis 2012). Clinical pharmacy specialists also participate in VA clinical research (Finley et al. 2003).

Comorbid Disorders Complicating Treatment

Several disorders are likely to occur in veterans and manifest symptoms that can confound the clinical presentation of schizophrenia-related psychoses or complicate their treatment. In particular, post-traumatic stress disorder (PTSD), Parkinson's disease, and delirium associated with intoxication or acute alcohol withdrawal can produce hallucinations, paranoia, and other experiences that are difficult to differentiate from those associated with the primary psychoses. Psychotic symptoms related to Parkinson's disease can be treated with antipsychotic medications, but psychosis reduction may require a trade-off with worsening extrapyramidal symptoms. When an acceptable balance between these opposing actions of routinely prescribed antipsychotic medications is not possible, clozapine should be considered because of its minimal extrapyramidal side effects (Seppi et al. 2011). In delirium, the underlying cause must be treated emergently because acute intoxication and withdrawal can be life threatening. In rare cases of acute intoxication with substances other than alcohol, psychotic symptoms may be so severe that treatment with antipsychotic medication must be considered, but generally this is not helpful, and treatment should focus on mitigating the physiologic effects of the intoxication.

PTSD poses a special challenge for clinicians treating veterans with schizophrenia or schizoaffective disorder because it is a chronic disorder that is highly prevalent in serious mental illness (Grubaugh et al. 2011), and psychotic symptoms are frequently reported by individuals who have experienced severe trauma as civilians or through combat exposure (Norredam et al. 2011). Moreover, suicide risk is elevated in veterans with comorbid PTSD and schizophrenia or schizoaffective disorder (Strauss et al. 2006). Hallucinations per se are not among the *DSM-5* diagnostic features of PTSD, but the involuntary reexperiencing of traumatic events can be so intense and vivid that it appears hallucinatory in nature (Brewin and Patel 2010). Individuals with PTSD-associated hyperarousal and hypervigilance can be so violently reactive and guarded that they appear paranoid, and severe dissociative episodes may suggest catatonia. Some (e.g., Braakman et al. 2009) have even advocated for designating a PTSD subtype, "PTSD with secondary psychotic features." Hallucinatory content in PTSD is overwhelmingly (71–100%) related to trauma (Braakman et al. 2009), and trauma-related dissociation may contribute to hallucinatory experiences (Anketell et al. 2010). Psychotic symptoms correlate positively with hyperarousal in Croatian combat veterans (Kaštelan et al. 2007).

Interpreting sensory symptoms as activated memories of real experiences is conceptually appealing and often helpful in distinguishing PTSD phenomena from psychosis-related hallucinations, but this distinction is not always clear because in both cases the source of the experience is perceived as being outside the individual, and hallucinations are both inherently complex (Stephane et al. 2003; McCarthy-Jones et al. 2014) and highly variable between individuals (Plaze et al. 2011). Veterans with either schizophrenia or PTSD score similarly on the positive and negative syndrome scale (PANSS), in particular with respect to hallucinations (Hamner et al. 2000), although it is not clear whether those authors attempted to exclude patients with subsyndromal schizophrenia or schizoaffective disorder, or schizotypal disorder, from the PTSD group. Veterans with both PTSD and either a schizophrenia-related psychosis or major depression with psychosis have significantly higher scores on positive symptoms (especially paranoid and violent ideation) and general psychopathology than do veterans with only one of these diagnoses (Sautter et al. 1999). Hamner et al. (2000) point out that PTSD symptom content can often be traced to actual experiences, in contrast to the bizarre features or disorganization that are more common in schizophrenia and schizoaffective disorder, and individuals with PTSD are usually aware of and distressed by the unreality of their symptoms, whereas patients with schizophrenia-related psychosis often are not (Hamner et al. 2000). A symbolic relationship between trauma experience and the content of psychotic symptoms has also been postulated in non-US combat veteran cohorts (Kozarić-Kovačić and Borovečki 2005).

There is also an emerging view that hallucinations in schizophrenia, at least in some cases, are rooted in earlier traumatic experiences that have been transformed through the reconstructive properties of memory into hallucinatory symptoms (McCarthy-Jones and Longden 2015). Noncombat trauma is highly prevalent (94%), and PTSD has a high rate of comorbidity (53%), in individuals diagnosed with a schizophrenia-related psychotic disorder (Kilcommons and Morrison 2005). A variety of symptoms routinely attributed to schizophrenia-related psychosis may be understood more accurately as representations of personal trauma (Muenzenbaier et al. 2010). In a nonpsychiatric sample of college students, negative beliefs about self and others and the reexperiencing of trauma appeared to mediate the emergence of psychotic symptoms (Gracie et al. 2007).

This is an evolving discourse, and the relationship between psychotic disorders and trauma experience is not yet settled. There is some evidence that veterans with comorbid PTSD and serious mental illnesss experience symptoms and utilize mental health services more intensely than veterans with either diagnosis alone, but research is limited (Grubaugh et al. 2011). A few studies that have examined antipsychotic medication treatment of PTSD report benefit, but most have failed to demonstrate this, and VA treatment guidelines for PTSD do not recommend their use. However, a very recently published study (Villareal et al. 2016) reported that quetiapine produced significant improvement in Positive and Negative Syndrome Scale (PANSS) positive symptom and general psychopathology scores as well as in a number of PTSD symptom measures.

Recovery

Psychosocial interventions and services can help individuals with schizophrenia and other psychoses recover fully from their illness episodes and return to satisfying roles within their families and communities. Recovery-oriented interventions can and should be included in the treatment plan as soon as the patient is able to utilize them, as early as the stabilization phase of the acute stage (Fig. 21.1). Whereas medications are critical in the most acute segment of the episode, recovery interventions and activities become increasingly important over the course of the illness. They reduce hospitalization, improve social and vocational functioning, and enhance quality of life and personal satisfaction (Lauriello et al. 1999). *Family intervention*, consisting of a prolonged (at least 9 months) psychoeducational and supportive family program, is an effective intervention for reducing risk of relapse, especially in families that are overly critical or hostile. There is no difference in outcome between a multifamily group intervention model and individual family treatment, and no evidence that more intensive family interventions have better outcomes. *Assertive community treatment* (ACT) is a care model in which multidisciplinary teams consisting of a case manager, social worker, psychiatrist, nurse, and other clinical staff are responsible for all the service needs of a small fixed caseload of patients. This team is on call 24/7 and operates in conventional care settings (clinics and hospitals) and the community. The team provides medication home delivery when needed, monitors mental and physical health, and provides social skills training in the patient's own environment. The most consistent benefits of assertive community treatment engagement are a reduction in hospital days and improved housing stability, especially for patients who are homeless and/or without families. However, these gains are not sustainable following assertive community treatment involvement without *social skills training* (SST) (Lauriello et al. 1999).

Social skills training entails hands-on work with patients to remediate problems in relationships, activities of daily living, employment, and leisure. Social skills training has several forms: basic, social problem-solving, and cognitive remediation. In basic social skills training, the therapist breaks down complex social behavioral repertoires into simpler steps and then models the correct behavior. Patients learn through practice. After all steps have been learned, they are recombined in the clinic and enacted in role-playing exercises. These rehearsed behaviors are then mastered through additional repetition in natural social situations, with therapist support as needed. Social problem-solving social skills training addresses information processing deficits that are believed to impair social skills and is the next step in building (or rebuilding) skills necessary for social adjustment. It focuses on medication and symptom management, basic conversation, recreation, and self-care and is designed to increase cognitive flexibility and the ability to generalize skills to novel situations. Cognitive remediation attempts to improve the attention, memory, and planning deficits that are core features of schizophrenia and are assumed to contribute to impaired social skills. One relatively well-known example uses computer games to improve specific cognitive abilities, followed by social problem-solving exercises that draw upon those abilities. All of these social skills training approaches have demonstrated improved social competence in research and clinic settings and may reduce relapse rate, but any gains tend to erode without "booster" sessions, and they have not been shown to increase competitive employment (Lauriello et al. 1999).

The rate of competitive employment for patients with schizophrenia is low (less than 20%). For patients with schizophrenia, vocational rehabilitation can help sustain jobs in agency-affiliated transitional or sheltered employment programs, but it does not increase success in securing or sustaining competitive employment. The modest effectiveness of sheltered employment led to the concept of *supported employment*, which aims to place a patient in a permanent regular non-agency job, based on an assessment of the patient's strengths and skills. Screening by a vocational rehabilitation professional is minimal, and there is no prevocational training; the specific skills needed are learned on the job with support from a job coach. Supported employment programs do increase competitive employment, but job tenure is relatively brief (about 6 months on average). Nonetheless, employment rates are higher at all intervals up to 2 years for individuals with serious mental illness who participate in supported employment, compared to those who are engaged in other forms of vocational rehabilitation (Ahmed et al. 2016). Cognitive impairment appears to be an important mediator of long-term employment success (Ahmed et al. 2016).

Finally, *cognitive behavioral therapy* (CBT) focuses on mitigating persistent symptoms through a variety of techniques that teach or improve cognitive strategies. Unlike intensive psychodynamically oriented psychotherapy, it does not have as a goal understanding the unconscious meaning of symptoms (Lauriello et al. 1999). Cognitive behavioral therapy promotes rational alternative perspectives to the problematic experiences with the aim of enhancing recognition of symptoms and early signs of relapse. Basic elements of this treatment include development of a shared understanding of the illness between patient and therapist, mutual identification of target symptoms, and the use of specific cognitive and behavioral strategies to cope with those symptoms (Shean 2009). Cognitive behavioral therapy can be delivered in individual or group formats and is associated with reductions in positive, negative, and mood symptoms as well as improved social functioning (Mueser et al. 2013).

Based on a review of the relevant literature, the Schizophrenia Patient Outcomes Research Team (PORT) formulated eight evidence-based psychosocial treatment recommendations (Dixon et al. 2010). That group generally confirmed the usefulness of the modalities previously endorsed by Lauriello and colleagues (assertive community treatment, supported employment, skills training, cognitive behavioral therapy, family-based services), but they did not find sufficient evidence to recommend the cognitive remediation form of social skills training. Evidence was also considered adequate to recommend the use of three additional interventions: *token economy* programs, psychosocial *interventions for alcohol and substance use disorders*, and psychosocial *interventions for weight management*. Token economies use contingent positive reinforcement schedules to help severely impaired individuals alter clearly defined target behaviors in the domains of personal hygiene, basic social interactions, and other activities essential for daily living. Interventions for patients with schizophrenia and alcohol or substance use disorders should be integrated with mental health care and include motivational enhancement techniques in addition to skills training for coping and relapse prevention. Psychosocial intervention for weight management is recommended for individuals with body mass index ≥25 and should be comprehensive in scope. Interventions that were reviewed but not recommended due to insufficient evidence were *peer support* and *peer-delivered services*, interventions that target *adherence to antipsychotic medications*, and psychosocial treatments tailored to recent onset schizophrenia (Dixon et al. 2010).

Mueser and colleagues (2013) focused on seven interventions in their comprehensive review of meta-analytic studies of psychosocial treatments for schizophrenia. They concluded that assertive community treatment improves stable community living but has limited impact on other outcomes; cognitive behavioral therapy reduces symptoms broadly, improves social functioning, and is well tolerated by patients with schizophrenia but is not clearly superior to other psychological interventions; cognitive remediation can improve social functioning but needs to be combined with psychiatric rehabilitation to be effective; family psychoeducation reduces relapses and hospitalization; social skills training improves certain aspects of social competence but may be limited by deficits in attention; and supported employment increases the rate of competitive employment. They noted that a recently developed technique of "attention shaping" offers some promise for enhancing the effectiveness of social skills training.

Illness self-management training is the seventh intervention for which Mueser and colleagues found evidence of effectiveness. Illness self-management focuses on educating patients about schizophrenia and its treatment to enable informed decision-making and teaching strategies for medication adherence, relapse prevention, and coping. This approach is also useful for managing comorbid medical disorders (Mueser et al. 2013). Two of the most recognized self-management interventions for individuals with schizophrenia are Illness Management and Recovery (IMR) and the Wellness Recovery Action Plan (WRAP). Illness Management and Recovery is usually delivered by traditional care providers (e.g., case managers, clinicians), whereas the Wellness Recovery Action Plan is usually provided by peer specialists (Ahmed et al. 2016).

Patients with schizophrenia often have experienced trauma, before and after illness onset. Posttraumatic stress disorder (PTSD) has an estimated prevalence of 25–50% in people with serious mental illness, compared to 8–12% in the general population (Mueser et al. 2013). Preliminary studies support the feasibility of adapting evidence-based PTSD treatments for use in patients with schizophrenia, including those that employ exposure or cognitive restructuring (Mueser et al. 2013). Other promising interventions that are not yet at the level of an evidence-based practice include peer support services, prodromal stage intervention, social cognition training, supported education, and supported housing (Mueser et al. 2013).

The utilization of peer-delivered services has expanded dramatically over the past three decades in response to a widening recognition of the relatively circumscribed benefits of medications alone and a cultural shift often referred to as "the consumer movement" which places the patient at the center of the illness discourse and reframes recovery as a nonlinear process or journey rather than a medically defined end state. However, there is some disagreement within the consumer movement regarding how peers should be included in the recovery process, and this has led to variations in practice (Ahmed et al. 2012). The incorporation of peers—individuals with "lived experience with mental illness"—into mental health programs is seen as an antidote for the devaluation and disenfranchisement often experienced by patients. Peers draw upon their own experiences with mental illness and its challenges to mentor patients in collaborative and mutual relationships. Peer services generally take the form of self-help groups; consumer-operated services, which are independent of traditional health systems; and peer support services, which can be offered within or outside of traditional health-care venues. In the first two instances, the relationships between peers are seen to be reciprocal in nature (i.e., some peers may be more skilled or experienced, but all participants are expected to benefit). Peer support is different in that it is asymmetrical— at least one of the individuals has experienced significant improvement in his/her psychiatric condition and is offering services or support to other individuals with serious mental illness who have not progressed as far in their own recovery (Davidson et al. 2006a). In most states Medicare and/or Medicaid reimburse for peer services within or outside of conventional care venues. Peer services have potential for increasing access to helpful interventions for patients, and enthusiasm for them continues to grow at many levels of our healthcare industry, but empirical evidence supporting their benefits is still limited (Ahmed et al. 2012).

A guiding principle of the consumer movement in mental health is the notion of recovery, which asserts that attainment of a meaningful and valued life, rather than symptom reduction is the basis of mental health (Mueser et al. 2013). Common to all definitions of recovery is the notion that "it is a process in which the individual strives to overcome the fact of mental illness and its impact on one's sense of self" (Bellack 2006). The recovery model redefines the parameters of psychiatric care rather than promoting particular treatment approaches (Ahmed et al. 2016). Recovery-oriented treatment goals are centered "on the promotion of the care recipient's wellness, independence, and the subjective experience of personalized experiential recovery" (Ahmed et al. 2016; p. 314). Recovery-based approaches and traditional psychiatric care share an important philosophical foundation in recognizing the importance of the individual's preferences, values, and informed decision-making. However, recovery-based care redefines outcome in terms of hope, optimism, empowerment, personal meaning, connectedness, and citizenship (Ahmed et al. 2016).

There is no precise historical turning point that marks the beginning of the consumer movement in the USA, but two federal government reports (one from the Office of the Surgeon General in 1999 and the other authored by the President's New Freedom Commission on Mental Health in 2003) gave it major impetus (Bellack 2006). In a national consensus statement formulated in 2004, the Substance Abuse and Mental Health Services Administration (SAMHSA) characterized recovery-oriented mental health services as self-directed, individualized and person-centered, empowering, holistic, nonlinear, strengths based, peer supported, respectful, fostering personal responsibility, and encouraging hope (Bellack 2006). Similar features are cited in other conceptualizations of recovery-oriented mental health care (Davidson et al. 2006b).

VA has established a spectrum of programs and services that provide evidence-based recovery-oriented interventions for veterans with schizophrenia and other psychotic disorders. In July 2011 Robert Petzel, M.D., VA under secretary for health, released a series of prescriptive documents mandating the establishment of programs and services for meeting the needs of veterans with serious mental illness,[7] including schizophrenia. The first of these, "Psychosocial Rehabilitation and Recovery Services" (VHA Handbook 1163.01), provided the expectations, procedures, and reporting requirements for these services under the auspices of Veteran Health Administration's Office of Mental Health Services. The scope of psychosocial rehabilitation and recovery (PSR&R) services was to include family services, local recovery coordinators, peer support, Psychosocial Rehabilitation and Recovery Centers (PRRC), skills training, and therapeutic and supported employment programs. Following publication of the President's New Freedom Commission on Mental Health in

[7] Serious mental illness (SMI) is defined by VA as a mental, behavioral, or emotional disorder that meets *Diagnostic and Statistical Manual of Mental Disorders* (DSM) diagnostic criteria (excluding cognitive and developmental disorders and disorders due to a general medical condition) and meets all of the following criteria: (1) Single unremitting episode of symptoms or with frequently recurring and/or prolonged episodes of symptoms; (2) Symptoms result in impairments in mood, thinking, family or other interpersonal relationships, behavior (often resulting in socio-legal consequences), and/or self-care which substantially interfere with or limit major life activities; and (3) The impact of these symptoms results in a functional impairment equivalent to a Global Assessment of Functioning (GAF) score of 50 or below (*VHA Handbook 1163.06*, January 7, 2016, p. 3).

2003, VA and other federal agencies participated in the development of the under secretary's Action Agenda entitled "Achieving the Promise, Transforming Mental Health Care in VA" (Bellack 2006). This work became the foundation for VA's Comprehensive Mental Health Strategic Plan approved by the Secretary of Veterans Affairs in 2004, which emphasizes the transformation of mental health services to a veteran-driven, recovery-oriented system of care. This plan, together with the Uniform Mental Health Services in VA Medical Centers (VAMC) and Clinics Handbook (1160.01) (September 11, 2008), provided the general authority for the Psychosocial Rehabilitation and Recovery Services Handbook.

The Psychosocial Rehabilitation and Recovery Services Handbook defines serious mental illness as a *DSM* Axis I disorder "resulting in significant functional impairment and/or disruption in major activities of daily living [and]…typically includes schizophrenia and other psychotic disorders, bipolar disorder, major depression, and severe Post-Traumatic Stress Disorder (PTSD)." The handbook identifies recovery as the paramount goal for mental health services and cites the Substance Abuse and Mental Health Services Administration (SAMHSA) 2004 national consensus statement for the purpose of defining this goal: "Mental health recovery is a journey of healing and transformation enabling a person with a mental health problem to live a meaningful life in a community of his or her choice while striving to achieve his or her full potential." It delineates responsibilities for this mission at each level of the organization, such as the responsibility of the facility mental health leader to appoint a *Local Recovery Coordinator* (LRC) to help focus efforts on the transformation to a recovery-oriented system of care. The Local Recovery Coordinator role includes training and consulting with facility leadership, staff, veterans, and family members regarding recovery-oriented services; helping to ensure that veterans have access to psychosocial rehabilitation and recovery services; promoting activities to eliminate stigma associated with mental illness; providing direct, recovery-oriented clinical services; working collaboratively with the other Local Recovery Coordinators in the regional VA network and nationally; and conducting an annual "reengagement outreach" effort to reestablish contact with veterans with serious mental illness who have been lost to follow up. Veterans with serious mental illness who were lost to follow up and successfully reengaged in care through outreach have substantially lower mortality than those for whom reengagement efforts fail (Davis et al. 2012).

Simultaneous with the release of the Psychosocial Rehabilitation and Recovery Services Handbook, the under secretary also released Veterans Health Administration Handbook 1163.03, "Psychosocial Rehabilitation and Recovery Centers (PRRC)," which laid out the procedures and expectations for developing new Psychosocial Rehabilitation and Recovery Centers or transforming existing day treatment, day hospital, and analogous programs to Psychosocial Rehabilitation and Recovery Centers. The handbook defines Psychosocial Rehabilitation and Recovery Centers as "outpatient transitional learning centers designed to support recovery and integration into meaningful self-determined community roles for veterans challenged with serious mental illness and severe functional impairment. Programming is curriculum-based and is specifically designed to teach the requisite skills that are necessary for defining and realizing veteran's self-chosen roles and goals in all domains of health and life." The Psychosocial Rehabilitation and Recovery Centers were explicitly intended to replace all existing day treatment centers (DTC), day hospitals, partial hospitals, and similar programs because they lacked a recovery orientation. Instead, those programs emphasized clinical stabilization and avoidance of rehospitalization and had "limited expectations for those in the program to recover or to be fully integrated into the community." This document mandated all VA medical centers with 1500 or more veterans in the VA National Psychosis Registry to establish a PRRC, and it strongly encouraged VA medical centers with 1000–1499 veterans included in the registry to establish a PRRC. In addition, all very large community-based outpatient clinics treating 10,000 or more unique veterans annually were encouraged to have a Psychosocial Rehabilitation and Recovery Center. Operational and staffing guidance for Psychosocial Rehabilitation and Recovery Centers was also provided by the handbook. Only time-limited day hospital programs closely associated with acute inpatient units were exempted from this transformation.

Finally, a third major element of psychosocial rehabilitation and recovery services was addressed with the release of Veterans Health Administration Handbook 1163.05, "Psychosocial Rehabilitation and Recovery Services: Peer Support" in July 2011. The document asserted that peer support "is a fundamental building block of recovery-oriented services … [and] … a promising best practice which provides role models for veteran consumers of the Department of Veterans Affairs (VA) mental health care program to engender hope, demonstrate recovery, and teach advocacy skills…"

Peer support positions were first funded by Veterans Health Administration in 2005, but the aim of incorporating peer specialists into mental health treatment programs received a major boost with the publication of the Peer Specialist Toolkit (2013), the product of a collaborative effort by VA Regional Mental Illness Research, Education, and Clinical Centers (MIRECC) in New England and Pennsylvania. This document explained the concept of peer support, reviewed supporting research, and provided a detailed how-to-hire manual for VA managers. Section 405 of Public Law 110–387, as codified in 38 USC. 7402(b)(13), establishes eligibility to be appointed to a peer specialist position. For this, the individual must (1) be a veteran who has recovered or is recovering from a mental health condition and (2) be certified by (a) a not-for-profit entity engaged in peer specialist training as having met such criteria as the secretary shall establish for a peer specialist position or (b) a state as having satisfied relevant state requirements for a peer specialist position. In addition, the individual must have spent a minimum of 1 year in personal recovery from a mental health condition (VA Handbook 5005/59, Appendix F3; July 17, 2012).

The limited research on peer support has tended to validate its usefulness. For example, peer support case management appears to be at least as effective as traditional case management (Davidson et al. 2006a). Vet to Vet is a consumer-operated peer education and support program designed by Moe Armstrong, a veteran with schizophrenia; veterans who participate in that program report more positive recovery-based outcomes, and these benefits were increased when peers were paid rather than working as volunteers (Ahmed et al. 2012).

VA Case Management Programs

Case management arose in state systems as a response to the failures of deinstitutionalization, which were caused by inadequate funding and fragmented, uncoordinated care in poorly developed community-based health-care systems unprepared for the exodus of long-hospitalized individuals with serious mental illness (Davidson et al. 2006b). The case manager's role was to help patients otherwise incapable—cognitively or logistically—of navigating this unwieldy patchwork of services. When it became clear that case managers working alone could not reliably ensure access to care, teams of mental health professionals were formed to provide the needed services themselves or to negotiate them with third parties. Barriers to care, including distance and limited transportation resources—common challenges in many VA health-care systems due to their geographic locations—reduce treatment retention in veterans with serious mental illness (McCarthy et al. 2007). The most rigorously articulated and evaluated team-based approach to intensive case management is assertive community treatment (ACT) (Davidson et al. 2006b).

Mental Health Intensive Case Management (MHICM), Rural Access Network for Growth Enhancement (RANGE), and Enhanced Rural Access Network for Growth Enhancement (E-RANGE)

In VA, the Intensive Community Mental Health Recovery (ICMHR) services programs include Mental Health Intensive Case Management

(MHICM), Rural Access Network for Growth Enhancement (RANGE), and Enhanced Rural Access Network for Growth Enhancement (E-RANGE). These programs adapt the well-known assertive community treatment (ACT) model to improve clinical outcomes for veterans with serious mental illness who are served by the VA mental health system. The mission of Intensive Community Mental Health Recovery programs is to provide intensive recovery-oriented mental health services to veterans with a serious mental illness that enable them to live meaningful lives in the community of their choosing. Intensive Community Mental Health Recovery programs fully embrace and incorporate the core principles of psychosocial rehabilitation and recovery in all interactions, interventions, and program development (VHA Handbook 1163.06, p. 4). In addition to Intensive Community Mental Health Recovery case management services, the community residential care (CRC) program helps veterans locate and maintain supervised living quarters in the community.

The primary target population for Intensive Community Mental Health Recovery services is veterans with severe psychosis, severe mood disorders, or severe PTSD whose functional status is severely impaired. Veterans who have one of these diagnoses are eligible for Intensive Community Mental Health Recovery services if they also meet the following criteria: they are inadequately served by conventional clinic-based outpatient treatment (i.e., they are unable to successfully maintain stable community integration with the use of conventional services, even when augmented with services such as Psychosocial Rehabilitation and Recovery Centers); they are high resource utilizers (e.g., frequent hospital use as defined by >30 days of inpatient mental health care or ≥3 episodes of mental health hospitalization over the past year); and they are clinically appropriate for an outpatient level of care.

Community Residential Care (CRC)

The community residential care (CRC) program (VHA Handbook 1140.01, 2014) consists of independent, privately owned and operated housing in the community for which veterans pay a negotiated rent in exchange for room and board. The housing available through this program ranges from a single bed in an owner-occupied home to aggregate owner-operated housing with a range of single and multiple occupancy rooms. The settings are also diverse and include urban as well as more rural or remote locations. Community residential care homes generally do not have professionally trained staff but most have the ability to provide assistance with activities of daily living. Most are able to supervise medication self-administration, and in some homes, one or more staff members are trained and state certified specifically for safe medication administration. All homes provide one or more meals every day, and some transportation to and from medical appointments. The VA's role is to identify good matches between a home's location and capabilities and an individual veteran's needs and financial resources; generally, homes that provide more support are also more expensive. The rent charged by each community residential care home must be approved by VA, which determines whether it is fair and reasonable. In addition to this mediating role, VA inspects each home annually to ensure that it continues to meet safety standards, including safe medication handling; homes that fail the inspection are given an opportunity to correct the deficiencies before being subjected to a formal adjudication process that may lead to removal from the program.

The vast majority of veterans who enter community residential care homes do so following an inpatient hospitalization. After a veteran has been placed in a community residential care home, a community residential care case manager maintains contact with the veteran for as long as he or she resides in the home. The case manager makes regular scheduled visits to the home to assess the veteran and the home environment, to provide ongoing emotional and logistical support (e.g., transportation) and for crisis intervention. The Community Residential Care program makes it possible for veterans with serious mental illness who would otherwise be consigned to long-term inpatient hospitalization to live for extended periods in the community while developing sustained and supportive relationships with the homeowner, home staff, and co-residents. It is not unusual for a veteran to remain in the same home for decades by choice. Although most veterans who reside in community residential care homes have a serious mental illness, the only requirement to participate in the program is that the veteran is willing and able to pay the rent and agrees to abide by the rules of the home and the program.

Housing for Homeless Veterans (HUD-VASH and VJO)

Homelessness can be a consequence of persistent psychosis, and VA has two programs designed specifically to address the needs of homeless veterans. The collaboratively administered Department of Housing and Urban Development-Veterans Affairs Supportive Housing (HUD-VASH) program provides housing subsidies to eligible veterans and their families for as long as this assistance is needed. Veterans enrolled in this program also receive case manager services to assist in locating and leasing the housing. This program is often crucial to the veteran's early success in navigating community reentry and obtaining further education or competitive employment. For veterans who need intensive recovery programming and/or vocational rehabilitation, VA has an extensive array of Domiciliary Residential and Rehabilitation Treatment Programs, which include basic residential care as well as programs that target certain disorders (e.g., post-traumatic stress disorder or substance use disorders).

It is now widely appreciated that individuals with psychotic disorders are often incarcerated inappropriately because they are unable to access adequate mental health care or because the health-care system is not equipped to manage their complex behavioral problems. Once an individual with a serious mental illness is incarcerated, it becomes even more difficult for her to access effective mental health treatment. In recognition of this problem, VA has created the Veterans Justice Outreach (VJO) case management program. According to a Veterans Health Administration white paper (McGuire and Clark 2009), the most recent (2002) data from the US Department of Justice indicate that 9.3% of people incarcerated in jails are veterans. The controlling offense for 70% of these veterans was a non-violent crime; 45% had served two or more state prison sentences, and at least 90,000 of the 9 million unique inmates annually released from US jails are veterans. A large majority (82%) is likely eligible for VA services, having been discharged either under honorable (65%) or general with honorable (17%) conditions. On May 27, 2009, the Deputy Under Secretary for Health for Operations and Management issued a memorandum requiring VA medical centers to provide outreach to justice-involved veterans in the communities they serve.

In communities where justice programs relevant to veterans exist (veterans courts, drug courts, mental health courts, and police crisis intervention teams), VA takes the initiative in building working relationships to ensure that eligible justice-involved veterans get needed care. In communities where no such programs exist, VA will reach out to potential justice system partners (judges, prosecutors, police, and jail administrators) to connect eligible justice-involved veterans with VA services. VA medical centers must also ensure that VA police located at their facilities receive training on veteran-specific issues. A Veterans Justice Outreach National Steering Committee provides counsel and direction for VA's involvement with justice system partners nationwide.

All of these case management programs provide critical outreach and support to veterans who are unable to access needed levels of health care and for whom this assistance may be literally lifesaving. Veterans with serious mental illness who are lost to follow up experience greater noninjury mortality, especially from cancer-related illness, and have shorter life spans (Bowersox et al. 2012).

Telehealth and Tele-Mental Health

Telehealth and tele-mental health technologies are now used in VA and Department of Defense to extend the capabilities of treatment facilities and improve access to services for veterans and service members (DoD/VA Report to the Congress 2014). Applications range from monitoring of basic parameters such as blood pressure and blood sugar to long distance expert consultation regarding more complex diagnostic and treatment challenges. These practices are still early in their development but appear likely to continue expanding.

Mental Health Treatment in VA Compared to Non-VA Systems

One study compared the quality of VA inpatient mental health care received between 1993 and 1997 with that accessed through private insurance (Leslie and Rosenheck 2000). The timing of this study was significant in that it occurred in the context of a major reorganization of VA services from independent medical centers and outpatient clinics into 22 regional care networks (Veterans Integrated Service Networks or VISNs), which was implemented in late 1995. The veteran sample differed from the private sector patients in that it was older, predominantly male, and more than twice as likely to be dually diagnosed; the prevalence of schizophrenia in the veteran inpatient sample was three times higher than in the private sector (16.4–18.1% vs. 5.6–5.9%), whereas the frequency of major depression and bipolar disorder was approximately fourfold higher in the privately insured patients. The authors found that the private sector outperformed VA "to a modest degree" on most of the quality outcome measures, but suggested this may have been accounted for by unmeasured differences in the patient groups. For example, they cite low average income, a high prevalence of disability, and a high frequency of homelessness as characteristics of veterans who are eligible for VA care (Leslie and Rosenheck 2000). They concluded that VA and private care quality were likely equivalent if adjusted for severity of illness and demographic cofactors.

Veterans with schizophrenia are more likely to be treated with an antipsychotic medication than are private sector patients, and prescribing of conventional agents was significantly more likely to conform to Schizophrenia Patient Outcomes Research Team (PORT) guidelines (Leslie and Rosenheck 2003). Veterans were more frequently prescribed antipsychotic medication doses exceeding Schizophrenia Patient Outcomes Research Team guidelines, whereas private patients were more frequently underdosed according to the same guidelines. Significantly greater rates of comorbid PTSD, substance use, and personality disorder in the veteran group may account for higher dosing of antipsychotic medications. Thus, on several measures veterans appeared to have better access to adequate treatment, but clozapine is underutilized in VA (Weissman 2002; Leslie and Rosenheck 2003), and antipsychotic polypharmacy is common with variability in rates between sites (Weissman 2002). There is also wide variation among VA medical centers in the use of SGAs (Owen et al. 2001).

Recently Watkins and colleagues (2016) used the VA National Patient Care Database and national private insurance administrative claims data to compare very large cohorts of veterans and privately insured individuals receiving mental health care with respect to how consistently the clinical services provided conformed to nationally accepted performance measures. The veteran cohort consisted of all veterans less than 65 years old who had at least one inpatient episode with a qualifying primary or secondary diagnosis or two outpatient encounters, at least one of which was for a qualifying primary or secondary diagnosis, between October 2006 and September 2007. There were 43 qualifying diagnoses, including schizophrenia, bipolar I disorder, PTSD, major depression, and substance use disorders. Each patient was assigned to only one diagnostic cohort on the basis of the modal frequency of diagnosis codes, except that dually diagnosed veterans were placed in both corresponding cohorts. Using this method of classification, a diagnosis of schizophrenia was greater than three times more prevalent in the veteran cohort (8.1% vs. 2.4%). VA outperformed private care by at least 30% for every measure. One of the largest differences was in the rate at which the medication lab tests indicator was met: adherence was 77% in VA, 13 times higher than in private plans (6%). This measure applied to antipsychotic medications as well as mood stabilizers and reflects the proportion of these patients who received all recommended blood level monitoring tests during the study period. Veterans with schizophrenia were also more than twice as likely to receive appropriate initial medication treatment. Those authors suggest that clinical support structures implemented by VA—such as a fully integrated electronic record, co-location of pharmacy and laboratory services near primary care and specialty clinics, online decision support tools, and automated clinical reminders—may account for some of the performance differences. Better coordination of care could help account for the fact that increased mortality risk is substantially attenuated (about half of what has been observed in studies using nonveteran samples) in individuals with those disorders who are treated within VA (Chwastiak et al. 2010).

Key Concepts

1. Mental disorders are the dominant source of medical and occupational morbidity among active-duty US military personnel. Schizophrenia and related psychotic disorders are often disabling conditions and, although less prevalent in active service members than in the general population, account for a substantial portion of psychiatric hospitalizations and medical retirements from active duty.
2. Antipsychotic medications are a mainstay of treatment for schizophrenia and related disorders. Although there is some disagreement regarding the specifics of medication selection, the consensus is that monotherapy is preferred over polypharmacy and that a clozapine trial should be attempted after two adequate treatment courses with non-clozapine antipsychotic medications have failed (i.e., treatment-resistant schizophrenia).
3. Approximately 30–60% of individuals with schizophrenia are treatment resistant and should receive a clozapine trial according to all widely accepted treatment guidelines, but clozapine is very substantially underutilized with respect to this treatment standard, both within and outside VA. The reasons for its widespread underutilization include logistical challenges for patients, prescriber factors, and misconceptions about its contribution to health-care costs.
4. Once the most acute and disabling psychotic symptoms have been attenuated with medication, the process of recovery should become the focus of treatment. There are many different components to a recovery-oriented plan of treatment; any of these elements that are available and appropriate to the patient's needs should be considered and, if the patient wishes, included in the plan. This practice embodies the principle that the recovery process must reflect the individual patient's hopes, aspirations, and meaningful life goals.
5. In many respects, VA treatment of schizophrenia and related disorders is as good as or better than what is available in other venues. Likely reasons for this quality difference include a fully integrated (across all VA facilities) electronic medical record that incorporates decision tools and automated reminders informed by current treatment guidelines; a comprehensive spectrum of evidence-based clinical services that can be tailored to the needs of individual veterans; and the tendency of veterans to remain within the VA system of care once enrolled, which facilities continuity of care.

References

Ahmed AO, Doane NJ, Mabe PA, Buckley PF, Birgenheir D, Goodrum NM (2012) Peers and peer-led interventions for people with schizophrenia. Psychiatr Clin N Am 35:699–715

Ahmed AO, Marino BA, Rosenthal E, Buckner A, Hunter KM, Mabe PA, Buckley PF (2016) Recovery in schizophrenia: what consumers know and do not know. Psychiatr Clin N Am 39:313–330

Aleman A, Kahn RS, Selten J-P (2003) Sex differences in the risk of schizophrenia: evidence from meta-analysis. Arch Gen Psychiatry 60:656–571

Allen MH, Currier GW, Hughes DH, Docherty JP, Carpenter D, Ross R (2003) Treatment of behavioral emergencies: a summary of the expert consensus guidelines. J Psychiatr Pract 9:16–38

American Psychiatric Association (2013) Diagnostic and statistical manual of mental disorders (DSM-5), 5th edn. American Psychiatric Publishing, Washington, DC

American Psychiatric Association, Steering Committee on Practice Guidelines (2004) Practice guideline for the treatment of patients with schizophrenia. Am J Psychiatry 161(suppl 2):1–56

Anketell C, Dorahy MJ, Shannon M, Elder R, Hamilton G, Corry M, MacSherry A, Curran D, O'Rawe B (2010) An exploratory analysis of voice hearing in chronic PTSD: potential associated mechanisms. J Trauma Dissoc 11:93–107

Barnes TRE and the Schizophrenia Consensus Group of the British Association for Psychopharmacology (2011) Evidence-based guidelines for the pharmacological treatment of schizophrenia: recommendations from the British Association for Psychopharmacology. J Psychopharmacol 25:567–620

Bauer MS, Lee A, Miller CJ, Bajor L, Li M, Penfold RB (2015) Effects of diagnostic inclusion criteria on prevalence and population characteristics in database research. Psychiatr Serv 66:141–148

Bellack AS (2006) Scientific and consumer models of recovery in schizophrenia: concordance, contrasts, and implications. Schizophr Bull 32:432–442

Blow FC, Zeber JE, McCarthy JF, Valenstein M, Gillon L, Bingham CR (2004) Ethnicity and diagnostic patterns in veterans with psychoses. Soc Psychiatry Psychiatr Epidemiol 39:841–851

Bobo WV, Hoge CW, Messina MA, Pavlovcic F, Levandowski D, Grieger T (2004) Characteristics of repeat users of an inpatient psychiatry service at a large military tertiary care hospital. Mil Med 169:648–653

Bowersox NW, Kilbourne AM, Abraham KM, Reck BH, Lai Z, Bohnert ASB, Goodrich DE, Davis CL (2012) Cause-specific mortality among Veterans with serious mental illness lost to follow-up. Gen Hosp Psychiatry 34:651–653

Braakman MH, Kortmann FAM, van den Brink W (2009) Validity of 'post-traumatic stress disorder with secondary psychotic features': a review of the evidence. Acta Psychiatr Scand 119:15–24

Brewin CR, Patel T (2010) Auditory pseudohallucinations in United Kingdom war veterans and civilians with posttraumatic stress disorder. J Clin Psychiatry 71:419–425

Brissos S, Veguilla MR, Taylor D, Balanzá-Martinez V (2014) The role of long-acting injectable antipsychotics in schizophrenia: a critical appraisal. Ther Adv Psychopharmacol 4:198–219

Buchanan RW, Kreyenbuhl J, Kelly DL, Noel JM, Boggs DL, Fischer BA, Himelhoch S, Fang B, Peterson E, Aquino PR, Keller W (2010) The 2009 Schizophrenia PORT psychopharmacological treatment recommendations and summary statements. Schizophr Bull 36:71–93

Buckley PF, Schooler NR, Goff DC, Kopelowicz A, Lauriello J, Manschreck TC, Mendelowitz A, Miller DD, Wilson DR, Ames D, Bustillo JR, Kane JM, Looney SW (2016) Comparison of injectable and oral antipsychotics in relapse rates in a pragmatic 30-month Schizophrenia Relapse Prevention Study. Psychiatr Serv Adv. https://doi.org/10.1176/appi.ps.201500466

Carpenter WT Jr (2016) The RDoC controversy: alternate paradigm or dominant paradigm? Am J Psychiatry 173:562–563

Chien WT, Yip ALK (2013) Current approaches to treatments for schizophrenia spectrum disorders, part I: an overview and medical treatments. Neuropsychiat Dis Treat 9:1311–1332

Christian R, Saavedra L, Gaynes BN, Sheitman B, Wines RCM, Jonas DE, Viswanathan M, Ellis AR, Woodell C, Carey TS (2012) Future research needs for first- and second-generation antipsychotics for children and young adults. Future Research Needs Paper No. 13. (Prepared by the RTI-UNC Evidence-based Practice Center under Contract No. 290 2007 10056 I.) Rockville: Agency for Healthcare Research and Quality; Feb 2012. www.effectivehealthcare.ahrq.gov/reports/final.cfm

Chwastiak LA, Rosenheck RA, Desai R, Kasis LE (2010) The association of psychiatric illness and all-cause mortality in the national Department of Veterans Affairs health care system. Psychosom Med 72:817–822

Clark NG (2004) Consensus development conference on antipsychotic drugs and obesity and diabetes. Diabetes Care 27:596–601

Coleman KJ, Stewart C, Waitzfelder BE, Zeber JE, Morales LS, Ahmed AT et al (2016) Racial-ethnic differences in psychiatric diagnoses and treatment across 11 health care systems in the mental health research network. Psychiatr Serv 67:749–757

College of Psychiatric and Neurologic Pharmacists (CPNP) (2016) https://cpnp.org/about/public/faq. Accessed 8/12/16

Cone SM, Brown MC, Stambaugh RL (2008) Characteristics of ambulatory care clinics and pharmacists in veterans affairs medical centers: an update. Am J Health Syst Pharm 65:631–635

Correll CU, Gallego JA (2012) Antipsychotic polypharmacy: a comprehensive evaluation of relevant correlates of a long-standing clinical practice. Psychiatr Clin North Am 35:661–681

Cowan DN, Weber NS, Fisher JA, Bedno SA, Niebuhr DW (2011) Incidence of adult onset schizophrenic disorders in the US military: patterns by sex, race and age. Schizophr Res 127:235–240

Crilly J (2007) The history of clozapine and its emergence in the U.S. market: a review and analysis. Hist Psychiatry 18:39–60

Davidson L, Chinman M, Sells D, Rowe M (2006a) Peer support among adults with serious mental illness: a report from the field. Schizophr Bull 32:443–450

Davidson L, Tondora J, Staeheli M, O'Connell M, Frey J, Chinman M (2006b) Recovery guides: an emerging model of community-based care for adults with psychiatric disabilities. In: Lightburn A, Sessions P (eds) Handbook of community-based clinical practice. Oxford University Press, London, pp 476–501. chapter 30

Davies LM, Drummond MF (1993) Assessment of costs and benefits of drug therapy for treatment-resistant schizophrenia in the United Kingdom. Br J Psychiatry 162:38–42

Davis CL, Kilbourne AM, Blow FC, Pierce JR, Winkel BM, Huycke E, Langberg R, Lyle D, Phillips Y, Visnic S (2012) Reduced mortality among Department of Veterans Affairs patients with schizophrenia or bipolar disorder lost to follow-up and engaged in active outreach to return for care. Am J Public Health 102:S74–S79

De Fazio P, Gaetano R, Caroleo M, Cerminara G, Maida F, Bruno A, Muscatello MR, Moreno MJJ, Russo E, Segura-García C (2015) Rare and very rare adverse effects of clozapine. Neuropsychiatr Dis Treat 11:1995–2003

de Leon J, Odom-White A, Josiassen RC, Diaz FJ, Cooper TB, Simpson GM (2003) Serum antimuscarinic activity during clozapine treatment. J Clin Psychopharmacol 23:336–341

DeVylder JE, Koyanagi A, Unick J, Oh H, Nam B, Stickley A (2016) Stress sensitivity and psychotic experiences in 39 low- and middle-income countries. Schizophr Bull ., e-pub ahead of print. https://doi.org/10.1093/schbul/sbw044

Dishman BR, Ellenor GL, Lacro JP, Lohr JB (1994) Pharmacists' role in clozapine therapy at a Veterans Affairs medical center. Am J Hosp Pharm 51:899–901

Dixon L, Perkins D, Calmes C (2009) Guideline watch (September 2009): practice guideline for the treatment of patients with schizophrenia. American Psychiatric Association, Washington, DC. http://psychiatryonline.org/pb/assets/raw/sitewide/practice_guidelines/guidelines/schizophrenia-watch.pdf

Dixon LB, Dickerson F, Bellack AS, Bennett M, Dickinson D, Goldberg RW, Lehman A, Tenhula WN, Calmes C, Pasillas RM, Peer J, Kreyenbuhl J (2010) The 2009 schizophrenia PORT psychosocial treatment recommendations and summary statements. Schizophr Bull 36:48–70

DoD/VA (2014) Report to the Congress in response to Senate Report 113–44, accompanying S.1197, the National Defense Authorization Act for Fiscal Year 2014

Elkis H, Buckley PF (2016) Treatment-resistant schizophrenia. Psychiatr Clin N Am 39:239–265

Every-Palmer S, Nowitz M, Stanley J, Grant E, Huthwaite M, Dunn H, Ellis PM (2016) Clozapine-treated patients have marked gastrointestinal hypomotility, the probable basis of life-threatening gastrointestinal complications: a cross sectional study. EBioMedicine in press. https://doi.org/10.1016/j.ebiom.2016.02.020

Falkai P, Wobrock T, Lieberman J, Glenthoj B, Gattaz WF, Möller H-J, WFSBP Task Force on Treatment Guidelines for Schizophrenia (2005) World Federation of Societies of Biological Psychiatry (WFSBP) guidelines for biological treatment of schizophrenia, part 1: acute treatment of schizophrenia. World J Biol Psychiatry 6:132–191

Finley PR, Crismon L, Rush AJ (2003) Evaluating the impact of pharmacists in mental health: a systematic review. Pharmacotherapy 23:1634–1644

Fleischhacker WW, Uchida H (2014) Critical review of antipsychotic polypharmacy in the treatment of schizophrenia. Int J Neuropsychopharmacol 17:1083–1093

Freudenreich O, Goff DC, Henderson DC (2016) Antipsychotic drugs. In: Stern TA, Fava M, Wilens TE, Rosenbaum JF (eds) Massachusetts General Hospital Psychopharmacology and Neurotherapeutics. Elsevier, New York. Chapter 7, pp 72–85

Gadelha A, Souza Noto C, De Jesus MJ (2012) Pharmacological treatment of schizophrenia. Int Rev Psychiatry 24:489–498

Galletly C, Castle D, Dark F, Humberstone V, Jablensky A, Killackey E, Kulkarni J, McGorry P, Nielssen O, Tran N (2016) Royal Australian and New Zealand College of Psychiatrists clinical practice guidelines for the management of schizophrenia and related disorders. Aust N Z J Psychiatry 50:410–472

Gardner DM, Baldessarini RJ, Waraich P (2005) Modern antipsychotic drugs: A critical review. Can Med Assoc J 172:1703–1711

Gopalakirshna G, Ithman MH, Lauriello J (2016) Update on new and emerging treatments for schizophrenia. Psychiatr Clin N Am 39:217–238

Gould CM (2012a) Psychopharmacologic treatment of acute agitation: part I. Psychopharm Rev 47:49–56

Gould CM (2012b) Psychopharmacologic treatment of acute agitation: part II. Psychopharm Rev 47:65–72

Gracie A, Freeman D, Green S, Garety PA, Kuipers E, Hardy A, Ray K, Dunn G, Bebbington P, Fowler D (2007) The association between traumatic experience, paranoia and hallucinations: a test of the predictions of psychological models. Acta Psychiatr Scand 116:280–289

Grubaugh AL, Zinzow HM, Paul L, Egede LE, Frueh BC (2011) Trauma exposure and posttraumatic stress disorder in adults with severe mental illness: a critical review. Clin Psychol Rev 31:883–899

Gunderson EKE, Hourani LL (1998) The epidemiology of mental disorders in the U.S. Navy: the psychoses. *Report No. 98–3*. Naval Health Research Center, San Diego and Naval Medical Research and Development Command, Bethesda

Gurrera RJ, Parlee AC, Perry NL (2016) Aspiration pneumonia: an underappreciated risk of clozapine treatment. J Clin Psychopharmacol 36:174–176

Hamner MB, Frueh BC, Ulmer HG, Huber MG, Towmey TJ, Tyson C, Arana GW (2000) Psychotic features in chronic posttraumatic stress disorder and schizophrenia: comparative severity. J Nerv Ment Dis 188:217–221

Herrell R, Henter ID, Mojtabai R, Bartko JJ, Venable D, Susser E, Merikangas KR, Wyatt RJ (2006) First psychiatric hospitalizations in the US military: the National Collaborative Study of Early Psychosis and Suicide (NCSEPS). Psychol Med 36:1405–1415

Hibbard KR, Propst A, Frank DE, Wyse J (2009) Fatalities associated with clozapine-related constipation and bowel obstruction: a literature review and two case reports. Psychosomatics 50:415–419

Hiemke C, Baumann P, Bergemann N, Conca A, Dietmaier O, Egberts K, Fric M, Gerlach M, Greiner

C, Gründer G, Haen E, Havemann-Reinecke U, Sirot EJ, Kirchherr H, Laux G, Lutz UC, Messer T, Müller MJ, Pfuhlmann B, Rambeck B, Riederer P, Schoppek B, Stingl J, Uhr M, Ulrich S, Waschgler R, Zernig G (2011) AGNP consensus guidelines for therapeutic drug monitoring in psychiatry: Update 2011. Pharmacopsychiatry 44:195–235

Hoge CW, Lesikar SE, Guevara R, Lange J, Brundage JF, Engel CC Jr, Messer SC, Orman DT (2002) Mental disorders among U.S. military personnel in the 1990s: association with high levels of health care utilization and early military attrition. Am J Psychiatry 159:1576–1583

Hoge CW, Castro CA, Messer SC, McGurk D, Cotting DI, Koffman RL (2004) Combat duty in Iraq and Afghanistan, mental health problems, and barriers to care. N Engl J Med 351:13–22

Jablensky A (2006) Subtyping schizophrenia: implications for genetic research. Mol Psychiatry 11:815–836

Jones PB, Barnes TRE, Davies L, Dunn G, Lloyd H, Hayhurst KP, Murray RM, Markwick A, Lewis SW (2006) Randomized controlled trial of the effect on quality of life of second- vs. first-generation antipsychotic drugs in schizophrenia. Cost utility of the latest antipsychotic drugs in schizophrenia study (CUtLASS 1). Arch Gen Psychiatry 63:1079–1087

Kapur S, Seeman P (2001) Does fast dissociation from the dopamine D2 receptor explain the action of atypical antipsychotics?: a new hypothesis. Am J Psychiatry 158:360–369

Karagianis JL, Phillips LC, Hogan KP, LeDrew KK (1999) Clozapine-associated neuroleptic malignant syndrome: two new cases and a review of the literature. Ann Pharmacother 33:623–630

Kaštelan A, Frančišković T, Moro L, Rončević-Gržeta I, Grković J, Jurcan V, Lesica T, Graovac M, Girotto I (2007) Psychotic symptoms in combat-related posttraumatic stress disorder. Mil Med 172:273–277

Khan AY, Preskorn SH (2005) Examining concentration-dependent toxicity of clozapine: role of therapeutic drug monitoring. J Psychiatr Pract 11:289–301

Kilcommons AM, Morrison AP (2005) Relationships between trauma and psychosis: an exploration of cognitive and dissociative factors. Acta Psychiatr Scand 112:351–359

Kishimoto T, Nitta M, Borenstein M, Kane JM, Correll CU (2013) Long-acting injectable versus oral antipsychotics in schizophrenia: a systematic review and meta-analysis of mirror-image studies. J Clin Psychiatry 74:957–965

Kishimoto T, Robenzadeh A, Leucht C, Leucht S, Watanabe K, Mimura M, Borenstein M, Kane JM, Correll CU (2014) Long-acting injectable vs. oral antipsychotics for relapse prevention in schizophrenia: a meta-analysis of randomized trials. Schizophr Bull 40:192–213

Kozarić-Kovačić D, Borovečki A (2005) Prevalence of psychotic comorbidity in combat-related posttraumatic stress disorder. Mil Med 170:223–226

Lambert BL, Cunningham FE, Miller DR, Dalack GW, Hur K (2006) Diabetes risk associated with use of olanzapine, quetiapine, and risperidone in Veterans Health Administration patients with schizophrenia. Am J Epidemiol 164:672–681

Lauriello J, Bustillo J, Keith SJ (1999) A critical review of research on psychosocial treatment of schizophrenia. Biol Psychiatry 46:1409–1417

Lee J, Bies R, Takeuchi H, Fervaha G, Bhaloo A, Powell V, Remington G (2016) Quantifying intraindividual variations in plasma clozapine levels: a population pharmacokinetic approach. J Clin Psychiatry 77:681–687

Lenzenweger MF, Lane MC, Loranger AW, Kessler RC (2007) DSM-IV personality disorders in the National Comorbidity Survey Replication. Biol Psychiatry 62:553–564

Leslie DL, Rosenheck RA (2000) Health care for public-sector and privately insured populations. Psychiatr Serv 51:650–655

Leslie DL, Rosenheck RA (2003) Benchmarking the quality of schizophrenia pharmacotherapy: a comparison of the Department of Veterans Affairs and the private sector. J Ment Health Pol Econ 6:113–121

Leucht C, Heres S, Kane JM, Kissling W, Davis JM, Leucht S (2011) Oral versus depot antipsychotic drugs for schizophrenia—a critical systematic review and meta-analysis of randomised long-term trials. Schizophr Res 127:83–92

Leucht S, Tardy M, Komossa K, Heres S, Kissling W, Salanti G, Davis JM (2012) Antipsychotic drugs versus placebo for relapse prevention in schizophrenia: a systematic review and meta-analysis. Lancet 379:2063–2071

Lewis S, Lieberman J (2008) CATIE and CUtLASS: can we handle the truth? Br J Psychiatry 192:161–163

Lewis SW, Barnes TRE, Davies L, Murray RM, Dunn G, Hayhurst KP, Markwick A, Lloyd H, Jones PB (2006) Randomized controlled trial of effect of prescription of clozapine versus other second-generation antipsychotic drugs in resistant schizophrenia. Schizophr Bull 32:715–723

Lieberman JA (1998) Maximizing clozapine therapy: managing side effects. J Clin Psychiatry 59(suppl 3):38–43

Lieberman JA, Stroup TS (2011) The NIMH-CATIE schizophrenia study: what did we learn? Am J Psychiatry 168:770–775

Lieberman JA, Stroup TS, McEvoy JP, Swartz MS, Rosenheck RA, Perkins DO, Keefe RSE, Davis SM, Davis CE, Lebowitz BD, Severe J, and Hsaio JK for the CATIE Investigators (2005) Effectiveness of antipsychotic drugs in patients with chronic schizophrenia. N Engl J Med 353:1209–1223

Lindenmayer J-P, Kaur A (2016) Antipsychotic management of schizoaffective disorder: a review. Drugs 76:589–564. [REFERENCE MUST BE PURCHASED]

Lobeck F, Traxler WT, Bobinet DD (1989) The cost-effectiveness of a clinical pharmacy service in an out-

patient mental health clinic. Hosp Comm Psychiatry 40:643–645
Malhi GS, Green M, Fagiolini A, Peselow ED, Kumari V (2008) Schizoaffective disorder: diagnostic issues and future recommendations. Bipol Disord 10:215–230
Marshall M, Rathbone J (2011) Early intervention for psychosis (review). Cochrane Databas Syst Rev (Issue 6):CD004718. https://doi.org/10.1002/14651858.CD004718.pub3
McCarthy JF, Blow FC, Valenstein M, Fischer EP, Owen RR, Barry KL, Hudson TJ, Ignacio RV (2007) Veterans Affairs health system and mental health treatment retention among patients with serious mental illness: evaluating accessibility and availability barriers. Health Serv Res 42:1042–1060
McCarthy S, Chinman M, Henze K, Sweeney P (2013) Peer specialist toolkit: implementing peer support services in VHA
McCarthy-Jones S, Longden E (2015) Auditory verbal hallucinations in schizophrenia and post-traumatic stress disorder: common phenomenology, common cause, common interventions? Front Psychol 6(12):1071
McCarthy-Jones S, Trauer T, Mackinnon A, Sims E, Thomas N, Copolov DL (2014) A new phenomenological survey of auditory hallucinations: evidence for subtypes and implications for theory and practice. Schizophr Bull 40:225–235
McEvoy JP, Meyer JM, Goff DC, Nasrallah HA, Davis SM, Sullivan L, Meltzer HY, Hsiao J, Scott Stroup T, Lieberman JA (2005) Prevalence of the metabolic syndrome in patients with schizophrenia: baseline results from the Clinical Antipsychotic Trials of Intervention Effectiveness (CATIE) schizophrenia trial and comparison with national estimates from NHANES III. Schizophr Res 80:19–32
McEvoy JP, Lieberman JP, Stroup TS, Davis SM, Meltzer HY, Rosenheck RA, Swartz MS, Perkins DO, Keefe RSE, Davis CE, Severe J, Hsiao JK, for the CATIE Investigators (2006) Effectiveness of clozapine versus olanzapine, quetiapine, and risperidone in patients with chronic schizophrenia who did not respond to prior atypical antipsychotic treatment. Am J Psychiatry 163:600–610
McGorry PD, Nelson B, Amminger P, Bechdolf A, Francey SM, Berger G, Riecher-Rossler A, Klosterkotter J, Ruhrmann S, Schultze-Lutter F, Nordentoft M, Hickie I, McGuire P, Berk M, Chen EYH, Keshavan MS, Young AR (2009) Intervention in individuals at ultra-high risk for psychosis: a review and future directions. J Clin Psychiatry 70:1206–1212
McGrath J, Saha S, Welham J, El Saadi O, MacCauley C, Chant D (2004) A systematic review of the incidence of schizophrenia: the distribution of rates and the influence of sex, urbanicity, migrant status and methodology. BMC Med 2:13. https://doi.org/10.1186/1741-7015-2-13
McGrath J, Saha S, Chant D, Welham J (2008) Schizophrenia: a concise overview of incidence, prevalence, and mortality. Epidemiol Rev 30:67–76
McGuire J, Clark S (2009) The veterans justice outreach initiative. White Paper, Department of Veterans Affairs. (downloaded 8/8/16). http://justiceforvets.org/sites/default/files/files/VJO%20White%20Paper.pdf
Meltzer HY, Matsubara S, Lee J-C (1989) Classification of typical and atypical antipsychotic drugs on the basis of dopamine D-1, D-2 and serotonin$_2$ pK_i values. J Pharmacol Exp Ther 251:238–246
Mews MR, Quante A (2013) Comparative efficacy and acceptability of existing pharmacotherapies for delusional disorder. J Clin Psychopharmacol 33:512–519
Meyer J, Loh C, Leckband SG, Boyd JA, Wirshing WC, Pierre JM, Wirshing D (2006) Prevalence of the metabolic syndrome in veterans with schizophrenia. J Psychiatr Pract 12:5–10
Miyamoto S, Miyake N, Jarskog LF, Fleischhacker WW, Leiberman JA (2012) Pharmacology treatment of schizophrenia: a critical review of the pharmacology and clinical effects of current and future therapeutic agents. Mol Psychiatry 17:1206–1227
Miyamoto S, Jarskog LF, Fleischhacker WW (2014) New therapeutic approaches for treatment-resistant schizophrenia: a look to the future. J Psychiatr Res 58:1–6
Mokhtari M, Rajarethinam R (2014) Early intervention and the treatment of prodrome in schizophrenia: a review of recent developments. J Psychiatr Pract 19:375–385
Mouaffak F, Tranulis C, Gourevitch R, Poirier M-F, Douki S, Olié J-P, Lôo H, Gourian D (2006) Augmentation strategies of clozapine with antipsychotics in the treatment of ultraresistant schizophrenia. Clin Neuropharmacol 29:28–33
Muenzenbaier K, Spei E, Gross DR (2010) Complex posttraumatic stress disorder in men with serious mental illness: a reconceptualization. Am J Psychother 64:257–268
Mueser KT, Deavers F, Penn DL, Cassisi JE (2013) Psychosocial treatments for schizophrenia. Ann Rev Clin Psychol 9:465–497
National Institute for Health and Clinical Excellence (NICE) (2014) Psychosis and schizophrenia in adults: prevention and management. Clinical guideline 178. https://www.nice.org.uk/guidance/cg178
Nielsen J, Damkier P, Lublin H, Taylor D (2011) Optimizing clozapine treatment. Acta Psychiatr Scand 123:411–422
Nielsen J, Correll CU, Manu P, Kane JM (2013) Termination of clozapine treatment due to medical reasons: when is it warranted and how can it be avoided? J Clin Psychiatry 74:603–613
Norredam M, Jensen M, Ekstrøm M (2011) Psychotic symptoms in refugees diagnosed with PTSD: a series of case reports. Nord J Psychiatry 65:283–288
Olivares JM, Sermon J, Hemels M, Schreiner A (2013) Definitions and drivers of relapse in patients with schizophrenia: a systematic literature review. Ann General Psychiatry 12:32. https://doi.org/10.1186/1744-859X-12-32

Owen RR, Feng W, Thrush CR, Hudson TJ, Austen MA (2001) Variations in prescribing practices for novel antipsychotic medications among Veterans Affairs hospitals. Psychiatr Serv 52:1523–1525

Palmer SE, McLean RM, Ellis PM, Harrison-Woolrych M (2008) Life-threatening clozapine-induced gastrointestinal hypomotility: an analysis of 102 cases. J Clin Psychiatry 69:759–768

Pearlson GD, Clementz BA, Sweeney JA, Keshavan MS, Tamminga CA (2016) Does biology transcend the symptom-based boundaries of psychosis? Psychiatr Clin N Am 39:165–174

Perkins DO, Gu H, Boteva K, Lieberman JA (2005) Relationship between duration of untreated psychosis and outcome in first-episode schizophrenia: a critical review and meta-analysis. Am J Psychiatry 162:1785–1804

Perry PJ, Miller DD, Arndt SV, Cadoret RJ (1991) Clozapine and norclozapine plasma concentrations and clinical response of treatment-refractory schizophrenic patients. Am J Psychiatry 148:231–235

Plaze M, Paillère-Martinot M-L, Penttilä J, Januel D, de Beaurepaire R, Bellivier F, Andoh J, Galinowski A, Gallarda T, Artiges E, Olié J-P, Mangin J-F, Martinot J-L, Cachia A (2011) "Where do auditory hallucinations come from?" – a brain morphometry study of schizophrenia patients with inner or outer space hallucinations. Schizophr Bull 37:212–221

Pollack S, Woerner MG, Howard A, Fireworker RB, Kane JM (1998) Clozapine reduces rehospitalization among schizophrenia patients. Psychopharmacol Bull 34:89–92

Remington G, Agid O, Foussias G, Ferguson L, McDonald K, Powell V (2013) Clozapine and therapeutic drug monitoring: is there sufficient evidence for an upper threshold? Psychopharmacology 225:505–518

Rosell DR, Futterman SE, McMaster A, Seiver LJ (2014) Schizotypal personality disorder: a current review. Curr Psychiatry Rep 16:452. https://doi.org/10.1007/s11920-014-0452-1

Rosenheck R, Cramer J, Allan E, Erdos J, Frisman LK, Xu W, Thomas J, Henderson W, Charney D, for the Department of Veterans Affairs Cooperative Study Group on Clozapine in Refractory Schizophrenia (1999) Arch Gen Psychiatry 56:565–572

Saha S, Chant D, Welham J, McGrath J (2005) A systematic review of the prevalence of schizophrenia. PLoS Med 2:e141. https://doi.org/10.1371/journal.pmed.0020141

Samara MT, Leucht C, Leeflang MM, Anghelescu I-G, Chung Y-C, Crespo-Facorro B, Elkis H, Hatta K, Giegling I, Kane JM, Kayo M, Lambert M, Lin C-H, Moller H-J, Pelayo-Teran JM, Riedel M, Rujescu D, Schimmelmann BG, Serretti A, Correll CU, Leucht S (2015) Early improvement as a predictor of later response to antipsychotics in schizophrenia: a diagnostic test review. Am J Psychiatry 172:617–629

Sautter FJ, Brailey K, Uddo MM, Hamilton MF, Beard MG, Borges AH (1999) PTSD and comorbid psychotic disorder: comparison with veterans diagnosed with PTSD or psychotic disorder. J Traum Stress 12:73–88

Seppi K, Weintraub D, Coelho M, Perez-Lloret S, Fox SH, Katzenschlager R, Hametner E-M, Poewe W, Rascol O, Goetz CG, Sampaio C (2011) The *Movement* Disorder Society evidence-based medicine review update: treatments for the non-motor symptoms of Parkinson's disease. Mov Disord 26(suppl 3):S42–S80

Sernyak MJ (2007) Implementation of monitoring and management guidelines for second-generation antipsychotics. J Clin Psychiatry 68(suppl 4):14–18

Shean GD (2009) Evidence-based psychosocial practices and recovery from schizophrenia. Psychiatry 72:307–320

Siskind D, McCartney L, Goldschlager R, Kisely S (2016) Clozapine v. first- and second-generation antipsychotics in treatment-refractory schizophrenia: systematic review and meta-analysis. Br J Psychiatry. e-pub ahead of print 1–8. https://doi.org/10.1192/bjp.bp.115.177261

Stephane M, Thuras P, Nasrallah H, Georgopoulos AP (2003) The internal structure of the phenomenology of auditory verbal hallucinations. Schizophr Res 61:185–193

Strauss JJ, Calhoun PS, Marx CE, Stechuchak KM, Oddone EZ, Swartz MS, Butterfield MI (2006) Comorbid posttraumatic stress disorder is associated with suicidality in male veterans with schizophrenia or schizoaffective disorder. Schizophr Res 84:165–169

Sun FF, Stock EM, Copeland LA, Zeber JE, Ahmedani BK, Morissette SB (2014) Polypharmacy with antipsychotic drugs in patients with schizophrenia: trends in multiple health care systems. Am J Health Syst Pharm 71:728–738

Suzuki T, Remington G, Mulsant BH, Uchida H, Rajji TK, Graff-Guerrero A, Mimura M, Mamo DC (2012) Defining treatment-resistant schizophrenia and response to antipsychotics: a review and recommendation. Psychiatry Res 197:1–6

Takeuchi H, Suzuki T, Uchida H, Watanabe K, Mimura M (2012) Antipsychotic treatment for schizophrenia in the maintenance phase: a systematic review of the guidelines and algorithms. Schizophr Res 134:219–225

Taylor DM, Smith L, Gee SH, Nielsen J (2012) Augmentation of clozapine with a second antipsychotic – a meta-analysis. Acta Psychiatr Scand 125:15–24

Teh CF, Kilbourne AM, McCarthy JF, Welsh D, Blow FC (2008) Gender differences in health-related quality of life for veterans with serious mental illness. Psychiatr Serv 59:663–669

Tranulis C, Mouaffak F, Chouchana L, Stip E, Gourevitch R, Poirier MF, Olié J-P, Lôo H, Gourion D (2006) Somatic augmentation strategies in clozapine resistance – what facts? Clin Neuropharmacol 29:34–44

Tsuang MT, Tohen M (2002) Textbook in psychiatric epidemiology, 2nd edn. Wiley-Liss. Chapter 15, New York, pp 365–387

U.S. Food and Drug Administration (2015) FDA drug safety communication: FDA modifies monitoring for neutropenia associated with schizophrenia medicine clozapine; approves new shared REMS program for all clozapine medicines (Sept. 15). http://www.fda.gov/Drugs/DrugSafety/ucm461853.htm

Uchida H, Suzuki T, Takeuchi H, Arenovich T, Mamo DC (2011) Low dose vs. standard dose of antipsychotics for relapse prevention in schizophrenia: meta-analysis. Schizophr Bull 37:788–799

Veterans Health Administration (2014) VHA handbook 1140.01: community residential care program. Available at: http://www.va.gov/vhapublications/publications.cfm?pub=2&order=asc&orderby=pub_Number

Villareal G, Hamner MB, Canive JM, Robert S, Calais LA, Durklaski V, Zhai Y, Qualis C (2016) Efficacy of quetiapine monotherapy in posttraumatic stress disorder: a randomized, placebo-controlled trial. Am J Psychiatry., (AJP in Advance). e-pub ahead of print. https://doi.org/10.1176/appi.ajp.2016.15070967

Walker E, Mittal V, Tessner K (2008) Stress and the hypothalamic pituitary adrenal axis in the developmental course of schizophrenia. Ann Rev Clin Psychol 4:189–216

Warnez S, Alessi-Severini S (2014) Clozapine: a review of clinical practice guidelines and prescribing trends. BMC Psychiatry 14:102

Watkins KE, Smith B, Akincigil A, Sorbero ME, Paddock S, Woodroffe A, Huang C, Crystal S, Pincus HA (2016) The quality of medication treatment for mental disorders in the Department of Veterans Affairs and in private-sector plans. Psychiatr Serv 67:391–396

Weissman EM (2002) Antipsychotic prescribing practices in the Veterans Healthcare Administration – New York metropolitan region. Schizophr Bull 28:31–42

Williams T, Purvis TL (2012) Development of an outpatient pharmacist-managed clozapine clinic. Am J Health Syst Pharm 69:1192–1195

Wilson ALG, Messer SC, Hoge CW (2009) U.S. military mental health care utilization and attrition prior to the wars in Iraq and Afghanistan. Soc Psychiatry Psychiatr Epidemiol 44:473–481

World Health Organization (2016) International Statistical Classification of Diseases and Related Health Problems, 10th Revision (ICD-10). Chapter V: "Mental and behavioral disorders", F20–F29 "Schizophrenia, schizotypal and delusional disorders"

Yee CM, Javitt DC, Miller GA (2015) Replacing DSM categorical analyses with dimensional analyses in psychiatry research: the research domain criteria initiative. JAMA Psychiatr 72:1159–1160

Yung AR, Phillips LJ, Yuen HP, Francey SM, McFarlane CA, Hallgren M, McGorry PD (2003) Psychosis prediction: 12-month follow up of a high-risk ("prodromal") group. Schizophr Res 60:21–32

Yusufi B, Mukherjee S, Flanagan R, Paton C, Dunn G, Page E, Barnes TRE (2007) Prevalence and nature of side effects during clozapine maintenance treatment and the relationship with clozapine dose and plasma concentration. Int Clin Psychopharmacol 22:238–243

22 Mental Health of the Older Veteran

Aazaz Ul Haq and Laura B. Dunn

The Aging of the Veteran Population

As the nation's 4.4 million World War II and Korean War veterans enter their 90s and the 7.5 million Vietnam War veterans enter their mid-60s and 70s, the majority of US veterans are now elderly (United States Department of Veterans Affairs n.d.). In 2013, there were 12.2 million veterans above age 60 in the United States, comprising 55% of the veteran population (United States Department of Veterans Affairs n.d.). However, unlike the civilian elderly population, for which a significant increase in number is expected in the coming decades, the elderly veteran population is projected to decrease to 10.9 million by 2023 and to 7.7 million by 2043, reflecting a trend of decreased number of veterans overall (United States Department of Veterans Affairs n.d.).

The mental health care needs of older veterans are best understood in the context of their generation's unique combination of specific military conflicts and cultural environment. The mass scale of psychiatric illness seen in World War II veterans, who were exposed to combat with greater destructiveness than ever seen before, led the United States Army to adopt the logo, "Every Man Has His Breaking Point" (Marlowe 2000). Postwar investigations of this group's psychiatric symptoms led to the formulation of the first edition of the *Diagnostic and Statistical Manual* (*DSM*) in 1952 (Grob 1991). Vietnam War veterans served while facing an antiwar political climate at home and a burgeoning drug epidemic in both Vietnam and the United States, unique challenges that predecessors from previous wars had not faced, and many bear ongoing scars from these experiences (Marlowe 2000). Lessons learned from these veterans about post-traumatic stress disorder (PTSD), substance abuse, and the importance of postwar societal integration will prove valuable as the veterans of more recent conflicts, such as those in Iraq and Afghanistan, age in the coming decades (Katz 2014).

Older veterans face psychiatric issues similar to those faced by the general population, including depression, neurocognitive disorders, and PTSD, but they have unique mental health care needs that require special considerations. Their older age confers greater frailty, medical and neuropsychiatric comorbidity, and unique psychosocial challenges, such as loss of spouses, retirement, and increased need for assistance with activities of daily living. Their veteran status confers a greater likelihood of the presence of certain mental illnesses, such as PTSD and

A.U. Haq
VA Palo Alto Healthcare System,
Palo Alto, CA, USA

L.B. Dunn (✉)
Stanford University, Palo Alto, CA, USA
e-mail: Laura.dunn@stanford.edu

L.W. Roberts, C.H. Warner (eds.), *Military and Veteran Mental Health*,
https://doi.org/10.1007/978-1-4939-7438-2_22

traumatic brain injury (TBI), and requires the clinician to carefully understand their particular military service experience. This chapter will discuss some considerations that should be kept in mind in the care of this unique population.

Case Study

Major (ret.) Joseph Allister (pseudonym) is a 64-year-old Vietnam War army veteran who is referred to the geriatric psychiatry clinic with a 6-month history of low mood, social withdrawal, and a 30-lb weight loss. He has been treated for 4 months with fluoxetine 40 mg daily by his primary care physician without benefit. A medical work-up by his primary care provider for the weight loss has been unrevealing. Major Allister lives alone in a one-bedroom apartment and has been requiring increasing assistance from his son to help with medications, finances, cooking, and groceries. Screening cognitive testing reveals a Montreal Cognitive Assessment (MoCA) score of 22/30, with deficits in executive functioning, complex attention, and memory. His Hamilton Depression Rating Scale (HAM-D) score is 35, indicating severe depression. On exam, he is seen to be rocking back and forth, moaning softly, and wringing his hands. He voices a desire to be dead and fears of being tortured at night. Major Allister is admitted to the inpatient geriatric psychiatry service. A basic lab work-up is unremarkable, and brain imaging shows mild-to-moderate microvascular changes but no other abnormalities. On the inpatient unit, he paces frequently, has disrupted sleep, and requires prompting by nursing staff to eat. Fluoxetine is switched to venlafaxine ER, which is titrated up to 300 mg daily with minimal response. Mirtazapine is added as a combination agent and titrated to 45 mg at bedtime, again with minimal response. Aripiprazole as an augmenting agent is poorly tolerated, and addition of lithium up to 450 mg daily produces no benefit. Major Allister is referred for electroconvulsive therapy. His antidepressant medications are discontinued, and a course of three times per week electroconvulsive therapy is started. He begins to show partial response after four treatments and has complete remission of symptoms after nine treatments, with HAM-D score of nine. With improvement of depression, his MoCA score improves to 28/30. His electroconvulsive therapy course is tapered to discontinuation after 13 treatments, and he is discharged home on venlafaxine XR 150 mg daily and mirtazapine 15 mg at bedtime. Involvement of social work helps him get in-home support services, which helps with household chores. He remains symptom-free when seen at 1-, 4-, and 12-week follow-up appointments in the geriatric psychiatry clinic.

Depression in Older Veterans

Depression in older veterans causes emotional suffering, increases all-cause mortality (Zivin et al. 2015), worsens the outcome of other medical and neuropsychiatric conditions (Byers et al. 2012; Byers and Yaffe 2014; Zivin et al. 2015), and increases risk for suicide (Pukay-Martin et al. 2012; Yi and Hong 2015). Depression in the elderly population is often underdiagnosed and undertreated, particularly in primary care settings (Allan et al. 2014). More than one-third (35.9%) of veterans aged 50+ who are diagnosed with depression over the previous year do not receive treatment with either medications or psychotherapy, and likelihood of being treated decreases with increasing age (Burnett-Zeigler et al. 2012). The presence of low mood, anhedonia, neurovegetative disturbances, psychomotor abnormalities, and/or suicidality in older veterans should trigger a thorough investigation into possibility of depression and discussion of treatment options.

Epidemiology

Depression in elderly veterans is common, but it is not an inevitable part of aging. Studies have reported rates of depressive symptoms in US veterans aged 65+ years of 25.8–31.0% (Selim et al. 2004; Hankin et al. 1999). These rates are comparable to the rate of depressive symptoms in the nonveteran elderly population (25.1–27.0%) (Forlani et al. 2014; Blazer 1987). After controlling for sociodemographic factors, such as age, ethnicity, education, and medical conditions, veteran status by itself is not associated with the presence of elevated depression or anxiety scores (Gould et al. 2015). Nearly 25% of veterans aged 65+ in VA Community Living Centers (CLCs) carry diagnoses of depression, and almost 50% of Community Living Center residents are prescribed an antidepressant (Hanlon et al. 2011).

Older veterans often carry multiple biological risk factors for depression, including comorbid medical and/or neurocognitive illnesses, uncontrolled pain, vascular risk factors, substance abuse, and insomnia (Chang and Chueh 2011). Psychosocial factors also have an important impact on depression. In one sample, 44% of veterans aged 60+ reported feeling lonely at least "some of the time," and 10.4% reported "often" feeling lonely (Kuwert et al. 2014). Other known psychosocial risk factors in the elderly include death of spouse, adverse life events, low socioeconomic status, functional impairment from illness, and nursing home residence (Bruce 2002).

Elderly age is a risk factor for suicide, and suicide rates increase gradually from age 60 until decreasing slightly in 90s (Shah et al. 2016) (Table 22.1). Of a sample of 1962 male US veterans over age 60, 6% reported suicidal ideation over the past week—with rates of 9.2% among combat veterans and 4.0% among noncombat veterans. This study also found that 2.6% of the respondents had attempted suicide in their lifetime, with major depression, PTSD, generalized anxiety disorder (GAD), and physical health difficulties being strong risk factors (Fanning and Pietrzak 2013). Another study of 10,238 Korean veterans from the Vietnam War (mean age 56.3) found that 41 of these men had committed suicide on 7.5-year follow-up, with the strongest risk factors being higher depression severity, very poor health, low education, and past drinking (Yi and Hong 2015).

Table 22.1 Risk and protective factors for suicidal ideation and attempts among older veterans

Risk factors
Combat veteran
Current physical complaints
Current probable major depression
Disability in instrumental activities of daily living (IADLs) or activities of daily living (ADLs)
Generalized anxiety disorder
Lifetime alcohol use disorder
Lifetime trauma exposure
Post-traumatic stress disorder (PTSD)
Protective factors
Conscientiousness
Curiosity
Emotional stability
Emotional/instrumental social support
Secure attachment
Sense of purpose
Social connectedness

References: Fanning and Pietrzak (2013) and Conwell et al. (2010)

Assessment

Screening tools for late-life depression, such as the Geriatric Depression Scale (GDS) (Yesavage et al. 1982), Patient Health Questionnaire (PHQ-9) (Kroenke et al. 2001), Cornell Scale for Dementia in Depression (Alexopoulos et al. 1988), and the Center for Epidemiologic Studies-Depression (CES-D) Scale (Radloff 1977), can be useful for detecting depression in older adults and monitoring treatment progress. As highlighted in Table 22.2, when depression is suspected in an elderly veteran, a thorough assessment should be conducted, including assessing past psychiatric history, substance and medication use, cognitive status, general health status and medical comorbidities, functional status, social functioning, and nutritional status. Screening labs (complete blood count, basic metabolic panel, urinalysis, thyroid testing, and vitamin B12/folate levels) should be obtained.

Table 22.2 Assessment of depression in the older veteran

Screening tests
Geriatric Depression Screen (GDS)
Patient Health Questionnaire (PHQ-9)
Cornell Scale for Depression in Dementia
Center for Epidemiologic Studies-Depression (CES-D) Scale
History
Past psychiatric history (previous episodes of depression and mania, previous medication trials, suicide attempts, hospitalizations)
Functional status (instrumental activities of daily living (IADLs) and activities of daily living (ADLs))
Cognitive status, including executive functioning
General medical history
Nutritional status
Social functioning
Family history
Substance and medication use
Labs/imaging
Complete blood count
Basic metabolic panel
Thyroid function tests
Urinalysis
Vitamin B12 and folate
Cholesterol panel
Head CT or MRI (if prominent cognitive deficits or atypical presentation)

Brain imaging (head CT or brain MRI) is not obtained routinely but should be considered if cognitive deficits are prominent, the patient is experiencing a first episode of depression, or the presentation is atypical.

Etiology/Mechanisms of Disease

Depression with first onset after age 60 is termed late-onset depression (LOD). Late-onset depression is more typically associated with accumulation of microvascular lesions in the frontal cortical-subcortical circuits ("vascular depression") (Hwang et al. 2010). Compared to early-onset depression (EOD), late-onset depression is associated with higher medical comorbidity, more prominent cognitive features, longer hospital stays, more residual symptoms at discharge, more frequent relapses, and negative family and past psychiatric histories (Conwell et al. 1989; Alexopoulos et al. 1988).

Psychotic depression in elderly adults is often present with particularly severe depressive symptoms, more psychomotor disturbance, more guilt preoccupation, worse prognosis, and more severe executive dysfunction (Gournellis et al. 2014). Catatonic features of stupor, mutism, and psychomotor retardation can accompany depression and may be misdiagnosed as advanced dementia (Fink and Taylor 2006). The presence of psychotic and/or catatonic features should prompt inpatient hospitalization and early consideration of electroconvulsive therapy.

Interventions

Psychopharmacology Antidepressants are efficacious for depression in the elderly (Tedeschini et al. 2011). Medications should be started at lower dosages than for younger patients, but full therapeutic dosages are often needed to achieve complete remission. Monotherapy is preferred, although augmentation with lithium, bupropion, or nortriptyline can be beneficial in treatment-resistant patients (Dew et al. 2007). Selective serotonin reuptake inhibitors (SSRIs) are considered first-line because of a favorable side effect profile, although serotonin/norepinephrine reuptake inhibitors (SNRIs), mirtazapine, bupropion, and tricyclic antidepressants can be used safely in the elderly population, with appropriate precautions.

Psychotherapy Psychotherapy has been shown to be effective in depressed elderly patients, particularly those with subthreshold depressive symptoms (Lee et al. 2012; Huang et al. 2014). In elderly veterans, several types of psychotherapies have been examined for efficacy in alleviating depressive symptoms, including cognitive behavioral therapy (Karlin et al. 2015), acceptance and commitment therapy (Karlin et al. 2013), problem-solving therapy (Kasckow et al. 2014), and group reminiscence therapy (Chueh and Chang 2014). While preliminary data are promising, larger studies are needed that are appropriately powered to evaluate for subgroup differences and for mediators of effects.

Electroconvulsive Therapy Electroconvulsive therapy (ECT) remains the most effective and rapid treatment for depression in the elderly and should be considered early for patients with psychotic features, catatonia, high suicidality, or treatment resistance (Kerner and Prudic 2014). Electroconvulsive therapy can also be particularly useful in the elderly population who may have difficulty tolerating medication side effects. In severely depressed older patients, neurocognitive performance often improves or does not change after ECT (Verwijk et al. 2014), although mild neurocognitive impairments in the acute post-ECT phase have been documented in a minority of patients (Dybedal et al. 2014). However, electroconvulsive therapy remains underutilized in the VA system nationwide. Of the 187,811 patients diagnosed with major depression in the VA between 1999 and 2004, only 307 (0.16%) received ECT (Pfeiffer et al. 2011).

Implications for the Future

Depression is not a normal part of aging in veterans. Efforts are needed to improve detection and treatment of depression in primary care settings, where up to 80% of cases of depression are seen (Kessler et al. 2010), to increase the number of mental health care providers focused on the elderly veteran population, and to increase the funding of research into the treatment of depression in this unique population.

Neurocognitive Disorders in Elderly Veterans

Neurocognitive disorders (NCDs) in elderly veterans are a major public health concern. There are currently more than 500,000 veterans in the United States with Alzheimer's disease (Sibener et al. 2014), and this number is expected to rise significantly in the coming decades with the aging of the veteran population. Among all patients above age 65 seen in the VA Healthcare System, major neurocognitive disorder (dementia) prevalence of 7.3% (5.8–9.4% across Veterans Integrated Service Networks) has been reported, and these rates were 50% higher among African Americans (Krishnan et al. 2005). Veterans with major neurocognitive disorder have greater inpatient service utilization and more outpatient visits (Krishnan et al. 2005), and major neurocognitive disorder contributes significantly to functional disability and health-care costs.

Epidemiology

There is now robust evidence for the role of a number of important factors, possibly specific to veterans, that increase the risk of developing major neurocognitive disorder (Sibener et al. 2014). Veterans with a history of traumatic brain injury (TBI) had a 1.6 times increased risk of major neurocognitive disorder over 9 years of follow-up compared to those without a history of TBI. Moreover, patients with TBI experience onset of major neurocognitive disorder an average of 2 years earlier than patients without TBI (Gardner et al. 2014). Additionally, posttraumatic stress disorder (PTSD) was shown to be associated with a 1.8 times increased risk of major neurocognitive disorder over 7 years of follow-up in a sample of older veterans (Yaffe et al. 2010). Consistent with the literature in the general older adult population, depression and/or dysthymia was associated with a 2.4 times higher risk of major neurocognitive disorder in older veterans over a 7-year follow-up (Byers et al. 2012).

Proposed mechanisms connecting depression with increased risk of major neurocognitive disorder among older veterans include the association of depression with increased vascular risk factors, changes in glucocorticoid steroids and hippocampal atrophy, increased deposition of amyloid plaques, inflammatory changes, and alteration of neurotrophic factors (Byers and Yaffe 2014).

Lifestyle and health-related risk factors for neurocognitive disorder, including vascular risk factors (i.e., diabetes, obesity, hypercholesterolemia, hypertension), tobacco and alcohol use, physical inactivity, and sleep disturbances, are also often increased in elderly veterans and contribute to cognitive decline (Yaffe et al. 2014; Veitch et al. 2013).

Diagnosis

The *DSM-5* introduced some significant changes in the conceptualization of neurocognitive disorders from its predecessors. For the first time, it defined six cognitive domains, i.e., complex attention, memory, executive functioning, perceptual-motor, language, and social cognition. Further, the new manual specifies that a deficit in any one or more of these domains is sufficient to meet criteria for neurocognitive disorders. This change reflects a movement to deprioritize the importance memory impairment as a requirement to diagnose neurocognitive disorder.

The *DSM-5* formalizes the concept of mild cognitive impairment (MCI) into mild neurocognitive disorder (mild NCD). Mild neurocognitive disorder is diagnosed when cognitive deficits are present but do not impair independent functioning in the instrumental activities of daily living (IADLs), such as management of finances and medications, cooking, cleaning, grocery shopping, and driving (Table 22.3). As improved neuroimaging and biomarker research promise earlier diagnosis of some type of neurocognitive disorders in the coming decades, this category is intended to allow for earlier counseling and treatment of patients who previously were not formally diagnosed (Blazer 2013), although there is also concern for a greater number of false positives. In a study of 131 veterans with mean age 74.8 ± 6.5 with "cognitive impairment, not dementia" (CIND)—a diagnosis analogous to minor neurocognitive disorder—16 (12%) progressed to major neurocognitive disorder; 88 (67%) remained stable with a diagnosis of "cognitive impairment, not dementia"; and 27 (21%) improved to normal cognition (Holsinger et al. 2015).

When cognitive impairment is severe enough to require assistance with one or more instrumental activities of daily living (IADLS), major neurocognitive disorder is diagnosed. When major neurocognitive disorder is mild in severity, only IADLs are affected. As the disorder progresses to a moderate stage, independent functioning in more basic activities of daily living (ADLs), such as bathing, dressing, ambulating, toileting, transfers, and feeding, becomes affected. At the severe stages, the patient is completely dependent on others for all aspects of functioning. Major neurocognitive disorder can be accompanied by behavioral disturbances, such as agitation, aggression, care refusal, wandering, vocalizations, or apathy, which can present management challenges to caregivers.

Etiology

Neurocognitive disorders in elderly veterans can be due to a variety of etiologies, and more than one etiology are often simultaneously present. The most common cause of neurocognitive disorder among veterans is Alzheimer's disease (Krishnan et al. 2005), which causes progressive impairment in multiple cognitive domains, often most prominently in memory. Neurocognitive disorder due to cerebrovascular disease, either in the form of single or multiple major strokes or cumulative microvascular disease, is also common in veterans. Traumatic brain injury (TBI), particularly due to blast or penetrating trauma, is another major issue in veterans, and history of TBI is associated with increased risk of major neurocognitive disorder later in life (Barnes et al. 2014). Veterans who have evidence of repeated trauma during their time in their service often have evidence of chronic traumatic encephalopathy (CTE), with personality and behavioral changes, as well as executive function and memory deficits that progress slowly over decades (McKee and Robinson 2014). Data specific to older veterans regarding neurocognitive disorder due to other causes (e.g., frontotemporal lobar degeneration, Lewy body disease, Parkinson's disease, Huntington disease, substance use, HIV infection, and other medical conditions) is lacking, but these should be considered in the differential diagnosis of cognitive decline. A careful work-up, including careful mental status and

Table 22.3 Evaluation of the older veteran with cognitive impairment

Screening tests
Mini Mental Status Exam (MMSE)
Montreal Cognitive Assessment (MoCA)
Frontal Assessment Battery (FAB)
The Executive Interview (EXIT-25)
Mini-Cog
General Practitioner Assessment of Cognition (GPCOG)
Memory Impairment Screen (MIS)
Clock-Drawing Test (CDT)
History
Recent memory changes (i.e., forgetting recent events or conversations; word-finding difficulties)
Recent executive functioning changes (i.e., problems with judgment, difficulty handling everyday arithmetic problems, difficulty following a story in a book or television)
Functional decline
Instrumental activities of daily living (IADLs): driving, managing finances, managing medications, grocery shopping, cooking, cleaning
Activities of daily living (ADLs): bathing, ambulating, transfers, toileting, changing clothes, eating
Behavioral disturbances (agitation, apathy, non-directed vocalization, aggression, sexual disinhibition, sleep disturbance)
Psychiatric symptoms (depression, psychosis, anxiety)
Nutritional status
Past psychiatric history
Medications and substance use
Past medical and surgical history
Family history of dementia
Psychosocial history
Military history
Labs/studies
Complete blood count
Basic metabolic panel
Vitamin B12 and folate levels
Hgb A1C
Cholesterol panel
HIV test
Thyroid function tests
RPR
Urinalysis
Head CT or brain MRI
PET with amyloid-binding agent such as florbetapir (may be helpful for atypical cases, or if frontotemporal dementia is suspected)

neurological exam, neuropsychological testing, neuroimaging, and lab work-up, should be conducted to differentiate among these etiologies.

Interventions

Nonpharmacologic Interventions All veterans over 60 with risk factors for neurocognitive disorders, such as history of PTSD, TBI, depression, or vascular disease, should be screened for cognitive impairment. Emphasis should be placed on identifying and addressing modifiable healthcare and lifestyle risk factors for cognitive decline. It has been estimated that up to half of all cases of Alzheimer's disease are contributed to by modifiable risk factors, and a 10–25% decrease in the prevalence of seven of these (i.e., diabetes, hypertension, obesity, depression, physical inactivity, smoking, and cognitive inactivity) could prevent 1.1–3.0 million of these cases worldwide (Barnes and Yaffe 2011). Psychosocial and functional challenges should be addressed, and adequate support for caregivers should be sought.

Pharmacologic Interventions for Cognitive Impairment The available medications for cognitive impairment in elderly veterans are used primarily to delay the progression of the symptoms. Studies of cholinesterase inhibitors, such as donepezil, rivastigmine, and galantamine, have shown statistically significant improvement on some measures of cognition and global function with use of these medications, although the clinical significance of these improvements has not been definitively demonstrated (Qaseem et al. 2008). Patients should be monitored for side effects of bradycardia, diarrhea, and nausea with these medications. Similarly, memantine, a glutamate NMDA-receptor antagonist, has been shown to provide statistically significant, but clinically unimportant, improvement in cognition scores in moderate-to-severe Alzheimer's disease, and there is limited evidence that it may improve quality of life, caregiver burden, and resource utilization (Qaseem et al. 2008).

Interventions for Behavioral Symptoms of Dementia In elderly veterans with major neurocognitive disorder, behavioral and psychiatric syndromes that cause distress or interfere with caregiving should be carefully defined, and nonpharmacologic approaches to address them should be tried first. If unsuccessful, pharmacologic approaches can be helpful. However, the smallest effective doses should be used.

Depression is common in patients with major neurocognitive disorder and often responds to standard pharmacologic treatments at low doses (Koenig et al. 2014). Apathy can be targeted with low-dose stimulants, with methylphenidate being the best studied for this indication (Dolder et al. 2010; Rosenberg et al. 2013). Psychotic symptoms and agitation may be targeted with antipsychotics. However, these medications should be used judiciously, given the black box warning regarding the increased risk of stroke and death with the use of these agents in elderly individuals with major neurocognitive disorder. Anticonvulsants, such as valproic acid, carbamazepine, and oxcarbazepine, are sometimes used to target agitation in major neurocognitive disorder, although evidence supporting their use for this indication remains inconclusive, and tolerability concerns remain (Sommer et al. 2009; Lonergan and Luxenberg 2009). Anxiety in major neurocognitive disorder can be targeted with SSRIs or SNRIs, and acute anxiety can be treated with low-dose benzodiazepines. However, benzodiazepines should be used judiciously in this population, for short periods of time and at low doses, due to increased risk of falls, cognitive impairment, and formation of dependence.

Future Directions

Increasingly, research is focused on efforts to diagnose neurocognitive disorders in preclinical or very mild stages. These efforts include the use of cerebrospinal fluid biomarkers, such as tau and amyloid β_{1-42}, and imaging modalities, such as the PET amyloid-binding agents (e.g., florbetapir). However, efforts to halt the progression of neurocognitive disorders have been frustrating so far. While numerous pharmaceutical companies are engaged in trials of monoclonal antibodies that bind soluble amyloid-β peptide, thus far no breakthrough has occurred, despite some encouraging findings (e.g., decreased amyloid plaque deposition). With the influx of veterans returning from the wars in Iraq and Afghanistan—many with multiple risk factors for neurocognitive disorders—ongoing efforts are needed to better understand and manage these conditions.

Post-traumatic Stress Disorder in Older Veterans

Post-traumatic stress disorder (PTSD) was introduced in the *DSM* in 1980. However, the symptoms of post-traumatic stress have been described by military historians and mental health professionals over the past century with a varied constellations of different names, including "soldier's heart," "battle fatigue," "shell shock," and "war psychoneurosis" (Turnbull 1998; Hoge 2015). Since the Vietnam War, and the postwar establishment of community counseling centers for combat veterans, the public has become increasingly aware of the impact of combat-related PTSD on veterans, families, and communities. However, the needs of older veterans with PTSD have received comparatively less attention than those of younger veterans, despite the large number of older veterans with PTSD.

Epidemiology

Although the public is increasingly aware of PTSD and its implications among the younger generations of returning veterans, data from the Veterans Administration indicate that, from 2001 to 2013, a larger number of Vietnam-era veterans were newly diagnosed with PTSD (615,500) compared to veterans from the Persian Gulf, Iraq, and Afghanistan conflicts (400,746) (Smith et al. 2015a, b).

In 1983, Congress mandated a study of PTSD and other psychological sequelae experience by

Vietnam veterans, resulting in the National Vietnam Veterans Readjustment Study (NVVRS). More than 30 years later, Marmar and colleagues conducted a follow-up study, called the National Vietnam Veterans Longitudinal Study (NVVLS), to investigate the longitudinal course of PTSD in a large sample (n = 1450) of surviving National Vietnam Veterans Readjustment Study participants (Marmar et al. 2015). The authors reported prevalence rates of 4.5% for current PTSD diagnosis among men and 6.1% among women based on clinician-rated criteria (10.8% and 8.7%, respectively, when subthreshold PTSD was included) and 11.2% and 6.6% via a self-reported symptom scale. The prevalence of comorbid major depression was 36.7% among those meeting full PTSD criteria and 30.9% among those with subthreshold PTSD. In contrast, comorbidity of alcohol and other drug abuse was low in this sample. These longitudinal prevalence rates were lower than those estimated by the National Vietnam Veterans Readjustment Study (15.2%), which utilized *DSM-II*-R criteria (as opposed to *DSM-5* criteria in the National Vietnam Veterans Longitudinal Study). While methodological differences, including different assessment tools and changes in *DSM* criteria, may account for at least part of this difference, the findings are also consistent with a previous study that reported decreased rates of PTSD over time (i.e., 14 years post-conflict) (Koenen et al. 2003).

PTSD in older veterans is associated with an increased risk of multiple medical comorbidities. A study of cardiovascular disease in veterans 55 and older found that veterans with PTSD had increased risk over an 8-year follow-up period for all four types of vascular disease studied, including myocardial infarction, congestive heart failure, cerebrovascular disease, and peripheral vascular disease, even after adjusting for demographic factors, as well as medical, substance use, and psychiatric comorbidities (Beristianos et al. 2014). Similarly, World War II prisoners of war with PTSD, compared to those without PTSD, were also found to have a higher likelihood of both cardiovascular disease and hypertension (Kang et al. 2006). Other studies have found that, among older veterans, current and lifetime PTSD were associated with a greater likelihood of being overweight or obese (Smith et al. 2015; in press).

Etiology

The neurobiological underpinnings of PTSD remain an active area of investigation. While much of the work conducted to date has focused on the role of stress hormones, genetic factors, and, more recently, epigenetic changes that may contribute to PTSD, relatively scant research has focused on the etiopathology of PTSD in older veterans, including identifying biological correlates and predictors of varying trajectories of PTSD symptoms over time.

A great deal of research has focused on the role of the hypothalamic-pituitary-adrenal axis in the development of PTSD. In this model, PTSD represents a hyperactive stress response, the classic "fight or flight" response, in which a stressful situation leads to the release of the corticotropin-releasing hormone (CRH) from the hypothalamus, in turn signaling the release of adrenocorticotropic hormone (ACTH) from the pituitary gland, which is followed by the release of glucocorticoids from the adrenal glands. However, subsequent work challenged this notion as conflicting findings emerged regarding cortisol levels in individuals with or without PTSD (Pizzimenti and Lattal 2015).

More recently, researchers have focused on brain circuits and epigenetic mediators of stress responses (Pizzimenti and Lattal 2015). Epigenetic modifications refer to stable changes to DNA (e.g., DNA methylation) that lead to changes in gene expression. This work, by demonstrating that even delayed activation of implicated circuits can contribute to anxiety and fear responses, is helpful in thinking clinically about older veterans with PTSD. Furthermore, a better understanding of fear circuitry and epigenetic modifications related to PTSD may eventually lead to improved treatments targeting these mechanisms.

Diagnosis

As the *DSM* has evolved through numerous iterations, the diagnosis of PTSD has also evolved. The most recent iteration, *DSM-5*, includes several major changes from *DSM-IV*. First, PTSD is now no longer classified as an anxiety disorder but is instead has been reclassified as a trauma- and stressor-related disorder. Whereas in *DSM-IV*, Criterion A (the stressor criterion) did not require specification of whether the traumatic event was experienced directly, experienced indirectly, or witnessed, *DSM-5* now requires this specification. Military personnel—even those who did not serve in combat directly—who witnessed traumatic events or graphic scenes may meet this criterion.

In addition, the *DSM-IV* subjective response criterion ("the person's response involved intense fear, helplessness, or horror") has been removed in *DSM-5*. It is possible that, particularly for older veterans who may not have reacted with fear or considered their exposure "traumatic," the removal of this criterion may result in greater rates of diagnosis, although this remains to be shown empirically. Moreover, while *DSM-IV* delineated three major symptom clusters (re-experiencing, avoidance/numbing, and arousal), *DSM-5* now includes four symptom clusters, based on recent studies that used factor analytic methods (Elhai and Palmieri 2011). Specifically, the avoidance/numbing cluster has now been divided into two categories—avoidance and persistent negative changes in cognitions and mood. These changes may be particularly relevant for older patients with PTSD, as older male veterans with PTSD tend to rate their numbing symptoms lower than younger veterans, whereas older female veterans were rated by clinicians as having significantly lower hyperarousal symptom severity (Lunney et al.). Thus, with the DSM-5 change in PTSD clusters, it will be crucial to examine the effects of these new clusters on both clinician and self-reported symptoms in older vs. younger veterans and in both men and women.

Accurate diagnosis is crucial for appropriate treatment in older veterans, even decades after traumatic events. In older veterans, the assessment of PTSD may be more challenging for a number of reasons (willingness to disclose, cognitive and sensory changes, and medical and psychiatric comorbidity), and the pattern of symptoms may be different (Lunney et al. 2014; Frueh et al. 2004). Several studies have shown that clinicians tend to rate older veterans' overall symptom severity lower than younger veterans (Lunney et al. 2014; Frueh et al. 2004), whereas older patients' self-rated symptom severity only differed (in one study) in terms of only one symptom (numbing) (Lunney et al. 2014). Lunney and colleagues suggested that these findings, taken together with those of other researchers, indicate that clinicians may underdiagnose PTSD symptoms particularly in older veterans.

Treatment

A recent study of the types of treatment received by older veterans with PTSD sheds light on the landscape of treatment of older veterans with PTSD. Based on a large VA database of administrative and pharmacy data on veterans 50 years or older who received a new diagnosis of PTSD between 2008 and 2011, Smith and colleagues (2015) reported that the majority (74%) of these veterans had at least one follow-up mental health visit after the PTSD diagnosis. However, increased age (those ages 65–79, as well as those 80 or older) was associated with lower likelihood of receiving mental health services, as well as lower likelihood of receiving combined pharmacotherapy and psychotherapy and longer wait times. Those veterans with PTSD who also had a comorbid mood or anxiety disorder were more likely to receive mental health treatment. The study did not examine the specific types of psychotherapy received by the sample. Nevertheless, these findings raise concerns about access to appropriate care and appropriateness of care and follow-up for PTSD among older veterans, particularly with increased age. These findings could reflect a lack of availability of geriatric mental health practitioners equipped to work with the older adult population, although that possibility was not explicitly investigated. Other barriers to receipt of care include geographic constraints, as well as functional limitations, particularly in those with medical comorbidities.

The gold standard for treatment of PTSD in the veteran population remains the combination of biological and psychological therapies. However, whether (and which) combination therapies are effective in older veterans with PTSD needs further study. In addition, specific forms of PTSD-focused psychotherapies (e.g., prolonged exposure therapy) have only recently begun to be studied for effectiveness in older veterans (Thorp et al. 2012).

In terms of pharmacotherapy for older veterans with PTSD, first-line therapies include SSRIs and SNRIs (Bernardy and Friedman 2015). Evidence regarding efficacy of these medications suggests that older veterans may not have as robust a response as younger veterans to these medications. However, findings are conflicting and may be confounded by cohort or conflict-specific effects (e.g., Vietnam-era veterans have been more treatment-resistant than younger veterans) (Bernardy and Friedman 2015). Benzodiazepines, in contrast, have not been shown to be effective for PTSD and are considered relatively contraindicated, particularly in older adults.

Additional pharmacologic treatments—often considered second-line, yet frequently used in real-world settings as part of combination strategies—include prazosin and atypical antipsychotic agents. Prazosin, an alpha-1 receptor blocker that is particularly helpful for recurrent nightmares, may increase total sleep and REM sleep time and may reduce alcohol cravings in those with alcohol use disorders (Writer et al. 2014). While the use of prazosin for PTSD remains off-label, encouraging findings thus far suggest it may be an effective adjunctive treatment particularly for patients with chronic PTSD or those who may seem treatment-resistant. Given the risk of orthostatic hypotension with prazosin, it should be used with caution in the elderly and titrated slowly, particularly when used with other medications with vasodilating properties (e.g., phosphodiesterase-5 inhibitors such as sildenafil).

Antipsychotics have some evidence of efficacy as augmenting agents for the treatment of PTSD, although their use for this indication remains off-label. Recent meta-analyses reported that atypical antipsychotics may be effective for PTSD symptoms, particularly intrusion and possibly hyperarousal and hypervigilance, although the number of studies and sample sizes have been small (Han et al. 2014).

General principles of geriatric pharmacotherapy, including use of lower dosage and slower titration, attention to polypharmacy and medicine interactions, awareness of comorbid medical conditions that may complicate therapy, and caution regarding side effects more common in older adults, such as delirium and falls, should be followed carefully in treating older veterans with PTSD.

Future Directions

Numerous important research questions regarding PTSD in older veterans warrant further study. These include the needs to (1) identify distinct trajectories of PTSD (and unique clusters of PTSD symptoms) among veterans over time; (2) evaluate the correlates and consequences of these symptom trajectories among older veterans, including effects on cognition and on specific domains of physical and psychological functioning and quality of life; (3) examine the biological mechanisms (e.g., genetic, epigenetic, and neural circuitry) mediating response to stress in older veterans; (4) identify and evaluate novel treatments for both newly emergent and chronic forms of PTSD in older veterans; and (5) understand and address the common comorbid medical and psychiatric conditions in older veterans in PTSD.

Conclusions

Old age in veterans is not synonymous with disease. Over 80% of veterans aged 60–96 reported in the National Health and Resilience in Veterans Study that they felt they were aging successfully (Pietrzak et al. 2014). However, aging does come with increased risk factors for various mental and physical ailments that require ongoing monitoring. Negative predictors of successful aging include substance abuse, physical difficulties, and emotional distress, while protective factors include resilience, a purpose in life, an active lifestyle, and social connectedness (Pietrzak et al. 2014). Ongoing research is needed to identify the most effective interventions targeting these factors, examine mediators of effectiveness, and develop optimal ways of engaging older veterans in these efforts.

Key Concepts

1. Depression, though relatively common, is not a normal or inevitable part of aging in veterans.
2. Suicide risk is increased in older veterans, with important risk factors including depression, anxiety, PTSD, combat veteran status, disability, and alcohol use disorders.
3. The numbers of veterans with Alzheimer's disease and other neurocognitive disorders (NCDs) is large and increasing, with higher prevalence rates among African Americans.
4. Veterans with major neurocognitive disorder have greater inpatient and outpatient service utilization, as well as greater functional disability.
5. PTSD in older veterans is associated with an increased risk of multiple medical comorbidities.
6. The gold standard treatment of PTSD is the combination of biological treatment (pharmacotherapy) and psychological therapies; however, further research is needed regarding which combinations are effective in older veterans with PTSD.

References

Alexopoulos GS, Young RC, Meyers BS, Abrams RC, Shamoian CA (1988) Late-onset depression. Psychiatr Clin North Am 11(1):101–115

Allan CE, Valkanova V, Ebmeier KP (2014) Depression in older people is underdiagnosed. Practitioner 258(1771):19–22. 12-13

Barnes DE, Yaffe K (2011) The projected effect of risk factor reduction on Alzheimer's disease prevalence. Lancet Neurol 10(9):819–828

Barnes DE, Kaup A, Kirby KA, Byers AL, Diaz-Arrastia R, Yaffe K (2014) Traumatic brain injury and risk of dementia in older veterans. Neurology 83(4):312–319

Beristianos MH, Yaffe K, Cohen B, Byers AL (2014) PTSD and risk of incident cardiovascular disease in aging veterans. Am J Geriatr Psychiatry 24:192

Bernardy NC, Friedman MJ (2015) Psychopharmacological strategies in the management of posttraumatic stress disorder (PTSD): what have we learned? Curr Psychiatry Rep 17(4):564

Blazer D, Hughes DC, George LK. The epidemiology of depression in an elderly community population. Gerontologist. 1987;27(3):281–7

Blazer D (2013) Neurocognitive disorders in DSM-5. Am J Psychiatry 170(6):585–587

Bruce ML (2002) Psychosocial risk factors for depressive disorders in late life. Biol Psychiatry. 52(3):175–84

Burnett-Zeigler I, Zivin K, Ilgen M, Szymanski B, Blow FC, Kales HC (2012) Depression treatment in older adult veterans. Am J Geriatr Psychiatry 20(3):228–238

Byers AL, Yaffe K (2014) Depression and dementias among military veterans. Alzheimers Dement 10(3 Suppl):S166–S173

Byers AL, Covinsky KE, Barnes DE, Yaffe K (2012) Dysthymia and depression increase risk of dementia and mortality among older veterans. Am J Geriatr Psychiatry 20(8):664–672

Chang TY, Chueh KH (2011) Relationship between elderly depression and health status in male veterans. J Nurs Res 19(4):298–304

Chueh KH, Chang TY (2014) Effectiveness of group reminiscence therapy for depressive symptoms in male veterans: 6-month follow-up. Int J Geriatr Psychiatry 29(4):377–383

Conwell Y, Nelson JC, Kim KM, Mazure CM (1989) Depression in late life: age of onset as marker of a subtype. J Affect Disord 17(2):189–195

Conwell Y, Duberstein PR, Hirsch JK, Conner KR, Eberly S, Caine ED (2010) Health status and suicide in the second half of life. Int J Geriatr Psychiatry 25(4):371–379

Dew MA, Whyte EM, Lenze EJ, Houck PR, Mulsant BH, Pollock BG, Stack JA, Bensasi S, Reynolds CF 3rd (2007) Recovery from major depression in older adults receiving augmentation of antidepressant pharmacotherapy. Am J Psychiatry 164(6):892–899

Dolder CR, Davis LN, McKinsey J (2010) Use of psychostimulants in patients with dementia. Ann Pharmacother 44(10):1624–1632

Dybedal GS, Tanum L, Sundet K, Gaarden TL, Bjolseth TM (2014) Cognitive side-effects of electroconvulsive therapy in elderly depressed patients. Clin Neuropsychol 28(7):1071–1090

Elhai JD, Palmieri PA (2011) The factor structure of posttraumatic stress disorder: a literature update, critique of methodology, and agenda for future research. J Anxiety Disord 25(6):849–854

Fanning JR, Pietrzak RH (2013) Suicidality among older male veterans in the United States: results from the National Health and Resilience in Veterans Study. J Psychiatr Res 47(11):1766–1775

Fink M, Taylor MA (2006) Catatonia: a Clinician's guide to diagnosis and treatment. Cambridge University Press, New York

Forlani C, Morri M, Ferrari B, Dalmonte E, Menchetti M, De Ronchi D, Atti AR (2014) Prevalence and gender differences in late-life depression: a population-based study. Am J Geriatr Psychiatry. 22(4):370–80

Frueh BC, Elhai JD, Hamner MB, Magruder KM, Sauvageot JA, Mintzer J (2004) Elderly veterans with combat-related posttraumatic stress disorder in specialty care. J Nerv Ment Dis 192(1):75–79

Gardner RC, Burke JF, Nettiksimmons J, Kaup A, Barnes DE, Yaffe K (2014) Dementia risk after traumatic brain injury vs nonbrain trauma: the role of age and severity. JAMA Neurol 71(12):1490–1497

Gould CE, Rideaux T, Spira AP, Beaudreau SA (2015) Depression and anxiety symptoms in male veterans and non-veterans: the Health and Retirement Study. Int J Geriatr Psychiatry 30(6):623–630

Gournellis R, Oulis P, Howard R (2014) Psychotic major depression in older people: a systematic review. Int J Geriatr Psychiatry 29(8):789–796

Green B (2014) Prazosin in the treatment of PTSD. J Psychiatr Pract 20(4):253–259

Grob GN (1991) Origins of DSM-I: a study in appearance and reality. Am J Psychiatry 148(4):421–431

Han C, Pae CU, Wang SM, Lee SJ, Patkar AA, Masand PS, Serretti A (2014) The potential role of atypical antipsychotics for the treatment of posttraumatic stress disorder. J Psychiatr Res 56:72–81

Hankin CS, Spiro A 3rd, Miller DR, Kazis L (1999) Mental disorders and mental health treatment among U.S. Department of Veterans Affairs outpatients: the Veterans Health Study. Am J Psychiatry 156(12):1924–1930

Hanlon JT, Wang X, Castle NG, Stone RA, Handler SM, Semla TP, Pugh MJ, Berlowitz DR, Dysken MW (2011) Potential underuse, overuse, and inappropriate use of antidepressants in older veteran nursing home residents. J Am Geriatr Soc 59(8):1412–1420

Hoge CW (2015) Measuring the long-term impact of war-zone military service across generations and changing posttraumatic stress disorder definitions. JAMA Psychiatry 72:861

Holsinger T, Plassman BL, Stechuchak KM, Burke JR, Coffman CJ, Williams JW Jr (2015) Stability of diagnoses of cognitive impairment, not dementia in a veterans affairs primary care population. J Am Geriatr Soc 63(6):1105–1111

Huang AX, Delucchi K, Dunn LB, Nelson JC (2014) A systematic review and meta-analysis of psychotherapy for late-life depression. Am J Geriatr Psychiatry 23:261

Hwang JP, Lee TW, Tsai SJ, Chen TJ, Yang CH, Lirng JF, Tsai CF (2010) Cortical and subcortical abnormalities in late-onset depression with history of suicide attempts investigated with MRI and voxel-based morphometry. J Geriatr Psychiatry Neurol 23(3):171–184

Kang HK, Bullman TA, Taylor JW (2006) Risk of selected cardiovascular diseases and posttraumatic stress disorder among former World War II prisoners of war. Ann Epidemiol 16(5):381–386

Karlin BE, Walser RD, Yesavage J, Zhang A, Trockel M, Taylor CB (2013) Effectiveness of acceptance and commitment therapy for depression: comparison among older and younger veterans. Aging Ment Health 17(5):555–563

Karlin BE, Trockel M, Brown GK, Gordienko M, Yesavage J, Taylor CB (2015) Comparison of the effectiveness of cognitive behavioral therapy for depression among older versus younger veterans: results of a national evaluation. J Gerontol B Psychol Sci Soc Sci 70(1):3–12

Kasckow J, Klaus J, Morse J, Oslin D, Luther J, Fox L, Reynolds C, Haas GL (2014) Using problem solving therapy to treat veterans with subsyndromal depression: a pilot study. Int J Geriatr Psychiatry 29(12):1255–1261

Katz IR (2014) Mental health needs of older veterans. Am J Geriatr Psychiatry. 22(6):527–30

Kerner N, Prudic J (2014) Current electroconvulsive therapy practice and research in the geriatric population. Neuropsychiatry (London) 4(1):33–54

Kessler RC, Birnbaum H, Bromet E, Hwang I, Sampson N, Shahly V (2010) Age differences in major depression: results from the National Comorbidity Survey Replication (NCS-R). Psychol Med 40(2):225–237

Koenen KC, Stellman JM, Stellman SD, Sommer JF Jr (2003) Risk factors for course of posttraumatic stress disorder among Vietnam veterans: a 14-year follow-up of American legionnaires. J Consult Clin Psychol 71(6):980–986

Koenig AM, Butters MA, Begley A, Ogbagaber S, Wahed AS, Reynolds CF 3rd (2014) Response to antidepressant medications in late-life depression across the spectrum of cognitive functioning. J Clin Psychiatry 75(2):e100–e107

Krishnan LL, Petersen NJ, Snow AL, Cully JA, Schulz PE, Graham DP, Morgan RO, Braun U, Moffett ML, Yu HJ, Kunik ME (2005) Prevalence of dementia among Veterans Affairs medical care system users. Dement Geriatr Cogn Disord 20(4):245–253

Kroenke K, Spitzer RL, Williams JB (2001) The PHQ-9: validity of a brief depression severity measure. J Gen Intern Med: Off J Soc Res Educ Prim Care Intern Med 16(9):606–613

Kuwert P, Knaevelsrud C, Pietrzak RH (2014) Loneliness among older veterans in the United States: results from the National Health and Resilience in Veterans Study. Am J Geriatr Psychiatry 22(6):564–569

Lee SY, Franchetti MK, Imanbayev A, Gallo JJ, Spira AP, Lee HB (2012) Non-pharmacological prevention of major depression among community-dwelling older adults: a systematic review of the efficacy of psychotherapy interventions. Arch Gerontol Geriatr 55(3):522–529

Lonergan E, Luxenberg J (2009) Valproate preparations for agitation in dementia. Cochrane Database Syst Rev 3:CD003945

Lunney CA, Schnurr PP, Cook JM (2014) Comparison of clinician- and self-assessments of posttraumatic stress symptoms in older versus younger veterans. J Trauma Stress 27(2):144–151

Marmar CR, Schlenger W, Henn-Haase C, Qian M, Purchia E, Li M, Corry N, Williams CS, Ho CL, Horesh D, Karstoft KI, Shalev A, Kulka RA (2015) Course of Posttraumatic Stress Disorder 40 Years After the Vietnam War: Findings From the National Vietnam Veterans Longitudinal Study. JAMA Psychiatry. Sep;72(9):875–81

Marlowe DH (2000) Psychological and psychosocial consequences of combat and deployment with special emphasis on the Gulf War, RAND. Available at: http://www.gulflink.osd.mil/library/randrep/marlowe_paper/index.html

McKee AC, Robinson ME (2014) Military-related traumatic brain injury and neurodegeneration. Alzheimers Dement 10(3 Suppl):S242–S253

Pfeiffer PN, Valenstein M, Hoggatt KJ, Ganoczy D, Maixner D, Miller EM, Zivin K (2011) Electroconvulsive therapy for major depression within the Veterans Health Administration. J Affect Disord 130(1–2):21–25

Pietrzak RH, Tsai J, Kirwin PD, Southwick SM (2014) Successful aging among older veterans in the United States. Am J Geriatr Psychiatry 22(6):551–563

Pizzimenti CL, Lattal KM (2015) Epigenetics and memory: causes, consequences and treatments for post-traumatic stress disorder and addiction. Genes Brain Behav 14(1):73–84

Pukay-Martin ND, Pontoski KE, Maxwell MA, Calhoun PS, Dutton CE, Clancy CP, Hertzberg MA, Collie CF, Beckham JC (2012) The influence of depressive symptoms on suicidal ideation among U.S. Vietnam-era and Afghanistan/Iraq-era veterans with posttraumatic stress disorder. J Trauma Stress 25(5):578–582

Qaseem A, Snow V, Cross JT Jr, Forciea MA, Hopkins R Jr, Shekelle P, Adelman A, Mehr D, Schellhase K, Campos-Outcalt D, Santaguida P, Owens DK, American College of Physicians/American Academy of Family Physicians Panel on D (2008) Current pharmacologic treatment of dementia: a clinical practice guideline from the American College of Physicians and the American Academy of Family Physicians. Ann Intern Med 148(5):370–378

Radloff LS (1977) The CES-D scale: a self-report depression scale for research in the general population. Appl Psychol Measur 1:385–401

Rosenberg PB, Lanctot KL, Drye LT, Herrmann N, Scherer RW, Bachman DL, Mintzer JE, Investigators A (2013) Safety and efficacy of methylphenidate for apathy in Alzheimer's disease: a randomized, placebo-controlled trial. J Clin Psychiatry 74(8):810–816

Selim AJ, Berlowitz DR, Fincke G, Cong Z, Rogers W, Haffer SC, Ren XS, Lee A, Qian SX, Miller DR, Spiro A 3rd, Selim BJ, Kazis LE (2004) The health status of elderly veteran enrollees in the Veterans Health Administration. J Am Geriatr Soc 52(8):1271–1276

Shah A, Bhat R, Zarate-Escudero S, DeLeo D, Erlangsen A (2016) Suicide rates in five-year age-bands after the age of 60 years: the international landscape. Aging Ment Health. 20(2):131–8

Sibener L, Zaganjor I, Snyder HM, Bain LJ, Egge R, Carrillo MC (2014) Alzheimer's disease prevalence, costs, and prevention for military personnel and veterans. Alzheimers Dement 10(3 Suppl):S105–S110

Smith NB, Cook JM, Pietrzak R, Hoff R, Harpaz-Rotem I (2015a) Mental health treatment for older veterans newly diagnosed with PTSD: a national investigation. Am J Geriatr Psychiatry 24:201

Smith BN, Tyzik AL, Neylan TC, Cohen BE (2015b; In press) PTSD and obesity in younger and older veterans: results from the mind your heart study. Psychiatry Res 229: 895

Sommer OH, Aga O, Cvancarova M, Olsen IC, Selbaek G, Engedal K (2009) Effect of oxcarbazepine in the treatment of agitation and aggression in severe dementia. Dement Geriatr Cogn Disord 27(2):155–163

Tedeschini E, Levkovitz Y, Iovieno N, Ameral VE, Nelson JC, Papakostas GI (2011) Efficacy of antidepressants for late-life depression: a meta-analysis and meta-regression of placebo-controlled randomized trials. J Clin Psychiatry 72(12):1660–1668

Thorp SR, Stein MB, Jeste DV, Patterson TL, Wetherell JL (2012) Prolonged exposure therapy for older veterans with posttraumatic stress disorder: a pilot study. Am J Geriatr Psychiatry 20(3):276–280

Turnbull GJ (1998) A review of post-traumatic stress disorder. Part I: historical development and classification. Injury 29(2):87–91

United States Department of Veterans Affairs National Center for Veterans Analysis and Statistics (n.d.)

Veitch DP, Friedl KE, Weiner MW (2013) Military risk factors for cognitive decline, dementia and Alzheimer's disease. Curr Alzheimer Res 10(9):907–930

Verwijk E, Comijs HC, Kok RM, Spaans HP, Tielkes CE, Scherder EJ, Stek ML (2014) Short- and long-term neurocognitive functioning after electroconvulsive therapy in depressed elderly: a prospective naturalistic study. Int Psychogeriatr 26(2):315–324

Writer BW, Meyer EG, Schillerstrom JE (2014) Prazosin for military combat-related PTSD nightmares: a critical review. J Neuropsychiatr Clin Neurosci 26(1):24–33

Yaffe K, Vittinghoff E, Lindquist K, Barnes D, Covinsky KE, Neylan T, Kluse M, Marmar C (2010) Posttraumatic stress disorder and risk of dementia among US veterans. Arch Gen Psychiatry 67(6):608–613

Yaffe K, Hoang TD, Byers AL, Barnes DE, Friedl KE (2014) Lifestyle and health-related risk factors and risk of cognitive aging among older veterans. Alzheimers Dement 10(3 Suppl):S111–S121

Yesavage JA, Brink TL, Rose TL, Lum O, Huang V, Adey M, Leirer VO (1982) Development and validation of a geriatric depression screening scale: a preliminary report. J Psychiatr Res 17(1):37–49

Yi SW, Hong JS (2015) Depressive symptoms and other risk factors predicting suicide in middle-aged men: a prospective cohort study among Korean Vietnam War veterans. Peer J 3:e1071

Zivin K, Yosef M, Miller EM, Valenstein M, Duffy S, Kales HC, Vijan S, Kim HM (2015) Associations between depression and all-cause and cause-specific risk of death: a retrospective cohort study in the Veterans Health Administration. J Psychosom Res 78(4):324–331

Traumatic Brain Injury Among US Service Members, Veterans, and Their Families

23

Treven Pickett, Lillian Stevens, Ajit Pai, and Nicholas Pastorek

Introduction

Traumatic brain injury (TBI) has been defined as "an alteration in brain function, or other evidence of brain pathology, caused by an external cause" (Menon et al. 2010). Given that the vast majority of TBI injuries are considered mild in accordance with established TBI injury severity criteria, this chapter focuses on mild TBI (mTBI), a term used interchangeably with "concussion." For the veteran seeking treatment in this chapter's case study, it would be important for clinicians to consider that the myriad of presenting, distressing symptoms reported may or may not be etiologically related to the mTBI (or history of multiple mTBIs). Regardless of etiology, presenting symptoms should be considered within the veteran's overall psychosocial context and the meaning they attribute to their symptoms.

Case Study

Staff Sergeant (ret.) Jonathan Williams (pseudonym) is a 35-year-old male, honorably discharged service member who recently registered with the Veterans Health Administration and presented to the Primary Care Clinic with a history of multiple mild traumatic brain injury (mTBI) events during deployments to Afghanistan and Iraq. Specifically, he described exposure to three

T. Pickett (✉)
McGuire VA Medical Center, Richmond, VA, USA

Department of Psychology, Virginia Commonwealth University, Richmond, VA, USA

Department of Psychiatry, Virginia Commonwealth University, Richmond, VA, USA

Departments of Physical Medicine and Rehabilitation, Virginia Commonwealth University, Richmond, VA, USA
e-mail: Treven.Pickett@va.gov

L. Stevens, Ph.D.
Department of Psychology, Virginia Commonwealth University, Richmond, VA, USA

Departments of Physical Medicine and Rehabilitation, Virginia Commonwealth University, Richmond, VA, USA

A. Pai
Mental Health Service, Hunter Holmes McGuire Veterans Affairs Medical Center, Richmond, VA, USA

Departments of Physical Medicine and Rehabilitation, Virginia Commonwealth University, Richmond, VA, USA

N. Pastorek
Michael E. DeBakey VA Medical Center, Rehabilitation and Extended Care Line, Baylor College of Medicine, Department of Physical Medicine and Rehabilitation, Houston, TX, USA

L.W. Roberts, C.H. Warner (eds.), *Military and Veteran Mental Health*,
https://doi.org/10.1007/978-1-4939-7438-2_23

detonations of improvised explosive devices (IEDs) during combat situations, following which he felt "dazed and confused," and one detonation after which he experienced positive loss of consciousness and subsequent evacuation to a field medical tent. He reported persisting symptoms including headaches, tinnitus, light sensitivity, and dizziness. Additionally, he reported "panic attacks" and occasional passive suicidal ideation in the context of no history of suicidal gestures or behaviors. He revealed increased alcohol consumption in the evenings, delayed sleep onset, and intermittent awakenings throughout the night secondary to nightmares (resulting in daytime fatigue). He attributed recent marital separation to these aforementioned symptoms and shared a sense of isolation and that he missed his wife, children, and dog. He described generalized "stress" related to financial strain with simultaneous interpersonal conflicts occurring at his job as a store manager, placing his job in jeopardy. He expressed interest in returning to college using GI Bill benefits while simultaneously doubting that he could succeed academically due to cognitive problems with attention and concentration and forgetfulness. He requested medications to relieve headache pain and improve sleep. On screening measures, responses raised concern that history of mTBIs might be contributing to current symptom presentation and for possible diagnosis of posttraumatic stress disorder (PTSD). The primary care physician placed consultations to the Polytrauma Network Site (PNS) program, a specialty interdisciplinary outpatient program that assesses and treats veterans with a history of TBI. Separately, consults were placed to the Mental Health Service given concerns about potential comorbid psychiatric conditions including PTSD, depression, and alcohol abuse.

Phenomenology

What is known to clinicians working with veterans with a history of mTBI sustained in combat situations—but may not be fully appreciated by clinicians working with individuals with predominantly stateside injuries—is that the context of the combat situation matters in a very real way when considering the veteran's later phenomenological experience of emotional and cognitive symptoms. For the veteran, mTBI event(s) and resulting symptoms themselves can take on symbolic meanings and direct associations with the military culture, the deployment process, and/or the deployment or combat environment. As one specific example, a common post-concussive symptom is headache. For the veteran who sustained a mTBI in a life-threatening combat situation where he/she witnessed others in their unit badly injured or dying while simultaneously fearing for their own life, the headache symptom may become strongly associated with that distressing series of memories. The veteran may then try desperately through unconscious and conscious means to avoid headache onset because in so doing he/she would be avoiding the onset of sensory pain (due to headache) and simultaneously the onset of emotional distress (headache-triggering flashbacks of distressing combat situations). From a phenomenological perspective, what may get lost in a bulk of literature concerning combat-related TBI is that, for veterans, the post-concussive symptoms can themselves take on profound symbolic significance. It may be that addressing post-concussive symptoms superficially bypasses many of the less obvious (but powerful) symbolic drivers that may conspire to strengthen post-concussive symptoms over time.

In short, a symptom may represent much more than a symptom to a veteran who has been injured in a military context. The astute clinician may achieve a deeper and more enduring healing relationship with a veteran if he/she is able to empathically inquire about the contextual significance, or symbolic meaning, of a post-concussive symptom(s) for that veteran. For instance, asking

"Does the symptom of headache take on any additional significance for you, in that you are a veteran and the concussion occurred in a combat situation?" In this chapter's case study, the emotional, cognitive, and physical symptoms were occurring at a pivotal life juncture for Staff Sergeant (ret.) Jonathan Williams, wherein he was simultaneously experiencing marital and family separation, financial stress, occupational stress, the feeling of having let down comrades by being injured, and a deep concern about his ability to successfully move forward in light of distressing symptoms and self-doubt.

An additional phenomenological consideration is the relative impact of the presenting post-concussive symptoms and the meaning of these in the context of the family system. To a point, and to the extent that the individual's clinical symptoms begin to interfere with established premorbid family roles, the family system can begin to experience the veteran as physically present while emotionally absent. There is risk that the veteran can become so consumed and overwhelmed by clinical symptoms that a new identity is formed around clinical symptoms, thereby resulting in the family system experiencing an incremental "loss" of the veteran they knew before the injury. Pauline Boss, PhD, has written much about the experience of "ambiguous loss" and the tension created between the physical presence and simultaneous psychological absence, of an individual secondary to a host of neurologic and psychiatric conditions (Boss 2016). It can be argued that a similar set of tensions can surface for family systems when a veteran presents for clinical care with a historical mTBI(s), especially when co-occurring psychiatric and persisting post-concussive symptoms begin to account for a larger proportion of the veteran's identity (Landau and Hissett 2008).

Epidemiological Evidence

Traumatic brain injury is a significant health issue for US military service members and veterans especially, as they are at increased risk of sustaining a TBI during both times of peace and war. Compared to civilian peers, active duty and reserve service members are at increased risk for TBI partly due to demographics (young men between ages of 18 and 24 are at great risk for TBI) and partly because service members are deployed to areas where they are at high risk of experiencing blast exposures. Additionally, according to the Defense and Veterans Brain Injury Center (DVBIC), active duty service members participate in routine operational and training activities, and leisure activities, that place them at higher risk for TBI (DVBIC 2014). A total of 357,048 service members, across all components of the Army, Air Force, Navy, and Marine Corps, received medical diagnoses of TBI since 2000, with 82.3% of these being mTBI injuries. In 2015 alone, 22,681 diagnoses of TBI occurred in the military, with 18,666 (82.3%) classified as mTBI (DVBIC 2017).

Historical Overview

Head injury treatment was documented over 3,000 years ago. However, literature from that time describes moderate to severe TBI rather than mTBI. Trepanation (burr hole) was utilized to reduce pressure on the brain by draining hematoma; however, it was believed to drain "pus" rather than blood. The Hippocratic corpus makes the first mention of the term "concussion" in historical texts; interestingly, it does not distinguish between concussion and other types of brain injury (Hippocrates 1950). It was not until 900 AD that Muhammad ibn Zakariya al-Razi first documented concussion (*commotio cerebri*; McCrory and Berkovic 2001). He described concussion as a transient physiologic state, which represented a pivotal moment in the history of head injury treatment in that the term distinguished concussion from severe TBI.

In the fourteenth through seventeenth centuries, many European physicians continued to document concussion. In 1687, the College of Physicians in London described concussion in a range of ways, including a singing of the ears after the wound is received, falling after the blow, swooning for a time, slumber after the wound is received, dazzling of the eyes, and a giddiness which passes rapidly (Read 1687). Yet, beyond the description of concussive symptoms, there was as yet no clear understanding of the pathophysiology of injury. A variety of hypotheses were posited to explain the pathology of concussion beginning in the sixteenth century. Early hypotheses suggested that the shaking of the brain resulted in brain tissue injury, secondary to damaging physical contact with the architecture of the skull. It was not until 1774, when Jean-Louis Petit documented that immediate loss of consciousness was attributable to concussion and subsequent loss of consciousness was due to brain tissue compression due to changes in blood, that a linkage of concussion to pathophysiology was posited (McCrory and Berkovic 2001). In 1792, Thomas Kirkland wrote that loss of consciousness from a blow is independent of any pathologic change in the brain (McCrory and Berkovic 2001). It was not until the late nineteenth century that the brain was examined under a microscope. In 1962 Symonds surmised that a concussive event could result in diffuse axonal injury (DAI), which was perhaps the first time this term was introduced in the medical literature (Symonds 1962). Later, in a review of extant literature, Gennarelli (1986) expanded upon this observation to conclude that many neuronal axons must be functionally impaired due to the wide range of symptoms after concussion.

During World War I, neurosurgical management strategies increased the rate of survival from severe TBI to approximately 35% (Boake 1989). Unfortunately, during WWI, morbidity rates attributable to concussion were poorly documented. Despite increased survival rates, there was only one TBI rehabilitation hospital in the USA (Boake 1989). The mortality rate from TBI dropped to 10–13% in World War II, thus requiring the creation of specialized TBI centers. Mortality rates continued to drop during the Korean and Vietnam wars (Cifu et al. 2013). With advanced weaponry used in the Persian Gulf War, 17% of fatalities were attributable to brain injury, and over 4,000 service members were admitted to military hospitals secondary to TBI. The Defense Veterans Head Injury Program (DVHIP) was created in 1992 to address the growing numbers of individuals surviving TBI with complex rehabilitative needs (Salazar et al. 2000). Later renamed the DVBIC, the organization represented a collaboration between Department of Defense (DoD), Department of Veterans Affairs (VA), and civilian partners, with the goals of providing clinical care, education, and research for TBI care across the three healthcare settings.

Since the late 1980s, a greater awareness and formal recognition of mTBI through war, and sports, has resulted in advances in research. OEF and OIF conflicts, along with legal cases in the National Football League, have brought an awareness of concussion into the home of the everyday, nonmedical person. As advanced equipment and sideline concussion evaluation protocols have been developed in the world of sports, similar parallel advances in battlefield protective equipment and concussion evaluation algorithms have developed in the post-9/11 combat theater. For example, in 2007, the DVBIC created the Military Acute Concussion Evaluation (MACE), which is an in-theater mTBI screening tool. Increased publicity and public awareness about concussion has resulted in large, national-level research efforts to characterize mTBI and successive mTBIs, as well as to advance treatment for TBI of all severities in both the military and civilian settings. One example of a national initiative is the 5-year, $62 million Chronic Effects of Neurotrauma Consortium (CENC), awarded in 2012 as part of a National Research Action Plan (NRAP). The Chronic Effects of Neurotrauma Consortium is a coordinated, multicenter collaboration linking basic science, translational, and clinical neuroscience researchers from the VA, military, and academia to establish a comprehensive understanding of the chronic sequelae associated with neurotrauma with a primary focus on mTBI/concussion.

TBI was designated the "signature wound" of OEF/OIF conflicts because over 60% of blast injuries resulted in TBI. In order to treat the large number of returning service members and separated veterans with TBI and comorbid complex, life-threatening injuries (e.g., burns, orthopedic injuries and amputations, infections), the US Congress allocated special purpose funding for VA to create the Polytrauma System of Care (PSC) in 2005. The Polytrauma System of Care is comprised of four components that either directly provide or formally link the lifelong needs of service members and veterans with TBI/polytrauma (and their families) to healthcare options. The Polytrauma System of Care uses a tiered system of rehabilitation, with regional referral centers known as Polytrauma Rehabilitation Centers (PRC) and Polytrauma Network Sites (PNSs) that provide post-acute rehabilitation and coordination of polytrauma services within the Veterans Integrated Service Network (VISN), Polytrauma Support Clinic Teams that provide outpatient interdisciplinary rehabilitation, and Polytrauma Point of Contacts that facilitate referrals to higher-level interdisciplinary Polytrauma System of Care programs. Additional Polytrauma Transitional Rehabilitation Programs have been created, and co-located with the Polytrauma Rehabilitation Center sites, in order to serve veterans with TBI/polytrauma history, who are judged to benefit from a more structured residential setting in the service of optimizing community integration and participation.

Mechanisms of the Disease

A traumatic brain injury is by definition a historical event that can occur in any variety of contexts. More recently it has been conceptualized as a chronic disease process insofar as data, especially for moderate-severe TBI, implicate the injury as causative for increased rates of mortality and as a risk factor for other medical conditions including Parkinsonism and dementia.

For military personnel, TBI can occur in deployment and non-deployment contexts. While perhaps surprising to some unfamiliar with base rates of TBI in military populations, a greater percentage of TBI injuries requiring healthcare services occur in non-deployment settings, as a consequence of stateside motor vehicle accidents, falls, or training accidents.

In combat situations, TBI has most commonly been the result of blast detonations (e.g., improvised explosive devices (IEDs), rocket-propelled grenades, mortars), and these events have resulted in high rates of mTBI. The environment in which the blast occurs (mounted within a vehicle, dismounted out of a vehicle, near water, open space, etc.), the type of materials used in the explosive (amount of trinitrotoluene (TNT) equivalents), the mechanism used to deliver the blast (improvised explosive device, artillery, etc.), and the distance between the person and blast are all important when considering the clinical effects of blast-related mTBI.

Blast injuries often have multiple mechanisms of injury. Primary blast injury results due to a change in air pressure in which an overpressure wave is followed by an under-pressure wave. This change can result in injures to fluid- or gas-filled organs such as the intestinal tract, eyes, ears, and lungs. One hypothesis also is that pressure transmitted through the abdomen or thorax can result in increased intracranial pressure, thereby resulting in brain injury. Secondary blast injuries can result as a consequence of projectiles from the blast that hit or penetrate an individual. This type of injury can result in blunt head trauma or penetrating brain injury. Tertiary blast injury results from an individual being thrown against another object, which can also independently result in blunt head trauma. Quaternary injury occurs from toxins that can cause hypoxia or burns, and other environmental threats after the blast can compound the number of injuries.

Whether a veteran has suffered a blast injury; a vehicular, sports-related injury; or injury of a separate mechanism, the hallmark sign of mTBI is some alteration of consciousness which may or may not include a frank loss of consciousness. Although McCrory et al. (2013) defined concussion in the setting of sport, their definition can be used in any setting of mTBI (see Table 23.1).

The Status of Interventions and the Relationship Between the Latest Interventions and Clinical Care

In the case of mTBI and persistent post-concussive symptoms, it is important to note the high level of symptom overlap with other commonly occurring conditions among post-9/11 veterans. While PTSD is the prototypical comorbid condition in veterans with a history of concussion, other conditions also co-occur such as insomnia and chronic pain—highly prevalent conditions that present with symptoms very similar to post-concussive disorder. As an example, post-concussive symptoms of attention and concentration problems, irritability, and fatigue also overlap with common symptoms of clinical depression or PTSD. This overlap creates a vexing differential diagnostic conundrum for clinicians who may feel compelled to attempt to delineate the etiology of presenting symptoms. While attempting to discriminate between comorbid conditions with largely non-specific symptoms presents an intimidating diagnostic challenge, Maguen et al. (2012) have identified symptoms that are specific to concussion history (i.e., dizziness/balance problems, light sensitivity, headaches, and memory problems) and PTSD (i.e., nightmares and avoidance) in veterans.

When working with veterans with a history of concussion, making accurate diagnoses regarding comorbid psychiatric conditions is critical to ensure that evidence-based treatments for these conditions are made available to these individuals, even if additional intervention for concussion-related symptoms is warranted. Aggressive management of comorbid conditions is ideal to reduce overall symptom burden in individuals with a history of concussion, as there is indication that the relation between history of concussion and negative health outcomes, including psychosocial and work-related difficulties, is mediated by the presence of co-occurring PTSD (Pietrzak et al. 2009). There is a strong case that the management of comorbidities, especially PTSD, may optimize a broad range of mTBI health-related outcomes.

Table 23.1 Definition of concussion (McCrory et al. 2013)

Cause	Concussion may be caused by a direct blow to the head, face, neck, or elsewhere on the body with an "impulsive" force transmitted to the head
Underlying pathology	Concussion may result in neuropathological changes, but the acute clinical symptoms largely reflect a functional disturbance rather than a structural injury, and, as such, no abnormality is seen on standard structural neuroimaging studies
Immediate sequelae	Concussion typically results in the rapid onset of short-lived impairment of neurological function that resolves spontaneously. However, in some cases, symptoms and signs may evolve over a number of minutes or hours
Symptom resolution	Concussion results in a graded set of clinical symptoms that may or may not involve loss of consciousness. Resolution of the clinical and cognitive symptoms typically follows a sequential course. However, it is important to note that in some cases symptoms may be prolonged

Due to the complex nature of these cases, frontline clinicians in the primary care environment are often confronted with the reality that the most prudent way forward, from a holistic perspective, is to refer the veteran to a specialty interdisciplinary team associated with the VA Polytrauma System of Care. These interdisciplinary teams are composed of medical specialists, rehabilitation nurses, care coordinators, and a variety of therapeutic disciplines that are well suited to identify the needs and implement treatment plans for veterans with a history of combat-related concussion. The level of coordinated care made available by interdisciplinary teams can help to overcome issues related to scope of practice and time constraints that might otherwise limit the effectiveness of providers working individually (Shultz et al. 2011).

Prior to OEF/OIF conflicts, treatment recommendations regarding the management of concussion-related symptoms were largely derived from the study of civilians recovering from motor vehicle collisions, falls, assaults, and sports injuries. Consistent with research indicating that expectation biases following concussion serve to magnify and perpetuate symptom report (e.g., Mittenberg et al. 1992), psychoeducational interventions were developed to normalize the presence of symptoms commonly reported in the weeks following concussion and to create an expectation of recovery and return to pre-injury social and role functioning. Following earlier success in reducing the prevalence of the abnormal persistence of symptoms after concussion (i.e., post-concussional disorder), this psychoeducational strategy has successfully been adapted for use in emergency rooms and via telehealth.

While the development of these interventions represents important advances in the prevention and management of post-concussional symptoms, the application of such evidence-based strategies in the VA Healthcare System is complicated by the fact that veterans typically present for initial evaluation and treatment years—rather than hours or days—after the injury (Belanger et al. 2009). Rather than preventing the development of post-concussional symptoms in a population of individuals who are hours to days post-injury, clinicians working with veterans are faced with managing chronic symptoms (i.e., post-concussion syndrome) in individuals who have lived through a host of severe—and potentially life-threatening—stressors between the time of their concussion and the moment they present for evaluation and treatment. Furthermore, rates of physical and psychiatric comorbidities are extremely high in the VA population, further confounding the use of straightforward psychoeducational strategies developed to manage concussion in civilians.

Numerous rationally and empirically developed recommendations are available for treating the myriad of cognitive, somatic/sensory, and emotional/behavioral symptoms often attributed to a history of concussion in veterans, such as poor concentration, headache, and vestibular deficits (e.g., Shultz et al. 2011). While management of individual symptoms is important, especially when the symptoms are believed to contribute directly to activity limitations and participation restrictions, the wide range of symptoms attributed to post-concussion syndrome would make a comprehensive review of such treatments unwieldy and premature.

In 2009, the Department of Veterans Affairs and the Department of Defense (VA/DoD) released a set of clinical practice guidelines with the goal of promoting evidence-based management of veterans with a history of concussion based on review of available literature and on consensus derived from leading brain injury experts from the VA, Department of Defense, and the private sector (VA/DoD 2009). These were updated in Version 2.0, published in 2016. Patient-centered education and symptom management lie at the core of the treatment strategies.

The role of education is to provide veterans with empirically based information about recovery following concussion. In cases where the education can be delivered hours or days following the injury, the goal is to reduce the likelihood that early post-concussive symptoms will persist beyond the usual recovery period (post-concussive syndrome/disorder), by normalizing the early post-concussive symptoms and creating an expectation for recovery. Further research is needed to determine the effectiveness of such education with veterans, however, since they typically present for clinical evaluation years after the concussion event. Nevertheless, the goal of education in this context is presumably to reduce anxiety about health-related concerns that are actually common in community-dwelling individuals according to base rates while also exploring the possibility that symptoms are being misattributed to remote history of concussion rather than to other existing conditions that may be easily treatable.

When veterans continue to report significant cognitive, somatic, and emotional/behavioral symptoms thought to be related to concussion after the implementation of education-based treatment strategies, the clinical practice guidelines offer empirically based and consensus-driven guidelines regarding the management of these presumed post-concussive symptoms using pharmacological and non-pharmacological treatment. Follow-up referrals to appropriate specialists are encouraged for otherwise intractable symptoms. The clinical practice guidelines highlight the importance of care management, especially in cases where multiple specialty providers are involved, to ensure that patients are able to follow through with their individualized care plan.

While assessment and management of self-reported symptoms are encouraged in the clinical practice guidelines for concussion (VA/DoD

2009), it is important to note that there is wide agreement that post-concussive symptoms, especially those that persist years post-injury, are largely non-specific. Indeed, endorsement of "post-concussive symptoms" has been found to be higher among veterans diagnosed with PTSD relative to veterans with a history of mTBI (Soble et al. 2014). The overlap of post-concussive symptoms with psychiatric disorders is especially problematic, given that approximately one-third of service members and veterans with history of concussion also meet clinical diagnostic criteria for PTSD and depression (Hoge et al. 2008).

Through the challenges inherent to differential diagnosis, a way forward to the appropriate treatment of these individuals is to arrive at individualized treatment planning that addresses four overarching areas of health: physical, cognitive, psychological, and spiritual. Achieving such an individualized treatment plan ultimately requires inclusion of the family system to the extent possible. Not surprisingly, the complex and functionally impairing symptoms associated with mTBI can result in marked family strain. For families, adjustment to the veteran's symptoms is experienced in the context of their collective experience of the pre-, peri-, and post-deployment stages (e.g., Collins and Kennedy 2008). There is a recognized need to provide care and support to family members of veterans with mTBI; however, there is very little scientific literature on evidence-based interventions for military families. Multifamily Group Treatment for Veterans with TBI (Perlick et al. 2013) has demonstrated promising preliminary results, with veterans reporting reduction in anger expression and increased social support and occupational activity, while their caregivers have reported decreased burden and increased empowerment. Future research and clinical efforts should be geared toward increased understanding of family functioning related to persistent, post-concussive symptoms. Further attention to perspectives from various family members beyond only the caregiver, as well as to cultural differences, may help better inform the need for, and content of, family interventions.

Implications for the Future

As with many aspects of healthcare in the twenty-first century, technology is changing how TBI is evaluated and managed. The Veterans Health Administration (VHA) has started providing concussion evaluation and treatment to veterans at community-based outpatient clinics and at the homes of veterans through the use of clinical video telehealth technologies. While the use of telehealth will irrefutably improve access to care—especially for veterans who do not live close to large medical centers—research is still needed to determine whether outcomes associated with telehealth versus in-person visits are equivalent. Rehabilitation professionals should see the ability to provide care within a veteran's local community as an opportunity to augment skill transfer to real-life settings, a process that is typically challenging when therapy is provided only in a formal treatment setting.

Similarly, mobile applications are now available to assist veterans and their providers in managing post-concussive symptoms and comorbid conditions. These applications provide means not only to deliver real-time therapeutic strategies to veterans but also to collect information about the severity, intensity, and duration of symptoms that can be shared with therapists. Mobile applications such as the Concussion Coach, developed by the Department of Veterans Affairs in 2013, provide basic assessment tools that help direct the user to the most appropriate intervention strategies based on their self-reported problems—a tailoring of treatment that is essential given the large universe of symptoms and treatment strategies potentially available for those recovering from concussion.

While technology has created exciting new avenues for providing contextualized intervention in real-life situations, the role of vocational rehabilitation services in assisting veterans to transfer skills into real-life situations has never been more important. Early interventional strategies after TBI that focus on symptom reduction and maximizing independence should ultimately yield to specific community reintegration goals, the most important of which may be a return to productive, meaningful activity regardless of disability severity (e.g., Wehman et al. 2009). The role of vocational rehabilitation, or specifically supported employment, has expanded rapidly in the VA healthcare system over the last 10 years. OEF/OIF veterans can benefit tremendously from these services, as they provide an important element of support for veterans who require additional assistance to adjust to the cognitive, emotional, or physical demands of a competitive workplace situation.

Lastly, there is broad consensus in the professional community that the vast majority of individuals suffering from a concussion experience should experience quantifiable cognitive changes within 3–12 months (Carroll et al. 2004). More recently, however, there has been increasing concern regarding the long-term health impact of concussion, especially repeated concussions. Theories have been put forth suggesting that repeated concussions may result in a unique neurodegenerative condition, called chronic traumatic encephalopathy (CTE), or that repeated brain injury may result in a reduction in cognitive reserve that allows for the earlier expression of age-related neurodegenerative disorders, such as Alzheimer's disease (Randolf and Kirkwood 2009). While the possibility that multiple concussions suffered in the line of duty may put veterans at increased risk of developing a neurodegenerative condition later in life is alarming, especially given rates of TBI in recent conflicts, multiple case studies have been published that do not draw a definitive causal link between concussions and neurodegenerative conditions (Karantzoulis and Randolph 2013). Prospective, longitudinal, multicenter studies of veterans are now underway to carefully explore the potential long-term consequence of multiple concussions. At present, however, clinicians should be cautious in discussing the potential relation between concussion (especially a single concussion) and neurodegenerative processes with patients and other healthcare professionals (Wortzel et al. 2013).

Large systems of care have been launched to address the complex assessment and treatment needs for service members and veterans who require specialized healthcare following TBI. In addition to the Polytrauma System of Care in the Department of Veterans Affairs, the National Intrepid Center of Excellence (NICoE) opened its doors in 2010 as a center designed to advance understanding of the "invisible wounds" from Iraq and Afghanistan. The NICoE has since this time established its role as a directorate within Walter Reed National Military Medical Center (WRNMMC) and as a key component within the Military Health System (MHS) TBI Pathway of Care. There is a collaboration between the NICoE and a developing network of "Intrepid Spirit Centers," localized TBI care facilities, to help address the continued challenge of TBI incidence in the MHS.

Conclusions

The incidence of concussion in military populations is well established. These rates have increased commensurate with increased recognition and awareness of the existence of mTBI, together with injuries sustained in combat and noncombat situations. The use of explosive devices through Operation Enduring Freedom/Operation Iraqi Freedom conflicts has further sensitized the medical community to the myriad physical and psychiatric sequelae of single or multiple mTBI events. Department of Defense, Veterans Health Administration, and university settings have developed interdisciplinary rehabilitation programs to provide comprehensive, lifelong care options for veterans with a history of TBI/polytrauma. The general consensus is that treating these individuals using a holistic, patient-centered approach requires some understanding of the context of the injury event and an appreciation for military culture and deployment-related mental health conditions. Team-based and early educational interventions hold promise in optimizing rehabilitation outcomes. Additional, scientifically informed intervention methods are needed to address the complexities of longer-term, persistent post-concussive symptoms, especially as these commonly present with comorbid psychiatric comorbidities. There is a need for the development of evidence-based interventions at both the patient and family systems levels for individuals with persisting post-concussive symptoms with and without accompanying psychiatric conditions.

Key Concepts

1. The vast majority of military traumatic brain injuries (TBIs) are mild, with 82% of the approximately 23,000 military TBIs reported in 2015 being classified as such.
2. A TBI has traditionally been defined as a historical event, though it has more recently been reconceptualized as a chronic disease due to the increased risk for developing other medical conditions following moderate to severe TBI.
3. Blast exposure, the most common cause of combat-related mild traumatic brain injury (mTBI), can cause direct and indirect neurological injury through multiple mechanisms, including rapid changes in pressure (primary), projectiles set in motion by the blast (secondary), being thrown against another object (tertiary), and exposure to toxins (quaternary).
4. Post-concussive symptoms are largely nonspecific and difficult to differentiate from the symptoms associated with other medical conditions common in persons with a history of mTBI.
5. Diagnosis and aggressive management of comorbid conditions are necessary to optimize outcome when treating veterans with a history of mTBI.
6. Education focused on normalization of symptoms and on creating an expectation of recovery is considered best practice for mTBI management, though more research is necessary to determine how best to apply this treatment strategy to veterans who are often first evaluated years post-injury.
7. Coordinated interdisciplinary care, including the family system, is sometimes needed to effectively manage persisting somatic, cognitive, and affective post-concussive symptoms.
8. Technology-driven advances in TBI care, including clinical video telehealth and mobile applications, hold promise for maximizing reintegration through delivery of services in real-life settings.

References

Belanger HG, Uomoto JM, Vanderploeg RD (2009) The Veterans Health Administration's (VHA's) polytrauma system of care for mild traumatic brain injury: costs, benefits, and controversies. J Head Trauma Rehabil 24(1):4–13

Boake C (1989) A history of cognitive rehabilitation of brain-injured patients, 1915–1980. J Head Trauma Rehabil 4:1–8

Boss P (2016) The context and process of theory development: the story of ambiguous loss. J Fam Theory Rev 8:269–286

Carroll LJ, Cassidy D, Peloso PM, Borg J, von Holst H, Holm L, Paniak C, Pepin M (2004) Prognosis for mild traumatic brain injury: results of the WHO collaborating centre task force on mild traumatic brain injury. J Rehabil Med Suppl 43:84–105

Cifu DX, Granier JP, Grimes J, Crowder T, Pai AB, Lew HL (2013) The history and evolution of traumatic brain injury rehabilitation in military service members and veterans in the United States. In: Amara J, Hendricks AM (eds) Military health care: from pre-deployment to post-separation. Routledge, New York, pp 163–176

Collins RC, Kennedy MC (2008) Serving families who have served: providing family therapy and support in interdisciplinary polytrauma rehabilitation. J Clin Psychol In Session 64:993–1003

Defense and Veterans Brain Injury Center (2014) TBI and the military. Retrieved from http://dvbic.dcoe.mil/tbi-military

Defense and Veterans Brain Injury Center. (2017) DoD TBI worldwide numbers since 2000. Retrieved from http://dvbic.dcoe.mil/dod-worldwide-numbers-tbi

Gennarelli T (1986) Mechanisms and pathophysiology of cerebral concussion. J Head Trauma Rehabil 1(2):23–29

Hippocrates (1950) Hippocratic writings. In: Lloyd GER, Chadwock J, Mann WN (eds) (trans: Chadwick J, Mann WN). Penguin Books, London

Hoge CW, McGurk D, Thomas JL, Cox AL, Engel CC, Castro CA (2008) Mild traumatic brain injury in U.S. soldiers returning from Iraq. N Engl J Med 358:453–463

Karantzoulis S, Randolph C (2013) Modern chronic traumatic encephalopathy in retired athletes: what is the evidence? Neuropsychol Rev 23:350–360

Landau J, Hissett J (2008) Mild traumatic brain injury: impact on identity and ambiguous loss in the family. Fam Syst Health 26(1):69–85. https://doi.org/10.1037/1091-7527.26.1.69

Maguen S, Lau KM, Madden E, Seal K (2012) Relationship of screen-based symptoms for mild traumatic brain injury and mental health problems in Iraq and Afghanistan veterans: distinct or overlapping symptoms? J Rehabil Res Dev 49(7):1115–1126

McCrory PR, Berkovic SF (2001) Concussion: the history of clinical and pathophysiological concepts and misconceptions. Neurology 57:2283–2289

McCrory P, Meeuwise WH, Aubry M, Cantu B, Dvorak J, Echemendia RJ et al (2013) Consensus statement on concussion in sport: the 4th international conference on concussion in sport held in Zurich, November 2012. Br J Sports Med 47:250–258

Menon DK, Schwab K, Wright DW, Maas AI (2010) Position statement: definition of traumatic brain injury. Arch Phys Med Rehabil 91:1637–1640

Mittenberg W, DiGuilio D, Perrin S, Bass A (1992) Symptoms following mild head injury: expectation as aetiology. J Neurol Neurosurg Psychiatry 55:200–204

Perlick DA, Straits-Troster K, Strauss JL, Norell D, Tupler LA, Levine B, Luo X et al (2013) Implementation of multifamily group treatment for veterans with traumatic brain injury. Psychiatr Serv 64(6):534–540

Pietrzak RH, Johnson DC, Goldstein MB, Malley JC, Southwick SM (2009) Posttraumatic stress disorder mediates the relationship between mild traumatic brain injury and health and psychosocial functioning in veterans of Operations Enduring Freedom and Iraqi Freedom. J Nerv Ment Dis 197:748–753

Randolf C, Kirkwood MW (2009) What are the real risks of sport-related concussion, and are they modifiable? J Int Neuropsychol Soc 15(4):512–520

Read A (1687) Chirurgorum comes, or the whole practice of chirurgery, begun by the learned doctor read; continued and completed by a member of the College of Physicians in London. C Wilkinson, London

Salazar AM, Zitnay GA, Warden DL, Schwab KA (2000) Defense and veterans head injury program: background and overview. J Head Trauma Rehabil 15:1081–1091

Shultz BA, Cifu DX, McNamee S, Nichols M, Carne W (2011) Assessment and treatment of common persistent sequelae following blast induced mild traumatic brain injury. NeuroRehabilitation 28:309–320

Soble JR, Silva MA, Vanderploeg RD, Curtiss G, Belanger HG, Donnell AJ, Scott SG (2014) Normative data for the neurobehavioral symptom inventory (NSI) and post-concussion symptom profiles among TBI, PTSD, and nonclinical samples. Clin Neuropsychol 28(4):614–632

Symonds C (1962) Concussion and its sequelae. Lancet 279(7210):1–5

VA/DoD (2009) VA/DoD clinical practice guideline for management of concussion/mild traumatic brain injury. J Rehabil Res Dev 46(6):CP1–C68

Wehman P, Gentry T, West M, Arango-Lasprilla JC (2009) Community integration: current issues in cognitive and vocational rehabilitation for individuals with ABI. J Rehabil Res Dev 46(6):909–918

Wortzel HS, Brenner LA, Arcineagas DB (2013) Traumatic brain injury and chronic traumatic encephalopathy: a forensic neuropsychiatric perspective. Behav Sci Law 31:721–738

Suicidal Behaviors in Military and Veteran Populations: Risk Factors and Strategies for Prevention and Intervention

24

Holly B. Herberman Mash, James A. Naifeh, Carol S. Fullerton, Joshua C. Morganstein, and Robert J. Ursano

Introduction

Over the past decade, suicide rates in the US Armed Forces have increased substantially, prompting considerable efforts to address this devastating public health concern. The effects of a suicide can echo through families, unit members, and the military community (Carr 2011). Better understanding of the epidemiology of suicidality among soldiers, and increased ability to identify factors that predict or protect from suicidal thoughts and behaviors, have important implications for risk assessment, case conceptualization, and treatment planning. However, these phenomena have multiple determinants, and the interactions among preexisting vulnerabilities, stressors, and protective factors are complex. This chapter briefly summarizes suicidal behaviors among military service members and veterans, including epidemiology and history, risk and protective factors, and prevention and treatment.

Case Study

Mike Browning (pseudonym) is a 24-year-old Private First Class in the US Army Reserve. He was admitted to an army medical center after his fiancée found him unconscious and unresponsive on their living room couch, with a nearly empty bottle of vodka in his lap and an empty bottle of oxycodone on the coffee table. After he was medically stable, a psychiatric consultation was requested. Mike reported experiencing anxiety and occasional panic attacks for the past 5 months, beginning 6 weeks after returning from his first deployment. Mike had insomnia due to frequent nightmares, which were often related to combat experiences in Afghanistan. During deployment, an improvised explosive device detonated within 10 yards of Mike's MRAP (mine-resistant ambush protected vehicle) and killed his buddy Joe. Mike struggled with grief and repeated intrusive thoughts about the incident. He initially began drinking a moderate amount of alcohol to help him sleep, but more recently began drinking to intoxication weekly. Upon returning home, Mike regularly interacted with friends and was happy

H.B.H. Mash (✉) • J.A. Naifeh • C.S. Fullerton
J.C. Morganstein • R.J. Ursano
Uniformed Services University of the Health Sciences, Bethesda, MD, USA
e-mail: Holly.herberman-mash.ctr@usuhs.edu

L.W. Roberts, C.H. Warner (eds.), *Military and Veteran Mental Health*,
https://doi.org/10.1007/978-1-4939-7438-2_24

to be living with his fiancée again. However, the anxiety he began to experience in public places led to increasingly isolative behavior. Mike also began to miss work and seemed more withdrawn and inattentive while there, resulting in a warning from his supervisor. Mike stopped going out with friends and rarely returned phone calls. Arguments with his fiancée became more frequent and intense, particularly those concerning finances. Mike denied previous suicide attempts or suicidal thoughts until 10 days before his hospitalization and reported serious suicidal thoughts 2 days prior. He acknowledged considering an overdose as the most accessible method, using oxycodone he had from a previous training injury. On the day of his hospitalization, Mike recalled watching television alone, feeling very angry, and drinking several shots of vodka.

Phenomenology of Suicidality and Classification of Suicidal Thoughts and Behavior

There are various types of suicidal thoughts and behaviors, which have different base rates, risk and protective factors, courses, and treatment outcomes (Brown et al. 2005; Kessler et al. 2005; Nock and Kessler 2006). Suicide ideation refers to thoughts about ending one's own life and is distinct from passive thoughts about death or dying. Service members and veterans who have been exposed to life-threatening situations and death during combat deployments may experience thoughts about their own mortality or death. Such thoughts are not classified as suicidal unless the content involves self-injury and/or a desire to die. A suicide plan is a strategy by which one intends to die (e.g., date, time, place, and method). A suicide attempt is a self-injurious behavior with intent to die. The degree of lethality and degree of intent may vary. Suicide refers to a self-inflicted injury with intent to die, resulting in death. Researchers have proposed additional distinctions for suicidal behaviors that may not fit cleanly into one of the above categories, including preparatory acts, aborted suicide attempts, and interrupted suicide attempts (Barber et al. 1998; Marzuk et al. 1997; Posner et al. 2007). For clinicians, understanding the intent and lethality is an important part of safety assessment.

Epidemiological Evidence

Suicide is the tenth leading cause of death in the USA, occurring at an annual rate of 12.6/100,000 people (CDC 2013). The lifetime prevalence of suicide ideation in the general population is 5.6–14.3%. History of developing a suicide plan is reported by 3.9% of the general population, and 1.9–8.7% report having made one or more suicide attempts (Nock et al. 2008).

Historically, US military service members have had a lower suicide rate than civilians of the same age and sex in the general population (Eaton et al. 2006). This discrepancy may have been due in part to the military's ability to screen out individuals with pre-enlistment mental health problems or criminality, both of which are related to increased suicide risk, and efforts to control access to weapons (Boardman et al. 1999; Harris and Barraclough 1997; Hill et al. 2006). The military's universal access to health care, steady employment, and community support may also have contributed to historically lower rates. However, following the commencement of Operation Iraqi Freedom (OIF), the suicide rate in the US Army began to increase (Nelson 2004), surpassing the matched general population rate for the first time (Kuehn 2009) (Fig. 24.1). Between 2001 and 2009, the suicide rate increased from 9.0/100,000 to 21.7/100,000 in the Army and from 16.7/100,000 to 22.3/100,000 in the Marine Corps. Air Force and Navy suicide rates climbed to a level similar to the matched civilian rate. Drug overdose was the most common method of attempted suicide (54.8%), followed by the use of a sharp or blunt object (12.2%) and hanging/asphyxiation (9.1%).

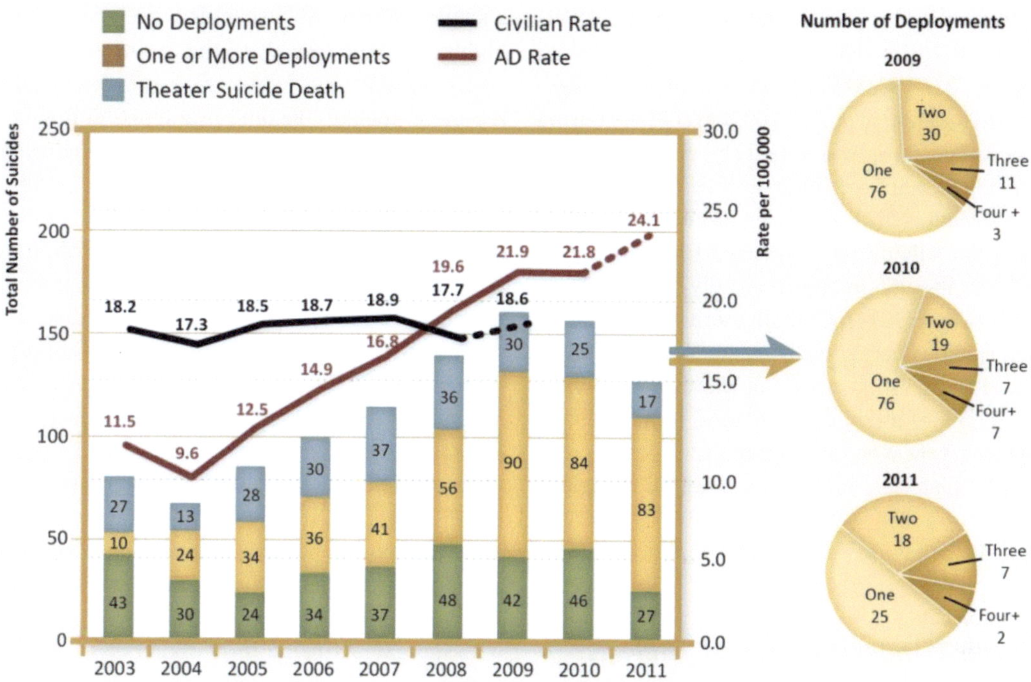

Fig. 24.1 Active duty suicide death rates in the US Army from 2003 to 2011 (Department of the Army 2012)

The three most common methods of suicide death were personal firearm/gun (48.9%), hanging/asphyxiation (22.9%), and military-issued firearm/gun (11.7%) (Corr 2014).

Methodological challenges have somewhat limited suicide research on veterans as a group (Kaplan et al. 2007). Most studies have utilized Department of Veterans Affairs (VA) health-care data, resulting in findings that are most representative of veterans who use VA services rather than all veterans. Nevertheless, evidence indicates that veterans are at increased risk for suicide relative to non-veterans (Kemp 2014; McCarthy et al. 2009), with male veterans in the general population found to be twice as likely to die by suicide as nonveterans (Kaplan et al. 2007). Despite the fact that veterans comprise 1% of the US population, they represent 20% of all suicide deaths annually (Department of Veterans Affairs 2010). Although an analysis of VA patient data from 2001 to 2005 indicated that the suicide rate among Operation Enduring Freedom (OEF) and Operation Iraqi Freedom veterans was not significantly higher than that of general population (Kang and Bullman 2008), a recent study of all veterans receiving VA care from 2000 to 2007 found that the suicide rate was significantly higher than that of the age- and gender-adjusted rates in the general US population (Blow et al. 2012).

Historical Overview of Suicide

Concerns about suicidal behavior among US military service members and veterans date back to at least the Civil War (Lande 2011), with recorded rates of suicide ranging from 8.74 to 14.54/100,000 among Union soldiers during the war and 30.4/100,000 for the year following the war (Frueh and Smith 2012). However, rates appeared to be lower during times of war versus peacetime. Comparable wartime suicide rates of 15/100,000 soldiers were found during World War I (WWI), reduced from 53/100,000 prior to the war (Menninger 1948). The Army suicide rate between WWI and WWII doubled, to 30/100,000 soldiers, and then decreased to

9/100,000 during the period around WWII (1940–1946), which was lower than the civilian rate of 19.3/100,000 in 1941 (Menninger 1948).

The suicide rate of 11/100,000 soldiers during the Korean War was relatively consistent with previous wars (Military Suicide Research Consortium 2016). However, during the Vietnam War, the suicide rate increased from 5/100,000 soldiers in 1965 to approximately 38/100,000 in 1971 (Camp 2014). Overall, there were a total of 382 suicides during the Vietnam War, at a rate of 16/100,000. Army troops in Vietnam accounted for 92.6% of all military suicides. It must be recognized, however, that methods of capturing data in past historical records may not be complete, and factors such as the stigma related to reporting suicidal behaviors may affect record accuracy.

Current Understanding of Etiology of Suicidal Behaviors in the Military

In the military as well as in the civilian world, a vulnerability-stress model can facilitate the understanding of how wide-ranging risk factors contribute to suicidal behaviors. Within this conceptual framework, predisposing factors (vulnerabilities) interact with environmental events (stressors) to trigger suicidal behaviors.

Vulnerability Factors

Mental Disorders Mental health diagnoses are among the most consistent risk factors for active duty military and veteran suicides, with the greatest risk conveyed by mood, anxiety, and substance use disorders (Bachynski et al. 2012; Bossarte et al. 2012; Hyman et al. 2012; LeardMann et al. 2013; Maguen et al. 2015). According to Department of Defense Suicide Event Report (DoDSER) records, 15% of suicides and 25% of suicide attempts involved a previous diagnosis of anxiety disorder, whereas 21% of suicides and 40% of attempts involved a previous mood disorder diagnosis. Further, soldiers with psychiatric diagnoses are more likely to have a history of multiple suicide attempts versus a single attempt (Kochanski-Ruscio et al. 2014), highlighting the severity of this association.

Up to 25% of US service members have reported mental health problems following Operation Iraqi Freedom/Operation Enduring Freedom deployments (Hoge et al. 2004, 2006). The counts and rates of incident mental disorder diagnoses increased by approximately 65% from 2000 to 2011, with 936,283 active component members receiving at least one mental disorder diagnosis (Armed Forces Health Surveillance Center 2012). This upward trend was primarily attributable to increased diagnoses of adjustment disorders, depressive disorders, and post-traumatic stress disorder (PTSD) and other anxiety disorders. PTSD is of particular relevance to armed forces populations, given its historical and empirical relationship to combat exposure. Although PTSD is independently associated with increased suicide risk, soldiers with PTSD and depression comorbidity were almost three times more likely to report past year suicidality (Ramsawh et al. 2014), and comorbidity with two or more other mental disorders increased suicidal ideation risk sevenfold in Army National Guard members (Calabrese et al. 2011). In veterans, anxiety disorders, depression, and functional decline were similarly associated with higher risk of suicide (Dobscha et al. 2014). Further, those with PTSD were over four times more likely to experience suicidality than veterans without PTSD (Calabrese et al. 2011; Jakupcak et al. 2009) and those who reported suicidality were more likely to meet *DSM-5* PTSD criteria for clusters C (avoidance) and D (negative alterations in cognitions and mood) (Legaretta et al. 2015).

Another potential risk factor, traumatic brain injury (TBI), is one of the "signature wounds" of Operation Iraqi Freedom/Operation Enduring Freedom, affecting many service members with blast injuries (Hoge et al. 2009; Schneiderman et al. 2008). Despite evidence of a strong univariate association between TBI and military suicide (Hyman et al. 2012), there have been mixed findings regarding the relationship between type and frequency of TBIs and suicidality. Although a recent case-control study found no association between suicide and type or frequency of TBI in this population (Skopp et al. 2012), the number of TBIs was found to be associated with increased incidence of suicidal thoughts and behaviors, even after adjusting for depression and PTSD symptoms in a deployed military sample in Iraq (Bryan and Clemans 2013). The relationship between TBI and other risk factors for suicidality, including mental disorders (Hoge et al. 2008; Schneiderman et al. 2008), and increased aggression, disinhibition, and impulsivity (Kim 2002; Rao and Lyketsos 2000) suggests that further research is needed. Although the polytrauma clinical triad of co-occurring PTSD, TBI, and chronic pain, experienced in 42% of veterans receiving polytrauma care, is associated with suicidality, this combination may not increase suicide risk to a greater degree than PTSD, depression, or substance abuse alone (Finley et al. 2015).

Previous Suicidal Behaviors Past suicidal behavior is a strong predictor of future suicide-related outcomes among military service members (Bryan et al. 2014b), and this association remains significant even after accounting for other well-established risk factors (Joiner et al. 2005). Service members and veterans with a previous suicide attempt are over six times more likely to attempt suicide after joining the military (Bryan et al. 2014b), and multiple previous suicide attempts are a particularly strong risk factor for future death by suicide in this population (Kochanski-Ruscio et al. 2014).

Psychological Factors Soldiers who exhibited suicide-related behaviors indicated that their primary reason for attempting suicide was to alleviate or escape aversive psychological states (Bryan et al. 2013). In particular, the manner in which soldiers and veterans perceive themselves and their wartime behaviors, which may involve guilt, shame, and self-hatred from committing or witnessing actions that violated their moral beliefs, is a critical focus for prevention and treatment (Bower 2015; Bryan et al. 2014a, 2015c; Rudd et al. 2015).

Demographic Factors Univariate analyses have revealed that suicide risk is associated with male gender (Black et al. 2011), junior enlisted rank (Bachynski et al. 2012), reduction in rank, and history of divorce or separation (Hyman et al. 2012). Examination of nonfatal suicide events among active duty Air Force service members found several significant risk factors that differed by gender (Snarr et al. 2010). Risk of past-year suicidal ideation was predicted by female gender, lower enlisted rank, and non-Christian religion. Being unmarried increased suicidal ideation risk among men, and attempt risk was increased for lower-ranking men and Hispanic women (Snarr et al. 2010).

Stressful Life Experiences Service members must often manage numerous military-specific stressors during deployment and as they transition between military and civilian life (Castro and Kintzle 2014), in addition to life stressors and traumatic events commonly experienced in the general population (Kuehn 2009). Suicidal behaviors among current and former military personnel often follow conflict with a family member or romantic partner, bereavement, and legal or disciplinary problems (Army Suicide Prevention Task Force 2010; Maguen et al. 2015; Skopp et al. 2016). Similarly, interpersonal stressors, such as harassment, during combat are associated with suicidal ideation (Lemaire and Graham 2010). Traumatic stressors experienced before or during military service, including sexual trauma and child abuse, are also related to increased suicide risk (Afifi et al. 2016; Bryan et al. 2015a; Gradus et al. 2012; Kimerling et al. 2015; Maguen et al. 2011; Perales et al. 2012; Pietrzak et al. 2010). However, mental health symptoms may influence the relationship between deployment stressors and suicidal ideation (Gradus et al. 2013). Although deployment has not consistently been associated with suicide risk (Kang et al. 2015; Leardmann et al. 2013; Schoenbaum et al. 2014), as will be discussed below, other service-related stressors, including early military separation (under 4 years) and dishonorable discharge have been associated with increased rate of suicide (Reger et al. 2015). Historically, the majority of traumatic deaths during basic training have been identified as suicides (Scoville et al. 2004), highlighting the challenging nature of this initial period of service.

Situational Factors Specific situations, such as ready access to lethal means (Anestis and Bryan 2012; Lester 1998), may interact with vulnerabilities and environmental stressors to further elevate suicidal behavior risk. Firearms are used in more suicides than homicides annually in the USA (Xu et al. 2016), and are the most common method of suicide across all military branches (Department of Defense Task Force on the Prevention of Suicide by Members of the Armed Forces 2010) and among veterans, accounting for 67% of all veteran suicides (McCarten et al. 2015). Acute alcohol use is another situational factor that greatly increases the risk and lethality of suicidal behavior (Sher 2006), likely due to disinhibitory effects on cognition and behavior, and has been found to be specifically associated with increased death by firearms among civilians (Branas et al. 2016).

Protective Factors

Identification of factors that protect against suicidal behaviors has received relatively less empirical attention but may suggest promising targets for intervention and future research.

Psychological Factors Psychological traits, such as stoicism, character strength, hardiness, positive worldview and self-esteem, and autonomy, have been associated with posttraumatic growth, an adaptive response to extreme stressors (Linley and Joseph 2004; Peterson et al. 2008) that may reduce risk of suicidal ideation in combat-exposed service members (Bush et al. 2011).

Social Support Perceived unit cohesion (e.g., supportive leadership, strong peer relations) may be protective against suicidal ideation (Mitchell et al. 2012) and other psychiatric symptoms (Brailey et al. 2007). In contrast, low levels of social support have been associated with suicidal ideation in veterans (Bossarte et al. 2012), particularly in the context of depressive and PTSD symptoms (DeBeer et al. 2014). Similarly, family support during deployment was associated with lower levels of suicidal ideation in veterans, although this relationship may be modified by depressive and PTSD symptoms (Gradus et al. 2015).

Mental Health Treatment Although access to mental health treatment is protective against suicidal behaviors (Mann et al. 2005), its effectiveness may be influenced by the type and adequacy of treatment, probability and speed of entering treatment, and perceived barriers to treatment (Hoge et al. 2004). Although a majority of individuals who die by suicide have contact with a primary care provider in the year before death (Luoma et al. 2002), most individuals with a history of suicidality never receive any type of mental health treatment (Bruffaerts et al. 2011). A service member's or veteran's willingness to seek care may be affected by both structural (e.g., financial constraints, lack of treatment availability) and perceptual barriers (e.g., mental health stigma, beliefs that treatment will be ineffective, concerns about confidentiality) (Hoge and Castro 2012; Kaskutas et al. 1997; Wang et al. 2008). Further, being young and male, characteristics that describe the majority of US military members, are factors associated with decreased help-seeking behavior in the general population (Wang et al. 2005). Although stoicism and autonomy—traits that are valued in military culture and encouraged throughout training—are generally viewed as protective, they may also diminish the likelihood that a service member or veteran will seek help. Addressing barriers to care is necessary to maximize the protective benefits of mental health treatment.

Recent Findings on Suicidality in the US Army

Although recent research has allowed us to better understand factors that are associated with suicide risk, suicidal behaviors are inherently difficult to study. As with other low base rate phenomena, large samples are required to generate meaningful findings and test complex risk and resilience models. The Study to Assess Risk and Resilience in service members-Longitudinal Study (STARRS-LS, www.starrs-ls.org), formerly Army STARRS, is the largest and most comprehensive study of mental health risk and resilience ever conducted in the US Army. STARRS-LS is expected to continue and extend the work of the original Army STARRS through 2020. In addition, the Millennium Cohort Study, a longitudinal, prospective study of the health effects of military service (www.millenniumcohort.org) and internal Department of Defense efforts, such as the National Center for Telehealth and Technology (T2; http://t2health.dcoe.mil), which develops and delivers technology solutions for military psychological health, have focused specifically on factors contributing to suicide risk. Further understanding of suicidality has also been a goal of research conducted through the VA's Epidemiology Program (www.publichealth.va.gov/epidemiology) and Mental Illness Research, Education, and Clinical Centers (MIRECC; www.mirecc.va.gov/). These efforts are an important step in improving the ability of organizations, policymakers, and health-care professionals to respond to this devastating public health issue.

STARRS-LS consists of several component studies (Ursano et al. 2014): (1) the Historical Administrative Data Study (HADS), which integrates 40 Army/Department of Defense data systems containing administrative records for all 1.6 million soldiers on active duty from 2004 to 2009 (over 1.1 billion records); (2) two retrospective case-control studies of fatal and nonfatal suicidal behaviors; (3) a study of new soldiers assessed just before beginning basic training (BT) with self-administered questionnaires, neurocognitive tests, and blood samples; (4) a cross-sectional study of soldiers representative of all other active duty soldiers (exclusive of basic training); and (5) a study of three brigade combat teams surveyed just prior to deploying to Afghanistan and again 1, 3, and 9 months post-deployment (Table 24.1). STARRS-LS has thus far surveyed over 100,000 soldiers. Its extensive databases will allow scientists to investigate a diverse combination of factors from demographic, psychological, biological, neurological, behavioral, and social domains (Table 24.2).

To date, STARRS-LS has generated a number of important findings regarding the epidemiology of suicidal behaviors among US Army soldiers and the influence of service-related factors and mental health history on suicidality. From 2004 to 2009, risk of suicide death was elevated among enlisted Regular Army soldiers deployed during their first year of service and those who were in more junior ranks than expected based on time in service (Gilman et al. 2014). Although generally still higher among male soldiers, the suicide rate increased more among women than men specifically during deployment (Street et al. 2015). Further, the suicide rate of currently deployed women (14/100,000 person-years) was 3.1–3.5 times the rate of never deployed or previously deployed female soldiers. However, the association between deployment and suicidal behaviors is complex. Although suicide rates increased most substantially in currently and previously deployed soldiers, rates also increased in soldiers who had never deployed (Schoenbaum et al. 2014; Ursano et al. 2014). Among infantrymen and combat engineers, two occupations with significantly elevated suicide rates, risk was highest in those who had never deployed, less so in those previously deployed, and not at all in those currently deployed (Kessler et al. 2015a). Suicide risk was not associated with time in current deployment, time since returning from deploy-

Table 24.1 Army STARRS component studies and approximate soldier sample size

Component study	Soldier sample size
Historical Administrative Data Study (HADS)	>1.6 million
Soldier Health Outcomes Study A (SHOS-A)	150 cases and 300 controls
Soldier Health Outcomes Study B (SHOS-B)	150 cases and 300 controls
New Soldier Study (NSS)	51,000
All Army Study (AAS)	35,000
Pre-Post Deployment Study (PPDS)	9,400
Pre-Post Separation Study (PPSS)	1,500

ment, number of deployments, or the time interval between most recent deployments (Gilman et al. 2014).

The nonfatal suicide attempt rate also rose sharply from 2004 to 2009. Most reported cases of suicidal ideation, plans, and attempts (47.0–58.2%) had pre-enlistment onsets (Nock et al. 2014). Nearly 99% of attempts were made by enlisted soldiers, with higher risk in those who had never and previously deployed than in those who were currently deployed. The differential effects of deployment on fatal versus nonfatal suicidal behaviors may indicate that exposure to deployed environments influences the lethality of self-injurious behaviors, although further research is needed. It is noteworthy that other large-scale studies, which included additional US military branches, found no association between deployment history and suicide death (LeardMann et al. 2013; Reger et al. 2015), highlighting the importance of methodological factors. A recent meta-analysis suggests that suicide risk may be influenced more by specific traumatic experiences in combat (e.g., killing) than deployment, per se (Bryan et al. 2015b).

Table 24.2 Clinical considerations for assessing future suicide risk

History of self-injurious thoughts and behaviors
Method
Presence of intent to die
Consequences of attempt (e.g., severity of injuries, hospitalization)
Severity of current or recent self-injurious thoughts
Presence of intent to die
Presence of a suicide plan
Articulation of a specific method
Lethality of the method
Availability of the means to carry out attempt
Any preparatory acts
Follow-up question about alternative methods the patient may have considered
Situational stressors
May include:
Family discord
Breakup of a romantic relationship
Financial concerns
Legal or disciplinary problems
Psychiatric symptoms
Including anxiety, depression, mania, psychosis
Psychological factors
Presence of hopelessness, impulsiveness, aggression
Observational, self-report from the patient
Historical evidence of impulsiveness (e.g., fights or other aggressive acts, risky sexual behavior) and behaviors that may increase disinhibition (e.g., frequency and intensity of drug and alcohol use)
Protective factors
Availability of social support and willingness to access it
Current treatment involvement and history of treatment compliance
Patient-identified reasons for living

Adapted from American Psychiatric Association (2003), Bryan and Rudd (2006)

Risk of nonfatal suicide attempts was also highest during soldiers' first year of service (Ursano et al. 2015b). Examination of soldiers during their first week of service revealed that the lifetime prevalence of pre-enlistment suicide ideation, plans, and attempts was 14.1%, 2.3%, and 1.9%, respectively (Ursano et al. 2015a), and most new soldiers with a pre-enlistment suicide attempt history reported a prior mental disorder (59.0%) (Nock et al. 2015). Prior mental health disorders, particularly major depression and intermittent explosive disorder, were the strongest predictors of self-reported suicidal behaviors (Ursano et al. 2014). These findings are consistent with STARRS-LS data from a representative survey of the Regular Army, in which approximately half of the lifetime suicidal outcomes first occurred prior to enlistment, and pre-enlistment mental disorders were associated with one-third of post-enlistment suicide attempts (Nock et al. 2014). However, these findings are in contrast with previous research that identified no association between early detected mental disorders and suicide in active duty soldiers (Ireland et al. 2012), perhaps due to methodological differences, such as the use of formal medical diagnosis with associated treatment instead of self-report measures, suggesting the need for further investigation.

Examination of service-related and demographic characteristics provides additional insight into subgroups of soldiers who may be at particular risk for suicidal behaviors. Soldiers who were demoted within the past 2 years

(Ursano et al. 2014), male (or female during deployment), White, and of junior enlisted rank were at increased suicide risk (Schoenbaum et al. 2014). Further, older age at army entry, younger current age, less education, and short length of service were associated with suicide attempt risk (Ursano et al. 2015b). Among officers, only sociodemographic characteristics, including female gender, older age at army entry, younger current age, and less education, and presence and recency of mental health diagnoses significantly predicted suicide attempt risk (Ursano et al. 2015b), suggesting unique risk profiles for enlisted soldiers and officers.

Examination of the prevalence of *DSM-IV* mental disorders in soldiers provides insight into the emergence of suicidal thoughts and behaviors, given the strong association of mental disorders and suicidality. Generalized anxiety, post-traumatic stress, and conduct disorders, as well as multi-morbidity, were significantly more common among new soldiers than civilians (Rosellini et al. 2015). Approximately 25% and 11.1% of non-deployed soldiers met criteria for any 30-day disorder and multiple disorders, respectively (Kessler et al. 2014). Further, 76.6% of cases reported pre-enlistment age of onset of at least one 30-day disorder. Post-enlistment first suicide attempts were predicted by (1) pre-enlistment panic disorder and PTSD, (2) post-enlistment depression, and (3) pre- and post-enlistment intermittent explosive disorder (Nock et al. 2014). These findings suggest that interventions to limit accession or increase resilience of new soldiers with pre-enlistment mental disorders might reduce prevalence of mental disorders and contribute to decreased suicide attempts (Kessler et al. 2014). However, only 21.3% of soldiers with any current disorder reported current treatment (Colpe et al. 2015). Factors including, being currently or previously married, not being non-Hispanic black, deployment history, diagnosis of PTSD, bipolar or panic disorder, and having any prolonged disorder predicted current treatment. Among soldiers who indicated that they needed treatment but did not initiate or continue treatment, attitudinal reasons (e.g., stigma-related concerns, desire to handle problems independently) were primary barriers to treatment (Naifeh et al. 2016). Analysis of modifiable barriers to treatment is needed to help strengthen outreach efforts.

Taken together, these findings support prevention efforts focused on enlisted soldiers in the early phases of their first tour of duty and those with a history of mental disorders. STARRS-LS is guided by this concentration of risk approach, which aims to produce actionable findings regarding when, where, and for whom suicidal behavior risk is greatest. This approach was represented in a STARRS-LS study using machine learning to predict suicides in the 12 months following psychiatric hospitalization, a high-risk period accounting for 12.0% of all US Army suicides. Nearly 53% of post-hospitalization suicides occurred among the 5% of discharged soldiers with highest predicted risk, who were also represented by significantly elevated proportions of subsequent hospitalizations, unintentional injury deaths, and suicide attempts (Kessler et al. 2015b). These findings correspond with previous research indicating that service members who experienced psychiatric hospitalization were five times more likely to die from suicide following discharge than the general active duty population and that this risk was 8.2 times higher in the first 30 days versus 1 year post-discharge (Luxton et al. 2013).

STARRS-LS provides a model for studying rare events of concern for public health and national security. The Department of Defense (DoD) recently funded a 5-year continuation of study that will include analysis of administrative records from 2010 to the present and longitudinal follow-up of the initial survey respondents as they progress through their army careers and transition back into civilian life. A number of STARRS-LS databases have been made available for secondary analysis through the Inter-university Consortium for Political and Social Research (http://www.icpsr.umich.edu/icpsrweb/ICPSR/studies/35197).

Status of Preventive and Intervention Programs, Relationship Between Latest Intervention and Clinical Care

Suicide Prevention Strategies and Programs

Increased focus on suicide prevention within the Department of Defense (DoD) and the Department of Veterans Affairs (VA) has led to the development of programs that target at-risk groups and encourage early detection, intervention, education, and communication, and may be tailored to specific deployment phases (Warner et al. 2011). Prevention programs vary in their scope and methods, ranging from universal (primary) to selected (secondary) and indicated prevention (Ramchand et al. 2011), and may include elements of more than one category. Universal programs are delivered to an entire population, selected programs are delivered to groups considered high risk, and indicated programs are delivered to people with detectable symptoms.

A multicomponent suicide plan designed for Israeli Defense Forces soldiers that included restricted weapon availability, reducing stigma associated with help-seeking behavior, increased training for commanders and soldiers targeting service time periods and suicidality risk factors, and integration of mental health service providers into units decreased the suicide rate by 57% among active duty soldiers (Shelef et al. 2016). The Army's ACE program (Ask, Care, Escort) is a valued preventive approach involving buddy care, in which service members receive training to identify at-risk peers and refer them for treatment. However, service members who act as gatekeepers still may feel inadequately prepared and reluctant to intervene, in part due to concerns regarding being held responsible if an at-risk service member dies by suicide. Perceptions of personal responsibility should be highlighted in prevention training to encourage appropriate referral of vulnerable service members (Ramchand et al. 2015).

The Applied Suicide Intervention Skills Training (ASIST) program has been used by the Army to teach chaplains, behavioral health professionals, and other gatekeepers to identify soldiers with suicidal thoughts, assess risk, create a safety plan, and follow-up (Ramchand et al. 2011). Targeting those who often come in contact with these professionals is selected prevention, and assessment and intervention with those who report suicidal thoughts is indicated prevention.

Many universal programs are implemented online and can be accessed via the DoD/VA Suicide Outreach website (www.dspo.mil). For example, the Marine Corps' suicide prevention website provides the National Suicide Prevention Lifeline telephone number and training videos to help supervisors identify and assist those at risk (www.mccsmcrd.com/MarineAndFamilyPrograms/BehavioralHealth/SuicidePrevention/index.html). Other universal programs are provided in person, including the Marine Corps' Entry Level Training in Suicide Prevention, which is given to all Marines at boot camp, officer candidate school, and basic school. For enlisted Marines, trainings on signs, symptoms, and resources are delivered by a drill instructor via two short courses and an interactive discussion. These programs teach basic information and/or skills broadly and at low cost (Ramchand et al. 2011).

As noted, prevention programs are often both selected and indicated because they target high-risk groups and intervene with those who have detectable symptoms. Assessing and Managing Suicide Risk (AMSR) is a 1-day Air Force training program for behavioral health clinicians, which focuses on competencies including approaches to working with at-risk individuals, collecting accurate assessment information, formulating risk, developing treatment plans, and documentation and legal and regulatory issues related to suicidality (http://www.sprc.org/training-institute/amsr). The multicomponent Air Force Suicide Prevention Program (AFSPP), also developed specifically for Air Force personnel, emphasizes community and leadership involvement (http://www.airforcemedicine.af.mil/suicideprevention).

Similarly, the VA has universal, selected, and indicated prevention programs. However, these programs only target health professionals, veterans, and veterans' families, because the VA does not have leadership or peers (e.g., fellow soldiers) who can be interventionists. The VA's Suicide Prevention website (http://www.mentalhealth.va.gov/suicide_prevention) offers practical resources which can be accessed by providers in the VA system and those working with veterans in other settings. Further, veterans are provided access to spiritual and pastoral care services at all VA medical centers from staff clinical chaplains upon request, which has been found to be an effective resource in suicide prevention efforts (Kopacz et al. 2016).

As noted, a number of education, identification, and intervention programs have been developed to address suicidal behaviors in service members and veterans. However, additional research is still needed to investigate the efficacy of these programs and determine which particular groups may benefit from their use. Multiple studies are currently underway that systematically evaluate the effectiveness of these preventive and intervention programs, which will help to determine which programs should be continued, further developed, or discontinued.

Interventions for Soldiers at Risk for Suicidal Behaviors

Hospitalization Given the strong association of mental disorders and multiple suicide attempts in soldiers (Kochanski-Ruscio et al. 2014), those who are admitted to an emergency department following self-injurious behavior need to be carefully evaluated for psychiatric and suicide-related behavior history. This assessment provides important information about past behavior patterns and informs the development of appropriate treatment plans prior to discharge.

Continuity of Care Planning of transitions to care providers and interventions following hospital discharge is critical, in light of the high risk of suicidality among service members and veterans during this period (Desai et al. 2005; Kessler et al. 2015b; Luxton et al. 2013; Valenstein et al. 2009). This effort may be complicated both by structural and communication barriers, and by service members' transitions between installations, units, and deployments, and from military to civilian life (Brenner and Barnes 2012; Department of Defense Task Force on the Prevention of Suicide by Members of the Armed Forces 2010). Outreach efforts may be necessary when patients do not follow up with treatment. For example, among veterans with serious mental illness who had dropped out of VA care, those who returned to treatment after being recontacted by the VA had a significantly lower mortality rate (Davis et al. 2012).

Similarly, because most individuals who die by suicide have had contact with a primary care but not with a mental health provider (Luoma et al. 2002), primary care presents an important opportunity to intervene with at-risk patients. The VA has incorporated primary care screening procedures for depression, PTSD, and substance abuse, offering mental health referral to those who screen positive. Beginning in 2013, the Department of Defense mandated that all new primary care patients, existing patients on an annual basis, and those at high-risk receive screening for depression and PTSD (http://www.dtic.mil/whs/directives/corres/pdf/649015p.pdf). In an effort to more broadly address mental health needs in the primary care setting, both the Department of Defense and Department of Veterans Affairs have embedded full-time mental health providers in all primary care clinics (http://www.mentalhealth.va.gov/docs/MHG_English.pdf, http://www.dtic.mil/whs/directives/corres/pdf/649015p.pdf).

Pharmacotherapy Pharmacotherapy is effective in treating many of the psychiatric conditions associated with suicidal thoughts and behaviors; however, its efficacy in preventing suicidal behaviors requires additional study. Although previous research has indicated that pharmacotherapy does not appear to prevent suicidal behaviors (Mann et al. 2005), the use of medications such as lithium, as a mood stabilizer and adjunctive antidepressant, and clozapine, for treatment of psychosis, has demonstrated reduction in suicide (Lewitzka et al. 2015; Meltzer et al. 2003) and may be considered for service members who require treatment for these disorders and are vulnerable to suicidal behaviors. However, observed increases in suicidal behavior risk after discontinuation of lithium in veterans merits particular attention in treatment planning (Smith et al. 2014). Clinicians prescribing psychotropic medications for a co-occurring disorder should be mindful of potential misuse. The risk of intentional overdose may be managed through controlling when and how medications are dispensed, including coordination with the patient's family. In some instances, injectable formulations may serve to prevent the use of medication for suicidal thoughts and behaviors as well as increase adherence.

Psychotherapy Psychological interventions aimed at improving factors such as problem-solving ability and distress tolerance have been found to reduce the likelihood of future suicide attempts in high-risk patients (Brown et al. 2005; Linehan et al. 2006). Similarly, active duty soldiers who either attempted suicide or reported suicidal ideation with intent to die were 60% less likely to attempt suicide up to 24 months following brief cognitive behavioral treatment as compared to those who participated in treatment as usual (Rudd et al. 2015). Short-term psychodynamic therapy that focuses on the guilt associated with past combat-related experiences has been identified as a promising approach for treating veterans with PTSD who are at risk for suicidality (Hendin 2014).

Weapons Management Ready access to weapons poses a safety threat for suicidal service members, with unsecured storage of privately owned, loaded firearms moderating the relationship between suicidal ideation and future attempts (Khazem et al. 2016). However, firearm possession in the military is not only common but may be an operational requirement. Clinicians should give thoughtful consideration before recommending the removal of a weapon as a means of preventing self-harm, as the resultant shame and stigma associated with the absence of a weapon may serve to enhance, rather than reduce, risk. For these service members, possible alternatives should be considered, such as removing the firing pin but allowing for continued possession of the weapon. These decisions must involve command leadership because of their operational impact. Access to others' weapons must also be considered and may require coordination with family members and unit leadership. Factors to consider when firearms are present in the home include whether they are or can be locked away, whether the gun is loaded or ammunition is readily available, and whether someone else is able and willing to take custody of the weapon. Clinical assessment should also help inform decisions regarding if and when weapon restrictions should be lifted.

Safety Planning When hospitalization is not clinically indicated, suicidal patients presenting to emergency departments and other acute care settings will typically be referred to outpatient mental health treatment (Allen et al. 2002). Unfortunately, many patients will not follow up on these referrals (Krulee and Hales 1988), creating a need for very brief interventions that are deliverable during acute care. SAFE VET, a brief safety planning intervention adapted for use with veterans (Stanley and Brown 2008), allows clinicians and patients to work collaboratively to identify internal and external warning signs that may trigger suicidal thoughts and behaviors and develop a hierarchical plan for managing warning signs and suicidal thoughts and a plan for restricting access to lethal means. The program was expanded to include both the safety plan intervention (SPI) (Stanley and Brown 2012) and safety follow-up (SFU), consisting of structured telephone calls that offer support, encourage treatment engagement, and mitigate risk (Knox et al. 2012). Veterans who received the safety plan intervention/safety follow-up intervention were more likely to attend outpatient behavioral health appointments 3 months following their participation versus treatment attendance following previous emergency department visits that did not involve similar intervention (Stanley et al. 2015).

Clinical Practice Guidelines Extended indicated clinical services for veterans who present with symptoms of high risk are being implemented through the use of the VA/DoD Clinical Practice Guidelines for the Assessment and Management of Patients at Risk for Suicide (http://www.healthquality.va.gov/guidelines/MH/srb/). Additionally, the Air Force Guide for Managing Suicidal Behavior offers Department of Defense-relevant guidance, as well as tools and resources for providers (http://afspp.afms.mil/).

Implications for the Future and Conclusions

Recent findings focused on risk and resilience factors for suicide in the military provide valuable insight into potentially vulnerable groups and preventive measures and opportunities to circumvent the progression from suicide ideation to attempts. This understanding is critical as service members and veterans continue to manage the psychological and behavioral effects of extended and multiple deployments and separate from the military and transition back to civilian life. Although only 25.5% of veterans are estimated to use Veterans Health Administration (VHA) health-care services (Department of Veterans Affairs 2015), suicide rates have been found to decrease among male VHA-user soldiers and increase among non-VHA users (Kemp 2014), highlighting its critical role in suicide prevention.

In order to address military suicide risk in service members and veterans, training opportunities in conducting accurate assessments are recommended for a broad range of clinicians (Doran et al. 2016; McCarthy et al. 2015; Office of the Surgeon General 2012), as well as research to improve the sensitivity of evaluations and better understand psychological and biological markers for suicide (Boudreaux and Horowitz 2014; Glenn and Nock 2014; Claasen et al. 2014). Other services, including the VA Mental Health Enhancement Initiative and Suicide Prevention Program, were developed to provide integrated, easily accessible care through a 24-h Veterans Crisis Line, availability of suicide prevention coordinators to monitor the progress and provide evidence-based treatment to at-risk patients at all VA medical centers, as well as implement awareness and educational campaigns (Hoffmire et al. 2015). Further, the DoD/VA Integrated Mental Health Initiative acts as an ongoing collaborative activity by enhancing delivery of mental health care across a broad range of services (www.mentalhealth.va.gov/docs/VA-DoD_IMHS_Action_Summaries_040814.pdf).

Increased outreach efforts by the VA, with a focus on suicide-means safety (including weapons, medications, environmental factors) and skills-building strategies to manage major life stressors, would address the needs of the veteran population within their community (Kemp 2014). Further, efforts to identify patients with increased suicide risk based on predictive models using variables extracted from electronic VA medical records are expected to expand screening capabilities and improve preventive services and clinical care (McCarthy et al. 2015). The Department of Defense and VA are also examining methods for using big data with predictive modeling to support treatment and assist clinicians working with those who may be at risk for suicidality (Kessler et al. 2015b, 2016; McCarthy et al. 2015). These comprehensive strategies are anticipated to provide appropriate, timely care to the military and growing veteran populations, potentially preventing suicidal behaviors and reducing suicide rates in this high-priority group of service members.

Key Concepts

1. Research efforts have begun to address the increase in suicide rates in service members and veterans following the commencement of Operation Iraqi Freedom and Operation Enduring Freedom, by examining possible risk and protective factors that may influence suicidal behaviors.
2. History of mental health diagnoses and previous suicidal behaviors, as well as military-specific and life stressors and exposure to traumatic events, are important risk factors that have been predictive of suicidality in service members and veterans.

3. Access to mental health treatment is protective against suicidal behaviors. Attention to barriers to care is a critical focus in suicide prevention within the Department of Defense (DoD) and Department of Veterans Affairs (VA). Programs that target at-risk groups and encourage early detection, intervention, education, and communication are being developed that involve leadership, peers, and mental health-care providers.
4. Increased outreach efforts by the VA with a focus on suicide means safety (e.g., weapons management, medication, and situational factors) and skills-building strategies to manage major life stressors would address the needs of the veteran population within their community.

Disclaimer The opinions expressed in the manuscript are those of the authors and, therefore, do not necessarily reflect the views of the Department of Defense and the Uniformed Services University of the Health Sciences.

References

Afifi TO, Taillieu T, Zamorski MA, Turner S, Cheung K, Sareen J (2016) Association of child abuse exposure with suicidal ideation, suicide plans, and suicide attempts in military personnel and the general population in Canada. JAMA Psychiat 73(3):229–238. https://doi.org/10.1001/jamapsychiatry.2015.2732

Allen MH, Forster F, Zealberg J, Currier G (2002) Report and recommendations regarding psychiatric emergency and crisis services: a review and model program descriptions. American Psychiatric Association Task Force on Psychiatric Emergency Services, Washington, DC

American Psychiatric Association (2003) Practice guideline for the assessment and treatment of patients with suicidal behaviors. Am J Psychiatr 160(11):1–60. erratum *American Journal of Psychiatry* 16(4): 776, 2004

Anestis MD, Bryan CJ (2012) Means and capacity for suicidal behavior: a comparison of the ratio of suicide attempts and deaths by suicide in the US military and general population. J Affect Disord 148(1):42–47. https://doi.org/10.1016/j.jad.2012.11.045

Army Suicide Prevention Task Force (2010) Army health promotion, risk reduction, suicide prevention: report 2010. Department of Defense, Washington, DC

Armed Forces Health Surveillance Center (2012) Mental disorders and mental health problems, active component, US Armed Forces, 2000-2011. MSMR 19(6):11–17

Bachynski KE, Canham-Chervak M, Black SA, Dada EO, Millikan AM, Jones BH (2012) Mental health risk factors for suicides in the US Army, 2007–8. Inj Prev 18:405–412

Barber ME, Marzuk PM, Leon AC, Portera L (1998) Aborted suicide attempts: a new classification of suicidal behavior. Am J Psychiatr 155(3):385. (3)an

Black SA, Gallaway MS, Bell MR, Ritchie EC (2011) Prevalence and risk factors associated with suicides of Army soldiers, 2001–2009. Mil Psychol 23:433–451

Blow FC, Bohnert ASB, Ilgen MA, Ignacio R, McCarthy JF, Valenstein MM et al (2012) Suicide mortality among patients treated by the Veterans Health Administration from 2000 to 2007. Am J Public Health 102(Suppl 1):S98–S104

Boardman AP, Grimbaldeston AH, Handley C, Jones PW, Willmott S (1999) The North Staffordshire Suicide Study: a case-control study of suicide in one health district. Psychol Med 29:27–33

Bossarte RM, Knox KL, Piegari R, Altieri J, Kemp J, Katz IR (2012) Prevalence and characteristics of suicide ideation and attempts among active military and veteran participants in a national health survey. Am J Public Health 102(Suppl. 1):S38–S40

Boudreaux ED, Horowitz LM (2014) Suicide risk screening and assessment: designing instruments with dissemination in mind. Am J Prev Med 47(3 Suppl 2): S163–SI69

Bower B (2015) As suicide rates increase, researchers separate thoughts from actions. Sci News. Accessed 28 Jan 2016

Brailey K, Vasterling JJ, Proctor SP, Constans JI, Friedman MJ (2007) PTSD symptoms, life events, and unit cohesion in US soldiers: baseline findings from the Neurocognition Deployment Health Study. J Trauma Stress 20:495–503

Branas CC, Han S, Wiebe DJ (2016) Alcohol use and firearm violence. Epidemiol Rev 38(1):32–45. https://doi.org/10.1093/epirev/mxv010

Brenner LA, Barnes SM (2012) Facilitating treatment engagement during high-risk transition periods: a potential suicide prevention strategy. Am J Public Health 102(Suppl 1):S12–S14

Brown GK, Ten Have T, Henriques GR et al (2005) Cognitive therapy for the prevention of suicide attempts: a randomized controlled trial. JAMA 294(5):563. (5)iv

Bruffaerts R, Demyttenaere K, Hwang I, Tat Chiu W, Sampson N, Kessler RC et al (2011) Treatment of suicidal people around the world. Br J Psychiatry 199(1):64–70

Bryan CJ, Clemans TA (2013) Repetitive traumatic brain injury, psychological symptoms, and suicide risk in a clinical sample of deployed military personnel. JAMA Psychiat 70(7):686–691

Bryan CJ, Rudd MD (2006) Advances in the assessment of suicide risk. J Clin Psychol 62(2):185–200

Bryan CJ, Rudd MD, Wertenberger E (2013) Reasons for suicide attempts in a clinical sample of active duty soldiers. J Affect Disord 144:148–152

Bryan CJ, Bryan AO, Ray-Sannerud BN, Etienne N, Morrow CE (2014a) Suicide attempts before joining the military increase risk for suicide attempts and severity of suicidal ideation among military personnel and veterans. Compr Psychiatry 55(3):534–541

Bryan AO, Bryan CJ, Morrow CE, Etienne N, Ray-Sannerud B (2014b) Moral injury, suicidal ideation, and suicide attempts in a military sample. Traumatology 20(3):154–160

Bryan CJ, Griffith JH, Pace BT, Hinkson K, Bryan AO, Clemans TA et al (2015a) Combat exposure and risk for suicidal thoughts and behaviors among military personnel and veterans: a systematic review and meta-analysis. Suicide Life Threat Behav 45(5):633–649

Bryan CJ, Bryan AO, Clemans TA (2015b) The association of military and premilitary sexual trauma with risk for suicide ideation, plans, and attempts. Psychiatry Res 227:246–252

Bryan CJ, Roberge E, Bryan AO, Clemans TA, Imel ZE (2015c) Guilt as a mediator of the relationship between depression and post-traumatic stress with suicide ideation in two samples of military personnel and veterans. International Journal of Cognitive Therapy 8(2):143–155. https://doi.org/10.1521/ijct.2015.8.2.143

Bush NE, Skopp NA, McCann R, Luxton DD (2011) Posttraumatic growth as protection against suicidal ideation after deployment and combat exposure. Mil Med 176(11):1215–1222

Calabrese JR, Prescott M, Tamburrino M, Liberzon I, Slembarski R, Goldmann E, Shirley E, Fine T, Goto T, Wilson K, Ganocy S, Chan P, Serrano MB, Sizemore J, Galea S (2011) PTSD comorbidity and suicidal ideation associated with PTSD within the Ohio Army National Guard. J Clin Psychiatry 72(8):1072–1078

Camp NM (2014) US Army psychiatry in the Vietnam war. Borden Institute, US Army Medical Department Center and School, Fort Sam Houston, pp 299–302

Carr RB (2011) When a soldier commits suicide in Iraq: impact on unit and caregivers. Psychiatry 74(2):95–106

Castro CA, Kintzle S (2014) Suicides in the military: the post-modern combat veteran and the Hemingway effect. Curr Psychiatry Rep 16:460–469. https://doi.org/10.1007/s11920-014-0460-1

Centers for Disease Control and Prevention (CDC) (2013) Web-based Injury Statistics Query and Reporting System (WISQARS) [Online]. National Center for Injury Prevention and Control, CDC (producer). Accessed from http://www.cdc.gov/injury/wisqars/index.html on January 29, 2016

Claasen CA, Harvilchuck-Laurenson JD, Fawcett J (2014) Prognostic models to detect and monitor the near-term risk of suicide state of the science. Am J Prev Med 47(3 suppl 2):S181–S185

Colpe LJ, Naifeh JA, Aliaga P, Sampson NA, Heeringa SG, Stein MB, Ursano RJ, Fullerton CS, Nock MK, Schoenbaum ML, Zaslavsky AM, Kessler RC (2015) Mental health treatment among soldiers with current mental disorders in the Army Study to Assess Risk and Resilience in Servicemembers (Army STARRS). Mil Med 180(10)

Corr WP (2014) Suicides and suicide attempts among active component members of the US Armed Forces, 2010–2012id methods of self-harm vary by major geographic region of assignment. MSMR 21(10):2–5

Davis CL, Kilbourne AM, Blow FC, Pierce JR, Winkel BM, Huycke E et al (2012) Reduced mortality among Department of Veterans Affairs patients with schizophrenia or bipolar disorder lost to follow-up and engaged in active outreach to return for care. Am J Public Health 102(Suppl 1):S74–S79

DeBeer BB, Kimbrel NA, Meyer EC, Gulliver SB (2014) Combined PTSD and depressive symptoms interact with post-deployment social support to predict suicidal ideation in Operation Enduring Freedom and Operation Iraqi Freedom veterans. Psychiatry Res 216(3):357–362

Department of Defense Task Force on the Prevention of Suicide by Members of the Armed Forces (2010) The challenge and the promise: strengthening the force, preventing suicide and saving lives. Department of Defense, Washington, DC

Department of the Army (2012) Army 2020: Generating health and discipline in the force. Ahead of the strategic reset. Report 2012: Accessed from https://www.army.mil/e2/c/downloads/232541.pdf on October 10, 2016

Department of Veterans Affairs (2010) Facts about veteran suicide. Veterans by selected period of service and state: 2010. Accessed from http://www.census.gov/compendia/statab/2012/tables/12s0520.pdf on January 28, 2016

Department of Veterans Affairs (2015) Unique veterans users report FY 2013. National Center for Veterans Analysis and Statistics. Accessed from http://www.va.gov/vetdata/docs/SpecialReports/Profile_Of_Unique_Veteran_Users.pdf on January 29, 2016

Desai RA, Dausey DJ, Rosenheck RA (2005) Mental health service delivery and suicide risk: the role of individual patient and facility factors. Am J Psychiatr 162:311–318

Dobscha SK, Denneson LM, Kovas AE, Teo A, Forsberg CW, Kaplan MS, Bossarte R, McFarland BH (2014) Correlates of suicide among veterans treated in primary care: case-control study of a nationally representative sample. J Gen Intern Med 29(Suppl 4):S853–S860

Doran N, DePeralta S, Depp C, Dishman B, Gold L, Marshall R, Miller D, Vitale S, Tiamson-Kassab M (2016) The validity of a brief risk assessment tool for predicting suicidal behavior in veterans utilizing VHA mental health care. Suicide Life Threat Behav 46(4):471–485

Eaton KM, Messer SC, Wilson ALG, Hoge CW (2006) Strengthening the validity of population-based suicide rate comparisons: an illustration using US military and civilian data. Suicide Life Threat Behav 36:182–191

Finley EP, Bollinger M, Noel PH, Amuan ME, Copeland LA, Pugh JA, Dassori A, Palmer R, Bryan C, Pugh MJV (2015) A national cohort study of the association between the polytrauma clinical triad and suicide-related behavior among US veterans who served in Iraq and Afghanistan. Am J Public Health 105(2):380–387

Frueh BC, Smith JA (2012) Suicide, alcoholism and psychiatric illness among union forces during the US Civil War. J Anxiety Disord 26:769–775

Gilman SE, Bromet EJ, Cox KL, Colpe LJ, Fullerton CS, Gruber MJ, Heeringa SG, Lewandowski-Romps L, Millikan-Bell AM, Naifeh JA, Nock MK, Petukhova MV, Sampson NA, Schoenbaum M, Stein MB, Ursano RJ, Wessely S, Zaslavsky AM, Kessler RC (2014) Socio-demographic and career history predictors of suicide and suicide mortality in the United States Army 2004–2009. Psychol Med 44(12):2579–2592

Glenn CR, Nock MK (2014) Improving the short-term prediction of suicidal behavior. Am J Prev Med 47(3 suppl 2):S176–S180

Gradus JL, Shipherd JC, Suvak MK, Giasson HL, Miller M (2012) Suicide attempts and suicide among marines: a decade of follow-up. Suicide Life Threat Behav 43(1):39–49

Gradus JL, Street AE, Suvak MK, Resick PA (2013) Predictors of suicidal ideation in a gender-stratified sample of OEF/OIF veterans. Suicide Life Threat Behav 43(5):574–588

Gradus JL, Smith BN, Vogt D (2015) Family support, family stress, and suicidal ideation in a combat-exposed sample of Operation Enduring Freedom/ Operation Iraqi Freedom veterans. Anxiety Stress Coping 28(6):706–715

Harris EC, Barraclough B (1997) Suicide as an outcome for mental disorder. A meta-analysis. British Journal of Psychiatry 170:205–228

Hendin H (2014) An innovative approach to treating combat veterans with PTSD at risk for suicide. Suicide Life Threat Behav 44(5):582–590

Hill JV, Johnson RC, Barton RA (2006) Suicidal and homicidal soldiers in deployment environments. Mil Med 171(3):228–232

Hoffmire CA, Kemp JE, Bossarte RM (2015) Changes in suicide mortality for veterans and nonveterans by gender and history of VHA service use, 2000-2010. Psychiatr Serv 66(9):959–965

Hoge CW, Castro CA, Messer SC, McGurk D, Cotting DI, Koffman RL (2004) Combat duty in Iraq and Afghanistan: mental health problems and barriers to care. N Engl J Med 351:13–22. https://doi.org/10.1056/NEJMoa040603

Hoge CW, Auchterlonie JL, Milliken CS (2006) Mental health problems, use of mental health services, and attrition from military service after returning from deployment to Iraq or Afghanistan. J Am Med Assoc 295:1023–1032

Hoge CW, McGurk D, Thomas JL, Cox AL, Engel CC, Castro CA (2008) Mild traumatic brain injury in U.S. Soldiers returning from Iraq. New Engl J Med 358:453–463

Hoge CW, Castro CA (2012) Preventing suicides in US service members and veterans: concerns after a decade of war. JAMA 308(7):671–672

Hyman J, Ireland R, Frost L, Cottrell L (2012) Suicide incidence and risk factors in an active duty US military population. Am J Public Health 102(Suppl 1):S138–S146

Ireland RR, Kress AM, Frost LZ (2012) Association between mental health conditions diagnosed during initial eligibility for military health care benefits and subsequent deployment, attrition, and death by suicide among active duty service members. Mil Med 177(10):1149–1156

Jakupcak M, Cook J, Imel Z, Fontana A, Rosenheck R, McFall M (2009) Posttraumatic stress disorder as a risk factor for suicidal ideation in Iraq and Afghanistan War veterans. J Trauma Stress 22:303–306

Joiner TE, Conwell Y, Fitzpatrick KK, Witte TK, Schmidt NB, Berlim MT et al (2005) Four studies on how past and current suicidality relate even when "everything but the kitchen sink" is covaried. J Abnorm Psychol 114(2):291–303. https://doi.org/10.1037/0021-843X.114.2.291

Kang HK, Bullman TA (2008) Risk of suicide among US veterans after returning from the Iraq or Afghanistan war zones. J Am Med Assoc 300:652–653

Kang HK, Bullman TA, Smolenski DJ, Skopp NA, Gahm GA, Reger MA (2015) Suicide risk among 1.3 million veterans who were on active duty during the Iraq and Afghanistan wars. Ann Epidemiol 25:96–100. https://doi.org/10.1016/j.annepidem.2014.11.020

Kaplan MS, Huguet N, McFarland BH, Newsom JT (2007) Suicide among male veterans: a prospective population-based study. J Epidemiol Community Health 61(7):619–624. https://doi.org/10.1136/jech.2006.054346

Kaskutas LA, Weisner C, Caetano R (1997) Predictors of help seeking among a longitudinal sample of the general population, 1984-1992. J Stud Alcohol 58(2):155–161

Kemp J (2014) Suicide rates in VHA patients through 2011 with comparisons with other Americans and other Veterans through 2010. Veterans Health Administration, Washington, DC

Kessler RC, Berglund P, Borges G, Nock M, Wang PS (2005) Trends in suicide ideation, plans, gestures, and attempts in the United States, 1990–1992 to 2001–2003. J Am Med Assoc 293(20):2487–2495. https://doi.org/10.1001/jama.293.20.2487

Kessler RC, Heeringa SG, Stein MB, Colpe LJ, Fullerton CS, Hwang I, Naifeh JA, Nock MK, Petukhova M, Sampson NA, Schoenbaum M, Zaslavsky AM, Ursano RJ (2014) Thirty-day prevalence of DSM-IV mental disorders among nondeployed soldiers in the US Army: results from the Army Study to Assess Risk and Resilience in Servicemembers (Army STARRS). JAMA Psychiat 71(5):504–513

Kessler RC, Warner CH, Ivany C, Petukhova MV, Rose S, Bromet EJ, Brown M 3rd, Cai T, Colpe LJ, Cox KL, Fullerton CS, Gilman SE, Gruber MJ, Heeringa

SG, Lewandowski-Romps L, Li J, Millikan-Bell AM, Naifeh JA, Nock MK, Rosellini AJ, Sampson NA, Schoenbaum M, Stein MB, Wessely S, Zaslavsky AM, Ursano RJ (2015a) Predicting suicides after psychiatric hospitalization in US Army soldiers: the Army Study to Assess Risk and Resilience in Servicemembers (Army STARRS). JAMA Psychiat 72(1):49–57

Kessler RC, Stein MB, Bliese PD, Bromet EJ, Chiu WT, Cox KL, Colpe LJ, Bell A, Naifeh JA, Nock MK, Petukhova MV, Rosellini AJ, Sampson NA, Schoenbaum M, Zaslavsky AM, Ursano RJ (2015b) Occupational differences in US Army suicide rates. Psychol Med 45(15):3293–3304. https://doi.org/10.1017/S0033291715001294

Kessler RC, Stein MB, Petukhova MV, Bliese P, Bossarte RM, Bromet EJ, Fullerton CS, Gilman SE, Ivany C, Lewandowski-Romps L, Millikan Bell A, Naifeh JA, Nock MK, Reis BY, Rosellini AJ, Sampson NA, Zaslavsky AM, Ursano RJ (2016) Predicting suicides after outpatient mental health visits in the Army Study to Assess Risk and Resilience in Servicemembers. Mol Psychiatry., epub ahead of print. https://doi.org/10.1038/mp.2016.110

Khazem LR, Houtsma C, Gratz KL, Tull MT, Green BA, Anestis MD (2016) Firearms matter: the moderating role of firearm storage in the association between current suicidal ideation and likelihood of future suicide attempts among United States military personnel. Mil Psychol 28(1):25–33

Kim E (2002) Agitation, aggression, and disinhibitory syndromes after traumatic brain injury. NeuroRehabilitation 17(4):297–310

Kimerling R, Makin-Byrd K, Louzon S, Ignacio RV, McCarthy JF (2015) Military sexual trauma and suicide mortality. American Journal of Preventive Medicine, epub ahead of print. https://doi.org/10.1016/j.amepre.2015.10.019

Knox KL, Stanley B, Currier GW, Brenner L, Holloway MG, Brown G (2012) An emergency department-based brief intervention for veterans at risk for suicide (SAFE VET). Am J Public Health 102(Suppl 1):S33–S37

Kochanski-Ruscio KM, Carreno-Ponce JT, DeYoung K, Grammer G, Ghahramanlou-Holloway M (2014) Diagnostic and psychosocial differences in psychiatrically hospitalized military service members with single versus multiple suicide attempts. Uniformed Services University of the Health Sciences, Paper 131. http://digitalcommons.unl.edu/usuhs/131

Kopacz MS, Morley SW, Wozniak BM, Simons KV, Bishop TM, Vance CG (2016) Religious well-being and suicide ideation in veterans- an exploratory study. Pastor Psychol 65:481–491

Krulee DA, Hales RE (1988) Compliance with psychiatric referrals from a general hospital psychiatry outpatient clinic. Gen Hosp Psychiatry 10(5):339–345

Kuehn BM (2009) Soldier suicide rates continue to rise: military, scientists work to stem the tide. J Am Med Assoc 301(11):1111–1113. https://doi.org/10.1001/jama.2009.342

Lande RG (2011) Felo de se: soldier suicides in America's Civil War. Mil Med 176:531–536

LeardMann CA, Powell TM, Smith TC, Bell MR, Smith B, Boyko EJ et al (2013) Risk factors associated with suicide in current and former US military personnel. J Am Med Assoc 310(5):496–506

Legarreta M, Graham J, North L, Bueler CE, McGlade E, Yurgelun-Todd D (2015) DSM-5 posttraumatic stress disorder symptoms associated with suicide behaviors in veterans. Psychol Trauma: Theory Res Pract Policy 7(3):277–285

Lemaire CM, Graham DP (2010) Factors associated with suicidal ideation in OEF/OIF veterans. J Affect Disord 130:231–238

Lester D (1998) Preventing suicide by restricting access to methods for suicide. Arch Suicide Res 4:7–24

Lewitzka U, Severus E, Bauer R, Ritter P, Muller-Oerlinghausen B, Bauer M (2015) The suicide prevention effect of lithium: more than 20 years of evidence- a narrative review. Int J Bipolar Disord 3(15):1–16

Linehan MM, Comtois KA, Murray AM, Brown MZ, Gallop RJ, Heard HL et al (2006) Two-year randomized controlled trial and follow-up of dialectical behavior therapy vs therapy by experts for suicidal behaviors and borderline personality disorder. Arch Gen Psychiatry 63(7):757–766. https://doi.org/10.1001/archpsyc.63.7.757

Linley PA, Joseph S (2004) Positive change following trauma and adversity: a review. J Trauma Stress 17(1):11–21. https://doi.org/10.1023/B:JOTS.0000014671.27856.7e

Luoma JB, Martin CE, Pearson JL (2002) Contact with mental health and primary care providers before suicide: a review of the evidence. Am J Psychiatr 159:909–916

Luxton DD, Trofilmovich L, Clark LL (2013) Suicide risk among US service members after psychiatric hospitalization, 2001–2011. Psychiatr Serv 64(7):626–629

Maguen S, Luxton DD, Skopp NA, Gahm GA, Reger MA, Metzler JJ et al (2011) Killing in combat, mental health symptoms, and suicidal ideation in Iraq war veterans. J Anxiety Disord 25:563–567

Maguen S, Skopp NA, Zhang Y, Smolenski DJ (2015) Gender differences in suicide and suicide attempts among US Army soldiers. Psychiatry Res 225(3):545–549

Mann JJ, Apter A, Bertolote J, Beautrais A, Currier D, Haas A et al (2005) Suicide prevention strategies: a systematic review. J Am Med Assoc 294(16):2064–2074. https://doi.org/10.1001/jama.294.16.2064

Marzuk PM, Tardiff K, Leon AC, Portera L, Weiner C (1997) The prevalence of aborted suicide attempts among psychiatric in-patients. Acta Psychiatr Scand 96(6):492–496

McCarten JM, Hoffmire CA, Bossarte RM (2015) Changes in overall and firearm veteran suicide rates by gender, 2001–2010. Am J Prev Med 48(3):360–364

McCarthy JF, Valenstein M, Kim HM, Ilgen M, Zivin K, Blow FC (2009) Suicide mortality among patients receiving care in the veterans health administration health system. Am J Epidemiol 169(8):1033–1038. https://doi.org/10.1093/aje/kwp010

McCarthy JF, Bossarte RM, Katz IR, Thompson C, Kemp J, Hannemann CM, Nielson C, Schoenbaum M (2015) Predictive modeling and concentration of the risk of suicide: implications for preventive interventions in the US Department of Veterans Affairs. Am J Public Health 105(9):1935–1942

Meltzer HY, Alphs L, Green AI, Altamura AC, Anand R, Bertoldi A, Bourgeois M, Chouinar G, Islam MZ, Kane J, Krishnan R, Lindenmayer JP, Potkin S, International Suicide Prevention Trial Study Group (2003) Clozapine treatment for suicidality in schizophrenia. Arch Gen Psychiatry 60(1):82–91

Menninger WC (1948) Psychiatry in a troubled world. The MacMillan Company, New York, pp 166–167

Military Suicide Research Consortium (2016) MSRC's David Rudd consulted: "Why modern soldiers are more susceptible to suicide." Accessed from: (https://msrc.fsu.edu/news/msrcs-david-rudd-consulted-why-modern-soldiers-are-more-susceptible-suicide) and (http://usnews.nbcnews.com/_news/2013/03/02/17148761-why-modern-soldiers-are-more-susceptible-to-suicide?lite) on January 29, 2016

Mitchell MM, Gallaway MS, Millikan AM, Bell MR (2012) Interaction of combat exposure and unit cohesion in predicting suicide-related ideation among post-deployment soldiers. Suicide Life Threat Behav 42:486–494

Naifeh JA, Colpe LJ, Aliaga PA, Sampson NA, Heeringa SG, Stein MB, Ursano RJ, Fullerton CS, Nock MK, Schoenbaum M, Zaslavsky AM, Kessler RC (2016) Barriers to initiating and continuing mental health treatment among soldiers in the Army Study to Assess Risk and Resilience in Servicemembers (Army STARRS). *Military Medicine 181*(9):1021–1032

Nelson R (2004) Suicide rates rise among soldiers in Iraq. Lancet 363(9405):300. https://doi.org/10.1016/S0140-6736(03)15428-1

Nock MK, Kessler RC (2006) Prevalence of and risk factors for suicide attempts versus suicide gestures: analysis of the National Comorbidity Survey. J Abnorm Psychol 115(3):616–623. https://doi.org/10.1037/0021-843X.115.3.616

Nock MK, Borges G, Bromet EJ, Cha CB, Kessler RC, Lee S (2008) Suicide and suicidal behavior. Epidemiol Rev 30:133–154. https://doi.org/10.1093/epirev/mxn002

Nock MK, Stein MB, Heeringa SG, Ursano RJ, Colpe LJ, Fullerton CS, Hwang I, Naifeh JA, Sampson NA, Schoenbaum M, Zaslavsky AM, Kessler RC (2014) Prevalence and correlates of suicidal behavior among soldiers: results from the Army Study to Assess Risk and Resilience in Servicemembers (Army STARRS). JAMA Psychiat 71(5):514–522

Nock MK, Ursano RJ, Heeringa SG, Stein MB, Jain S, Raman R, Sun X, Chiu WT, Colpe LJ, Fullerton CS, Gilman SE, Hwang I, Naifeh JA, Rosellini AJ, Sampson NA, Schoenbaum M, Zaslavsky AM, Kessler RC (2015) Mental disorders, comorbidity, and pre-enlistment suicidal behavior among new soldiers in the US Army: results from the Army Study to Assess Risk and Resilience in Servicemembers (Army STARRS). Suicide Life Threat Behav 45(5). https://doi.org/10.1111/sltb.12153

Office of the Surgeon General and National Action Alliance for Suicide Prevention (2012) 2012 National Strategy for suicide prevention: goals and objectives for action. US Department of Health and Human Services, Washington, DC

Perales R, Gallaway S, Forys-Donahue KL, Speiss A, Millikan AM (2012) Prevalence of childhood trauma among US Army soldiers with suicidal behavior. Mil Med 177(9):1034–1040

Peterson C, Park N, Pole N, D'Andrea W, Seligman ME (2008) Strengths of character and posttraumatic growth. J Trauma Stress 21(2):214–217. https://doi.org/10.1002/jts.20332

Pietrzak RH, Goldstein MB, Malley JC, Rivers AJ, Johnson DC, Southwick SM (2010) Risk and protective factors associated with suicidal ideation in veterans of Operations Enduring Freedom and Iraqi Freedom. J Affect Disord 123:102–107

Posner K, Oquendo MA, Gould M, Stanley B, Davies M (2007) Columbia Classification Algorithm of Suicide Assessment (C-CASA): classification of suicidal events in the FDA's pediatric suicidal risk analysis of antidepressants. Am J Psychiatr 164(7):1035–1043. https://doi.org/10.1176/appi.ajp.164.7.1035

Rao V, Lyketsos C (2000) Neuropsychiatric sequelae of traumatic brain injury. Psychosomatics 41(2):95–103

Ramchand R, Acosta J, Burns RM, Jaycox LH, Pernin CG (2011) The war within: preventing suicide in the US military. RAND Corporation, Santa Monica

Ramchand R, Ayer L, Geyer L, Kofner A, Burgette L (2015) Noncommissioned officers' perspectives on identifying, caring for, and referring soldiers and marines at risk of suicide. Psychiatr Serv 66:1057–1063

Ramsawh HJ, Fullerton CS, Mash HBH, Ng TH, Kessler RC, Stein MB, Ursano RJ (2014) Risk for suicidal behaviors associated with PTSD, depression, and their comorbidity in the US Army. J Affect Disord 161:116–122. https://doi.org/10.1016/j.jad.2014.03.016

Reger MA, Smolenski DJ, Skopp NA, Metzger-Abamukang MJ, Kang HK, Bullman TA, Perdue S, Gahm GA (2015) Risk of suicide among US military service members following Operation Enduring Freedom or Operation Iraqi Freedom deployment and separation from the US military. JAMA Psychiat 72(6):561–569

Rosellini AJ, Heeringa SG, Stein MB, Ursano RJ, Chiu WT, Colpe LJ, Fullerton CS, Gilman SE, Hwang I, Naifeh JA, Nock MK, Petukhova M, Sampson NA, Schoenbaum M, Zaslavsky AM, Kessler RC (2015) Lifetime prevalence of *DSM-IV* mental disorders among new soldiers in the US Army: results from the Army Study to Assess Risk and Resilience in Servicemembers (Army STARRS). Depression Anxiety 32:13–24

Rudd MD, Bryan CJ, Wertenberger EG, Peterson AL, Young-McCaughan S, Mintz J, Williams SR, Arne KA, Breitbach J, Delano K, Wilkinson E, Bruce TO (2015) Brief cognitive-behavioral therapy effects on post-treatment suicide attempts in a military sample: results of a randomized clinical trial with 2-year follow-up. Am J Psychiatr 172:441–449. https://doi.org/10.1176/appi.ajp.2014.14070843

Schneiderman AI, Braver ER, Kang HK (2008) Understanding sequelae of injury mechanisms and mild traumatic brain injury incurred during the conflicts in Iraq and Afghanistan: persistent postconcussive symptoms and posttraumatic stress disorder. Am J Epidemiol 167(12):1446–1452

Schoenbaum M, Kessler RC, Gilman SE, Colpe LJ, Heeringa SG, Stein MB, Ursano RJ, Cox KL (2014) Predictors of suicide and accident death in the Army Study to Assess Risk and Resilience in Servicemembers (Army STARRS). JAMA Psychiat 71(5):493–503

Scoville SL, Gardner JW, Potter RN (2004) Traumatic deaths during US armed forces basic training, 1977-2001. Am J Prev Med 26(3):194–204

Shelef L, Tatsa-Laur L, Derazne E, Mann JJ, Fruchter E (2016) An effective suicide prevention program in the Israeli Defense Forces: a cohort study. Eur Psychiatry 31:37–43

Sher L (2006) Alcohol consumption and suicide. QJM 99(1):57–61. https://doi.org/10.1093/qjmed/hci146

Skopp NA, Trofimovich L, Grimes J, Oetjen-Gerdes L, Gahm GA (2012) Relations between suicide and traumatic brain injury, psychiatric diagnoses, and relationship problems, active component, US Armed Forces, 2001–2009. MSMR 19(2):7–11

Skopp NA, Smolenski DJ, Sheppard SC, Bush NE, Luxton DD (2016) Comparison of suicide attempters and decedents in the US Army: a latent class analysis. Suicide Life Threat Behav. https://doi.org/10.1111/sltb.12227

Smith EG, Austin KL, Kim HM, Miller DR, Eisen SV, Christiansen CL, Kilbourne AM, Sauer BC, McCarthy JF, Valenstein M (2014) Suicide risk in Veterans Health Administration patients with mental health diagnoses initiating lithium or valproate: a historical prospective cohort study. BMC Psychiatry 14:357

Snarr JD, Heyman RE, Slep AM (2010) Recent suicidal ideation and suicide attempts in a large-scale survey of the US Air Force: prevalences and demographic risk factors. Suicide Life Threat Behav 40(6):544–552

Stanley B, Brown GK (2008) The safety plan treatment manual to reduce suicide risk: veteran version. United States Department of Veterans Affairs, Washington, DC. http://www.mentalhealth.va.gov/docs/va_safety_planning_manual.pdf. Accessed 29 Jan 2016

Stanley B, Brown GK (2012) Safety planning intervention: a brief intervention to mitigate suicide risk. Cogn Behav Pract 19(2):256–264

Stanley B, Brown GK, Currier GW, Lyons C, Chesin M, Knox KL (2015) Brief intervention and follow-up for suicidal patients with repeat emergency department visits enhances treatment engagement. Am J Public Health 105(8):570–1572

Street AE, Gilman SE, Rosellini AJ, Stein MB, Bromet EJ, Cox KL, Colpe LJ, Fullerton CS, Gruber MJ, Heeringa SG, Lewandowski-Romps L, Little RJA, Naifeh JA, Nock MK, Sampson NA, Schoenbaum M, Ursano RJ, Zaslavsky AM, Kessler RC (2015) Understanding the elevated suicide risk of female soldiers during deployments. Psychol Med 45:717–726

The Assessment and Management of Risk for Suicide Working Group (2013) VA/DoD clinical practice guidelines for assessment and management of patients at risk for suicide. Version 1.0. Veterans Health Administration and Department of Defense, Washington, D.C.

Ursano RJ, Colpe LJ, Heeringa SG, Kessler RC, Schoenbaum M, Stein MB (2014) The Army study to assess risk and resilience in Servicemembers (Army STARRS). Psychiatry 77(2):107–119

Ursano RJ, Heeringa SG, Stein MB, Jain S, Raman R, Sun X et al (2015a) Prevalence and correlates of suicidal behavior among new soldiers in the US Army: results from the Army Study to Assess Risk and Resilience in Servicemembers (Army STARRS). Depress Anxiety 32:3–12

Ursano RJ, Kessler RC, Stein MB, Naifeh JA, Aliaga PA, Fullerton CS, Sampson NA, Kao T-C, Colpe LJ, Schoenbaum M, Cox KL, Heeringa SG (2015b) Suicide attempts in the US Army during the wars in Afghanistan and Iraq, 2004 C. S. JAMA Psychiatry 72(9):917–926. https://doi.org/10.1001/jamapsychiatry.2015.0987

Valenstein M, Kim HM, Ganoczy D, McCarthy JF, Zivin K, Austin KL, Hoggatt K, Eisenberg D, Piette JD, Blow FC, Olfson M (2009) Higher-risk periods for suicide among VA patients receiving depression treatment: prioritizing suicide prevention efforts. J Affect Disord 112(1–3):50–58

Wang PS, Berglund P, Olfson M, Pincus HA, Wells KB, Kessler RC (2005) Failure and delay in initial treatment contact after first onset of mental disorders in the National Comorbidity Survey Replication. Arch Gen Psychiatry 62(6):603–613. https://doi.org/10.1001/archpsyc.62.6.603

Wang PS, Gruber MJ, Powers RE, Schoenbaum M, Speier AH, Wells KB et al (2008) Disruption of existing mental health treatments and failure to initiate new treatment after hurricane Katrina. Am J Psychiatr 165(1):34–41. https://doi.org/10.1176/appi.ajp.2007.07030502

Warner CH, Appenzeller GN, Parker JR, Warner C, Diebold CJ, Grieger T (2011) Suicide prevention in a deployed military unit. Psychiatry 74(2):127–141

Xu J, Murphy SL, Kochanek KD (2016) Deaths: final data for 2013. Natl Vital Stat Rep 64(2):1–119

The Role of Sleep in Mental Illness in Veterans and Active Service Members

25

Lisa Talbot, Elizabeth Klingaman,
Michelle Primeau, Makoto Kawai, Sophia Pirog,
Joshua Jordan, and Ruth O'Hara

Sleep in Veteran and Service Member Populations

Sleep problems are increasingly recognized as a key feature of mental health in active and retired military service members. Impaired sleep in active service members and veterans is of significant distress to both patient and caregiver and may lead to or exacerbate the cognitive and behavioral core symptoms of psychiatric disorders. Sleep disturbances can be a sign of additional comorbid sleep disorders, many of which can be alleviated with a range of effective treatment approaches. The most common sleep disorders in this population include insomnia, obstructive sleep apnea (OSA), insufficient sleep syndrome, shift work sleep disorder, nightmare disorder, and parasomnias such as sleepwalking and dream-enacting behaviors.

Studies have generally found obstructive sleep apnea and insomnia to be two of the most prevalent sleep dysfunctions in veterans. In a sample of 2,866 veterans who completed the National Veterans Sleep Survey (Polley et al. 2013), the average amount of sleep reported was 5.6–1.1 h fewer than the average US citizen. Of these veterans, 74.3% "reported meeting general clinical criteria for insomnia." Insufficient sleep was attributed

L. Talbot
Stanford University School of Medicine, Palo Alto, CA, USA
e-mail: lisa.talbot@gmail.com

E. Klingaman
Department of Psychiatry, U.S. Department of Veterans Affairs Capitol Healthcare Network (VISN 5) Mental Illness Research, Education, and Clinical Center (MIRECC), University of Maryland School of Medicine, Baltimore, MD, USA
e-mail: Elizabeth.Klingaman@va.gov

M. Primeau
Stanford University School of Medicine, Palo Alto, CA, USA

Palo Alto Medical Foundation, Sunnyvale, CA, USA
e-mail: mprimeau@stanford.edu

M. Kawai • S. Pirog
Stanford University School of Medicine, VA Palo Alto Health Care System, Palo Alto, CA, USA
e-mail: mkawai71@stanford.edu; sapirog@stanford.edu

J. Jordan
California School of Professional Psychology at Alliant International University, San Francisco, CA, USA

Stanford University School of Medicine, VA Palo Alto Health Care System, Palo Alto, CA, USA
e-mail: jtjordan@stanford.edu

R. O'Hara (✉)
Department of Psychiatry and Behavioral Sciences, Stanford University School of Medicine, Palo Alto, CA, USA

Stanford University School of Medicine, VA Palo Alto Health Care System, Palo Alto, CA, USA
e-mail: roh@stanford.edu

L.W. Roberts, C.H. Warner (eds.), *Military and Veteran Mental Health*,
https://doi.org/10.1007/978-1-4939-7438-2_25

to a variety of factors, including difficulty falling or staying asleep (70%), poor sleep quality (53%), "being too busy with work or family responsibilities" (13%), "being a night owl" (12%), and "liking to watch television late at night" (8%).

Polysomnographic studies conducted on military personnel have found that, of 761 participants, 27.2% suffered from mild obstructive sleep apnea, 24.7% had insomnia, 24.7% had moderate to severe obstructive sleep apnea, and 11.2% suffered from behaviorally induced insufficient sleep (BIIS). However, it is important to also examine these sleep dysregulations in the context of comorbid psychiatric disorders. For example, those diagnosed with insomnia were more likely to have previously received a diagnosis of anxiety (23.4%), depression (31.4%), post-traumatic stress disorder (PTSD) (20.7%), or "two or more comorbid diagnoses" (31.9%) (Mysliwiec et al. 2013) and were more likely to be taking prazosin, pain medications, antidepressants, and nonbenzodiazepine receptor agonists (NBDRAs). These data highlight the importance of understanding not only the prevalence of sleep dysfunction within veteran and service member populations but also the function of such sleep dysfunctions in the context of comorbid psychiatric disorders and their treatments—pharmacological or therapeutic.

Case Study

Officer James Gonzalez (pseudonym) is a 25-year-old male officer who was deployed on multiple tours of duty, during which he was exposed to three improvised explosive device (IED) explosions. Officer Gonzalez had suffered symptoms of post-traumatic stress disorder (PTSD) and traumatic brain injury during his service, but has never revealed them because he did not want to be barred from further tours of duty. In some ways, returning to combat became a relief to him because his PTSD symptoms were more tolerable in that context. He has served valiantly and has been decorated for his heroism. Coming from a long line of military family members, this honor is important to him, as is behaving in ways that are always seen as righteous and above any reproach.

Officer Gonzalez has very recently returned from a tour of duty and was ordered to see the psychiatrist at the base because he was experiencing severe insomnia—he has difficulty falling asleep, staying asleep, and awakening early. In addition, his PTSD symptoms were noted by his commanding officer. He does not do well when he returns to his home on base—he misses the respect and adulation of his subordinates during combat. He starts to drink alcohol at home until he falls asleep, which he never does during tours because he fears it will slow his reaction time. He often has headaches and has trouble concentrating and remembering details. He denies any suicidal or homicidal ideation or plans and any depressed feelings, saying, "I am not that type of guy." He feels he hardly knows his wife and two young children, who were both born when he was overseas. He wants to play with his children, but he is usually irritable. He is also sensitive to sound and is quite easily upset by the noise made by his children. The children sometimes do not obey him when he tells them to quiet down or to stop what they are doing, and, on four occasions, his wife saw him hit the older son with his hand. He told his wife that he was very sorry and would not hit his son ever again. Officer Gonzalez did not think he needed to mention the hitting incidents during the psychiatric evaluation, but he feels so extremely guilty that he mentions it when asked about symptoms of guilt.

Insomnia

Prevalence of Insomnia in Veterans and Military Populations

Insomnia is defined as "difficulty falling asleep, staying asleep, and/or waking up too early, with next-day impairment, at least three times per week over the past three months" (American Psychiatric Association 2013). Insomnia symptoms appear more commonly in military populations: whereas the prevalence of insomnia in the general population is 6% (Ohayon 2002), in Operation Enduring Freedom/Operation Iraqi Freedom (OEF/OIF) military personnel assessed pre-deployment, the prevalence of insomnia is 17% (Gehrman et al. 2013). Additionally, the prevalence of insomnia in active component forces has increased almost 20-fold from 2000 to 2009 (Armed Forces Health Surveillance Center 2010). In deployed military populations, insomnia is one of the most frequent reasons for mental health evaluation (Cozza et al. 2004), and combat-related experiences increase the likelihood of sleep difficulties (Seelig et al. 2010). Insomnia was also the most common complaint of returning Operation Enduring Freedom/Operation Iraqi Freedom veterans (McLay et al. 2010). Interestingly, while the National Veterans Sleep Survey found that 74.3% of veterans report difficulty falling or staying asleep, three times a week for at least a month (Polley et al. 2013), an evaluation of those receiving care through the VA showed that only 3.4% were actually given a diagnosis of insomnia (Hermes and Rosenheck 2014).

Consequences of Insomnia

It has been shown that insomnia symptoms increase the risk for the development of psychiatric disorders. For example, in military personnel assessed pre-deployment, pre-existing insomnia increased the risk for the development of PTSD, depression, and anxiety post-deployment (Gehrman et al. 2013; Koffel et al. 2013; McLay et al. 2010). The presence of insomnia symptoms can also exacerbate co-occurring psychiatric conditions. In a prospective study by Wright et al. (2011), returning Iraq combat veterans were assessed for depression, PTSD, and insomnia post-deployment and followed for a year after returning home. While depression, PTSD, and insomnia symptoms were all correlated, insomnia symptoms at 4 months post-deployment predicted depression and PTSD symptoms at 12 months, but depression and PTSD severity did not predict insomnia symptoms. Further, in a longitudinal observational study of Operation Enduring Freedom/Operation Iraqi Freedom veterans recruited from Department of Veterans Affairs (VA) primary care clinics, patients with insomnia had higher baseline severity depression, PTSD, and alcohol use. Insomnia at baseline predicted higher depression and PTSD severity at 6 months (Pigeon et al. 2013). In this sample, while depression and PTSD symptoms declined over time, insomnia symptoms remained relatively stable (Pigeon et al. 2013).

Suicide Sleep disturbance and insomnia symptoms have been shown to be a risk factor for suicidality (Pigeon et al. 2012). In one retrospective chart review of veterans presenting to VA primary care clinics, suicidal ideation was associated with prolonged sleep latency and wake after sleep onset, as well as reduced sleep quality. When entered in a multivariate model, however, only reduced sleep quality remained significant for suicidal ideation (Chakravorty et al. 2014). In a study of young adults in the military, Ribeiro et al. (2012) found that insomnia symptoms significantly predicted suicidal ideation even after controlling for hopelessness, depression, PTSD, anxiety, and alcohol or drug abuse. They additionally found that, after controlling for baseline insomnia, depression, and hopelessness, insomnia symptoms predicted subsequent suicide attempts, suggesting that insomnia is a powerful—albeit treatable—risk factor for suicide.

Pathophysiology of Insomnia

The "3P" model—predisposing, precipitating, and perpetuating factors—has been widely used for conceptualizing psychiatric diagnoses, as well as insomnia (Spielman and Glovinski 1991). Deployed military and veteran populations may have novel characteristics that predispose them to insomnia. Predisposing factors may be genetic or related to some earlier experience. For example, adverse childhood experiences such as abuse or home instability have been shown to predict insomnia in adulthood (Kajeepeta et al. 2015), and in volunteer-era military men, adverse childhood experiences are twice as prevalent as in men without military service (Blosnich et al. 2014). The stressors of deployment—travel to a foreign location, constant threat to life, inconsistent sleep-wake schedules—can certainly precipitate insomnia. Perpetuating factors, such as maintaining the insomnia after the precipitating stressor has been removed, can be targeted in treatment, such as through cognitive behavioral therapy for insomnia (CBT-I), and can be grouped into physiologic hyperarousal, behavioral, and cognitive processes.

Hyperarousal refers to the concept of the individual having tonically heightened sympathetic activation. Individuals with insomnia may have a predisposition to the hyperaroused state, which is physiologic and measurable (Bonnet and Arand 2010), and hyperarousal may be triggered by the extreme conditions of deployment (e.g., fear for one's life, standing watch). Hyperarousal is a hallmark feature of PTSD, a frequent consequence of military-related traumas (American Psychiatric Association 2013). Veterans with greater daytime stressors also report more nightmares and longer sleep latency; worse PTSD severity predicts awakenings, shorter total sleep time, and longer sleep latency (Gehrman et al. 2015). Behavioral processes that interfere with sleep may include actions that disrupt the physiology of sleep from occurring. For example, a veteran who has not slept sufficient hours one night may drink large amounts of caffeine throughout the day to remain vigilant, not realizing that doing so can interfere with sleep the following night and thus perpetuate the cycle of inadequate rest.

Cognitive processes are the thought processes that can interfere with sleep and, in service members or veterans, may tie into the hyperarousal system. For example, there may be a compulsion to remain awake during the normal sleep period because of a feeling that it is essential they stand watch for their family. Veterans and active service members who have seen combat are almost twice as likely to feel that the need to be "on guard" interferes with sleep when compared to their peers who have not seen combat (Polley et al. 2013).

Treatment of Insomnia

Pharmacologic agents can be used for the treatment of insomnia. These typically include sedative hypnotics such as benzodiazepines or the nonbenzodiazepine "z-drugs." Off-label prescribing of sedating antidepressants, such as trazodone or doxepin; antihistamine agents, such as diphenhydramine; or sedating antipsychotics, such as quetiapine, is increasingly being used. The VA reported an increase in the use of quetiapine, an antipsychotic used off-label to treat insomnia, by more than 700% between 2001 and 2010, making it the second largest single medication expenditure in 2010. Despite this dramatic increase in off-label prescribing, only 53.1% of those diagnosed with insomnia in 2010 received a prescription for a sedative hypnotic medication (Hermes and Rosenheck 2014). These data not only suggest that insomnia is underdiagnosed in VA populations but also bring into question the appropriateness of current prescribing practices.

It is important to note that medications are not recommended for the long-term treatment of insomnia (Schutte-Rodin et al. 2008). Rather, psychological and behavioral therapies are recommended as best practice. Additionally, behavioral interventions for insomnia tend to be preferred by clinical populations (Hughes et al. 2013) and their healthcare providers (Epstein et al. 2013), making them a logical and effective approach in the treatment of insomnia.

Cognitive behavioral therapy for insomnia (CBT-I) is a highly efficacious treatment for insomnia (Trauer et al. 2015) and has been identified by the American Academy of Sleep Medicine as the first-line treatment for insomnia (Schutte-Rodin et al. 2008). Not only is CBT-I effective for insomnia, but it has also been shown to be effective in treating insomnia in patients with co-occurring depression, PTSD, and pain and in improving the symptoms of the co-occurring condition. The VA has recognized the value of CBT-I and has undertaken training mental health providers across the nation in the practice of CBT-I (Manber et al. 2012). This training program has successfully trained social workers, psychologists, psychiatrists, and nurses, working in primary care or mental health settings, in the implementation of CBT-I (Karlin et al. 2013). Previous research has shown that over the course of six sessions, newly trained clinicians are able to reduce the subjective severity of insomnia (as rated by the Insomnia Severity Index [ISI]) by approximately 50%, from moderate insomnia to subthreshold symptoms (Karlin et al. 2013). This program has been shown to reduce depression and improve quality of life, with a large effect size (d = 2.3; Trockel et al. 2014). Additionally, this CBT-I program is equally effective for older (age >65 years) veterans, who also demonstrate improvements in depression and quality-of-life scales when treated with CBT-I (Karlin et al. 2015).

Suicidal ideation can also be reduced using CBT-I. Among 405 veterans presenting for the initial wave of CBT-I treatment, 32% reported suicidal ideation, which was reduced to 21% by the end of treatment—a 33% change (Trockel et al. 2015). Furthermore, for each 7-point reduction in insomnia severity, there was a 65% reduction in the odds of suicidal ideation, even when controlling for age, gender, education level, and baseline severity of insomnia and depression. Although there was no treatment as usual to which to compare the effects of CBT-I, this study's results are promising since the decline in suicidal ideation was accelerated when compared with previous studies with no intervention at all (Trockel et al. 2015). Considering the real challenge that suicide presents to mental health practitioners, particularly those in the VA system, CBT-I offers an important prevention tool.

CBT-I has been shown to be effective for veterans with co-occurring conditions, including PTSD (Talbot et al. 2014a; Ulmer et al. 2010), and when combined with behavioral sleep medicine interventions for nightmares, it can effectively address the range of sleep disturbances experienced with PTSD (Germain et al. 2012). These behavioral interventions targeting sleep disturbances are effective at reducing PTSD symptoms as well (Margolies et al. 2013).

While research suggests that CBT-I is effective in treating comorbid psychiatric disorders, less is known about the effectiveness of CBT-I with insomnia and co-occurring sleep disorders. One review has found that combination therapy—combined cognitive behavioral therapy (CBT) and obstructive sleep apnea (OSA) treatment—is more effective in treating insomnia than cognitive behavioral therapy or obstructive sleep apnea treatment as stand-alone interventions (Luyster et al. 2010). This finding stresses the importance of understanding how the occurrence and treatment of insomnia may be affected by a co-occurring sleep disorder such as obstructive sleep apnea, especially since both occur with high frequency in the veteran population.

Sleep-Disordered Breathing

Obstructive sleep apnea syndrome (OSAS) is by far the most common form of sleep-disordered breathing (SDB) and is defined by frequent episodes of obstructed breathing during sleep. Specifically, it is characterized by complete (apneas) or partial (hypopneas) upper airway obstruction during sleep, with a characteristic association of snoring and excessive daytime sleepiness (Gastaut et al. 1965). Hypoxia is a defining feature of obstructive sleep apnea syndrome. Investigators have long suggested a model in which the neuronal injury resulting from hypoxia results in OSAS-associated cognitive impairment. Hypoxia impacts cerebral metabolism and induces inflammatory response and apoptosis, resulting in both reversible cell damage and cell death.

In a recent mouse model of sleep apnea, Xu et al. (2004) observed chronic intermittent hypoxia to be associated with both an increase in reactive oxygen species and cortical neuronal cell apoptosis. They concluded that increased oxidative stress contributes to hypoxia-mediated neuronal apoptosis, which subsequently leads to the neurocognitive dysfunction associated with obstructive sleep apnea syndrome. Indeed, a recent investigation found that intermittent hypoxic exposure during the sleep phase in aged rats resulted in significantly greater levels of neuronal apoptosis and substantially more spatial learning deficits than in young rats. Thus, the basic theoretical model is that OSAS-related cognitive impairment is primarily due to hypoxic events, with some additional impairment resulting from sleep fragmentation and daytime sleepiness. This theory is supported by the fact that cognitive impairment in human subjects is not always corrected after treatment, suggesting that daytime sleepiness alone cannot fully explain these deficits (Matthews and Aloia 2011). Despite the evidence pointing to a neuropathological basis for the cognitive-related effects of sleep apnea, to date few studies have used neuroimaging to examine the cerebral changes associated with obstructive sleep apnea syndrome. Those studies that have utilized neuroimaging techniques have tended to focus on different areas of the brain and have yielded mixed results.

Sharafkhaneh et al. (2005) reviewed data from 1998 to 2001 and identified veteran patient records with ICD-9 codes that indicated sleep apnea and various psychiatric conditions. Of 4,060,504 cases, 118,105 (2.91%) were identified with a diagnosis of sleep apnea, with a mean age of 57.6 years at time of diagnosis. There was significant psychiatric comorbidity among veterans with sleep apnea. Compared with matched veterans without a diagnosis of sleep apnea, they noted that significantly greater prevalence was found for depression (21.8%), anxiety (16.7%), PTSD (11.9%), psychosis (5.1%), and dementia (2.13%) in patients with sleep apnea.

In an active duty population referred for a sleep evaluation, over half of patients with PTSD (56.6%) were diagnosed with obstructive sleep apnea syndrome. Patients with PTSD and obstructive sleep apnea syndrome had lower quality of life and more somnolence than those without either OSAS or PTSD (Lettieri et al. 2016). Considering that obstructive sleep apnea affects cognition and mental health and that it can be reduced and treated through the use of continuous positive airway pressure (CPAP), identifying obstructive sleep apnea in veterans early on may be particularly helpful in lengthening and improving quality of life through the lifespan. Unfortunately, patients with PTSD demonstrated significantly lower adherence and response to CPAP therapy. Resolution of sleepiness occurred in 82% of patients with obstructive sleep apnea syndrome alone, compared with 62.5% of CPAP adherent and 21.4% of nonadherent PTSD + OSAS patients. Similarly, significantly improved quality-of-life scores were seen in 72% of obstructive sleep apnea syndrome patients treated with CPAP, compared to only 56.3% of PTSD + OSAS patients who were CPAP adherent and 26.2% who were nonadherent ($p < 0.03$).

Psychiatric Disorders and Sleep

Post-traumatic Stress Disorder (PTSD) and Sleep

Sleep disturbance is the most frequently reported PTSD symptom, even when nightmares are excluded (Roszell et al. 1991). A survey of Vietnam combat veterans with PTSD showed that 59–73% report insomnia and nonrestorative sleep (Mellman et al. 1995). Similarly, a large study of US Afghanistan/Iraq-era veterans (20% women) observed that both short and long sleep duration and poor sleep quality are all associated with PTSD (Swinkels et al. 2013).

While many veterans with PTSD report nightmares, insomnia is more common, and the insomnia associated with PTSD may have unique features. For example, there may be an increased fear of sleep and the dark and increased safety behaviors such as checking the environment including locks on doors (for a review, see Pigeon and Gallegos 2015). Moreover, some individuals have an association between trauma and the bed. Indeed, perhaps related to this association, a recent study observed that insomnia is more prevalent and severe in veterans with military sexual trauma compared to veterans without (Jenkins et al. 2015).

In addition to insomnia and nightmares, veterans with PTSD frequently experience sleep-disordered breathing. A study of 48 Vietnam veterans with PTSD over 3 years observed that sleep-disordered breathing worsened over time, which is particularly concerning given that earlier studies have shown a high prevalence of sleep-disordered breathing in PTSD and that it is associated with cognitive decline (Yesavage et al.

2014). Younger veterans with PTSD (i.e., Operation Enduring Freedom, Operation Iraqi Freedom, and Operation New Dawn veterans) also demonstrate a higher risk of obstructive sleep apnea compared to those in the civilian community (Colvonen et al. 2015).

In terms of sleep architecture, a meta-analysis of 20 polysomnography studies comparing sleep in people with and without PTSD showed that those with PTSD had more stage 1 sleep, less slow-wave sleep (SWS), and greater rapid eye movement density compared to people without PTSD (Kobayashi et al. 2007; Neylan et al. 2003). These differences are notable given that slow-wave sleep is the most physically restorative stage of sleep and reductions in slow-wave sleep are associated with a range of negative health outcomes (e.g., Rao et al. 2009). Moreover, it is hypothesized that disturbed rapid eye movement (REM) sleep may affect emotional memory processing, potentially contributing to either the initiation or maintenance of PTSD (Walker and van der Helm 2009).

Relationship Between Sleep Disturbance and Overall Symptoms and Functioning in PTSD

In addition to experiencing poor sleep as disturbing, individuals with PTSD may suffer from numerous sleep-related consequences. For example, there is a worse course of PTSD in the context of poor sleep, and PTSD is less likely to remit when insomnia is present (e.g., Marcks et al. 2010). Physical health problems also co-occur with sleep disturbance in PTSD. For example, a recent study of Operation Enduring Freedom/Operation Iraqi Freedom veterans with and without minor traumatic brain injuries (mTBIs) suggested that PTSD symptoms influence pain and that sleep problems may exacerbate this relationship (Powell et al. 2015). Moreover, given the high rates of metabolic syndrome in PTSD (e.g., 43% of older veterans; Heppner et al. 2009), and the substantial epidemiological and laboratory evidence that sleep disturbance may contribute to metabolic risk in healthy samples (e.g., Xi et al. 2013), it is possible that sleep contributes to the increased metabolic problems and higher rates of obesity in PTSD. There may also be sleep-related behavioral pathways to these metabolic and weight issues; a recent study of over 700 veterans with PTSD observed that worse sleep quality predicted lower physical activity 1 year later (Talbot et al. 2014b).

Sleep disturbance in PTSD is associated with declined overall functioning in veterans (Neylan et al. 1998). Interestingly, circadian factors may also contribute to this functioning; those with an eveningness chronotype have been observed to exhibit greater lifetime PTSD symptoms, more disturbed sleep, and more frequent and intense nightmares (Hasler et al. 2013).

Sleep as a Predictor of the Development of PTSD

In addition to the apparent exacerbation of PTSD symptoms and health issues from sleep disturbance, it is notable that a burgeoning literature suggests that sleep is a risk factor for the development of PTSD. One study observed that pre-deployment sleep complaints in National Guard troops contributed significantly to the prediction of PTSD up to 2 years after deployment (Koffel et al. 2013), and another study of over 15,000 individuals similarly observed that pre-deployment insomnia was associated with higher odds of the development of both PTSD and other anxiety and depression (Gehrman et al. 2013). A third study observed that pre-deployment nightmares were associated with an increased risk of the development of PTSD (van Liempt et al. 2013). Taken together, these studies suggest that pre-deployment sleep screening and treatment is warranted.

Treatment of Sleep Disturbance in PTSD

Sleep disturbance should be targeted in PTSD, as it may improve both recovery from PTSD and overall functioning. There are several appealing reasons for using sleep-specific cognitive behavioral therapy (CBT) in PTSD, primarily cognitive behavioral therapy for insomnia (CBT-I). Most notably, poor sleep persists in approximately 50% of patients following current available trauma-based cognitive behavioral therapy treatments for PSTD (Zayfert and DeViva 2004; Belleville et al. 2011b). Moreover, CBT-I is a short-term intervention with long-term clinical gains, frequently improves non-sleep symptoms in other disorders (e.g., depression), and may offer a non-stigmatizing entry into mental health treatment (Gilbert et al. 2015). Indeed, a recent meta-analysis, mostly comprised of veteran samples, examined 11 randomized controlled trials comparing sleep-specific cognitive behavioral therapy with waitlist control groups. Results indicated that sleep-specific cognitive behavioral therapy is highly efficacious for improving sleep diary-reported symptoms. There were also more moderate observed improvements in self-reported PTSD symptoms and depression (Ho et al. 2016).

Imagery rehearsal (IR) for nightmares in PTSD has been shown to be effective for the treatment of chronic nightmares (e.g., Krakow and Zadra 2006; for a review, see Schoenfeld et al. 2012). However, imagery rehearsal may be specific to a subgroup of patients with PTSD with repetitive nightmares, and those without these nightmares may be unlikely to benefit.

In terms of pharmacological treatment, Clinical Practice Guidelines issued by the VA and the Department of Defense (DoD) recommend prazosin for sleep disturbance/nightmares for veterans with PTSD. One study of 67 active duty soldiers returned from Iraq and Afghanistan observed that prazosin was well tolerated and effective for trauma nightmares, sleep quality, overall functioning, and PTSD symptoms (Raskind et al. 2013). However, the study investigators noted that there were substantial residual symptoms and suggested that combining behavioral treatments with this pharmacological treatment could be beneficial. A recent meta-analysis of six randomized controlled trials of prazosin for adults with PTSD and sleep disturbances, most of whom were male veterans, also showed that prazosin improved both overall PTSD symptoms and sleep disturbance (Khachatryan et al. 2015). In terms of other medications, antidepressants are frequently prescribed for overall PTSD symptoms, but the effects on sleep have not been well examined. Benzodiazepines are frequently prescribed for sleep disturbance but do not have long-term benefits, and antipsychotic agents are also prescribed but have significant adverse effects (Williams et al. 2015).

Anxiety and Sleep

In the general population, it is well established that anxiety disorders frequently co-occur with insomnia (e.g., Ohayon and Roth 2003) and with sleep apnea, yet the prevalence rates for the latter vary substantially (11–70%; Saunamaki and Jehkonen 2007). However, very little is known regarding anxiety and sleep in veterans. Although veterans experience anxiety disorders at rates higher than those observed in the general population (e.g., Fiedler et al. 2006), research has not focused on anxiety disorder or the intersection of anxiety and sleep in veterans. Factors that contribute to the limited research on anxiety and sleep in veterans are the poor diagnostic specificity of anxiety disorders in veterans (Barrera et al. 2014), the scarcity of research on anxiety disorders in veterans, and the focus of past research on anxiety within the context of PTSD in veterans. Here, we draw from research findings in the general population to identify what is known about two anxiety disorders that often affect veterans: generalized anxiety disorder and panic disorder. Generalized anxiety disorder affects 12% of VA primary care patients, and panic disorder affects 8.3% (Gros et al. 2011; Milanak et al. 2013). We exclude specific phobia and social anxiety disorder, as far less is known about sleep disturbance in the context of these disorders.

Generalized anxiety disorder (GAD), a disorder marked by frequent and difficult-to-control worry, has been shown to affect approximately 9.7% of Vietnam veterans, 6.0% of Gulf War veterans, and as many as 15% of Iraq and Afghanistan veterans (Fiedler et al.

2006; Hoge et al. 2004; Phillips et al. 2009). Some of the most common sleep complaints among individuals with generalized anxiety disorder are difficulty initiating and maintaining sleep (e.g., Bélanger et al. 2004). In fact, "trouble sleeping" may afflict approximately 60–70% of individuals with generalized anxiety disorder (for a review, see Papadimitriou and Linkowski 2005). These subjective sleep complaints are consistent with the high rates of co-occurrence of insomnia in individuals with generalized anxiety disorder (Monti and Monti 2000), yet the subjective sleep complaints do not correspond with consistent evidence of disturbance in sleep architecture (Monti and Monti 2000). In their review, Papadimitriou and Linkowski (Papadimitriou and Linkowski 2005) report that individuals with generalized anxiety disorder spend a high percentage of time in stage 2 sleep and less time in slow-wave sleep, consistent with elevated physiological arousal in generalized anxiety disorder. Thus, the majority of sleep-related complaints in generalized anxiety disorder focus on subjective sleep complaints that characterize insomnia.

Panic disorder (PD) often has been studied in conjunction with PSTD in veterans (e.g., Woodward et al. 2002). With regard to sleep, panic disorder is associated with not only nocturnal panic attacks but also longer sleep latency, diminished sleep efficiency, restless sleep, and complaints of difficulty breathing (Papadimitriou and Linkowski 2005; Stein et al. 1993). Nocturnal panic attacks occur during non-REM sleep, primarily stage 2 or 3 (Stein et al. 1995), and afflict between 18% and 45% of individuals with panic disorder (Papadimitriou and Linkowski 2005). Individuals with nocturnal panic attacks may also develop conditioned fears related to falling asleep and experience somatic symptoms at higher rates than those individuals with panic disorder without nocturnal panic attacks (see Papadimitriou and Linkowski 2005). Thus, sleep disturbance in panic disorder consists of both subjective and objective sleep complaints and should include careful assessment for nocturnal panic attacks as these nocturnal attacks may suggest the need for specific treatment considerations.

Treatment of Sleep Disturbance in Anxiety Disorders

The presence of anxiety disorders or symptoms among veterans with sleep disorders is important to consider because of the treatment implications. Treatment for anxiety improves sleep, and treatment for sleep disturbance improves anxiety symptoms. With regard to insomnia, the gold standard treatment recommended by the American Academy of Sleep Medicine, cognitive behavioral therapy for insomnia (CBT-I), has yielded moderate improvements for anxiety symptoms in addition to improvements in sleep outcomes (Belleville et al. 2011a). Additionally, sleep quality has shown to be improved following cognitive behavioral therapy treatment for panic disorder (PD) or generalized anxiety disorder (GAD) (Ramsawh et al. 2015). Yet, findings demonstrate that anxiety should be assessed, as the presence of elevated anxiety symptom severity has been associated with poor continuous positive airway pressure (CPAP) treatment adherence for sleep apnea (Kjelsberg et al. 2005). Smith et al. (2005) caution against using sleep restriction in patients with panic disorder without full consideration of and monitoring for increases in daytime panic. Taken together, these findings suggest that treatments for anxiety may improve sleep; however, clinicians should tailor sleep disorder treatments for individuals with anxiety to optimize both sleep and anxiety outcomes.

Sleep and Psychosis in Veterans

Up to 80% of people with psychotic disorders experience sleep disturbances. Polysomnography, actigraphy, and subjective sleep assessments reveal many sleep alterations among people both treated and untreated with antipsychotic medication, including circadian rhythm disturbance, less total sleep time, reduced sleep efficiency, and increased sleep latency, awakenings, and naps (Chouinard et al. 2004; Anderson and Bradley 2013; Monti et al. 2013). Although the exact mechanism is unknown, sleep alterations appear to play an important role in the severity and pathophysiology of psychotic illness (Lunsford-Avery and Mittal 2013; Benson 2015; Davies et al. 2016). Disturbed sleep is associated with greater illness severity, particularly delusions, hallucinations, and disorganized thinking, and behavior and is a key predictor of impending psychotic episodes in both chronic and first-episode psychosis (Lunsford-Avery and Mittal 2013). Furthermore, depriving the sleep of healthy individuals produces effects that are similar to the clinical presentation of those with psychotic disorders. These include perceptual alterations, hallucinations, and paranoia (West et al. 1962; Babkoff et al. 1989), increased proinflammatory cytokine production (Mullington et al. 2010), significant alterations in cortisol and melatonin levels (Goh et al. 2001), severe cognitive impairments (Killgore et al. 2010; Brown et al. 2012), and reduced frontal cortical and thalamic metabolism (Thomas et al. 2000) and functional connectivity (De Havas et al. 2012).

Even after adjusting for psychiatric symptom severity and medication side effects, insomnia symptoms remain strongly associated with many functional difficulties experienced by people with psychotic disorders. Poor sleep quality is associated with dissatisfaction with social relationships, daily activities, emotional functioning, and overall quality of life among those with psychosis (Hofstetter et al. 2005; Xiang et al. 2009; Brissos et al. 2013). Chronic insufficient sleep also causes deficits in cognitive functioning (Basner et al. 2013), and people with schizophrenia in particular experience impairments in sleep-dependent cognitive processes (Manoach and Stickgold 2009; Bromundt et al. 2011), such as memory consolidation (Manoach et al. 2004; Seeck-Hirschner et al. 2012; Wamsley et al. 2012; Goder et al. 2015). The functional difficulties associated with poor sleep are particularly relevant to the active military and veteran population. Disturbed sleep plays a significant role in obesity and cardiovascular illness (Czeisler 2011), both of which are highly prevalent in those with psychotic disorders (Mitchell et al. 2013), including veterans (Nelson 2006; Chwastiak et al. 2011; US Department of Veterans Affairs 2014). Insomnia is one of the most frequent reasons for mental health referrals in the Veterans Health Administration, and there is substantial evidence that insomnia causes considerable distress for veterans (Bramoweth and Germain 2013). However, the extant literature on sleep disorder prevalence and treatment efficacy for veterans with psychosis is sparse. Therefore, information from studies conducted within the general population of individuals with psychosis is presented with clinical and research implications specific to the veteran population.

An important development in the latest edition of the *Diagnostic and Statistical Manual* (*DSM-5*) was removal of the requirement that insomnia be coded as a secondary disorder in the presence of another psychiatric condition; in such circumstances, insomnia can now be coded as a primary disorder (American Psychiatric Association 2013). This means that insomnia can and should be treated simultaneously to treatment for psychotic disorders. The rate of insomnia among those with psychotic disorders ranges from 44% to 54%, with 30% additionally scoring at subthreshold levels (Freeman et al. 2009; Palmese et al. 2011). Pharmacological treatments are typically used to treat insomnia among people with psychotic disorders (Kantrowitz et al. 2009). However, they are not fully effective at improving sleep and involve important risks including dependence and a range of significant side effects (Buysse 2013). Furthermore, research indicates that people with mental illness often prefer taking fewer medications (Peacey et al. 2012) and instead have expressed interest in behavioral sleep interventions (Huthwaite et al. 2014).

Several pilot trials have used cognitive behavioral therapy for insomnia (CBT-I) with people with psychotic disorders. These suggest CBT-I reduces insomnia, fatigue, and psychotic symptoms and improves their sleep quality and quality of life (Dopke et al. 2004; Myers et al. 2011; Freeman et al. 2015). No clinical trials have examined its efficacy among veterans with psychotic disorders. As the largest integrated healthcare system in the United States, the Veterans Health Administration has impressively initiated the largest training and dissemination program of CBT-I in the nation. The Veterans Health Administration has its own CBT-I manual tailored to the needs and challenges of the veteran population (Manber et al. 2014). Although this manual does not specifically exclude veterans with psychotic disorders, it states that "some aspects of treatment may need to be avoided or cautiously applied" with this population (p. 13) and does not currently offer guidance as to how this should be done. Indeed, the aforementioned preliminary studies have documented the need for guidelines on how to adapt CBT-I to the challenges experienced by those with psychotic disorders (Dopke et al. 2004; Myers et al. 2011; Freeman et al. 2015), both to ensure client safety and to ensure effective treatment (see Dopke et al. 2004; Myers et al. 2011; Freeman et al. 2015; Klingaman et al. 2015 for more information on the rationale for and examples of potential guidelines). One small pilot study revealed that the use of CBT-I with veterans with psychosis was rare (Klingaman et al. 2015). Currently, guidelines are being developed and tested for veterans with psychosis (Klingaman et al. 2015). These guidelines will be disseminated nationally and will improve uptake and reach within VA by encouraging VA evidence-based psychotherapy (EBP) trainers to begin recommending use of CBT-I with veterans with psychosis and enabling VA clinicians to feel more prepared to use it.

Circadian Rhythm Sleep Disorders

To date, there exist no large-scale prevalence estimates of the rates of circadian rhythm sleep disorders (CRSD) among those with schizophrenia, although recent reviews have documented prevalent circadian misalignments that significantly detract from quality of life (Monti et al. 2013). In one recent small-scale study of 20 clinically stable people with schizophrenia and sleep complaints, two distinct subgroups were identified: one-half of the sample had severe delayed or both delayed and free-running sleep phases, while the other half showed prolonged, irregular, or fragmented sleep but no circadian or melatonin cycle abnormalities (Wulff et al. 2012). These results, coupled with the fact that many veterans must adjust from erratic sleep/wake or shift work schedules after returning from service, indicate the importance of screening veterans with psychotic disorders for circadian rhythm sleep disorders.

Melatonin supplements may be effective in the management of circadian rhythm sleep disorders among those with psychotic disorders (Shamir et al. 2000; Kumar et al. 2007). Harvey and colleagues have developed a transdiagnostic treatment approach to sleep disorders to address the needs of people with multiple co-occurring sources of sleep disturbance, including circadian rhythm sleep disorders (Harvey et al. 2011). This approach has not yet been tested in individuals with schizophrenia but is promising in its potential as an efficient psychotherapy designed to target multiple sleep disturbances at once. This could be especially fitting to the needs of the Veterans Health Administration, a system actively working to improve access to care via efficient use of resources already in place (Sarmiento et al. 2015).

Obstructive Sleep Apnea

In the few studies that have examined both psychosis and obstructive sleep apnea (OSA), approximately half of those with schizophrenia have OSA (Winkelman 2001; Naqvi et al. 2014). Risk factors echo those of the general population, including being older, male, and overweight. As noted above, obesity is highly prevalent among veterans with psychotic disorders, due to the obesogenic properties of antipsychotic medications, poor access to healthy food, and barriers to engaging in physical activity (Klingaman et al. 2014). Additionally, antipsychotics may independently predict obstructive sleep apnea above and beyond their obesogenic properties (Rishi et al. 2010). Larger trials are needed to replicate this finding; one avenue for future research would be to examine the prevalence of obstructive sleep apnea among veterans of normal weight who take antipsychotics. People with psychotic disorders can and do successfully use continuous positive airway pressure (CPAP) at home (Boufidis et al. 2003; Karanti and Landen 2007) and should be considered for this treatment, or oral devices, as warranted. Because obesity promotes obstructive sleep apnea, the VA national weight management program (MOVE!®) should be discussed with clients, and referrals to MOVE! should be made as a preventative strategy or treatment option for those who are overweight or obese and not interested in CPAP use.

Restless Legs Syndrome

The prevalence of restless legs syndrome (RLS) in those with schizophrenia is estimated to be twice that of healthy controls; one study found that 21.4% had RLS and almost half met at least one of the International Restless Legs Syndrome Study Group (IRLSSG) diagnostic criteria (Kang et al. 2007). That restless legs syndrome is a side effect of antipsychotic agents due to its antidopaminergic receptor profile (Benson 2015) may help explain this high rate, and one potential treatment for RLS includes use of dopamine agonists. However, prescribers should not use this standard treatment for veterans with psychosis because it has the potential to worsen hallucinations and delusions. Other medications such as gabapentin or pregabalin could be considered, and routine evaluation for iron deficiency is recommended (Benson 2015). Among non-medication treatments, leg massage, warm baths, and sequential compression devices have been studied with some success (Bega and Malkani 2016). Unfortunately, even among those without mental illness, there is little evidence for the efficacy of behavioral treatments of restless legs syndrome.

It is critical to ensure that veterans prescribed with antipsychotic agents are systematically screened and regularly monitored for symptoms of restless legs syndrome; early detection and treatment could prevent or lessen its detrimental consequences on sleep quality and psychiatric recovery.

Sleep and the Aging Veteran

There are several known changes that occur in sleep with aging. Sleep in older adults, compared to younger adults, has more nocturnal awakenings and decreased efficiency (Bliwise 1993). There is also an increase in daytime napping and fatigue reported in older adults (Bliwise 1993; Ohayon et al. 2004). It is also noted that circadian rhythm measured with core body temperature shows phase advance and decreased change in amplitude (Monk et al. 1997). There is evidence that sleep quality is related to cognition in older adults. A study based on questionnaires regarding sleep quality showed a correlation of sleep and cognition (Nebes et al. 2009; Potvin et al. 2012; Yaffe et al. 2014). Among sleep quality measurements, self-reported or actigraphy-based sleep duration is reportedly associated with cognition in older adults (Potvin et al. 2012; Yaffe et al. 2014; Blackwell et al. 2011).

For sleep duration, several studies consistently show that ideal sleep duration for older adults is around 7–9 h (Hirshkowitz et al. 2015). Both longer sleep duration and shorter sleep duration are associated with poor cognition (Yaffe et al. 2014). Cognitive impairment in shorter sleep duration is most likely due to sleep deprivation. However, long sleep duration shows association with poorer cognition consistently (Potvin et al. 2012; Yaffe et al. 2014; Blackwell et al. 2011). Involving populations with longer sleep to compensate subclinical, undiagnosed, or untreated sleep disorders is likely the mechanism of association of longer sleep duration with cognitive impairment. It should not be interpreted as long sleep duration "causes" cognitive impairment.

Sleep-disordered breathing (SDB) is common in older adults. The incidence ranges from 9% to 60% and depends on target population, definition of age limit for "older adults," and definition of SDB (Ancoli-Israel et al. 1991; Peppard et al.

2013). For example, some studies use apnea-hypopnea index (AHI) >5 events per hour, and others use AHI >15. Many studies indicate increased prevalence of sleep-disordered breathing among veterans, but the incidence is dramatically increased with age. Since there is increased recognition that sleep-disordered breathing increases the risk for dementia, increased screening for and treatment of sleep-disordered breathing in the older veteran may become an important way to ameliorate or delay cognitive decline and onset of dementia.

Conclusion

Despite a growing attention to the etiology, prevalence, and treatment options for sleep disorders comorbid with psychiatric disorders in the veteran population, much research remains to be conducted. Patients with psychiatric disorders are not routinely screened for sleep disorders in the Veterans Health Administration. It is also unclear how many seek care outside the Veterans Health Administration, whether they receive treatments offered, and the effectiveness of these treatments. A recent nationwide inventory of sleep resources available at VA Medical Centers revealed that many sleep programs are understaffed for their workload and that Veterans Health Administration is actively seeking innovative techniques to ensure access to sleep services (Sarmiento et al. 2015). As the Veterans Health Administration makes these changes, it will be important to monitor access to and effectiveness of screening and treatment within psychiatric populations. Now that standardized stop codes are used to track sleep workload (Sarmiento et al. 2015), VA administrative databases could be used for this purpose. Furthermore, as new treatment options are developed for people with psychiatric disorders, it will be important to assess both veterans' and providers' knowledge of and willingness to use these interventions. Such information could be used to target education and training programs and to raise awareness of the utility of treating sleep disorders of veterans who have comorbid psychiatric disorders. Compared to specialty treatment settings, integrating interventions into mental health settings has been a particularly successful approach for other areas of behavioral health among veterans with other mental health disorders (McFall et al. 2007). Research is needed on the effectiveness of integrating sleep treatment services within clinics and settings where veterans with psychiatric disorders already seek care. Treating sleep dysregulation presents a key opportunity to alleviate core psychopathological symptoms and improve functional status. One of the many strengths of the Veterans Health Administration is its ability to implement innovative programs on a large scale; the Veterans Health Administration is aptly poised to enhance the quality of life of veterans who experiences a disproportionate burden of chronic and comorbid disease.

However, just as further research must be conducted on sleep disorders comorbid with psychiatric disorders to better diagnose and treat mental illness, additional research is also needed to explore the effects of these and previously discussed disorders on an aging veteran population so that we may better understand what can be attributed to sleep alterations and deficits associated with getting older. Until such research is conducted, we once again turn to the general population for answers.

The importance of sleep as a combat multiplier is increasingly recognized. The military culture that assumes inadequate sleep as an unavoidable consequence of the profession is being challenged, but the balance between promotion of a healthy sleep-wake routine and the demand of military duty is a difficult leadership challenge. Once a maladaptive sleep pattern is established on active duty, it is often continued once the service member transitions to civilian life. The Veterans Health Administration and Department of Defense are continuing to conduct research to determine the extent to which inadequate sleep propagates impairments in other functional areas. Service-specific programs such as the Army Performance Triad promote a leader- and peer-driven awareness in the same way that the VA and Department of Defense have done for suicide prevention. As these programs mature and bear fruit, it will be interesting to see what impact they may also have on long-term veteran health.

Key Concepts

1. The prevalence of insomnia and sleep-disordered breathing is higher in veterans than in the general population.
2. Difficulties with sleep (e.g., insomnia) facilitate the development of and/or exacerbate the symptoms of psychiatric disorders and can also affect cognitive functioning (i.e., sleep-disordered breathing).
3. Cognitive behavioral therapy for insomnia (CBT-I) has received extensive support in treating insomnia and reducing psychiatric symptom severity, and continuous positive airway pressure (CPAP) is effective in treating sleep-disordered breathing.
4. Older veterans are at an increased risk for developing sleep-disordered breathing, which is associated with a greater likelihood of developing dementia.
5. Despite the greater prevalence of sleep difficulties in the veteran population, it is not routinely screened for in veterans with psychiatric disorders. The Veterans Health Administration is working to improve access to sleep services.

References

American Psychiatric Association (2013) Diagnostic and statistical manual of mental disorders, 5th edn. American Psychiatric Publishing, Arlington

Ancoli-Israel S et al (1991) Sleep-disordered breathing in community-dwelling elderly. Sleep 14(6):486–495

Anderson KN, Bradley AJ (2013) Sleep disturbance in mental health problems and neurodegenerative disease. Nat Sci Sleep 5:61–75. https://doi.org/10.2147/NSS.S34842

Armed Forces Health Surveillance Center (2010) Medical surveillance monthly report

Babkoff H et al (1989) Perceptual distortions and hallucinations reported during the course of sleep deprivation. Percept Mot Skills 68(3 Pt 1):787–798

Barrera TL et al (2014) Diagnostic specificity and mental health service utilization among veterans with newly diagnosed anxiety disorders. Gen Hosp Psychiatry 36(2):192–198

Basner M et al (2013) Sleep deprivation and neurobehavioral dynamics. Curr Opin Neurobiol 23(5):854–863

Bélanger L, Morin CM, Langlois F, Ladouceur R (2004) Insomnia and generalized anxiety disorder: effects of cognitive behavior therapy for gad on insomnia symptoms. J Anxiety Disord 18(4):561–571

Bega D, Malkani R (2016) Alternative treatment of restless legs syndrome: an overview of the evidence for mind-body interventions, lifestyle interventions, and neutraceuticals. Sleep Med 17:99–105. https://doi.org/10.1016/j.sleep.2015.09.009

Belleville G, Cousineau H et al (2011a) Meta-analytic review of the impact of cognitive-behavior therapy for insomnia on concomitant anxiety. Clin Psychol Rev 31(4):638–652

Belleville G, Guay S, Marchand A (2011b) Persistence of sleep disturbances following cognitive-behavior therapy for posttraumatic stress disorder. J Psychosom Res 70(4):318–327

Benson KL (2015) Sleep in schizophrenia: pathology and treatment. Sleep Med Clin 10(1):49–55

Blackwell T et al (2011) Association of sleep characteristics and cognition in older community-dwelling men: the MrOS sleep study. Sleep 34(10):1347–1356

Bliwise DL (1993) Sleep in normal aging and dementia. Sleep 16(1):40–81. Available at: http://dx.doi.org/

Blosnich JR et al (2014) Disparities in adverse childhood experiences among individuals with a history of military service. JAMA Psychiatry 71(9):1041–1048

Bonnet MH, Arand DL (2010) Hyperarousal and insomnia: state of the science. Sleep Med Rev 14(1):9–15

Boufidis S et al (2003) Treatment outcome of obstructive sleep apnea syndrome in a patient with schizophrenia: case report. Int J Psychiatry Med 33(3):305–310

Bramoweth AD, Germain A (2013) Deployment-related insomnia in military personnel and veterans. Curr Psychiatry Rep 15(10):401

Brissos S et al (2013) Satisfaction with life of schizophrenia outpatients and their caregivers: differences between patients with and without self-reported sleep complaints. Schizophr Res Treat 2013:502172

Bromundt V et al (2011) Sleep-wake cycles and cognitive functioning in schizophrenia. Br J Psychiatry 198(4):269–276

Brown RE, Basheer R, McKenna JT, Strecker RE, McCarley RW (2012) Control of sleep and wakefulness. Physiol Rev 2092(3):1087–1187. https://doi.org/10.1152/physrev.00032.2011

Buysse DJ (2013) Insomnia. J Am Med Assoc 309(7): 706–716

Chakravorty S et al (2014) Suicidal ideation in veterans misusing alcohol: relationships with insomnia

symptoms and sleep duration. Addict Behav 39(2): 399–405
Chouinard S et al (2004) Sleep in untreated patients with schizophrenia: a meta-analysis. Schizophr Bull 30(4):957–967
Chwastiak LA, Rosenheck RA, Kazis LE (2011) Association of psychiatric illness and obesity, physical inactivity, and smoking among a national sample of veterans. Psychosomatics 52(3):230–236
Colvonen PJ et al (2015) Obstructive sleep apnea and posttraumatic stress disorder among OEF/OIF/OND veterans. J Clin Sleep Med 11(5):513–518
Cozza S et al (2004) Topics specific to the psychiatric treatment of military personnel, 2nd edn. In: Schnurr P, Cozza S (eds) National Center for PTSD and Department of Defense, Washington, D.C
Czeisler CA (2011) Impact of sleepiness and sleep deficiency on public health – utility of biomarkers. J Clin Sleep Med 7(5 Suppl):S6–S8
Davies G et al (2016) A systematic review of the nature and correlates of sleep disturbance in early psychosis. Sleep Med Rev. Available at: https://doi.org/10.1016/j.smrv.2016.01.001
De Havas JA et al (2012) Sleep deprivation reduces default mode network connectivity and anti-correlation during rest and task performance. NeuroImage 59(2):1745–1751
Dopke CA, Lehner RK, Wells AM (2004) Cognitive-behavioral group therapy for insomnia in individuals with serious mental illnesses: a preliminary evaluation. Psychiatr Rehabil J 27(3):235–242
Epstein DR et al (2013) Feasibility test of preference-based insomnia treatment for Iraq and Afghanistan war veterans. Rehabil Nurs 38(3):120–132
Fiedler N et al (2006) Military deployment to the Gulf War as a risk factor for psychiatric illness among US troops. Br J Psychiatry 188:453–459
Freeman D, Pugh K, Vorontsova N, Southgate L (2009) Insomnia and paranoia. Schizophr Res 108(1–3): 280–284
Freeman D et al (2015) Efficacy of cognitive behavioural therapy for sleep improvement in patients with persistent delusions and hallucinations (BEST): a prospective, assessor-blind, randomised controlled pilot trial. Lancet Psychiatry 2(11):975–983. Available at: http://dx.doi.org/10.1016/s2215-0366(15)00314-4
Gastaut H, Tassinari C, Duron B (1965) Polygraphic study of diurnal and nocturnal (hypnic and respiratory) manifestations of Pickwick syndrome episodal. Rev Neurol 112(568–569)
Gehrman P et al (2013) Predeployment sleep duration and insomnia symptoms as risk factors for new-onset mental health disorders following military deployment. Sleep 36(7):1009–1018
Gehrman PR, Harb GC, Cook JM, Barilla H, Ross RJ (2015) Sleep diaries of Vietnam War veterans with chronic PTSD: the relationships among insomnia symptoms, psychosocial stress, and nightmares. Behav Sleep Med 13:255–264. https://doi.org/10.1080/15402002.2014.880344
Germain A et al (2012) Placebo-controlled comparison of prazosin and cognitive-behavioral treatments for sleep disturbances in US Military Veterans. J Psychosom Res 72(2):89–96
Gilbert KS et al (2015) Sleep disturbances, TBI and PTSD: implications for treatment and recovery. Clin Psychol Rev 40:195–212. Available at: http://dx.doi.org/10.1016/j.cpr.2015.05.008
Goder R et al (2015) Impairment of sleep-related memory consolidation in schizophrenia: relevance of sleep spindles? Sleep Med 16(5):564–569. Available at: http://dx.doi.org/10.1016/j.sleep.2014.12.022
Goh VH et al (2001) Effects of one night of sleep deprivation on hormone profiles and performance efficiency. Mil Med 166(5):427–431
Gros DF, Frueh BC, Magruder KM (2011) Prevalence and features of panic disorder and comparison to posttraumatic stress disorder in VA primary care. Gen Hosp Psychiatry 33(5):482–488
Harvey AG et al (2011) Sleep disturbance as transdiagnostic: consideration of neurobiological mechanisms. Clin Psychol Rev 31(2):225–235
Hasler BP et al (2013) Evening-type military veterans report worse lifetime posttraumatic stress symptoms and greater brainstem activity across wakefulness and REM sleep. Biol Psychol 94(2):255–262
Heppner PS et al (2009) The association of posttraumatic stress disorder and metabolic syndrome: a study of increased health risk in veterans. BMC Med 7:1
Hermes E, Rosenheck R (2014) Prevalence, pharmacotherapy and clinical correlates of diagnosed insomnia among Veterans Health Administration service users nationally. Sleep Med 15(5):508–514
Hirshkowitz M et al (2015) National Sleep Foundation's updated sleep duration recommendations: final report. Sleep Health 1(4):233–243. Available at: http://www.sciencedirect.com/science/article/pii/S2352721815001606
Ho FY, Chan CS, Tang KN (2016) Cognitive-behavioral therapy for sleep disturbances in treating posttraumatic stress disorder symptoms: a meta-analysis of randomized controlled trials. Clin Psychol Rev 43:90–102
Hofstetter JR, Lysaker PH, Mayeda AR (2005) Quality of sleep in patients with schizophrenia is associated with quality of life and coping. BMC Psychiatry 5:13
Hoge CW et al (2004) Combat duty in Iraq and Afghanistan, mental health problems, and barriers to care. N Engl J Med 351(1):13–22
Hughes J et al (2013) Insomnia and symptoms of post-traumatic stress disorder among women veterans. Behav Sleep Med 11(4):258–274
Huthwaite M et al (2014) Dysfunctional cognitions about sleep in psychiatric patients. J Psychiatr Pract 20(3):188–195
Jenkins MM et al (2015) Prevalence and mental health correlates of insomnia in first-encounter veterans with and without military sexual trauma. Sleep 38(10):1547–1554. Available at: https://doi.org/10.5665/sleep.5044

Kajeepeta S et al (2015) Adverse childhood experiences are associated with adult sleep disorders: a systematic review. Sleep Med 16(3):320–330

Kang SG et al (2007) Characteristics and clinical correlates of restless legs syndrome in schizophrenia. Prog Neuro-Psychopharmacol Biol Psychiatry 31(5):1078–1083

Kantrowitz J, Citrome L, Javitt D (2009) GABA(B) receptors, schizophrenia and sleep dysfunction: a review of the relationship and its potential clinical and therapeutic implications. CNS Drugs 23(8):681–691

Karanti A, Landen M (2007) Treatment refractory psychosis remitted upon treatment with continuous positive airway pressure: a case report. Psychopharmacol Bull 40(1):113–117

Karlin BE et al (2013) National dissemination of cognitive behavioral therapy for insomnia in veterans: therapist- and patient-level outcomes. J Consult Clin Psychol 81(5):912–917

Karlin BE et al (2015) National evaluation of the effectiveness of cognitive behavioral therapy for insomnia among older versus younger veterans. Int J Geriatr Psychiatry 30(3):308–315

Khachatryan D et al (2015) Prazosin for treating sleep disturbances in adults with posttraumatic stress disorder: a systematic review and meta-analysis of randomized controlled trials. Gen Hosp Psychiatry 39:46–52

Killgore WD, Killgore DB, Grugle NL, Balkin TJ (2010) Odor identification ability predicts executive function deficits following sleep deprivation. Int J Neurosci 120(5):328–334. https://doi.org/10.3109/00207450903389396

Kjelsberg FN, Ruud EA, Stavem K (2005) Predictors of symptoms of anxiety and depression in obstructive sleep apnea. Sleep Med 6(4):341–346

Klingaman EA et al (2014) Strategies, barriers, and motivation for weight loss among veterans living with schizophrenia. Psychiatr Rehabil J 37(4):270–276

Klingaman EA et al (2015) Sleep disorders among people with schizophrenia: emerging research. Curr Psychiatry Rep 17(10):79

Kobayashi I, Boarts JM, Delahanty DL (2007) Polysomnographically measured sleep abnormalities in PTSD: a meta-analytic review. Psychophysiology 44(4):660–669

Koffel E, Polusny MA, Arbisi PA, Erbes CR (2013) Pre-deployment daytime and nighttime sleep complaints as predictors of post-deployment PTSD and depression in National Guard troops. J Anxiety Disord 27(5): 512–519. https://doi.org/10.1016/j.janxdis.2013.07.003

Krakow B, Zadra A (2006) Clinical management of chronic nightmares: imagery rehearsal therapy. Behav Sleep Med 4(1):45–70

Kumar S, Kumar D, Paranjpe DA, Akarsh CR, Sharma VK (2007) Selection on the timing of adult emergence results in altered circadian clocks in fruit flies Drosophila melanogaster. J Exp Biol 210:906–918

Lettieri C, Williams S, Collen J (2016) OSA syndrome and posttraumatic stress disorder: clinical outcomes and impact of positive airway pressure therapy. Chest 149(2):483–490

van Liempt S et al (2013) Impact of impaired sleep on the development of PTSD symptoms in combat veterans: a prospective longitudinal cohort study. Depress Anxiety 30(5):469–474

Lunsford-Avery J, Mittal V (2013) Sleep dysfunction prior to the onset of schizophrenia: A review and neurodevelopmental diathesis–stress conceptualization. Clin Psychol Sci Prac 20:291–320

Luyster FS, Buysse DJ, Strollo PJ (2010) Comorbid insomnia and obstructive sleep apnea: challenges for clinical practice and research. J Clin Sleep Med 6(2):196–204. Available at: http://dx.doi.org/

Manber R et al (2012) Dissemination of CBTI to the non-sleep specialist: protocol development and training issues. J Clin Sleep Med 8(2):209–218

Manber R et al (2014) Cognitive behavioral therapy for insomnia in veterans: therapist manual. U.S. Department of Veterans Affairs, Washington, DC

Manoach DS, Stickgold R (2009) Does abnormal sleep impair memory consolidation in schizophrenia? Front Hum Neurosci 3:21

Manoach DS et al (2004) A failure of sleep-dependent procedural learning in chronic, medicated schizophrenia. Biol Psychiatry 56(12):951–956

Marcks BA et al (2010) The relationship between sleep disturbance and the course of anxiety disorders in primary care patients. Psychiatry Res 178(3):487–492

Margolies SO et al (2013) Efficacy of a cognitive-behavioral treatment for insomnia and nightmares in Afghanistan and Iraq veterans with PTSD. J Clin Psychol 69(10):1026–1042

Matthews EE, Aloia MS (2011) Cognitive recovery following positive airway pressure (PAP) in sleep apnea. Prog Brain Res 190:71–88. Review

McFall M et al (2007) Integrating smoking cessation into mental health care for post-traumatic stress disorder. Clin Trials 4(2):178–189

McLay R, Klam W, Volkert S (2010) Insomnia is the most commonly reported symptom and predicts other symptoms of posttraumatic stress disorder in U.S. service members returning from military deployments. Mil Med 175(10):759–762

Mellman TA et al (1995) Sleep events among veterans with combat-related posttraumatic stress disorder. Am J Psychiatry 152(1):110–115

Milanak ME et al (2013) Prevalence and features of generalized anxiety disorder in Department of Veteran Affairs primary care settings. Psychiatry Res 209(2):173–179

Mitchell AJ et al (2013) Prevalence of metabolic syndrome and metabolic abnormalities in schizophrenia and related disorders – a systematic review and meta-analysis. Schizophr Bull 39(2):306–318

Monk TH et al (1997) Circadian rhythms in human performance and mood under constant conditions. J Sleep Res 6(1):9–18

Monti JM, Monti D (2000) Sleep disturbance in generalized anxiety disorder and its treatment. Sleep Med Rev 4(3):263–276

Monti JM et al (2013) Sleep and circadian rhythm dysregulation in schizophrenia. Prog Neuro-Psychopharmacol Biol Psychiatry 43:209–216

Mullington JM et al (2010) Sleep loss and inflammation. Best Pract Res Clin Endocrinol Metab 24(5):775–784
Myers E, Startup H, Freeman D (2011) Cognitive behavioural treatment of insomnia in individuals with persistent persecutory delusions: a pilot trial. J Behav Ther Exp Psychiatry 42(3):330–336
Mysliwiec V et al (2013) Sleep disorders and associated medical comorbidities in active duty military personnel. Sleep 36(2):167–174. Available at: http://dx.doi.org/10.5665/sleep.2364
Naqvi HA et al (2014) Sleep-disordered breathing and psychiatric disorders. Curr Psychiatry Rep 16(12):519
Nebes RD et al (2009) Self-reported sleep quality predicts poor cognitive performance in healthy older adults. Ser B Psychol Sci Soc Sci 64(2):180–187
Nelson KM (2006) The burden of obesity among a national probability sample of veterans. J Gen Intern Med 21(9):915–919
Neylan TC et al (1998) Sleep disturbances in the Vietnam generation: findings from a nationally representative sample of male Vietnam veterans. Am J Psychiatry 155(7):929–933
Neylan TC et al (2003) Delta sleep response to metyrapone in post-traumatic stress disorder. Neuropsychopharmacology 28(9):1666–1676
Ohayon MM (2002) Epidemiology of insomnia: what we know and what we still need to learn. Sleep Med Rev 6(2):97–111
Ohayon MM, Roth T (2003) Place of chronic insomnia in the course of depressive and anxiety disorders. J Psychiatr Res 37(1):9–15
Ohayon MM et al (2004) Meta-analysis of quantitative sleep parameters from childhood to old age in healthy individuals: developing normative sleep values across the human lifespan. Sleep 27(7):1255–1273. Available at: http://dx.doi.org/
Palmese LB et al (2011) Insomnia is frequent in schizophrenia and associated with night eating and obesity. Schizophr Res 133(1–3):238–243
Papadimitriou GN, Linkowski P (2005) Sleep disturbance in anxiety disorders. Int Rev Psychiatry 17(4):229–236
Peacey J et al (2012) Sleep medication in acute psychiatric illness: patient's knowledge and prescription patterns in New Zealand. J Nerv Ment Dis 200(1):83–87
Peppard PE et al (2013) Increased prevalence of sleep-disordered breathing in adults. Am J Epidemiol 177(9):1006–1014
Phillips AC et al (2009) Generalized anxiety disorder, major depressive disorder, and their comorbidity as predictors of all-cause and cardiovascular mortality: the Vietnam experience study. Psychosom Med 71(4):395–403
Pigeon WR, Gallegos AM (2015) Posttraumatic stress disorder and sleep. Sleep Med Clin 10(1):41–48
Pigeon WR, Pinquart M, Conner K (2012) Meta-analysis of sleep disturbance and suicidal thoughts and behaviors. J Clin Psychiatry 73(9):e1160–e1167
Pigeon WR et al (2013) Longitudinal relationships of insomnia, nightmares, and PTSD severity in recent combat veterans. J Psychosom Res 75(6):546–550
Polley M, Frank D, Smith M (2013) National veterans sleep survey: results and findings. Available at: www.MyVetAdvisor.com. Accessed 12 Feb 2016
Potvin O et al (2012) Sleep quality and 1-year incident cognitive impairment in community-dwelling older adults. Sleep 35(4):491–499
Powell MA et al (2015) Sleep quality and reexperiencing symptoms of PTSD are associated with current pain in U.S. OEF/OIF/OND veterans with and without mTBIs. J Trauma Stress 28(4):322–329. Available at: https://doi.org/10.1002/jts.22027
Ramsawh HJ et al (2015) Sleep quality improvement during cognitive behavioral therapy for anxiety disorders. Behav Sleep Med:1–12. Available at: https://doi.org/10.1080/15402002.2014.981819
Rao MN et al (2009) Association between sleep architecture and measures of body composition. Sleep 32(4):483–490. Available at: http://dx.doi.org/
Raskind MA et al (2013) A trial of prazosin for combat trauma PTSD with nightmares in active-duty soldiers returned from Iraq and Afghanistan. Am J Psychiatry 170(9):1003–1010
Ribeiro JD et al (2012) Sleep problems outperform depression and hopelessness as cross-sectional and longitudinal predictors of suicidal ideation and behavior in young adults in the military. J Affect Disord 136(3):743–750
Rishi MA et al (2010) Atypical antipsychotic medications are independently associated with severe obstructive sleep apnea. Clin Neuropharmacol 33(3):109–113
Roszell DK, McFall ME, Malas KL (1991) Frequency of symptoms and concurrent psychiatric disorder in Vietnam veterans with chronic PTSD. Hosp Community Psychiatry 42(3):293–296
Sarmiento K et al (2015) The state of Veterans Affairs sleep medicine programs: 2012 inventory results. Sleep Breathing 20(1):379–382
Saunamaki T, Jehkonen M (2007) Depression and anxiety in obstructive sleep apnea syndrome: a review. Acta Neurol Scand 116(5):277–288
Schoenfeld FB, Deviva JC, Manber R (2012) Treatment of sleep disturbances in posttraumatic stress disorder: a review. J Rehabil Res Dev 49(5):729–752
Schutte-Rodin S et al (2008) Clinical guideline for the evaluation and management of chronic insomnia in adults. J Clin Sleep Med 4(5):487–504
Seeck-Hirschner M, Baier PC, Weinhold SL, Dittmar M, Heiermann S, Aldenhoff JB, Goder R (2012) Declarative memory performance is associated with the number of sleep spindles in elderly women. Am J Geriatr Psychiatry 20:782–788
Seelig AD et al (2010) Sleep patterns before, during, and after deployment to Iraq and Afghanistan. Sleep 33(12):1615–1622
Shamir E et al (2000) Melatonin improves sleep quality of patients with chronic schizophrenia. J Clin Psychiatry 61(5):373–377
Sharafkhaneh A et al (2005) Association of psychiatric disorders and sleep apnea in a large cohort. Sleep 28(11):1405–1411

Smith MT, Huang MI, Manber R (2005) Cognitive behavior therapy for chronic insomnia occurring within the context of medical and psychiatric disorders. Clin Psychol Rev 25(5):559–592

Spielman AJ, Glovinski PB (1991) Introduction: the varied nature of insomnia. In: Hauri PJ (ed) Case studies in insomnia. Plenum Publishing Corporation, New York

Stein MB, Chartier M, Walker JR (1993) Sleep in non-depressed patients with panic disorder: I. Systematic assessment of subjective sleep quality and sleep disturbance. Sleep 16(8):724–726

Stein MB, Millar TW, Larsen DK, Kryger MH (1995) Irregular breathing during sleep in patients with panic disorder. Am J Psychiatry 152(8):1168–1173

Swinkels CM et al (2013) The association of sleep duration, mental health, and health risk behaviors among U.S. Afghanistan/Iraq Era Veterans. Sleep 36(7):1019–1025

Talbot LS, Maguen S et al (2014a) Cognitive behavioral therapy for insomnia in posttraumatic stress disorder: a randomized controlled trial. Sleep 37(2):327–341

Talbot LS, Neylan TC et al (2014b) The mediating effect of sleep quality on the relationship between PTSD and physical activity. J Clin Sleep Med 10(7):795–801

Thomas M et al (2000) Neural basis of alertness and cognitive performance impairments during sleepiness. I. Effects of 24 h of sleep deprivation on waking human regional brain activity. J Sleep Res 9(4):335–352

Trauer JM et al (2015) Cognitive behavioral therapy for chronic insomnia: a systematic review and meta-analysis. Ann Intern Med 163(3):191–204. Available at: https://doi.org/10.7326/m14-2841

Trockel M et al (2014) Cognitive behavioral therapy for insomnia with veterans: evaluation of effectiveness and correlates of treatment outcomes. Behav Res Ther 53:41–46

Trockel M, Karlin BE, Taylor CB, Brown GK, Manber R (2015) Effects of cognitive behavioral therapy for insomnia on suicidal ideation in veterans. Sleep 38(2):259–265. https://doi.org/10.5665/sleep.4410

U.S. Department of Veterans Affairs (2014) Ischemic heart disease QUERI: revised goals and new projects. Available at: www.queri.research.va.gov/about/impact_updates/IHD.pdf. Accessed 29 Jan 2016

Ulmer CS et al (2010) A brief intervention for sleep disturbance in PTSD: pilot study findings. J Gen Intern Med 25:206

Walker MP, van der Helm E (2009) Overnight therapy? The role of sleep in emotional brain processing. Psychol Bull 135(5):731–748

Wamsley EJ et al (2012) Reduced sleep spindles and spindle coherence in schizophrenia: mechanisms of impaired memory consolidation? Biol Psychiatry 71(2):154–161

West LJ et al (1962) The psychosis of sleep deprivation. Ann N Y Acad Sci 96:66–70

Williams SG, Collen J, Orr N, Holley AB, Lettieri CJ (2015) Sleep disorders in combat-related PTSD. Sleep Breath 19(1):175–182

Winkelman JW (2001) Schizophrenia, obesity, and obstructive sleep apnea. J Clin Psychiatry 62(1):8–11

Woodward SH, Leskin GA, Sheikh JI (2002) Movement during sleep: associations with posttraumatic stress disorder, nightmares, and comorbid panic disorder. Sleep 25(6):681–688

Wright KM et al (2011) Insomnia as predictor versus outcome of PTSD and depression among Iraq combat veterans. J Clin Psychol 67(12):1240–1258

Wulff K et al (2012) Sleep and circadian rhythm disruption in schizophrenia. Br J Psychiatry 200(4):308–316

Xi B, He D, Zhang M, Xue J, Zhou D (2013) Short sleep duration predicts risk of metabolic syndrome: A systematic review and meta-analysis. Sleep Med Rev 18(4):293–297. https://doi.org/10.1016/j.smrv.2013.06.001.

Xiang YT, Weng YZ, Leung CM, Tang WT, Lai KYC, Ungvari GS (2009) Prevalence and correlates of insomnia and its impact on quality of life in Chinese schizophrenia patients. Sleep 32(1):105–109. PMCID: PMC2625313

Xu W et al (2004) Increased oxidative stress is associated with chronic intermittent hypoxia-mediated brain cortical neuronal cell apoptosis in a mouse model of sleep apnea. Neuroscience 126(2):313–323

Yaffe K, Falvey CM, Hoang T (2014) Connections between sleep and cognition in older adults. Lancet Neurol 13(10):1017–1028. Available at: http://www.thelancet.com/article/S1474442214701723/fulltext. Accessed 9 Sept 2015

Yesavage JA et al (2014) Longitudinal assessment of sleep disordered breathing in Vietnam veterans with post-traumatic stress disorder. Nat Sci Sleep 6:123–127

Zayfert C, DeViva JC (2004) Residual insomnia following cognitive behavioral therapy for PTSD. J Trauma Stress 17:69–73

Part IV

Clinical Cases and Self-Study Questions on Mental Health Needs of Military and Veteran Populations

Clinical Cases and Self-Study Review for the Mental Health of Military and Veteran Populations

26

Alan K. Louie, Honor Hsin, Kim Bullock, Margaret May, Chase Warren, and Laura Weiss Roberts

Clinical Case Study 1

A 22-year-old male soldier with a diagnosis of major depressive disorder is seen by a military psychiatrist for a routine follow-up visit for his selective serotonin reuptake inhibitor (SSRI) antidepressant treatment. The patient has had two major depressive episodes prior to joining the military, which developed quickly under stress, were severe, and resulted in two near-lethal suicide attempts. He began to have a third episode that was triggered by the stress of basic training. This episode was prevented by restarting his SSRI with aggressive increase to a relatively high dose. Since then he has been quite stable and euthymic stateside. He does not use illicit drugs or alcohol. He appears to have been adherent with his medications, despite the side effects of sexual dysfunction and excessive sweating and overheating with exertion—he fainted twice during calisthenic even though the weather was cool.

The soldier explains that he is excited that he will be deployed any day now on the "frontlines." He asks if he should be worried about being deployed to a hot climate where he will be wearing heavy gear. He will also likely be on missions that will be as rigorous as basic training, and he is concerned about possible relapse of his depression. He does not want to endanger his squad if he is unable to function due to depression. He denies current suicidal or homicidal ideation or plans.

Self-Study Review

A. Discuss your clinical reasoning and what you will tell the soldier regarding his risk of depressive relapse under combat stress and the side effects of his SSRI in a hot climate.

B. The soldier is honest about his concern that he will endanger his squad if he has a depressive relapse. Analyze how you would decide if this soldier should be deployed or not, for his own sake and that of his squad. Outline what you would decide if his current symptoms included mild sad mood or occasional passive suicidal ideation.

A.K. Louie
Stanford University School of Medicine, Palo Alto VA Health Care System, Palo Alto, CA, USA
e-mail: louiemd@stanford.edu

H. Hsin • K. Bullock • M. May • C. Warren
Stanford University, Palo Alto, CA, USA

L.W. Roberts (✉)
Department of Psychiatry and Behavioral Sciences, Stanford University School of Medicine, Palo Alto, CA, USA
e-mail: robertsl@stanford.edu

L.W. Roberts, C.H. Warner (eds.), *Military and Veteran Mental Health*,
https://doi.org/10.1007/978-1-4939-7438-2_26

C. Outline the confidentiality of protected health information in military psychiatry, what falls under mandated reporting, and when confidentiality may be breached in order to protect the welfare of fellow soldiers who may be put at risk by a patient's mental illness. How do military psychiatrist get involved with "fitness-for-duty" determinations?

Clinical Case Study 2

A 67-year-old male Vietnam veteran is brought to the outpatient mental health clinic by his daughter, because "his house is unlivable." According to his daughter, the patient has lived in this house for most of his adult life since his discharge from the military. His wife died many years ago from cancer. He has always worked as a supervisor at a bank, until he chose to retire voluntarily 2 years ago. His daughter recently moved to the area and lives near him now. Upon entering his home, she found all sorts of household items (old lamps, old computers), consumable products (detergents, toothpaste), and periodicals (newspapers, magazines) stacked precariously around the home, and there is little space to walk. The garage was packed with "junk" and he parks his care outside. The daughter has tried to clear this clutter, but the patient is unwilling to part with anything. Exasperated, she managed to reach an agreement with him to attend today's appointment instead. The patient acknowledges he has experienced "nerves" about his current living situation, but describes even greater anxiety at the thought of disposing his household objects. He estimates he has felt this way more and more during his adult life. He also describes a need to check things like his stove and locks for >1 h.

The veteran denies nightmares or flashbacks. He reports his mood is "fair," although he acknowledges that his energy, sleep, motivation, and appetite have decreased since his retirement. He denies delusions, hallucinations, and any suicidal or homicidal ideation or plans and denies owning a firearm. His thought process is linear, but he acknowledges progressive problems with memory and difficulty doing his bills and taxes over the last 3 years. The patient has a history of a transient ischemic attack 5 years ago, for which he was prescribed an antithrombotic agent and a lipid-lowering agent, but was lost to medical follow-up.

Self-Study Review

A. Outline how to apply cognitive and behavioral psychotherapy for this patient's symptoms.
B. Analyze whether this vignette may raise a question of a public health hazard and, if so, how this should be handled.
C. Discuss whether criteria are met for the following diagnoses and what additional history one might need to determine this.
   - Hoarding disorder
   - Major neurocognitive disorder
   - Obsessive-compulsive disorder
   - Obsessive-compulsive personality disorder
   - Psychiatric disorder due to another general medical condition

Clinical Case Study 3

A 30-year-old single male veteran presents to a methadone clinic for pre-screening in order to join a motivational enhancement therapy group. He describes having used heroin over the past 4 years since his discharge. He had sustained multiple back injuries during his service, and he went to his internist who prescribed opiate pain medication and physical therapy and recommended he attend a pain management class through the behavioral medicine clinic. The physical therapy and class conflicted with his work schedule so he never attended them. He started to take more and more pain medicationas it became less effective over time. He started to see multiple doctors to get multiple prescriptions of opioids and began to drink alcohol to excess to help him sleep. He lost his job and began seeking treatment at the VA. Clinicians at the VA refused to prescribe opioid pain medications for him, referring him instead to pain management classes, which he found "useless."

Then, he began to use intravenous heroin, which he had tried in high school, to treat his back pain and, eventually, just to get high. He found a place that would give him clean needles and syringes in a harm reduction program. His habit was expensive and he committed petty crimes to pay for it. Eventually, he was arrested and was referred to the VA drug court and drug rehabilitation. He tells of several attempts to quit prior to getting on methadone maintenance, which has helped him stay clean and sober for his longest period of time. Initially he was hesitant to get on methadone maintenance because his military buddies in Opiates Anonymous said that abstinence was the only way to go. Some of his military friends, who used heroin in the service, were able to return home and just stop using opioids—they were also different in that they did not have pain syndromes. He reports being depressed about his situation, but denies any suicidal or homicidal ideation or plans and denies owning a firearm.

Self-Study Review

A. This veteran was seen through the VA drug court and was diverted to drug rehabilitation. Explain the VA drug court program.

B. Describe the challenges in treating patients with pain syndromes, who become addicted to opioid medications and present to physicians seeking opioid prescription. How does one differentiate the use of an opioid for the treatment of pain from addictive behavior?

C. Discuss the tension between abstinence and harm reduction approaches to opioid addiction, and how military culture and Opiates Anonymous may influence the choice of approach.

Clinical Case Study 4

A 30-year-old woman attends a VA mental health clinic on a regular basis for medication management. She endorses a history of multiple military sexual traumas. These include several experiences of nonconsensual sexual intercourse during her military training, events that occurred between her and fellow officers. Then, during one of her deployments, she reported being forced to engage once in sexual contact with one of her superiors. When she mentioned this experience to other female and male officers, she felt the responses were non-supportive. She feels angry about these experiences but also guilty that she acted in some way to bring them about.

Since coming to the clinic, she has been managed on a selective serotonin reuptake inhibitor or serotonin norepinephrine reuptake inhibitor antidepressant for several years with moderate remission of her symptoms, which include depressed mood, low motivation, irritability, hypersomnia, low energy, and "panic attacks" around stressful events such as perceived rejections or slights. She also struggles with several chronic pain conditions including fibromyalgia, headaches, and back pain. She refuses strong analgesics because she does not want to become a "junkie." She has been able to maintain a job as a teacher, but she notes that her romantic life is chaotic as she goes in and out of a relationship with an older man, whom she feels is kind, but emotionally distant and relatively asexual. She denies a childhood history of sexual abuse or trauma. She denies any suicidal or homicidal ideation or plans and denies owning a firearm. She has recently become more open to seeing a therapist regularly to discuss some of these issues.

Self-Study Review

A. This veteran experienced multiple military sexual traumas involving fellow officers and a superior and found colleagues unsupportive when she told them about it. Describe what is known about the incidence of military sexual trauma and how this has been handled by the military.

B. The veteran subsequently reports multiple symptoms, physical and psychological, and relational problems. Discuss how one would explore any connection between the military sexual traumas and these symptoms and whether the patient has post-traumatic stress disorder (PTSD) from sexual trauma.

C. Discuss whether criteria are met for the following diagnoses and what additional history one might need to determine this.
   - Generalized anxiety disorder
   - Major depressive disorder
   - Panic disorder
   - Personality disorder
   - Post-traumatic stress disorder

Clinical Case Study 5

A 70-year-old male Vietnam-era veteran, with a long-standing diagnosis of schizophrenia, has been stable on antipsychotic medication for many years and presents to a VA mental health clinic for his regularly scheduled follow-up appointment. He is also followed for diabetes, morbid obesity, hypertension, gastric reflux, benign prostatic hypertrophy, and hypocholesteremia. He says that his delusions and hallucinations continued to be manageable and denies any suicidal or homicidal ideation or plans and ownership of a firearm. He notes, however, that he has been feeling particularly "upset" after a visit from his niece for whom he has been a godfather. At the conclusion of the visit, the niece asked the veteran for financial assistance; though he has limited resources, he reluctantly provided some funds. One month later, the veteran received a phone call from the niece, who suggested that he use his service-connected pension to relocate to where she lives in the southern part of the state. She said that she could take care of him as he gets older, especially since his memory and ability to deal with his financial affairs has been declining.

The patient's psychiatrist has known him for many years and reminds him that he does not do well with change, which has led to hospitalizations in the past. As the visit concludes, the veteran agrees that he does not want to move and is comfortable where he is now. Nevertheless, the veteran leaves a voicemail 1 month later, stating that his niece has, without his consent, hired a moving van to move him to her place. He said he does not know what to do, adding that she has a bad temper and he does not want to anger her, so he is going to go along with her plan even though he feels coerced. He said, "Besides, I already paid for the moving van." She says she will not cook for him and help him keep his medications straight if he is not "good."

Self-Study Review

A. Discuss the possible causes of the apparent decline in memory and in ability to handle financial matters in this veteran.
B. Enumerate the vulnerabilities that this veteran possesses that may make him susceptible to financial abuse or victimization. Outline the definition of elder abuse and the reporting requirements for physicians.
C. This veteran has a severe and persistent mental illness. List modalities of support, both logistical and therapeutic, that may be offered to aid the veteran in decision-making processes.
D. Explain briefly how service-connected pensions are determined for patients with severe and persistent mental illness.

Clinical Case Study 6

A recently trained military psychiatrist is stationed at a military treatment facility that is relatively close to hostile action. A squad of soldiers was caught in an ambush and pinned down for several hours. The combat was fierce and several of the squad members were critically injured or killed. The surviving soldiers were evacuated by helicopter to the psychiatrist's military treatment facility, and the psychiatrist was called because this combat experience was extremely traumatic for these soldiers.

Self-Study Review

A. Discuss the current recommendations for the acute psychiatric management of patients exposed to life-threatening trauma, in the immediate aftermath. What psychiatric procedures to mitigate the psychological consequences of trauma does the military have in place for this type of scenario?

B. Outline the epidemiological findings concerning the risk of post-traumatic stress disorder, acute stress disorder, and adjustment disorder following this type of trauma in the military.

C. Are some soldiers at greater risk for developing post-traumatic stress disorder? Are there ways to train soldiers so their risk is reduced?

Clinical Case Study 7

A 68-year-old male Vietnam-era veteran is referred by his primary care provider to an outpatient mental health clinic for depressed mood. He states that he is reluctant to seek treatment with a mental health provider because "I'm not a nut case." He voluntarily retired from a white-collar job 6 months ago and has struggled to find daytime activities to occupy his time. Three months ago he attended a funeral for a close former military buddy and has felt increasingly irritable and "hopeless" ever since. He finds little to enjoy in life and spends most days sitting on the couch watching television. He sleeps 4 h nightly, with difficulty falling asleep while he thinks about all his friends who have died. His appetite has been less than usual, and he lost 15 lb during this period. He denies any suicidal or homicidal ideation or plans, but sometimes has passive suicidal thoughts. He denies hallucinations or unusual experiences. This is the first time he has felt "so negative and hopeless." He owns one firearm for sport purposes.

Upon his retirement, he began drinking one to two glasses of wine with dinner every night, but after the funeral he began drinking a half bottle of wine daily. Sometimes now he will wake up in the morning with panic attacks and sweats, and drinks a beer and smokes a cigarette upon waking to minimize these symptoms. His niece feels that his irritability is worse after he drinks and she would like him to stop, but he does not think his drinking is a problem because he is not a "drunk." One time he drove home while intoxicated, but he denies any legal history. He has never seen a psychiatrist before and has never taken any psychiatric medication. His medical history includes hypertension, for which he takes a beta-blocker, coronary artery disease, and gastric reflux. He lives in a small town near his niece and lives on social security and retirement benefits. He has never married.

Self-Study Review

A. This veteran does not want to see a psychiatrist and does not want to be considered to be "a nut case." Discuss how to handle the stigma associated with psychiatric treatment and how behavioral health embedded in primary care may be part of a solution.

B. The veteran reports symptoms particularly since he attended a funeral of a fellow soldier. Discuss to what extent his presentation may involve a grief reaction.

C. Outline what you know about the relationship between the veteran's mood symptoms and substance use and what additional relevant history you need.

D. Describe how you would assess this patient's risk of suicide.

E. Discuss whether criteria are met for the following diagnoses and what additional history one might need to determine this.
   - Major depressive disorder
   - Major neurocognitive disorder
   - Persistent complex bereavement disorder
   - Psychiatric disorder due to another general medical condition
   - Substance use disorder

Clinical Case Study 8

A 32-year-old male Operation Iraqi Freedom/ Operation Enduring Freedom veteran presents to a mental health clinic with his mother who accompanies him, seeking help for "PTSD." The veteran immediately positions himself in the room facing the door with his back to the wall, saying very little. His mother explains that he served three tours and that, since returning from his last tour, he has been isolative, distancing himself from family and friends. She notes that approximately 1 month after returning home he began having difficulty sleeping, waking up several nights per week covered in sweat, yelling for help, and breathing heavily. He usually feels emotionally numb and cut off from others. He denies owning a firearm, having problems with anger, or substance/alcohol misuse. Eight months after returning, the veteran had to move to a small house owned by his parents in the mountains, because he feels better if he is away from a lot of people. The veteran's mother expresses concern that "things cannot continue this way," and the veteran begrudgingly remarks that "I just need more time to transition into civilian life; talking about it won't help." The veteran says he does not know why he bothered to come in for the appointment, because he lives many hours away and therefore would not be able to pursue any treatment, even if it would be helpful. Additionally, he gets anxious when he approaches populated areas. He denies any suicidal or homicidal ideation or plans.

After the clinical interview, the psychiatrist informs the veteran and his mother that telepsychiatry, wherein a patient receives for a mental health condition (including PTSD) from a provider by video from a remote location, is rapidly becoming more common for those in underserved areas. A quick search finds that there is a VA telehealth clinic only 1 h away from the veteran's residence. The veteran is open to the idea of telepsychiatry and says that he really cannot accept treatment under any other conditions.

Self-Study Review

A. The veteran is having difficulty with access to treatment because he lives in a remote area and does not want to enter the populated area where the VA clinic is located due to anxiety. Discuss the pros and cons of telepsychiatry, and under what conditions it might be useful and under what conditions it might not be prudent.

B. Outline the types of treatment that might be deliverable via telepsychiatry. If the patient becomes ready for prolonged exposure treatment for PTSD, how would this treatment be administered?

C. Describe how you would assess this veteran's risk of suicide, including dynamic (changeable) and static (unchangeable) risk factors. Discuss the contingency plan if the patient later says he is actively suicidal or homicidal during a telepsychiatry session.

Clinical Case Study 9

A 36-year-old male veteran is referred by his neurologist for evaluation by an addiction psychiatrist at the VA. The neurologist follows the patient for symptoms secondary to his traumatic brain injury that was sustained by exposure to a blast wave from an improvised explosive device at close range. His injury was closed and, based on the Glasgow Coma Scale, was moderate. He is primarily disabled by cognitive impairment. His attention is decreased to the extent that he cannot do paperwork, his processing speed is slowed, and his working memory is impaired. He has trouble with decision-making, being quite indecisive, and he does not pick up on social cues. He does not report being particularly depressed, but this is in the context of not being able to describe much with regard to his feelings. He suffers from chronic dizziness and headaches and various waxing and waning neurological symptoms. He has not had a seizure and he denies any suicidal or homicidal ideation or plans and ownership of a firearm.

Prior to his injury, he had occasionally experimented with marijuana and drank alcohol with occasional drunkenness. Since his discharge, he has used marijuana to help him relax and sleep and also began to use stimulants, cocaine and then methamphetamine, to help him "think more clearly and concentrate." He usually takes oral stimulants, but has smoked crack on several occasions. Currently, the veteran often uses marijuana and alcohol daily and uses methamphetamine in binges for a few days at a time, two to three times per month.

Self-Study Review

A. This veteran suffered a traumatic brain injury and presents with many symptoms that are probably related. Discuss the typical presentation of traumatic brain injury several years after the injury and the likely course and prognosis.
B. Describe the possible interactions of substances of abuse and traumatic brain injury symptoms.
C. Outline treatments, psychopharmacologic and psychotherapeutic, used for psychiatric symptoms secondary to traumatic brain injuries. Do these differ from the treatments used for similar symptoms that are not secondary to traumatic brain injury?

Clinical Case Study 10

A 27-year-old male Operation Iraqi Freedom/Operation Enduring Freedom veteran is brought by police to the emergency room after he cut his arm with a sharp object during an argument with his boyfriend and his boyfriend had called 911. Upon arrival in the emergency room, the patient was assessed by the on-call trauma surgeon, who stitched the laceration and recommended outpatient follow-up wound care. The patient's physical exam was otherwise unremarkable, and his labs were notable for a blood alcohol level of zero and urine toxicology positive for cannabis. The patient states he smokes one joint of marijuana twice a week, when he feels empty, and he drinks one glass of wine each night, but he had not used anything before or during the argument. He denies smoking cigarettes or other illicit substances. He works in retail and says that substance use does not interfere with his work performance.

On interview, the patient shares that he cut himself without the intention to die, but rather because he felt "so desperate that I didn't know what to do." He had suspected his boyfriend of 4 months was cheating on him, and his confrontation led to the argument. At one point he threatened to end the relationship because he couldn't bear the possibility that his boyfriend might leave him first. His mood is "all over the place" over the course of a single day, but overall he has felt "hollow inside." He has a history of self-harm attempts by cutting or pill overdose, which has resulted in several psychiatric hospitalizations and one medical hospitalization. Sleep is poor, with frequent nightmares of his combat experience, where he witnessed several comrades critically wounded and maimed from improvised device explosions. He has avoided anything that reminds him of the military and does not really want to talk about his military service. Instead he has "consumed" himself with a string of tumultuous relationships, one right after another. He feels quite distraught that he is in the emergency room now, thinking that he is "destine to be alone." He denies any homicidal ideation or plans and denies owning a firearm. He is unclear about any suicidal ideation or plans at the time of the interview.

Self-Study Review

A. This veteran reports that he thinks he is probably gay and "came out of the closet" when he left the military. Describe what further history you would take about his sexual orientation and how LGBTQI issues may affect his treatment.
B. This veteran is presenting in an emergency department. Concerning his psychiatric care, discuss your clinical reasoning about the various options for follow-up care and the optimal level of care.
C. Describe how you would assess this patient's risk of suicide and your treatment plan to manage this risk in the future.
D. Discuss whether criteria are met for the following diagnoses and what additional history one might need to determine this.
    - Borderline personality disorder
    - Bipolar disorder
    - Histrionic personality disorder
    - Post-traumatic stress disorder
    - Substance use disorder

Clinical Case Study 11

A 30-year-old female veteran is being seen regularly by her psychiatrist after returning from a tour of duty. During her deployment she was injured in an encounter with an improvised explosive device (IED) and was evacuated by helicopter to receive treatments for her injuries. She had to have three fingers amputated from her nondominant hand, and she has scarring from third-degree burns on the left side of her face. She is now working in a job that does not involve contact with the public. Following this event, she has experienced nightmares that involve scenes from the day of the IED explosion. She reports daily anxiety and a tendency to always be scanning her environment for dangers. Because large crowds seem to offer more potential for danger and chaos, she prefers to avoid them, but this has limited some of her previously enjoyable outings in public with her significant other.

While she was amenable to seeing a psychiatrist after her return and has maintained an ongoing relationship with a mental health team, she was initially reluctant to be on medication, noting that she preferred to deal with her symptoms "with complementary and alternative medicine" and that she feared medication would change her personality. Eventually, she agreed to try a medication to address the nightmares and found after a dose titration that it was effective at lessening her sense of anxiety when she awoke. However, she and her significant other would like to start a family, and she wants to stop her medication if she plans to get pregnant. Additionally, she has begun to experience higher levels of anxiety at the thought of having a baby, finding her mind constantly ruminating on the changes in her body that accompany pregnancy. She denies any suicidal or homicidal ideation or plans and denies owning a firearm.

Self-Study Review

A. Many veterans suffer bodily disfiguration and dismemberment. Analyze how this veteran's experience of permanent bodily disfigurement may relate to her fear that medications will "change her personality" or to her fear of pregnancy.
B. Describe how the VA health-care system approaches the management of the psychological effects of bodily injury and permanent disabilities in veterans.
C. This veteran desires to start a family, but is concerned about the risks during pregnancy of taking medications for PTSD versus the risks of untreated PTSD. Describe the conversation you would have with her about this concern and outline the evidence base for the treatment of PTSD during pregnancy.
D. Discuss whether criteria are met for the following diagnoses and what additional history one might need to determine this.
    - Agoraphobia
    - Generalized anxiety disorder
    - Major depressive disorder
    - Panic disorder
    - Post-traumatic stress disorder

Clinical Case Study 12

A 63-year-old male veteran presents to a psychiatrist at a VA, upon referral from a primary physician for the treatment of depression. The veteran has been on a selective serotonin reuptake inhibitor antidepressant for a year with no improvement. He primarily complains of difficulty with concentrating at work and insomnia; both have gradually worsened over the past 5 years. Now he has begun to worry that he may need to retire because he cannot concentrate on all the details of his desk job. He loves his job, and the prospect of retirement has resulted in depressed mood, poor self-esteem, and even loss of interest in going to work. He denies suicidal or homicidal ideation or plans and ownership of a firearm. He doesn't know what he will do at home all day during retirement. Although he says things are "not bad" at home, he stopped having sex with his wife about 7 years ago, around the time she started sleeping in another room due to his snoring. He drinks alcohol only during celebrations and does not use illicit drugs.

He has slowly gained considerable weight (BMI is now 30) and has had poor energy; these changes all began before his depression, about 10 years ago, and he thought they were just part of aging. His primary care physician has treated his hypertension and adult-onset diabetes with antihypertensive and oral antidiabetic agents, respectively, for several years. He has tried several programs to lose weight, but none seemed to work. He has had a trial of cognitive behavioral therapy for insomnia and this was not effective. He continues to smoke and has not really tried to quit. He figures that his weight, insomnia, and poor concentration are enough to contend with for now and has heard from friends that he may get more depressed if he tries to stop smoking.

Self-Study Review

A. The veteran's main complaints are poor concentration and insomnia. Discuss the pros and cons of obtaining specialized testing, e.g., neuropsychological testing, polysomnography, brain imaging, and specialized laboratory testing. Outline your differential diagnosis for these complaints.

B. Describe what you would tell the veteran about whether quitting smoking might make him more depressed and whether you recommend treatment to quit smoking at this time.

C. Discuss whether criteria are met for the following and what additional history one might need to determine this.
   - Adjustment disorder
   - Neurocognitive disorder
   - Normal aging
   - Depressive disorders
   - Sleep-wake disorder

Clinical Case Study 13

A 25-year-old Operation Iraqi Freedom/ Operation Enduring Freedom male veteran arrives for intake at a VA outpatient mental health clinic. He was brought by his cousin to an outpatient mental health clinic 2 months earlier to establish care, due to concern that he was isolating himself and losing significant weight ever since discharge from the military 2 years ago. His outpatient psychiatrist diagnosed him with PTSD and started him on a selective serotonin reuptake inhibitor, but he stopped taking medication after 1 week due to sexual side effects.

Upon presentation at this intake, the patient frequently stares straight ahead at a neighboring window. He states that he was gregarious and outspoken prior to his service, but is no longer like this—ever since he witnessed many combat casualties during his service. His friends now say that he is if often mentally "out to lunch." He denies blast exposure. He endorses frequent flashbacks and nightmares; however, he cannot recall specific details of his experiences. Ever since his return from deployment, he has experienced repeated episodes where he has felt "detached" from his own body. He denies hallucinations or delusions. He reports depressed mood, loss of interest in pleasurable activities, pervasive feelings of guilt as the only survivor of his squad, low energy, and poor appetite. He endorses frequent thoughts of "not existing" but denies any active suicidal or homicidal ideation or plans and denies owning a firearm. His thought process is linear although his speech is slowed.

Self-Study Review

A. This veteran is being seen at a VA outpatient mental health clinic. Explain how his symptom of feeling "detached" influences his diagnosis and treatment plan.

B. The veteran has frequent thoughts of "not existing" but denies any active suicidal plan or intent. Describe your assessment of his risk for suicide.

C. Discuss whether criteria are met for the following diagnoses and what additional history one might need to determine this.
   - Dissociative disorder
   - Major depressive disorder
   - Major neurocognitive disorder
   - Post-traumatic stress disorder
   - Substance use disorder

Clinical Case Study 14

A 65-year-old male veteran began experiencing paranoid delusions and auditory hallucinations in his twenties while enlisted. The symptoms and subsequent hospitalizations eventually led to a medical discharge from the military. For many years the patient was in and out of treatment with VA providers, both inpatient hospitalizations and outpatient clinic visits. He has had trials on several antipsychotics, but has had difficulty adhering to his medication regimen and has often discontinued medications for reasons including side-effect burden, belief that he did not need them, and paranoia about their contents. He has had housing instability. Initially his family helped to care for him, but as they have aged they have been less able to do so, and he has experienced homelessness at times. In his 50s, after a series of prolonged psychiatric hospitalizations that were complicated by medical issues, he was assigned an outpatient mental health-care treatment team, and significant efforts were made to ensure more stable housing.

After stabilizing the worst of his psychotic symptoms during a hospitalization, he became more amenable to this treatment approach and was discharged to a local group home. His comprehensive treatment team includes a nurse practitioner who helps manage his blood pressure, gastric reflux, and diabetes medications and does home visits as necessary; a mental health social worker who visits him weekly (or more if needed) to appraise his psychiatric symptom control; a community liaison who helps to connect him to local resources and go on group outings; a psychiatrist and psychologist who see him at the local clinic; and a case manager who provides longitudinal coordination of the team. After several years of improved stability, the patient is now needing to move out of his current group home because it is closing, and he is increasingly anxious about this change. He expresses several concerns that his next living situation will be "bugged" by his enemies. He denies any suicidal or homicidal ideation or plans and denies owning a firearm. Though he denies it, there is concern that he has started missing doses of his medications. His blood pressure and blood sugar have been higher than usual on the nurse visits as well.

Self-Study Review

A. Outline the services provided by the VA that are crucial to the care of people suffering from chronic schizophrenia.
B. Describe the role and responsibilities of a psychiatrist in the context of a treatment team for an outpatient suffering from chronic schizophrenia, both generally and during a period of crisis (e.g., loss of housing).
C. This veteran developed symptoms of schizophrenia during active military service. Most likely he would have developed these symptoms even if he had not joined the military. Outline how it is determined whether a diagnosis is "service connected" and whether a veteran will pay for treatment of such a diagnosis at a VA.
D. Discuss whether criteria are met for the following diagnoses and what additional history one might need to determine this.
   - An anxiety disorder
   - Delusional disorder
   - Major depressive disorder
   - Schizoaffective disorder
   - Schizophrenia

Clinical Case Study 15

A 25-year-old male officer was deployed on multiple tours of duty, during which he was exposed to three improvised explosive device explosions. He had suffered symptoms of PTSD and traumatic brain injury during his service, but has never revealed them because he did not want to be barred from further tours of duty. In some ways, returning to combat became a relief to him because his PTSD symptoms were more tolerable in that context. He has served valiantly and has been decorated for his heroism. Coming from a long line of military family members, this honor is important to him, as is behaving in ways that are always seen as righteous and above any reproach.

He has very recently returned from a tour of duty and was ordered to see the psychiatrist at the base because his PTSD symptoms were noted by his commanding officer. He does not do well when he returns to his home on base—he misses the respect and adulation of his subordinates during combat. He starts to drink alcohol at home until he falls asleep, which he never does during tours because he fears it will slow his reaction time. He often has headaches and has trouble concentrating and remembering details. He denies any suicidal or homicidal ideation or plans and any depressed feelings, saying, "I am not that type of guy." He feels he hardly knows his wife and two young children, who were both born when he was overseas. He wants to play with his children, but he is usually irritable. He is also sensitive to sound and is quite easily upset by the noise made by his children. The children sometimes do not obey him when he tells them to quiet down or to stop what they are doing, and, on four occasions, his wife saw him hit the older son with his hand. He told his wife that he was very sorry and would not hit his son ever again. The patient did not think he needed to mention the hitting incidents during the psychiatric evaluation, but he feels so extremely guilty that he mentions it when asked about symptoms of guilt.

Self-Study Review

A. Discuss the possible reluctance, as in this case, of active military personnel to reveal psychiatric symptoms to their physicians.
B. Returning from deployment to his home and family, this officer has hit his son on four occasions. Describe the multiple biological, psychological, and social factors that may be contributing to the hitting of his son.
C. Outline how the military defines and handles child abuse, what the psychiatrist should say to the patient, and she what should do administratively (e.g., reporting requirements). Outline the same for spouse or partner violence.
D. Discuss whether criteria are met for the following diagnoses and what additional history one might need to determine this.
   - Alcohol use disorder
   - Antisocial personality disorder
   - Narcissistic personality disorder
   - Post-traumatic stress disorder
   - Traumatic brain injury

Clinical Case Study 16

A 70-year-old male Vietnam-era veteran is transported to the VA hospital from a local emergency room and arrives sedated after receiving emergent antipsychotic medication 4 h earlier. The patient is too sleepy to cooperate with a psychiatric interview, including determining if he is suicidal or homicidal at this time. The psychiatrist talks to the patient's sister who called the police because the patient had spent the entire night in a shed in their backyard. The veteran patient had been afraid to go inside the house, stating it was "under surveillance." The patient lives alone in a rural area near his sister, and he had become increasingly irritable and agitated for the last several months, ever since a new family moved in across from his house lot. He would frequently guard the edges of their property at night with his shotgun. His sister states he has been "always on guard" ever since being discharged from the military, but had been able to work as a security guard until he voluntarily retired at age 63. She does not know any details about his combat experience in Vietnam, as he has always refused to discuss it. He had never seen a mental health professional before.

She states he typically consumes one beer a night, but in the last 3 months has been consuming one to two six packs nightly. He has a 30 pack-year history of smoking cigarettes. She is not aware of any illicit drugs he might be taking. He has a medical history of coronary artery disease, hypertension, and hypocholesteremia. He last saw a primary care physician 10 years ago and is not taking any medications for these conditions. Urine toxicology screen in the emergency room was negative. Blood alcohol level and other preliminary blood tests are pending at the time of evaluation.

Self-Study Review

A. This veteran owns firearms. Discuss how firearm ownership influences the risk of suicide.
B. Describe how dangerousness to others and the Tarasoff ruling are relevant to this vignette.
C. Describe how treatment planning may differ when caring for a veteran who lives in a rural area.
D. Outline VA guidelines concerning asking patients about gun ownership and where veterans may obtain free gunlocks.
E. Discuss the psychiatrist's differential diagnosis and how to pursue the work-up of the following:
   - Delusional disorder
   - Major neurocognitive disorder
   - Post-traumatic stress disorder
   - Psychiatric disorder due to another general medical condition
   - Substance use disorder

Clinical Case Study 17

A 65-year-old man is being seen at the spinal cord injury unit for his biannual medical care visit. He is brought to the visit by his son after a long-distance drive from their hometown. The patient has a history of a thoracic spine injury secondary to combat in the military. At first he primarily experienced lower extremity weakness, but recently his weakness and sensation loss have been progressive to the point that he is now paraplegic with loss of bowel and bladder function; however, his progression of symptoms is somewhat mysterious to the neurologists who have seen him over the years, and they do not fully understand why his symptoms would be progressive in nature. This perspective is reconfirmed by the neurology consultants who examined the patient and viewed the imaging during the current visit.

The patient utilizes a nonelectric wheelchair and his upper extremities are of normal strength, but, according to the son, he is dependent on his family (including wife, grown children, and other extended family) for most activities of daily living. The patient has struggled significantly with pain management issues and has undergone spinal stimulator placement, epidural steroid injections, physical therapy, multiple lumbar fusion surgeries, and finally placement of an intrathecal pump that delivers several opioid and non-opioid pain medications. In addition to his medical and spinal cord issues, the patient carries a diagnosis of depression for which he has had several trials of antidepressants. On his current regimen, his mood remains low and he reports irritability, frustration, anhedonia, fatigue, and mild hopelessness. The medical team decides to request a psychiatry consult, because the patient will not be able to return soon for a mental health evaluation. When the consult team arrives, the patient gives the above history but is somewhat withdrawn. He also appears confused and somnolent at times and his history is vague. He has difficulty following some of the questions and wishes to end the interview after 30 min. When the question of pain medications arises, he becomes irritable and insists that he is not getting enough pain medication coverage. He denies any suicidal or homicidal ideation or plans and denies owning a firearm.

During the consult, the patient's son describes that at home the patient's progressive symptoms have increasingly placed a caretaking burden on the entire family that has become nearly unsustainable. He describes that the patient has become more irritable, confused, demanding, and withdrawn. All other medical issues have been cleared during this visit, but the son feels that the patient's mental state is not being adequately addressed. Furthermore, the neurology team has shared that they cannot find a physiologic rationale to explain the patient's progressive symptoms and have suggested that an element of his presentation is "all psychological" in nature, which has confused and distressed the patient and his family.

Self-Study Review

A. The veteran's presentation is complex and with multiple comorbid conditions. Outline the broad differential diagnosis relevant to his current mental status, including acute and chronic diagnoses.

B. Discuss the approach to patients with chronic pain who state that they continue to be in pain and are not getting enough pain medication.
C. The psychiatrist has been asked to provide a consultation extemporaneously during a biannual medical care visit for an outpatient veteran. Outline the objectives and action plan that this psychiatrist should establish in this medical outpatient setting to best serve this veteran going forward.
D. Outline VA/Department of Defense Clinical Practice Guidelines for Opioid Therapy for Chronic Pain.
E. Discuss whether criteria are met for the following diagnoses and what additional history one might need to determine this.
   - Delirium
   - Major depressive disorder
   - Major neurocognitive disorder
   - Somatic symptom disorder
   - Substance-/medication-induced disorder
   - Substance use disorder

Clinical Case Study 18

A 35-year-old male veteran is being seen for the first time by a psychiatrist at a VA mental health clinic. The veteran reports various paranoid delusions and ideas of reference. He has experienced these delusions on and off for a couple of years and they now seem to be more frequent. When he is less paranoid, he gains insight into the possibility that he is not perceiving reality accurately. For instance, he will think that a coworker is talking about him and will later check with his friends and find out that there is no evidence of this and will then question his original suspicions. He also has trouble motivating himself. All he can do is to get himself to work and to try to complete his desk work. Otherwise he stays at home, watches television, and smokes "weed." He only socializes with people who come over to use marijuana with him. He smokes several joints each evening and almost continuously on the weekends. He sees himself as a sort of connoisseur of "really potent" hashish. He denies suicidal or homicidal ideation or plans and ownership of a firearm.

The veteran experimented with marijuana in middle school and used almost daily in high school. He never really got into any other types of illicit drugs and never liked alcohol. He joined the military because he could not get any other job after dropping out of high school. In the military, he was able to sometimes get marijuana and smoke with his fellow soldiers. He enjoys marijuana, does not think it is the cause of his anxiety or paranoia, has been smoking on a daily basis, and sees no reason to stop. He has no history of psychiatric disorders other than his substance use and has no family history of psychiatric disorders, including psychotic ones, or substance use disorders.

Self-Study Review

A. The veteran is reporting symptoms of psychosis and uses potent marijuana on a daily basis. Discuss the current literature on psychotic symptoms and marijuana use.
B. Based on the current evidence base, describe what you would specifically say to the veteran about the risks of continuing to use marijuana, especially with regard to his psychotic symptoms and lack of motivation.
C. Outline how you might proceed with motivational interviewing with this patient.
D. The veteran reports using marijuana in the military. Describe how the military addresses misuse/addiction with regard to substances of abuse in active duty personnel and the role of "zero tolerance," "random drug testing," and the stigma of addiction in the military. Consider this especially for marijuana, but also for alcohol, tobacco, and prescription opioid addictions.

Clinical Case Study 19

A 34-year-old female officer is seen by a psychiatrist. The officer's military career is going well and she is highly decorated for her accomplishments and service. She says that she has become involved with a commanding officer who would frequently request that she accompany him on various trips. She states that during these trips he pressured her to engage in oral copulation and other forms of sexualized interactions. She has threatened to report this behavioral but she has not done so yet over the past 2 years, stating that female service members who complain about being sexually harassed are labeled as "pathetic." In the service she has had a series of emotionally, sexually, and physically abusive relationships with enlisted soldiers. She has broken off the relationships whenever she became worried that they would be discovered.

The officer describes frequent nightmares of being sexually abused, feelings of rage, mood swings, rejection sensitivity, and moments of depressions and emptiness. She denies any suicidal or homicidal ideation or plans. She says she drinks too much alcohol at times and has used opiates, prescribed for headaches, to numb her feelings and to sleep. As a child, she was neglected, often left at home alone, and physically abused by a brother. Cutting herself as a teenager distracted her from emotional pain. After college, she joined the military for a new start in life.

Self-Study Review

A. This active duty officer is seeking care from a military psychiatrist. Is the information she divulges confidential or does the psychiatrist need to report anything, e.g., ongoing sexual harassment, military sexual trauma, and past relationships between an officer and enlisted personnel?
B. How does the officer's developmental history affect her interpersonal functioning and your psychosocial case formulation?
C. Outline a long-term treatment plan for this officer.
D. Explain what the Uniform Code of Military Justice is and if it is relevant to sexual harassment and military sexual trauma.
E. Discuss whether criteria are met for the following diagnoses and what additional history one might need to determine this.
   - Bipolar disorder
   - Borderline personality disorder
   - Histrionic personality disorder
   - Major depressive disorder
   - Post-traumatic stress disorder

Clinical Case Study 20

A 27-year-old male patient is being seen at a VA outpatient mental health clinic. He reports no psychiatric history prior to his deployment and denies a history of childhood abuse. During boot camp, he drank a lot of beer with his buddies but did not engage in other substance use. During his last deployment, his squad was trapped and several members of his squad were critically injured. They were taken as prisoners for a period of 10 days, during which he witnessed a soldier shot at point-blank range and was sexually assaulted by a male combatant before they escaped. Though an evaluation was performed and counseling was offered to him following the event, he expressed that he did not want to talk about it.

In the months following his discharge, his alcohol intake escalated to daily use, at first up to two or three six-packs per evening and eventually adding hard liquor on top of this amount. He also started smoking marijuana to help him sleep. Despite these measures he reported his sleep was poor: he continued to experience nightmares several times a week and would often avoid going to sleep, resulting in his being under-rested during the day. Upon returning home he felt progressively alienated from his friends and family, and even from fellow squad members with whom he was previously very close. He was unable to maintain steady employment due to his tendency to be late getting to work and having hangovers. Three years after discharge, he is finally seeking treatment at the outpatient VA clinic because his girlfriend says she was going to leave him, which he reports is in large part because of his difficulty engaging in affection and physical intimacy with her since his return. His girlfriend is also not happy about his drinking and his yelling outbursts. He eventually opens up that he feels guilt that he can no longer perform sexually with her, though he is able to masturbate, and about his fellow squad member's death. He denies any suicidal or homicidal ideation or plans and denies owning a firearm.

Self-Study Review

A. This veteran, like many, was exposed to multiple traumas related to his service. He was in combat, witnessed his fellow soldiers critically wounded and killed, and was sexually assaulted. Any one of these constitutes a major trauma. Discuss the effects of multiple traumas in combat. Outline VA/Department of Defense Clinical Practice Guidelines for PTSD.
B. This veteran declined support and to talk about the combat traumas immediately afterward and only later revealed deep guilt about the fate of his fellow soldiers. Discuss the studies regarding discussion about traumas in the immediate aftermath and the prevalence of survivor guilt among veterans. Discuss the veteran's reluctance to discuss his feelings, barriers in the veteran/military culture, and ways to overcome these barriers.
C. The case notes that the veteran was sexually assaulted, but makes no mention of his reaction to this experience, except that he experienced sexual dysfunction later. Discuss the effects of sexual assault on men and possible mechanisms for his subsequent sexual dysfunction.
D. Outline the evidence base for the following psychotherapies for PTSD:
   - Cognitive processing
   - Eye movement desensitization and reprocessing
   - Prolonged exposure
   - Stress inoculation
   - Virtual reality exposure therapy
E. Discuss whether criteria are met for the following diagnoses and what additional history one might need to determine this.
   - Intermittent explosive disorder
   - Major depressive disorder
   - Male hypoactive sexual desire disorder
   - Post-traumatic stress disorder
   - Substance use disorder

Clinical Case Study 21

A 37-year-old male Operation Iraqi Freedom/Operation Enduring Freedom veteran presents for his compensation and pension examination by a VA psychiatrist. He served in the military for 6 years and deployed to Iraq three times until his honorable discharge 1 year ago. At his last deployment, he was exposed to blast waves from three different improvised device explosions and lost consciousness for 3 h after one of them and 10 min after another. He reports that ever since these incidents he has experienced problems with concentration, multitasking, and short-term memory, to the point that he has only been able to hold a job since his discharge from service. He also reports frequent nightmares about the aftermath of the blasts and has generally avoided talking about his deployment. He describes his mood as "irritable," and he is always vigilant for danger, especially in public.

While the veteran is in bed for many hours, he really only sleeps a few hours per night and says that "I never wake up refreshed." He reports that his energy is variable and his concentration is poor. He denies racing thoughts, guilty ruminations, delusion of grandeur, or changes in appetite, but he has put on some weight recently. He reports frequent thoughts of wishing he were dead, but firmly denies suicidal plans because "I would not do that to my family." He owns three firearms at home for protection from possible home invasions, where he lives with his wife and new baby daughter. He denies homicidal ideation or plans.

Self-Study Review

A. This veteran suffered traumatic brain injury documented in his medical record. Describe the symptoms of traumatic brain injury and how they relate to his symptoms of mood and anxiety disorders.

B. The veteran will have a compensation and pension exam by a VA physician. Outline how this exam will be similar to and different from a clinical interview, and the role of this exam relative to receiving VA benefits.
C. Describe how you would assess this patient's risk of suicide and manage it on an outpatient basis.
D. Discuss whether criteria are met for the following diagnoses and what additional history one might need to determine this.
   - Major depressive disorder
   - Major neurocognitive disorder due to traumatic brain injury
   - Somatic symptom disorder with predominant pain
   - Post-traumatic stress disorder
   - Psychiatric disorder due to another general medical condition

Clinical Case Study 22

A 72-year-old male veteran is brought to the emergency room by ambulance with progressive weakness and inability to care for himself. He generally appears to be in very poor shape medically with multiple lab abnormalities, an abnormal neurological exam, and a disheveled appearance with soiled clothing. He is admitted to the hospital and found to have metastatic cancer throughout his body, including on his spinal cord. During his hospital stay, his primary team has had an extraordinarily difficult time developing rapport with this patient. He stays in his room, refuses to speak more than a few words with anyone (including nurses, chaplains, doctors, or other support staff), does not have any visitors, and does not seem to acknowledge the gravity of his current condition. He denies any suicidal or homicidal ideation or plans and denies owning a firearm.

When asked about his wishes for treatment, including palliative care options, he simply refuses to engage and cries out, "Leave me alone!" The primary team and social worker are unable to identify any family members or friends, either local or remote, as the patient appears to have been fairly reclusive. Decisions about treatment and disposition have been held up due to the difficulties of eliciting the patient's preferences. Psychiatry is called to consult on the case to help determine whether the patient possesses capacity and to help facilitate an understanding of the patient's wishes. During the initial consultation phone call, the primary team member voiced considerable exasperation over this "frustrating patient."

Self-Study Review

A. The number of geriatric veterans is expanding and some will present with issues relating to capacity. Outline the components of a capacity assessment and specific evidence on exam that one should document.
B. State what series of questions you would pose to the patient to determine his understanding of his illness and what he wishes for treatment.
C. For veterans who are determined to lack support of family or friends, as in this vignette, describe when you would involve the hospital ethics board and how they might be able to help.
D. Outline what percentage of current veterans are from the Vietnam era, their age range, and their likely mental health needs.
E. Discuss whether criteria are met for the following diagnoses and what additional history one might need to determine this.
   - Delirium
   - Delusional disorder
   - Major depressive disorder
   - Major neurocognitive disorder due to another general medical condition
   - Unspecified neurocognitive disorder

Clinical Case Study 23

A 22-year-old male soldier is participating in a 12-week anger management outpatient group held on the military base. He keeps going to the anger management group, but he is not sure it helps and he finds it exceedingly boring. He reports vacillating between his usual state of being "without any feelings" to episodes of "deep rage." During periods of rage, which commonly come upon him suddenly, he will feel a rush of adrenaline that can often be accompanied by shortness of breath, hyperventilation, and palpitations. He denies any suicidal or homicidal ideation or plans, problems with anxiety or depression, or current use of drugs or alcohol. Fellow soldiers generally describe him as "strong but silent" and deep down having good intentions. He is not hyperactive or hyperverbal. He is somewhat impulsive and is willing to do most things on a dare. He wants to do his duties well and wants to be promoted, but he is easily distracted; often, he does not complete tasks because he starts to do another task and never returns to complete the original task. His distractions have caused him to be written up several times. He has never been in combat.

As a child, he had many run-ins with law enforcement, was often suspended from school, and was given a choice of incarceration or joining the military. He reports a history of misusing alcohol, inhalants, methamphetamine, cocaine, and marijuana, but he got clean and sober in boot camp and has stayed that way due to newfound religion. He remembers that methamphetamine helped him to feel alert and on guard. His parents were told he had attention-deficit/hyperactivity disorder, but they never took him for treatment. He had a concussion and lost consciousness during a fight as a teen and was taken to an emergency room, but again his parents did not follow up with care thereafter.

Self-Study Review

A. How do you understand this soldier's attacks of rage, and what additional history would help you in understanding?
B. Does this soldier have adult attention-deficit/hyperactivity disorder? Assuming he does, how would you treat this with medications and/or psychotherapy?
C. How does the officer's developmental history help you understand his current history, and what do you make of his report of being clean and sober since boot camp?
D. Discuss whether criteria are met for the following diagnoses and what additional history one might need to determine this.
   - Attention-deficit/hyperactivity disorder
   - Bipolar disorder, mania/hypomania only
   - Intermittent explosive disorder
   - Substance use disorder
   - Traumatic brain injury

Clinical Case Study 24

A 50-year-old female spouse of an active duty officer presents to a psychiatric outpatient evaluation on the military base. She says that over the past year and a half she has begun taking benzodiazepines regularly for insomnia—mainly for difficulty falling asleep and staying asleep—and for increased anxiety. Although she has had clinicians recommend non-medication techniques for symptoms, she has found that her insomnia responds best to taking a pill. She tried improved sleep hygiene measures, but felt that they were not helpful. Her primary care physician will not give her a refill if she runs out of pills early, so she has started to consume up to one to two bottles of wine on some nights to tide her over to her prescription renewal. She recalls that many years ago she was prescribed benzodiazepines for insomnia by her primary care physician, but began using these to excess during the day and eventually tapered them.

She describes a long-standing history of anxiety starting in childhood and states that feelings of anxiety have plagued her ever since. She has consistently worried about all types of things and possible bad outcomes. When she starts to worry about an upcoming event, her anxiety will build over a couple hours and then she will have a panic attack. She denies agoraphobia, significant depression, or suicidal or homicidal ideation or plans. She never was much of a drinker of alcohol until 1 year ago and is surprised how much she is now drinking. She has never used illicit drugs—she would be too afraid to take anything like that. In recent years, her child left the home and she has had more marital strife with her often-absent husband, and they now sleep in different rooms for unclear reasons.

Self-Study Review

A. This spouse of an active duty officer describes problems with insomnia. What would you ask her in order to determine if she meets criteria for insomnia disorder? Outline non-medication techniques you might prescribe, besides improved sleep hygiene. List condition(s) relating to physical health that might be contributing to her insomnia.

B. Explain how you understand the fact that the patient never used alcohol previously in her life, but is now drinking up to two bottles of wine per night. Is this an alcohol use disorder with onset later in life?

C. Analyze how the patient's marital situation and sleeping in separate bedrooms figure into your clinical formulation.

D. Analyze whether this patient would benefit from psychotherapy and discuss the type(s). Do the TRICARE mental health benefits differ for military service members and authorized dependents, such as the wife of an officer?

E. Discuss whether criteria are met for the following diagnoses and what additional history one might need to determine this.
   - Alcohol use disorder
   - Anxiety due to another medical condition
   - Generalized anxiety disorder
   - Panic disorder
   - Sedative, hypnotic, or anxiolytic use disorder

Index

L.W. Roberts, C.H. Warner (eds.), *Military and Veteran Mental Health*,
https://doi.org/10.1007/978-1-4939-7438-2

M

MIX
Papier aus verantwortungsvollen Quellen
Paper from responsible sources
FSC® C105338

If you have any concerns about our products,
you can contact us on
ProductSafety@springernature.com

In case Publisher is established outside the EU,
the EU authorized representative is:
Springer Nature Customer Service Center GmbH
Europaplatz 3, 69115 Heidelberg, Germany

Printed by Libri Plureos GmbH
in Hamburg, Germany